Endometriosis

Camran R. Nezhat   Gary S. Berger
Farr R. Nezhat   Veasy C. Buttram, Jr.
Ceana H. Nezhat

Editors

Endometriosis

Advanced Management and Surgical Techniques

Managing Editor, Gary S. Berger
Foreword by Robert L. Barbieri
Foreword by Mary Lake Polan

With 112 Figures, 26 in Color

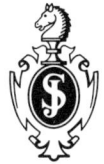

Springer-Verlag
New York Berlin Heidelberg London Paris
Tokyo Hong Kong Barcelona Budapest

Camran R. Nezhat, M.D., Department of Obstetrics and Gynecology, Mercer University School of Medicine, Macon, GA 31207; Department of Obstetrics and Gynecology, Department of Surgery, Stanford University School of Medicine, Stanford, CA 94305; and Center for Special Pelvic Surgery, Atlanta, GA 30342, and Palo Alto, CA 94304, USA

Gary S. Berger, M.D., Department of Obstetrics and Gynecology, University of North Carolina School of Medicine; Department of Maternal and Child Health, University of North Carolina School of Public Health; and Chapel Hill Fertility Center, Chapel Hill, NC 27514, USA

Farr R. Nezhat, M.D., Department of Obstetrics and Gynecology, Mercer University School of Medicine, Macon, GA 31207; Department of Obstetrics and Gynecology, Stanford University School of Medicine, Stanford, CA 94305; and Center for Special Pelvic Surgery, Atlanta, GA 30342, and Palo Alto, CA 94304, USA

Veasy C. Buttram, Jr., M.D., Department of Obstetrics and Gynecology, Baylor College of Medicine, Houston, TX 77054, USA

Ceana H. Nezhat, M.D., Department of Obstetrics and Gynecology, Mercer University School of Medicine, Macon, GA 31207; Department of Obstetrics and Gynecology, Stanford University School of Medicine, Stanford, CA 94305; and Center for Pelvic Surgery, Atlanta, GA 30342, and Palo Alto, CA 94304, USA

On the cover: Laparoscopic extraction of endometrial cyst from left ovary. Painted by Robert Gordon, MFA, CMI.

Library of Congress Cataloging-in-Publication Data
Endometriosis : advanced management and surgical techniques / Camran Nezhat . . . [et al.].
   p.   cm.
  Includes bibliographical references and index.
  ISBN 0-387-94243-2.—ISBN 3-540-94243-2
  1. Endometriosis—Surgery. 2. Endometriosis. I. Nezhat, Camran.
  [DNLM: 1. Endometriosis—surgery. WP 390 M691 1994]
RG483.E53M65 1994
618.1—dc20
                                     94-19130

Printed on acid-free paper.

Production coordinated by Chernow Editorial Services, Inc., and managed by Francine McNeill; manufacturing supervised by Jacqui Ashri.
Typeset by Best-set Typesetter Ltd., Hong Kong.
Printed and bound by Edwards Brothers, Inc., Ann Arbor, MI.
Printed in the United States of America.

9 8 7 6 5 4 3 2 1

ISBN 0-387-94243-2 Springer-Verlag New York Berlin Heidelberg
ISBN 3-540-94243-2 Springer-Verlag Berlin Heidelberg New York

To
Meredith White
and
all women with endometriosis

Foreword

The first known report concerning endometriosis was written by Rokitansky in 1860. Yet as late as 1920, fewer than twenty published manuscripts concerning endometriosis were available in world literature. In 1921, Sampson published the first report describing his theory of retrograde menstruation and implantation as a causative factor for the disease. This report was a creative milestone that excited great interest in the disease. During the past decade, a new and broader surge of interest in endometriosis has resulted in numerous important advances in patho-physiology, diagnosis, and treatment. This renaissance is the subject of the text *Endometriosis: Advanced Management and Surgical Techniques.*

A scientific renaissance is often characterized by the convergence of a unique historical opportunity and a group of creative pioneers who generate a burst of vigorous discovery. Major advances in the molecular and cell biology of the endo-metrium and simultaneous advances in surgical instrumentation were critical historical elements that fostered the endometriosis renaissance.

The development of advanced surgical techniques by an innovative group of clinicians has truly opened a new world of treatment options. In this text, the editors and contributors have taken time to stop and review these advances, which have reshaped our approach to the treatment of endometriosis. The result is a remarkably coherent text that concisely reviews the important advances of the last decade.

Each chapter in the text serves an important purpose. The majority of chapters document the surgical advances that have occurred during the endometriosis renaissance. These range from a better recognition of the visual presentation of the disease to innovative treatment modalities, especially those involving minimally invasive surgical techniques. The remaining chapters help to properly orient these surgical advances within the broader context of our improved understanding of the biology of endometriosis. Of great importance is that every chapter has been written by a pioneer, each of whom can be clearly credited with opening important territory in this new world. The illustrious and accomplished group of contributors makes this text a coherent, convincing, and complete survey of the key events in the endometriosis renaissance. Regarding the surgical treatment of endometriosis, we are clearly at the end of the middle ages and the beginning of modern times.

Robert L. Barbieri

Foreword

Continuum *n*: an uninterrupted, ordered sequence
Webster's Dictionary

Endometriosis is a continuum of changes that begins at the cellular level and is fully expressed as a debilitating, painful disease. Reflux of endometrial cells into the peritoneal cavity sometimes results in implantation of cells that continue to cycle in response to hormonal stimuli. Growth factors and cytokines permit intraperitoneal endometrial growth that results in the clinical presentation of pain, associated infertility, and structural damage to pelvic organs. Endocrinological suppressive strategies can temporarily halt these destructive anatomic processes, but cannot completely reverse them. Ultimately, endometriosis may progress to a stage where only surgical intervention can reverse its ravages. Thus, the continuum begins at a cellular, hormone/cytokine-driven level and ends with an intricate pathology that only sophisticated surgical procedures can address. The beginning and end of this continuum represent two important yet different frontiers for controlling endometriosis.

Both endometrial (epithelial) and stroma (mesenchymal) cells implant in the peritoneal cavity and secrete a variety of growth factors and cytokines. These secretory products interact with macrophages and other immune cells already within the peritoneal cavity and elicit an augmented cellular immune response. Elevated levels of cytokines and growth factors in the peritoneal cavity of endometriosis patients have been documented as has the secretory capability of peritoneal macrophages; however, little is known about the interactions between immune cells and endometrial tissue, or the mechanisms by which intraperitoneal endometrial growth is encouraged. The cellular basis for the pathophysiology resulting in the clinical syndrome demands careful examination. A clear understanding of the molecular response patterns would direct the design of therapeutic interventions early in the disease process—before severe anatomic destruction occurs. We are, unfortunately, far from such an understanding. Currently, physicians must deal with the end-stage reality of pelvic adhesions.

The surgical approach to endometriosis has advanced dramatically over the last decade, with new endoscopically based procedures. Endoscopic surgery was born in 1805, when Bozzini first visualized the urethral mucosa. Advances in urethral and bladder visualization continued throughout the nineteenth century, until Kelling used pneumoperitoneum to visualize the peritoneal cavity of dogs in 1901. The first human laparoscopic procedure was performed in 1910 by Jacobaeus in Sweden.

Laparoscopy was little used for fifty years until the early 1960s, when the intro-duction of fiberoptics and more powerful light sources advanced the technique. Twenty years later, in the early 1980s, the introduction of videolaparoscopy and videolaseroscopy by Nezhat allowed the involvement of the entire operating team in the surgery. Team participation and the development of multiple new specialized instruments expanding the range of procedures have, to a large extent, allowed many conservative endometriosis procedures to be approached endoscopically, with all the attendant benefits for patient recovery.

Laparoscopic surgery has matured slowly over nearly two decades. The recent explosion of knowledge of growth factors, cytokines, and their paracrine and autocrine interactions is in its infancy compared with the long history of endoscopic technology. We can expect an equivalent expansion of our knowledge of cellular and molecular biologic interactions in a shorter time frame. Thus, with this new under-standing of molecular events, we may someday be able to prevent the destructive sequelae of this disease.

This book, edited by Drs. Nezhat, Berger, Nezhat, Buttram, and Nezhat catalogs the state of the art in endometriosis pathophysiology, therapy, and surgical inter-vention. It is hoped that an equivalent expansion of our knowledge of basic cellular and molecular biologic mechanisms for initiating and stimulating the growth of inappropriate implantation will introduce modalities that will prevent and treat early disease, making current medical and surgical therapies of historical interest.

Mary Lake Polan

Preface

There are several books about endometriosis in print. This book is different. *Endometriosis: Advanced Management and Surgical Techniques* presents detailed descriptions and illustrations of the most current treatment methods, with special emphasis on advanced operative techniques used by the foremost experts. This book, however, is neither an atlas nor a "cookbook." It reviews the scientific background on which modern treatment methods are based as well as the clinical literature regarding effectiveness and complications of the various treatment methods described.

As a book written by many authors, different opinions are given regarding the best methods and tools to use in a particular situation. These differences are clearly stated. They enrich the manuscript by acknowledging the complexity of the issues at hand. It is up to the individual gynecologic surgeon, for whom this book is intended, to weigh the advantages and disadvantages of the various approaches discussed here. Each physician must choose the techniques most suitable to the clinical situation, taking into account his or her own training, skills, and experience. The surgeon's tremendous responsibilities in the operating theater, and the rapid developments in surgical technique that are taking place, demand a continuing reassessment of one's skills at all times. Careful reading of this book will enhance the quality of care that gynecologic surgeons can provide to their patients.

Camran R. Nezhat
Gary S. Berger
Farr R. Nezhat
Veasy C. Buttram, Jr.
Ceana H. Nezhat

Acknowledgments

We would like to thank all of the authors; without their superb contributions, this book would never have been possible. We would also like to express our appreciation to the artists for their superior work and attention to detail. And last, we would like to express our gratitude to our staff who have devoted endless hours of energy, dedication, and thoughtfulness. Those in special mention are "Miss Mary" Trowell, Audrey Jacoby, Mary Ann Bumgardner, Judy Leet, Kit Ayers, Terry Ledbetter, Rebekah Dowd, Sandra Carter, Vicki Craven, Susan Tripp, and Mary Hale. We also thank our O.R. staff at both the Atlanta clinic and the Stanford University clinic.

Camran R. Nezhat
Gary S. Berger
Farr R. Nezhat
Veasy C. Buttram, Jr.
Ceana H. Nezhat

Contents

Contributors

DAHLIA ADMON, M.D., Department of Obstetrics and Gynecology, Sheba Medical Center, Tel Hashomer, Israel

GUOMUNDUR ARASON, M.D., Department of Obstetrics and Gynecology, The University of Connecticut Health Center, Farmington, CT 06030, USA

MARY LOU Ballweg, President, Endometriosis Association, Milwaukee, WI 53223, USA

ROBERT L. BARBIERI, M.D., Department of Obstetrics, Gynecology, and Reproductive Biology; Department of Obstetrics and Gynecology, Brigham and Women's Hospital, Harvard Medical School, Boston, MA 02181, USA

GARY S. BERGER, M.D., Department of Obstetrics and Gynecology, University of North Carolina School of Medicine; Department of Maternal and Child Health, University of North Carolina School of Public Health; and Chapel Hill Fertility Center, Chapel Hill, NC 27514, USA

STEFANO BIANCHI, M.D., Research Fellow in Obstetrics and Gynecology, University of Milano School of Medicine, 20122 Milano, Italy

IVO BROSENS, M.D., Department of Obstetrics and Gynecology, University Hospital St. Rafael-Gasthuisberg, B-3000 Leuven, Belgium

MAURICE ANTOINE BRUHAT, M.D., Department of Obstetrics, Gynecology, and Reproductive Medicine, Polyclinique de L'Hôtel Dieu, Centre Hospitalier Universitaire, 63003 Clermont-Ferrand, France

VEASY C. BUTTRAM, JR., M.D., Department of Obstetrics and Gynecology, Baylor College of Medicine, Houston, TX 77054, USA

GIOVANNI B. CANDIANI, M.D., Department of Obstetrics and Gynecology, University of Milano School of Medicine, 20122 Milano, Italy

MICHEL CANIS, M.D., Department of Obstetrics, Gynecology, and Reproductive Medicine, Polyclinique de L'Hôtel Dieu, Centre Hospitalier Universitaire, 63003 Clermont-Ferrand, France

FRANÇOISE CASANAS-ROUX, Biologist, Department of Gynecology, Catholic University of Louvain, University Hospital St. Luc, 1200 Brussels, Belgium

MICHAEL J.W. COOPER, M.D., Department of Obstetrics, Gynecology, and Reproductive Medicine, Polyclinique de L'Hôtel Dieu, Centre Hospitalier Universitaire, 63003 Clermont-Ferrand, France

ALAN B. COPPERMAN, M.D., Fellow in the Division of Reproductive Endocrinology, The Mount Sinai Medical Center, New York, NY 10029, USA

MARK A. DAMARIO, M.D., Department of Obstetrics and Gynecology, Emory University School of Medicine, Atlanta, GA 30303, USA

JAN DEPREST, M.D., Center for Surgical Technologies, Faculty of Medicine, Katholieke Universiteit, Leuven, Belgium

PAUL DEVROEY, M.D., AZ-VUB Centre for Reproductive Medicine, 1090 Brussels, Belgium

W. PAUL DMOWSKI, M.D., Ph.D., Professor of Obstetrics and Gynecology, Rush Medical College, and Institute for the Study and Treatment of Endometriosis, Chicago, IL 60614, USA

JACQUES DONNEZ, M.D., Department of Gynecology, Catholic University of Louvain, University Hospital St. Luc, 1200 Brussels, Belgium

LUIGI FEDELE, M.D., Professor of Obstetrics and Gynecology, University of Milano School of Medicine, 20122 Milano, Italy

ROBERT R. FRANKLIN, M.D., Department of Clinical Obstetrics and Gynecology, Baylor College of Medicine, Houston, TX 77054, USA

GEORGE M. GRUNERT, M.D., Department of Clinical Obstetrics and Gynecology, Baylor College of Medicine, Houston, TX 77054, USA

LISA A. HASTY, M.D., Department of Obstetrics and Gynecology, Emory University School of Medicine, Atlanta, GA 30303, USA

MARY CASEY JACOB, Ph.D., Departments of Psychiatry and Obstetrics and Gynecology, The University of Connecticut Health Center, Farmington, CT 06030, USA

ANTHONY A. LUCIANO, M.D., Department of Obstetrics and Gynecology, The University of Connecticut Health Center, Farmington, CT 06030, USA

HUBERT MANHES, M.D., Department of Obstetrics, Gynecology, and Reproductive Medicine, Polyclinique de L'Hôtel Dieu, Centre Hospitalier Universitaire, 63003 Clermont-Ferrand, France

SANFORD M. MARKHAM, M.D., Division of Reproductive Endocrinology, Georgetown University Medical Center, Department of Obstetics and Gynecology, Washington, DC 20007, USA

DAN MARTIN, M.D., Department of Obstetrics and Gynecology, University of Tennessee, Memphis, TN 38103; and Reproductive Surgeon, Baptist Memorial Hospital, Memphis, TN 38103, USA

DEBORAH METZGER, M.D., Ph.D., Departments of Psychiatry and Obstetrics and Gynecology, The University of Connecticut Health Center, Farmington, CT 06030, USA

KAMRAN MOGHISSI, M.D., Division of Reproductive Endocrinology, Department of Obstetrics and Gynecology, Wayne State University, Hutzel Hospital, Detroit, MI 48201, USA

ANA A. MURPHY, M.D., Department of Obstetrics and Gynecology, Emory University School of Medicine, Atlanta, GA 30303

CAMRAN R. NEZHAT, M.D., Department of Obstetrics and Gynecology, Mercer University School of Medicine, Macon, GA 31207; Department of Obstetrics and Gynecology, Department of Surgery, Stanford University School of Medicine, Stanford, CA 94305; and Center for Special Pelvic Surgery, Atlanta, GA 30342, and Palo Alto, CA 94304, USA

CEANA H. NEZHAT, M.D., Department of Obstetrics and Gynecology, Mercer University School of Medicine, Macon, GA 31207; Department of Obstetrics and Gynecology, Stanford University School of Medicine, Stanford, CA 94305; and Center for Pelvic Surgery, Atlanta, GA 30342, and Palo Alto, CA 94304, USA

FARR R. NEZHAT, M.D., Department of Obstetrics and Gynecology, Mercer University School of Medicine, Macon, GA 31207; Department of Obstetrics and Gynecology, Stanford University School of Medicine, Stanford, CA 94305; and Center for Special Pelvic Surgery, Atlanta, GA 30342, and Palo Alto, CA 94304, USA

MICHELLE NISOLLE, M.D., Department of Gynecology, Catholic University of Louvain, University Hosptial St. Luc, 1200 Brussels, Belgium

DAVID OLIVE, M.D., Section of Reproductive Endocrinology and Fertility, Yale University School of Medicine, New Haven, CT 06510, USA

MARY LAKE POLAN, M.D., Ph.D., Department of Obstetrics and Gynecology, Stanford University Medical School, Stanford, CA 94305, USA

JEAN LUC POULY, M.D., Department of Obstetrics, Gynecology, and Reproductive Medicine, Polyclinique de L'Hôtel Dieu, Centre Hospitalier Universitaire, 63003 Clermont-Ferrand, France

PATRICK PUTTEMANS, M.D., Department of Obstetrics and Gynecology, St. Elisabeth Hospital, Brussels, Belgium

DAVID B. REDWINE, M.D., Endometriosis Institute of Oregon, Bend, OR 97701, USA

JOHN A. ROCK, M.D., Department of Obstetrics and Gynecology, Emory University School of Medicine/Grady Memorial Hospital, Atlanta, GA 30303, USA

GLORIA VASQUEZ, M.D., Ph.D., Department of Obstetrics and Gynecology, University Hospital St. Rafael-Gasthuisberg, B-3000 Leuven, Belgium

GUY VERHULST, M.D., AZ-VUB Center for Reproductive Medicine, 1090 Brussels, Belgium

ARNAUD WATTIEZ, M.D., Department of Obstetrics, Gynecology, Reproductive Medicine, Polyclinique de L'Hôtel Dieu, Centre Hospitalier Universitaire, 63003 Clermont-Ferrand, France

Color Insert

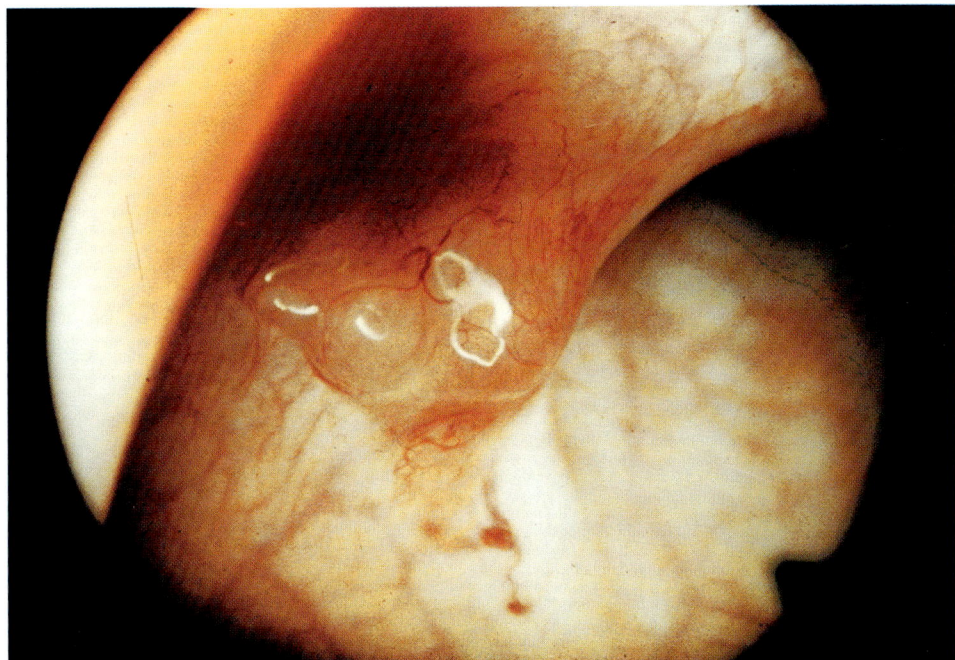

Figure 2.5A. Early peritoneal lesion: papular type. (Lesion represents distended endometrial gland. Note pattern of fine vascularization and absence of bleeding and fibrosis.)

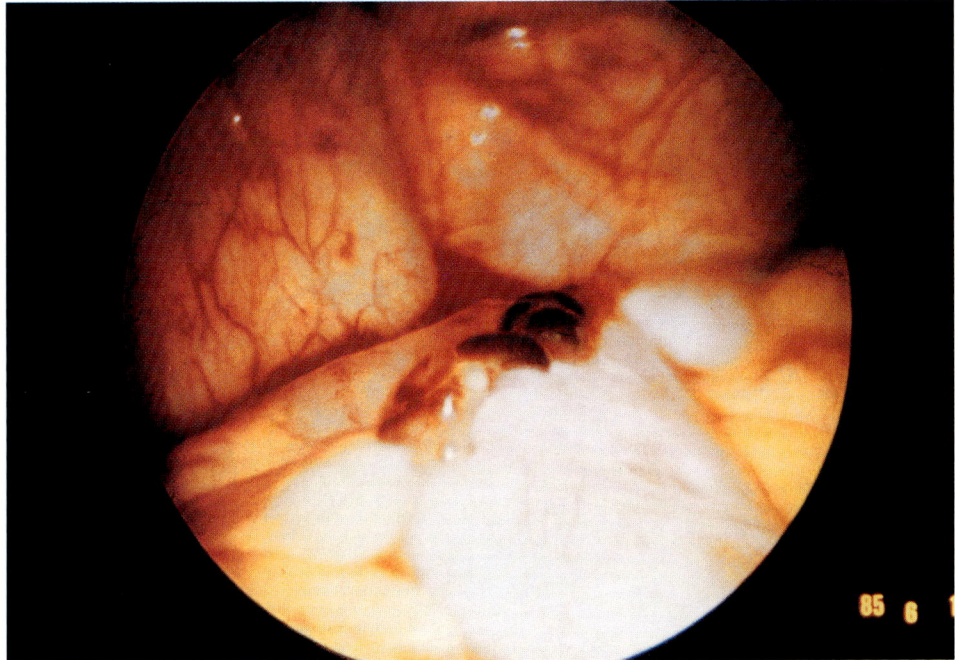

Figure 2.5B. Early peritoneal lesion: sero-hemorrhagic type. (Lesion represents an active implant. Note absence of fibrosis.)

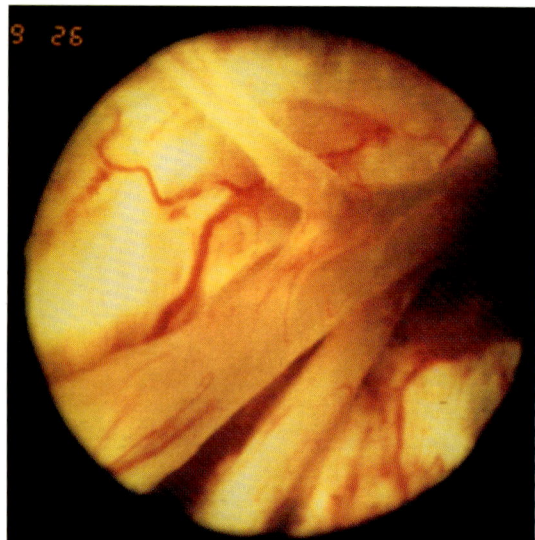

Figure 2.9. Ovarioscopy of endometrial cyst. Note the area of adhesion and retraction of the inverted ovarian cortex at the site of hemorrhagic endometrial implant.

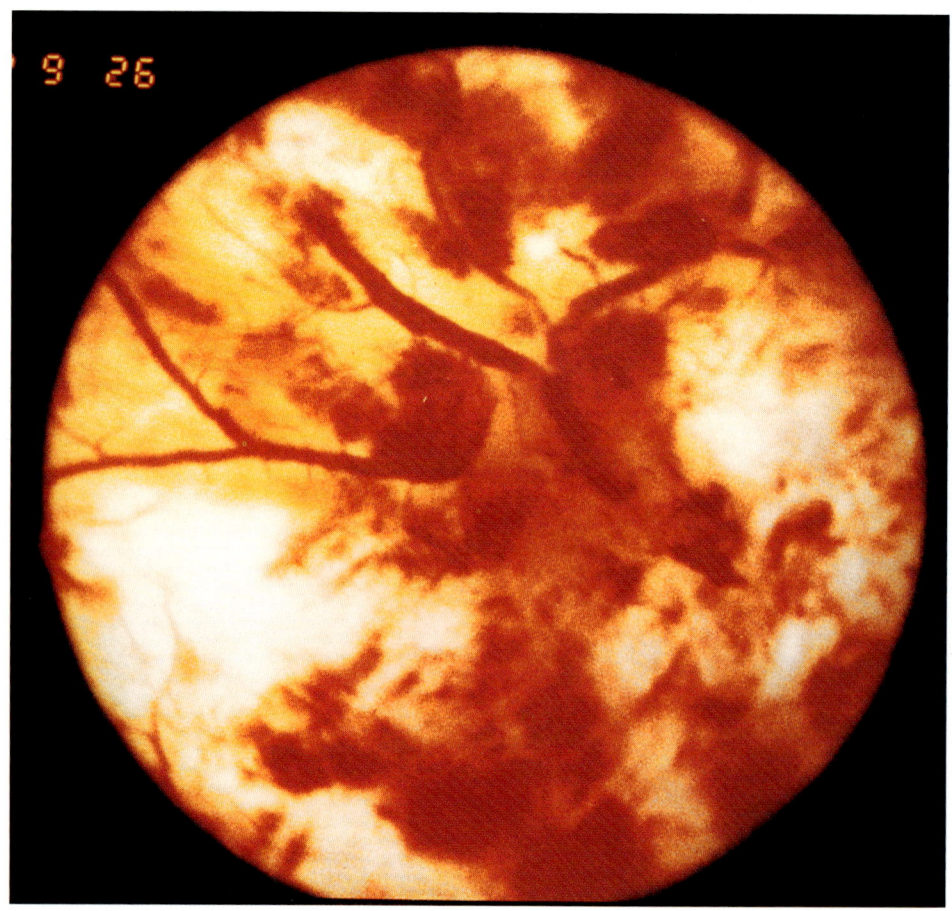

Figure 2.10. Ovarioscopy of endometrial cyst. The implants are scattered over surface of inverted cortex.

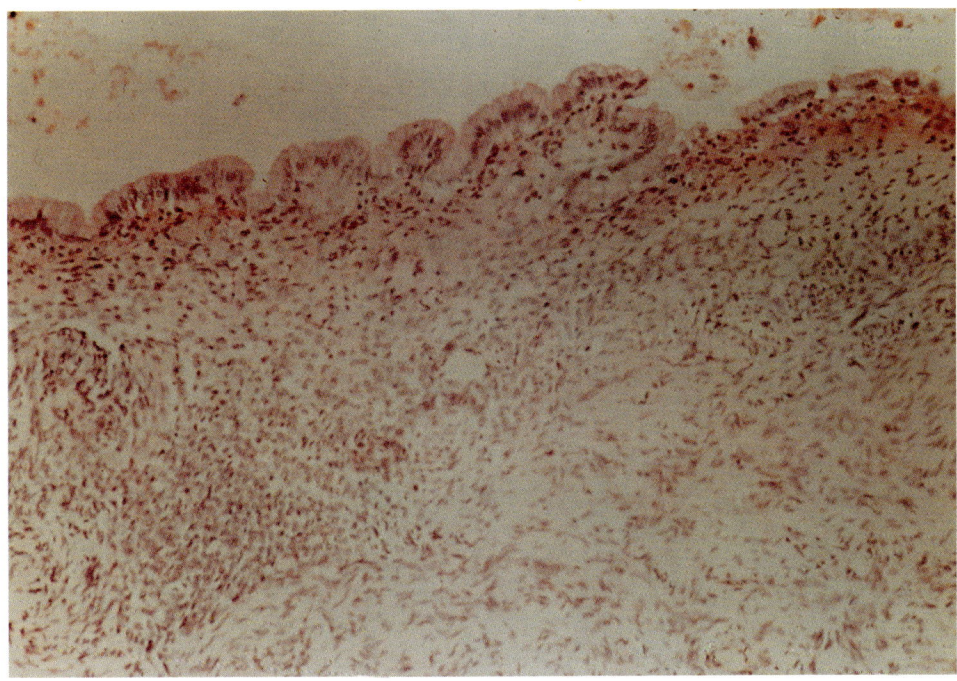

Figure 2.11. Biopsy of endometrial cyst. Specimen shows superficial endometrial tissue growing on the ovarian cortex.

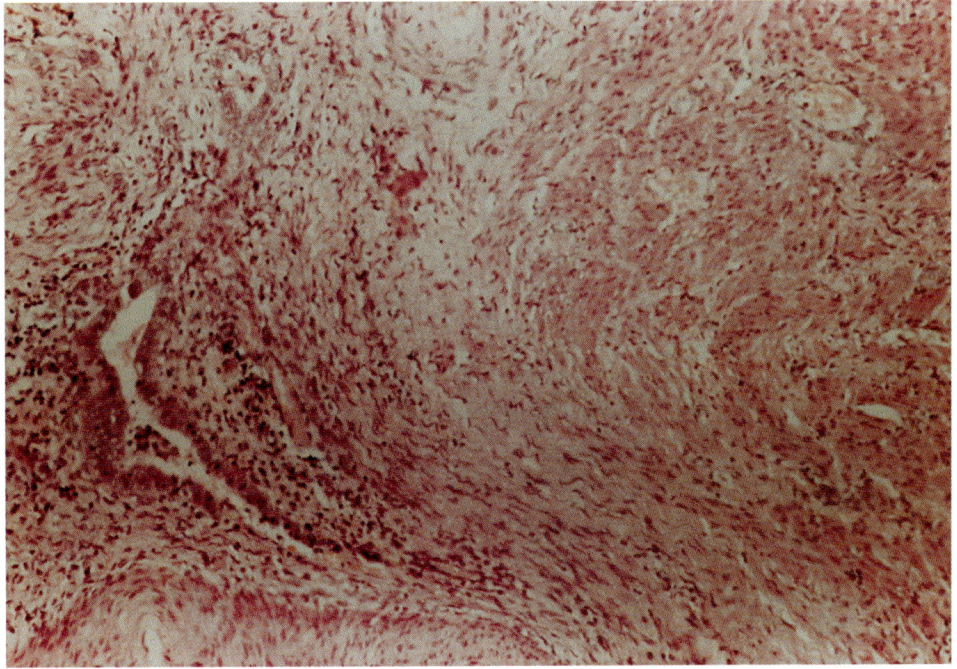

Figure 2.12. Endometriosis of rectovaginal septum. Lesion is characterized by a fibro-muscular nodule with fingerlike extensions of endometrial tissue (adenofibromyosis).

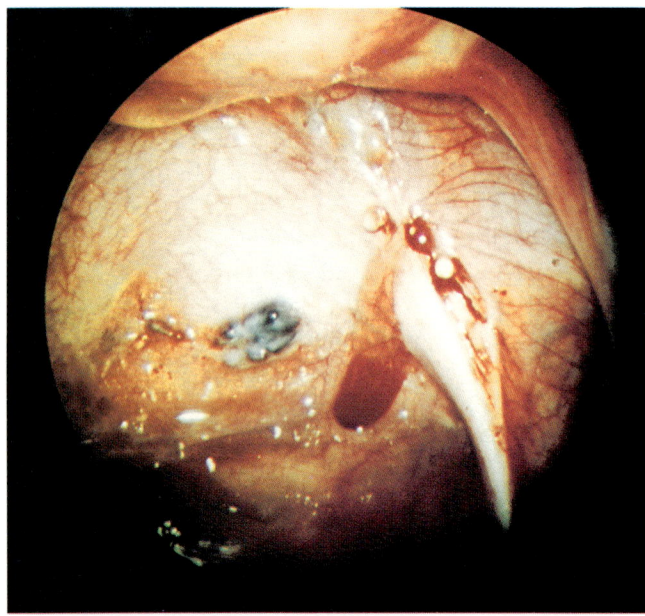

A

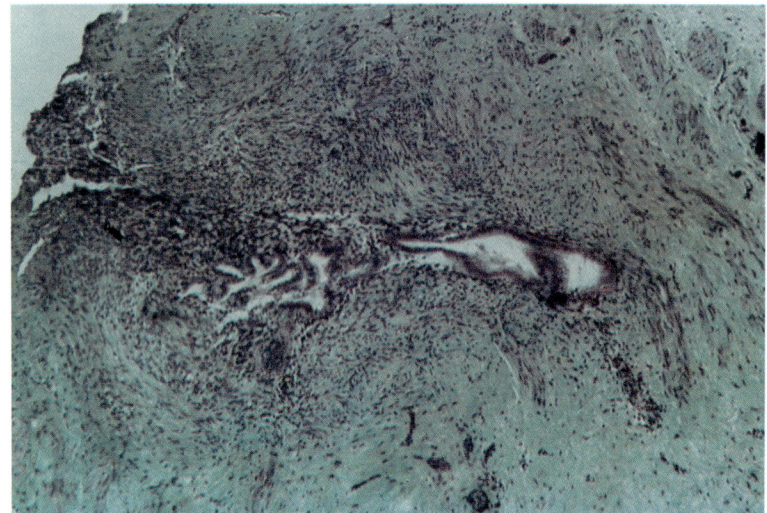

B

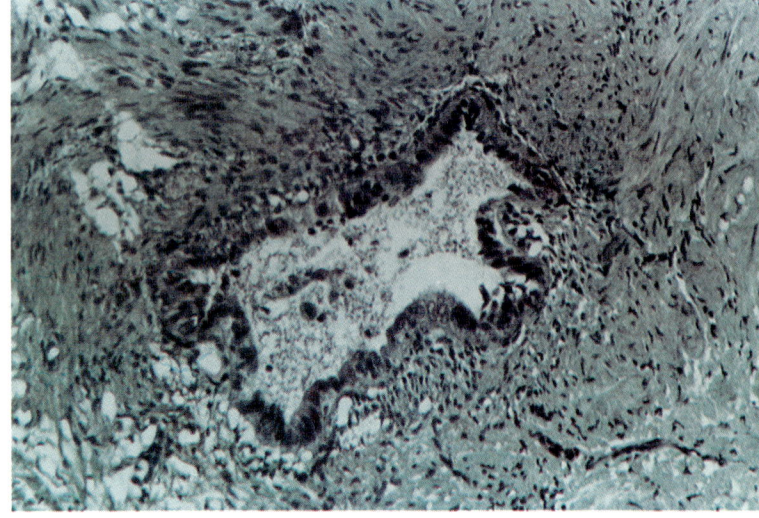

C

Figure 3.1. Typical puckered black lesion. **A**. Laparoscopic appearance: close to the black lesion, other types (red) are seen. **B**. Gomori's Trichrome at ×25 magnification shows combination of endometrial glands and typical stroma. **C**. Higher magnification (×56) of lesion shows intraluminal debris.

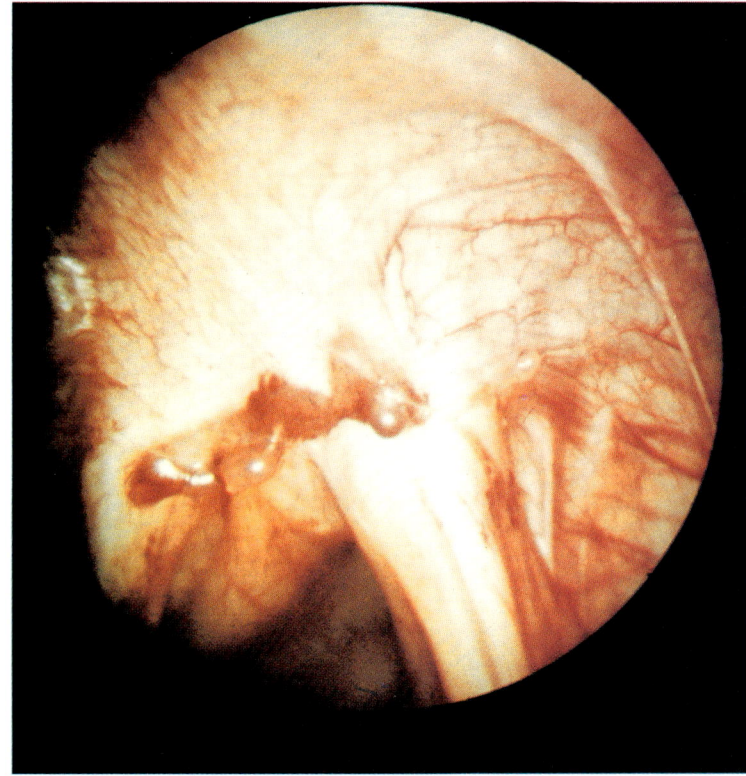

Figure 3.2. Laparoscopic appearance of red flamelike lesion.

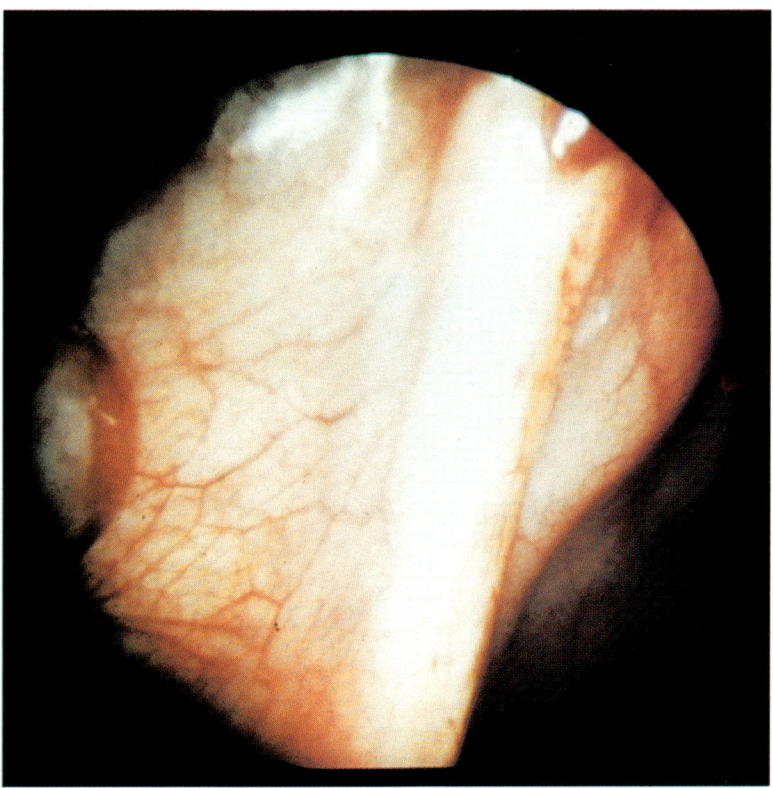

Figure 3.3. Laparoscopic appearance of white opacification of the peritoneum.

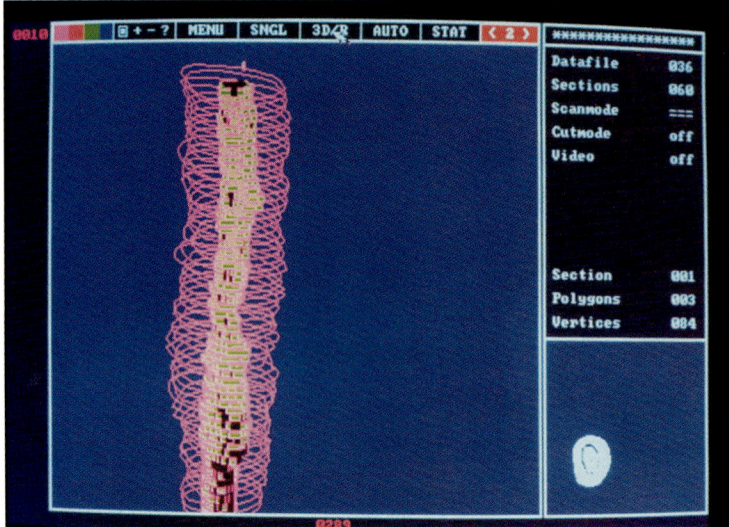

Figure 3.4. 3-D image models displayed as a transparent structure show cylinder-like gland and regular distribution of the glandular epithelium in the stroma.

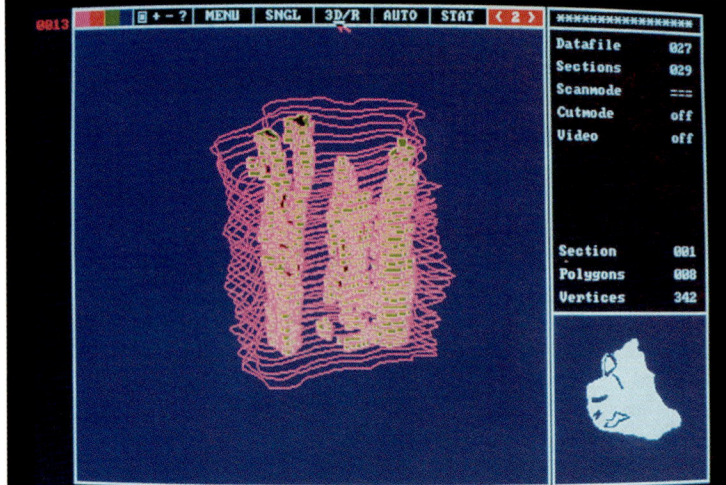

Figure 3.5. 3-D image models displayed as a transparent structure show glands with ramifications and interconnection of structures.

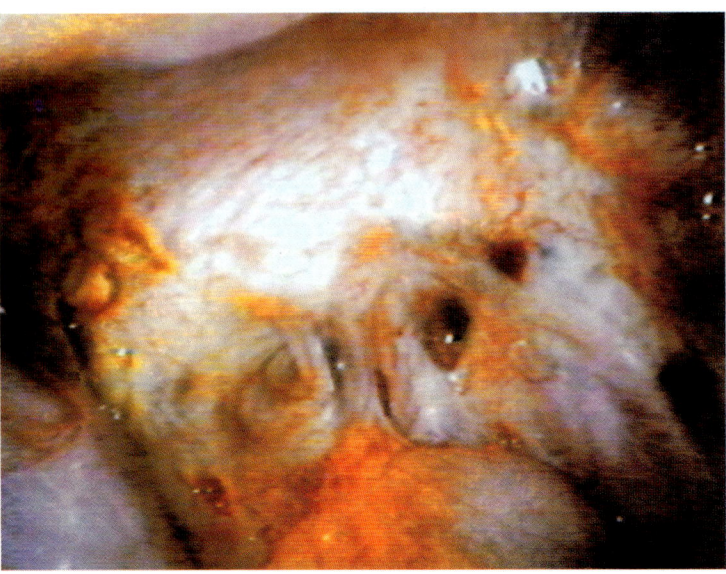

Figure 10.1. Atypical peritoneal implants and partial obliteration of the posterior cul-de-sac.

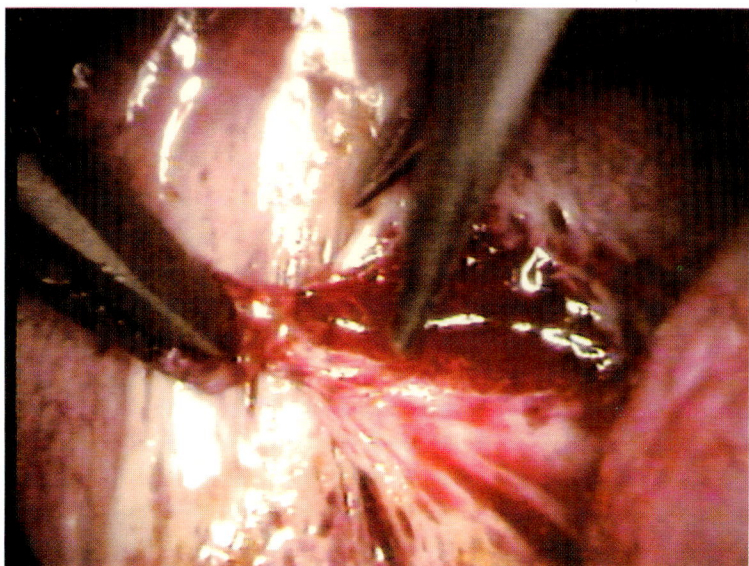

Figure 10.2. Excision of superficial peritoneal implants of the right broad ligament is performed with a grasping forceps and scissors.

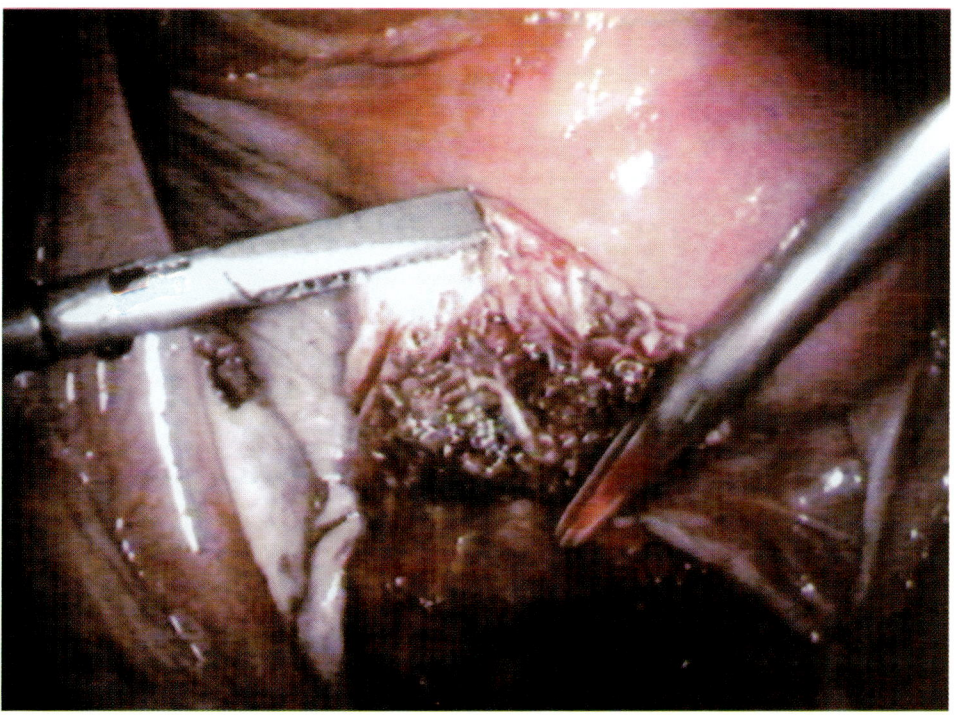

Figure 10.3. Excision of a large nodule (>2 cm in diameter) of the rectovaginal septum.

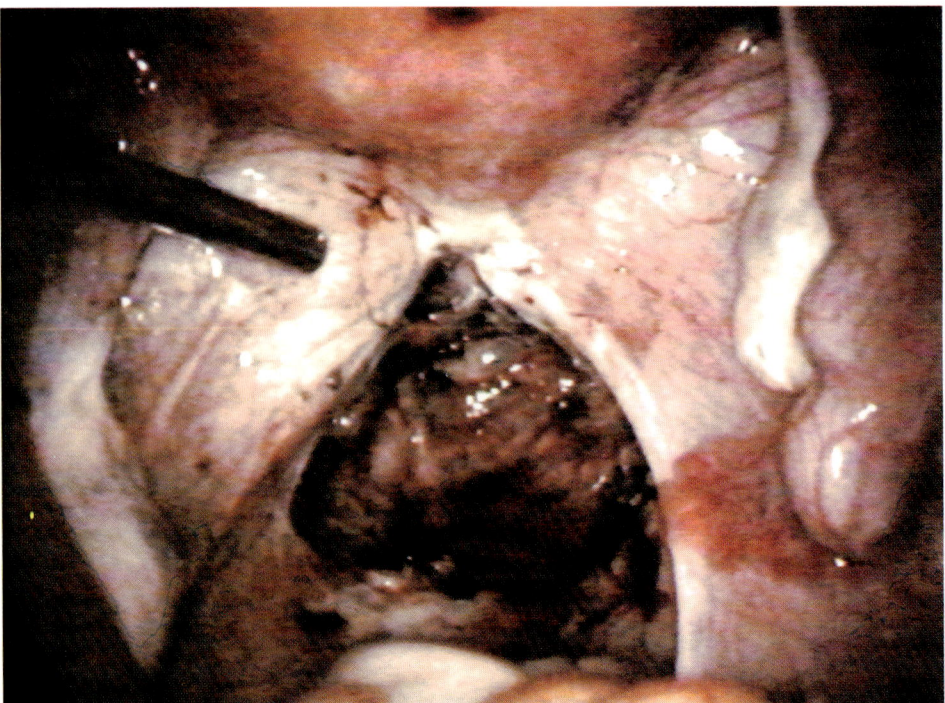

Figure 10.4. Final view after excision of nodule of the rectovaginal septum.

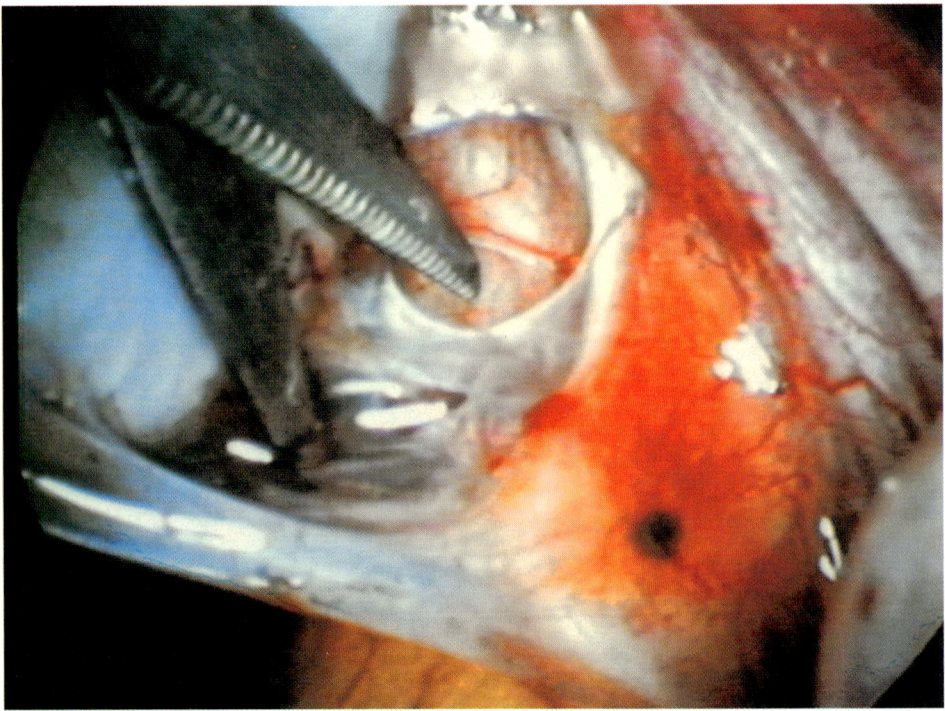

Figure 10.5. Laparoscopic ovariolysis obtained with scissors; subovarian endometriotic adhesions are visible on broad ligament.

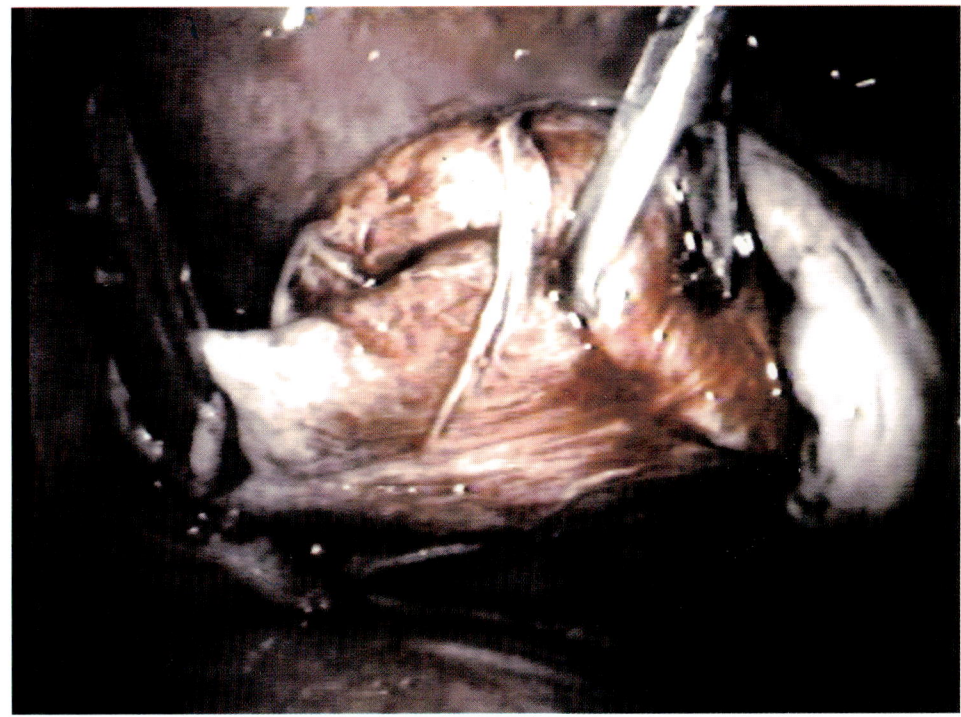

Figure 10.6. Laparoscopic ovarian cystectomy; the red fibrotic tissue on the surface of the cyst wall suggests that one should get closer to the cyst wall to identify the cleavage plane.

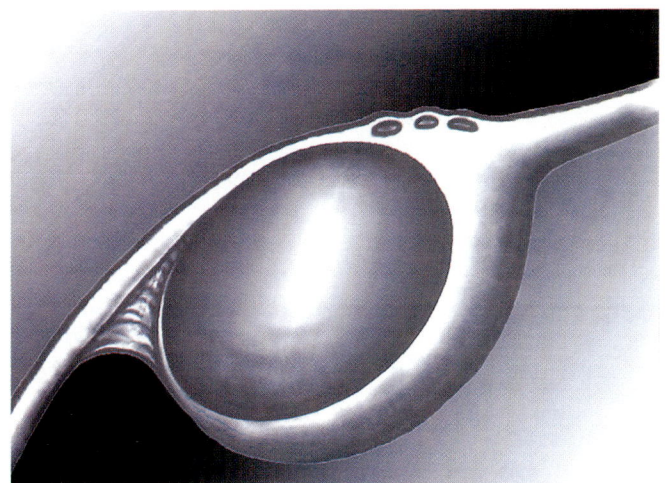

Figure 10.7. Representation of a left ovarian endometrioma fixed to the broad ligament. As suggested by Hughesdon in 1957, the cyst wall is an inverted anterior ovarian cortex fixed to the broad ligament.

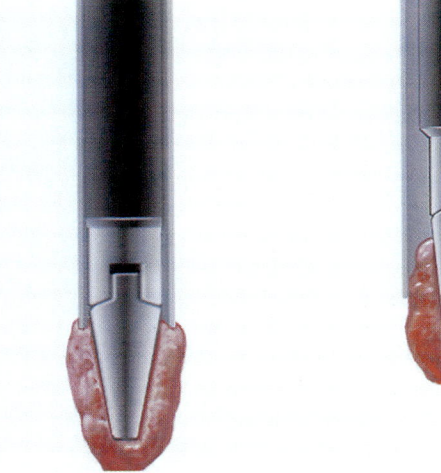

Figure 10.8. On the right, a fragment of the cyst wall is easily removed from the abdomen using a 10-mm trocar and a 5-mm forceps, but it would be cut by the trocar sleeve when removed with a 10-mm forceps, as shown on the left.

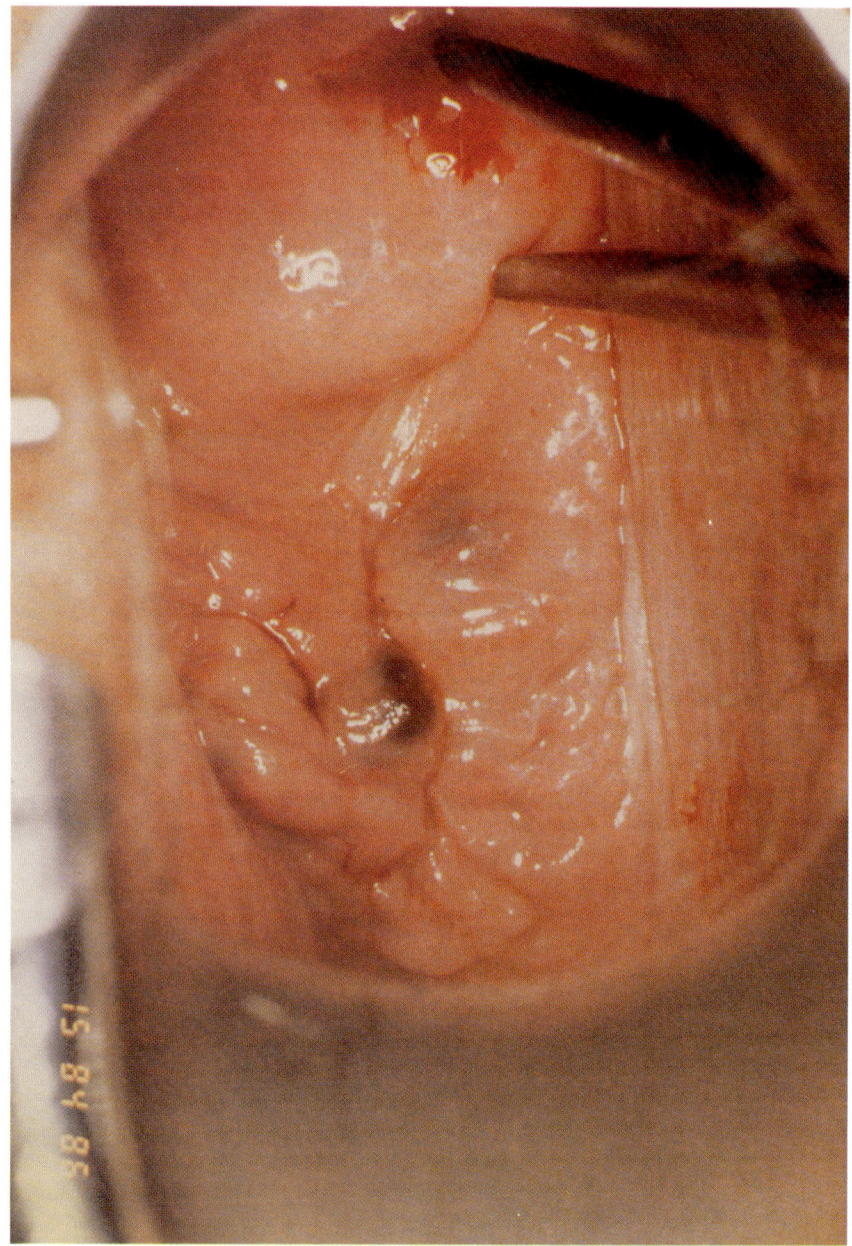

Figure 12.1. Discoloration of the posterior fornix is associated with mucosal invasion by a nodule of endometriosis of the rectovaginal septum. This abnormality was hidden by the posterior blade of a bivalve speculum on a previous pelvic examination.

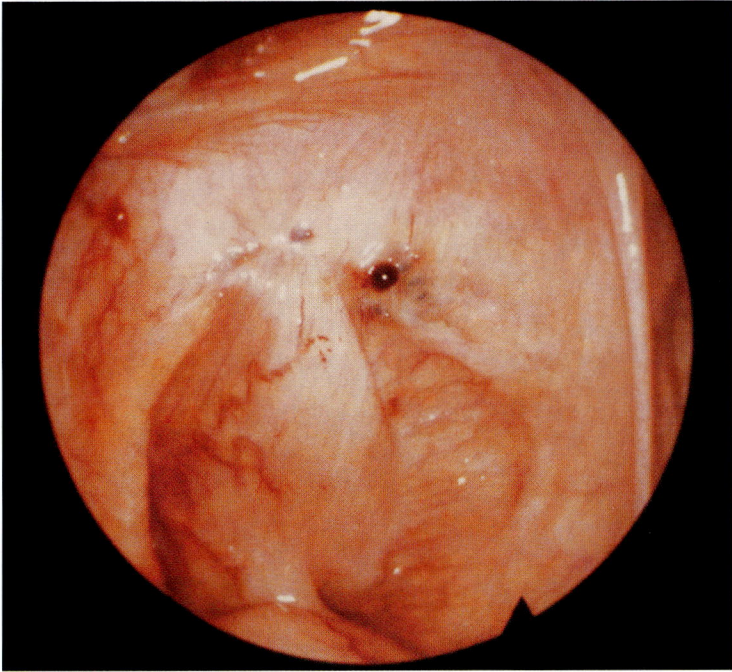

Figure 12.2. The rectosigmoid colon is adherent to the left uterosacral ligament, producing partial obliteration of the cul-de-sac. A significant nodule was palpable in this region on the pelvic examination.

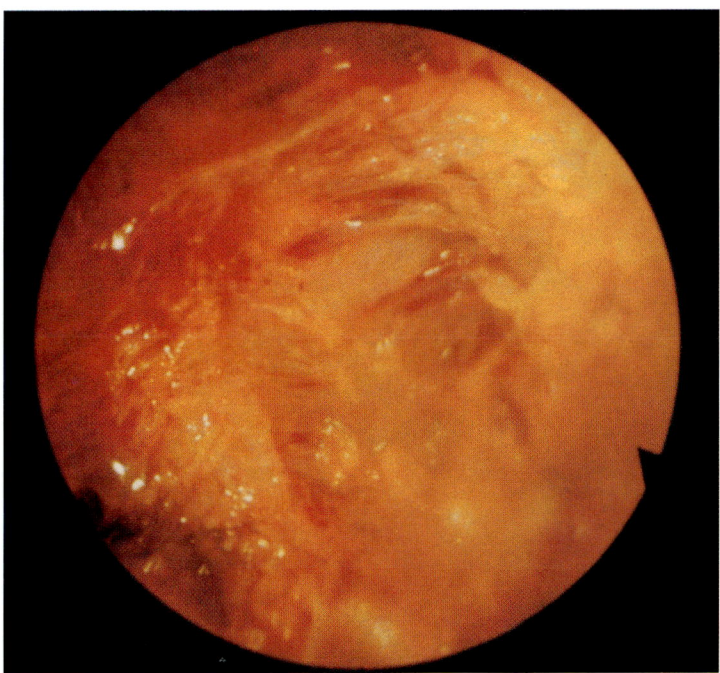

Figure 12.3. The peritoneum of the right side of the cul-de-sac has been excised. The vessels supplying the bowel wall can be seen lying within the retroperitoneal fatty tissue and along the bowel wall. These vessels can be tented up and injured during resection of even superficial cul-de-sac endometriosis. Efforts to control the bleeding with electrocoagulation may lead to damage to the adjacent rectum.

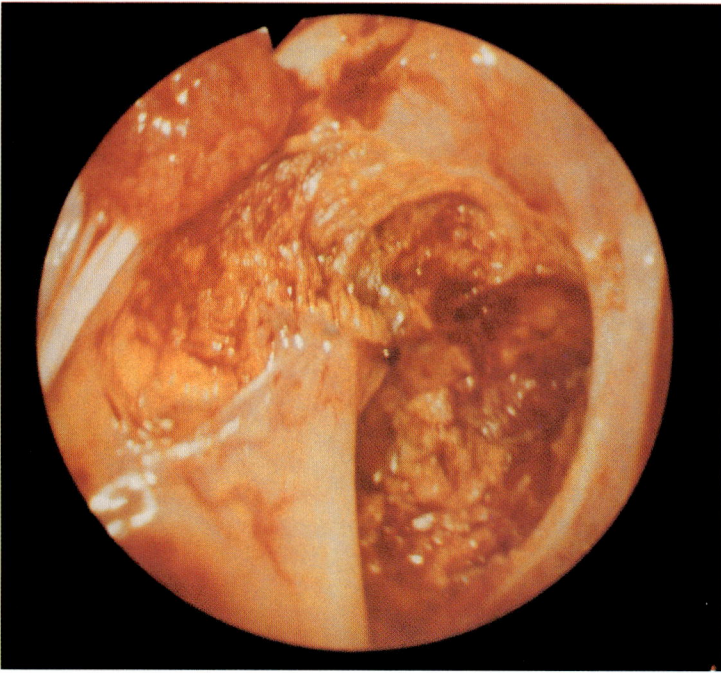

Figure 12.4. The left uterosacral ligament has been isolated by a lateral peritoneal incision and a medial incision in uninvolved peritoneum of the cul-de-sac. An intrafascial dissection down the left side of the posterior cervix has allowed the uterosacral ligament to be transected at its insertion into the posterior cervix. The invasive endometriosis of the left uterosacral and adjacent left posterior cervix and the attached rectosigmoid colon are falling posteriorly away from the cervix. The normal right uterosacral ligament is still intact.

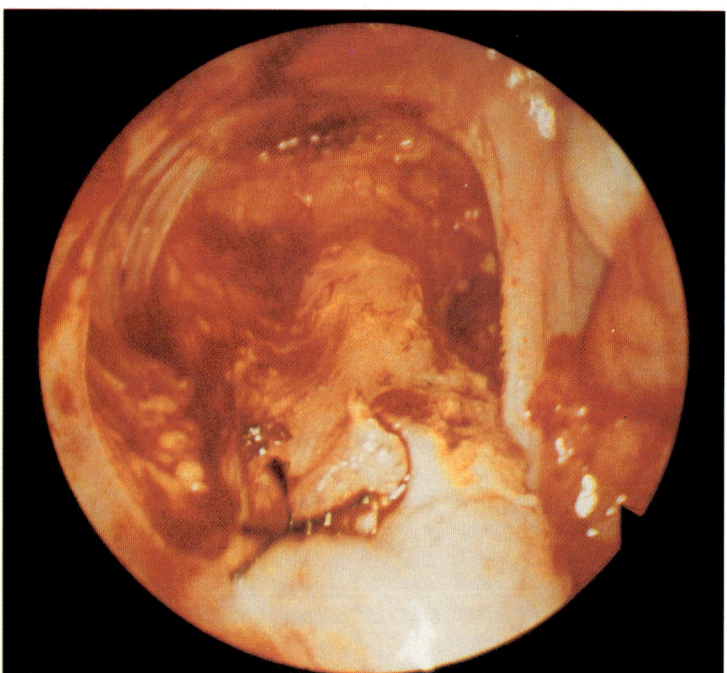

Figure 12.5. The rectal nodule of endometriosis has been removed by partial-thickness bowel resection (mucosal skinning). The seromuscularis has been closed with a single 3-0 silk suture.

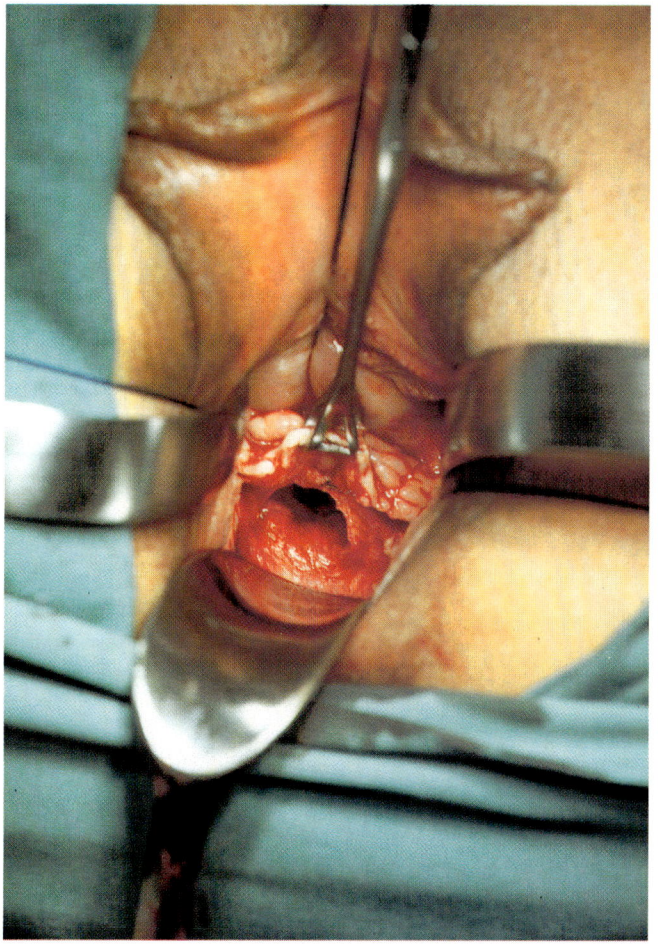

A

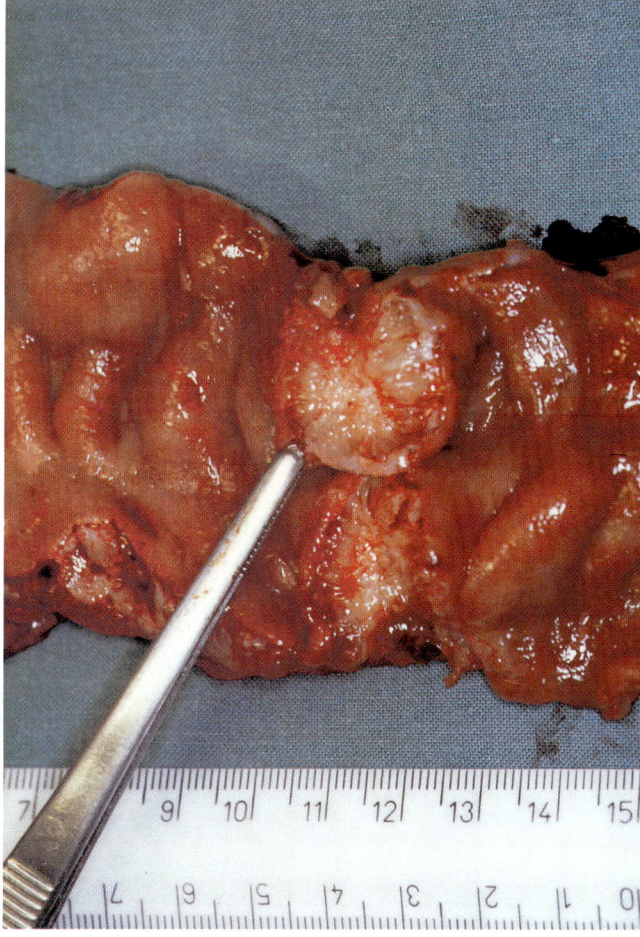

B

Figure 16.2. A 30-year-old nullipara underwent enucleation of left ovarian endometrioma at laparotomy, and after 18 months had a term delivery. Five years later, rectal pain, rectal bleeding, and deep dyspareunia developed, all closely related to the menstrual cycle. Posterior vaginal fornix and colorectal endometriosis was diagnosed. Vaginoabdominal surgery was performed with segmental removal of the posterior fornix and low anterior rectosigmoid resection with end-to-end anastomosis. **A.** The vaginal implants are removed. **B.** Rectosigmoid endometriosis.

(continued)

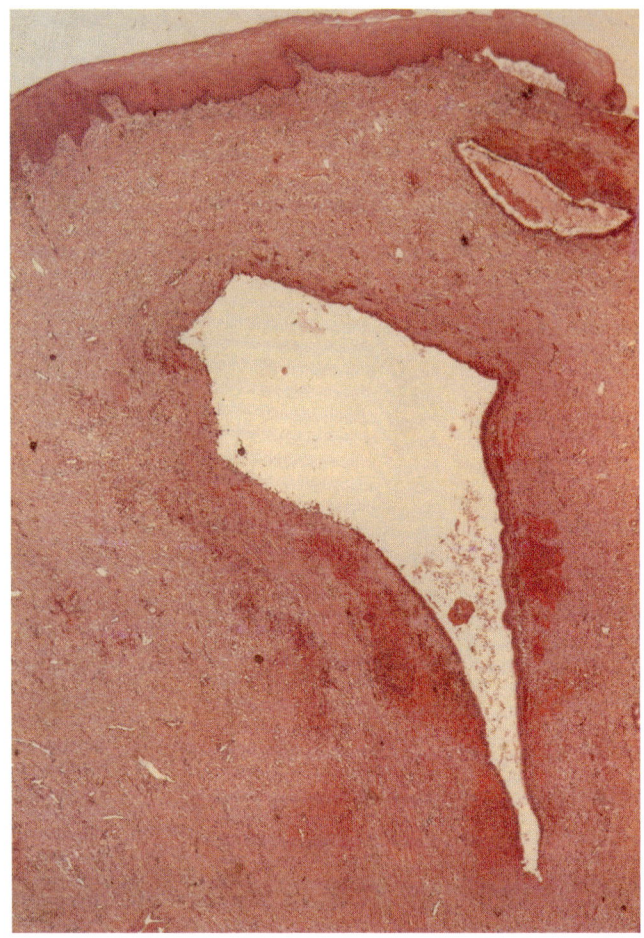

C(a)

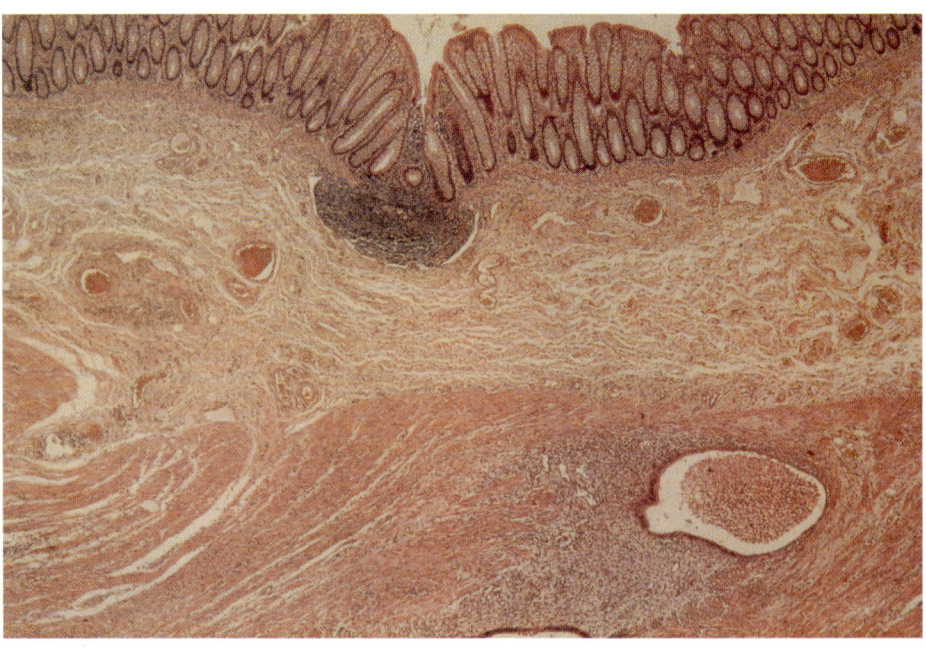

C(b)

C

Figure 16.2 (*continued*). **C.** Histologic results reveal: (a) vaginal endometriosis and (b) rectosigmoid endometriosis.

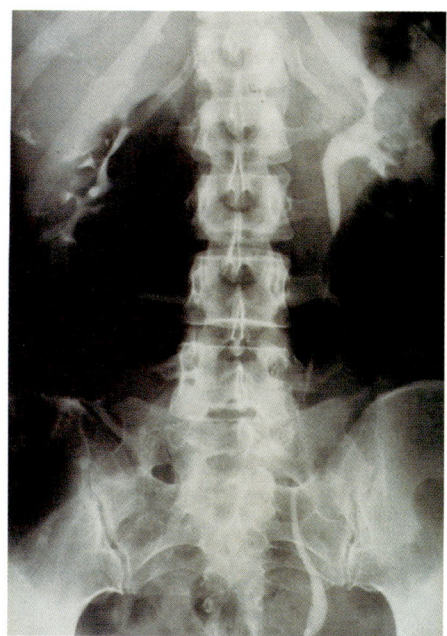

A

Figure 16.3. A multipara, aged 41, previously underwent right adnexectomy for rupture of an endometrioma with peritoneal irritation at age 28. Six years later, she developed severe left pelvic pain and hematuria. Vaginal and rectal examination revealed extensive thickening of the left parametrium, and complete resection of the left parametrium, partial resection of the left angle of the vesical dome and ureteral implantation according to Landbetter-Politano was performed. **A.** Preoperative pyelogram shows left ureteral obstruction with moderate hydronephrosis.

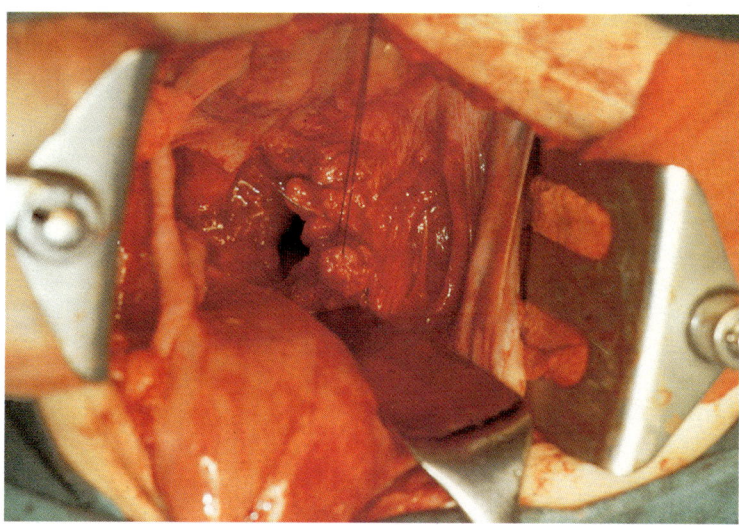

B

B. Endometriotic nodule of parametrium appears after surgical exposure.

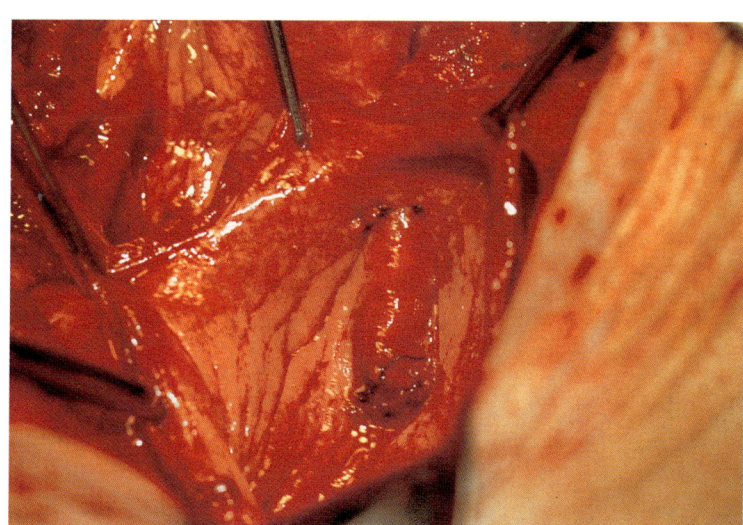

C

C. View of ureteral implantation after partial resection of the vesical dome.

(continued)

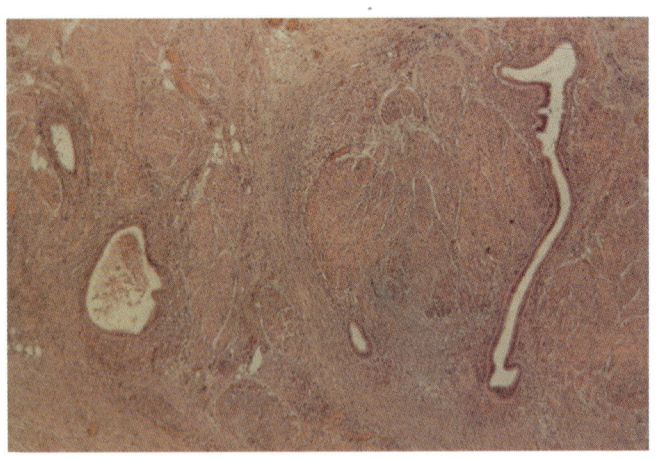

D(a)

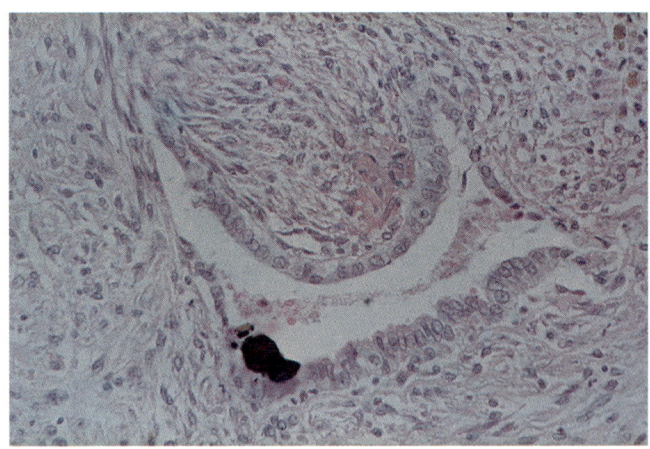

D(b)

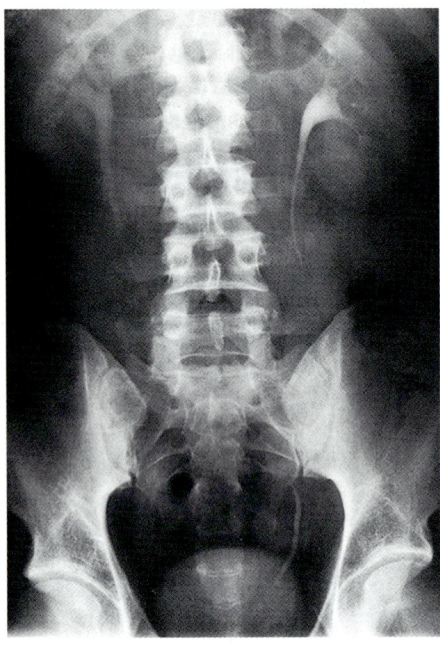

E

Figure 16.3 (*continued*). **D.** Histologic findings shown are of: (a) detrusor muscle, and (b) parametrial specimens. Note the presence of endometrial glands. **E.** Postoperative pyelogram shows restored left ureteral patency and resolution of left hydronephrosis.

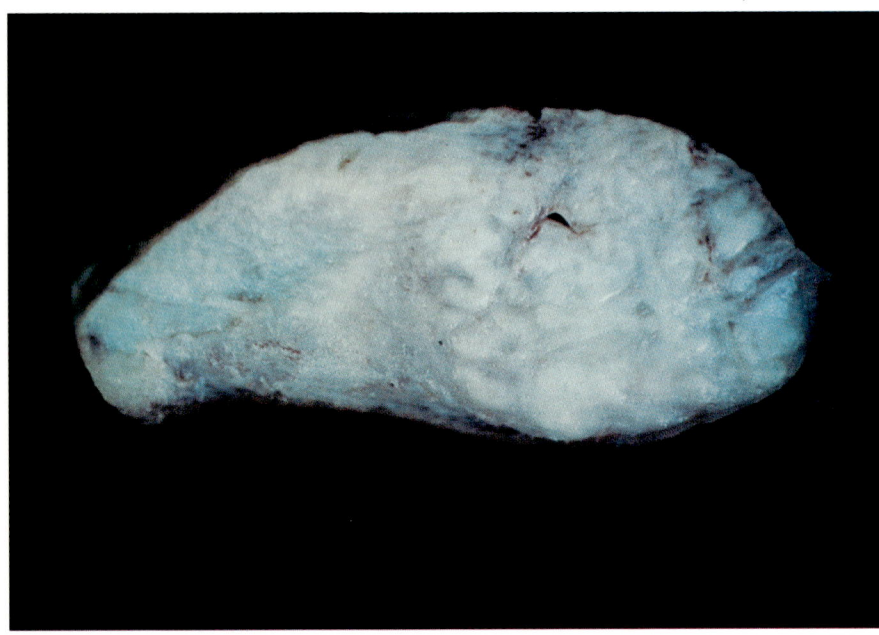

Figure 26.2. Cut surfaces of a uterus with diffuse and focal adenomyosis.

Part 1
Basic Issues

1

Epidemiology of Endometriosis

Gary S. Berger

Endometriosis is a disease which afflicts women of reproductive age. It is one of the most common causes of pelvic pain and infertility; an estimated 5 million women in the U.S. are affected.[1] Despite its apparent widespread occurrence, there are no national or international surveillance systems to determine how many suffer from this disease. Since there is no noninvasive test that is highly selective and specific for endometriosis, studies of its prevalence and incidence have been limited to women undergoing gynecologic operations.

Prevalence Studies

Table 1.1 lists endometriosis prevalence rates reported in various uncontrolled clinical studies.[2] The extraordinarily wide range of rates (1% to 53%) reflects inherent differences in the groups of women entered into the different studies ("selection bias"). The prevalence rates range from a low percentage, among parous women (who are at least risk of having endometriosis) undergoing either surgical sterilization or sterilization reversal, to over 50% of teenagers with pelvic pain severe enough to warrant laparoscopic investigation. These studies indicate that endometriosis affects from a few women to more than half of women depending upon age, parity, history of pelvic pain, and other factors that determine the chance of undergoing pelvic surgery. It is difficult to know how to apply these widely varying rates to the general female population.

In a group of case-control clinical studies, prevalence rates of endometriosis among women who underwent laparoscopy for evaluation of infertility were compared with rates for women laparoscopically sterilized (Table 1.2).[3-7] In these studies, 21% to 47% of infertile women were found to have endometriosis compared

with 1% to 5% of fertile "controls." These rates are difficult to apply to the general female population. We lack information about the prevalence of endometriosis among women with undetermined fecundity (those using contraception or not sexually active) or among infertile women who have not undergone laparoscopic evaluation. The absence of information about these groups is a significant limitation, since they make up over half of the female population of reproductive age.

A few epidemiologic studies have evaluated the prevalence of endometriosis in large population groups (Table 1.3). In a review of U.S. Army hospital inpatient records, 104,129 women aged 13 to 59 had undergone laparoscopy or laparotomy during 1980 to 1985; 6,456 (6.2%) of these women were diagnosed as having endometriosis.[8] One cannot simply apply this rate to the general female population, the majority of whom do not undergo laparotomy or laparoscopy. The prevalence of endometriosis is likely to be higher in women whose symptoms led to pelvic surgery. The prevalence of endometriosis among asymptomatic women, however, is unknown.

In a separate epidemiologic study of hospital discharge records from nonfederal acute care hospitals in the U.S. in 1980, endometriosis was listed as the primary diagnosis in 5.6% and as any diagnosis in 7.9% among nonpregnant women aged 15 to 64 with genital disorders.[9] In contrast to the U.S. Army study, the denominators for calculating these prevalence rates were hospital admissions rather than surgical procedures. These rates cannot be applied to the general population of nongravid women, most of whom have not been hospitalized with disorders of the genital tract.

The data in Table 1.4 are from the only epidemiologic studies of incidence cases of endometriosis. The study by Houston and co-workers included women aged 15 to

Table 1.1. Endometriosis prevalence rates in uncontrolled clinical studies.

Surgery (indication)	Total number	Women with endometriosis	
		Number	Rate
Tubal anastomosis	1,860	19	1%
Tubal sterilization	3,060	61	2%
Vaginal hysterectomy	858	69	8%
Abdominal hysterectomy	5,511	606	11%
Diagnostic laparoscopy (infertility)	724	116	16%
Operative laparoscopy	2,065	619	30%
Diagnostic laparoscopy (teenagers' pelvic pain)	140	74	53%

Adapted from Wheeler.[2]

Table 1.3. Endometriosis prevalence rates in epidemiologic studies.

Author	Population studied	Total number	Women with endometriosis	
			Number	Rate
Boling et al[8]	US Army Personnel & Dependents Inpatient Surgical Records	104,129	6,456	6.2%
Haupt & Graves[9]	Acute Nonfederal Hospitals Discharge Records		106,000	5.6%*
Candiani et al[7]			293,000	7.9%†

* 1st listed diagnosis for women hospitalized with genital disorders other than pregnancy.
† Any listed diagnosis for women hospitalized with genital disorders other than pregnancy.

59 in Rochester, Minnesota, during 1970 to 1979.[10] Incidence rates of endometriosis were calculated based on the following criteria: (1) histopathologic confirmation alone; (2) surgically visualized cases without histopathologic confirmation; (3) "clinically probable" cases, as defined by the presence of symptoms and palpable nodularity on pelvic exam; and (4) "clinically possible" cases defined by palpable nodularity on exam but absence of typical symptoms. Based on a total of 157,135 woman-years of observations, the overall annual rate of newly diagnosed cases was 0.11 to 0.25 per 1,000 woman-years, depending on the diagnostic criteria. The prevalence rate can be calculated by multiplying the incidence rate by the duration of disease. Assuming a range of 20 to 30 years for the duration of endometriosis, the overall prevalence rate would be in

Table 1.2. Endometriosis prevalence rates in case-control studies.

Author	Infertile women		
	Total Number	Women with endometriosis	
		Number	Rate
Hasson[3]	66	16	24%
Drake & Grunert[4]	38	18	47%
Strathy et al[5]	100	21	21%
Verkauf[6]	143	55	38%

Author	Fertile women		
	Total Number	Women with endometriosis	
		Number	Rate
Hasson[3]	296	4	1%
Drake & Grunert[4]	43	2	5%
Strathy et al[5]	200	4	2%
Verkauf[6]	251	13	5%

Adapted from Candiani et al.[7]

the range of 2.2% to 7.5%. Applying this range of prevalence rates to the U.S. population of women aged 15 to 54 in 1991 (approximately 75 million), an estimated 1.7 to 5.6 million women are affected.[11] Since the information in the study was collected before laparoscopy was commonly used as a diagnostic method, this is undoubtedly an underestimate of the true prevalence of endometriosis in the general population.

The most recently published epidemiologic study of endometriosis was performed among a cohort of 17,032 English women who entered the Oxford Family Planning Association study during the years 1968 to 1974.[12] These women were married, aged 25 to 39, and using a birth control method for 5 months or more upon entry into the study. The definition of a case of endometriosis was derived from hospital discharge information of women who had undergone either laparotomy or laparoscopy. Incidence rates were calculated only for fertile women with the principal diagnosis of endometriosis (cases in which endometriosis was listed secondary to another diagnosis were excluded).

While the trend in incidence rates by age was similar to the Minneapolis study (rates increasing to age 40 to 44, then declining), they were higher in most cases for similar age-specific groups than in the Minneapolis study. This was the finding despite the exclusion of cases in which endometriosis was listed as other than the primary diagnosis. The report from the Oxford Family Planning Association has been criticized because fewer than one third of the cases in this study were diagnosed at laparoscopy (the majority were diagnosed at laparotomy). This suggests that only the most severe cases of endometriosis were detected.[13] A similar type of bias ("detection bias") is present in the epidemiologic studies involving U.S. women as well.

In each of these studies, surgical cases were derived only from in-hospital procedures, primarily laparotomy. No epidemiologic study has yet been reported on a large

Table 1.4. Endometriosis incidence rates in epidemiologic studies.*

Age group (years)	Histopathologically confirmed cases		Rochester, Minnesota[a] Surgically visualized cases		Clinically probable cases		Clinically possible cases		Oxford family planning assoc.[b]	
	Number	Rate	Number	Rate	Number	Rate	Number	Rate	Number	Rate
15–19	5	0.02	8	0.03	20	0.07	20	0.07	—	—
20–24	13	0.04	21	0.06	56	0.16	59	0.17	—	—
25–29	25	0.09	47	0.18	83	0.31	87	0.33	3	0.13
30–34	28	0.13	41	0.19	65	0.30	69	0.32	14	0.28
35–39	35	0.21	55	0.32	64	0.38	67	0.40	42	0.60
40–44	40	0.29	51	0.36	55	0.34	56	0.40	58	0.81
45–49	25	0.18	29	0.21	30	0.22	30	0.22	18	0.51
≥50	—	—	—	—	—	—	—	—	—	—
Total	171	0.11	252	0.16	373	0.24	388	0.25	—	—

* Rates per 100 woman-years.
— Not given.
[a] Houston et al.[10]
[b] Vessey et al.[12]

population regarding the occurrence of endometriosis among women undergoing outpatient laparoscopies.

Is Endometriosis Increasing?

In the absence of accurate population-based statistics, it is unclear whether the occurrence of endometriosis is changing in the population. Data from the National Center for Health Statistics (NCHS) regarding hysterectomies performed in the U.S. between 1965 and 1984 provide some insight into this question.[14]

During 1965 to 1984, approximately 2 million U.S. women with the diagnosis of endometriosis underwent hysterectomies. Most of the women were between the ages of 25 and 54 (Fig. 1.1). The annual number of hysterectomies for endometriosis increased steadily throughout the 20-year period (Fig. 1.2). This trend did not simply reflect an increasing number of hysterectomies in general, but was specific to endometriosis. This is evident from the fact that the proportion of hysterectomies performed because of endometriosis, compared with the total number of hysterectomies for all reasons, rose steadily throughout this period (Fig. 1.3). This trend was observed for women of all age groups except those over 44 years of age, when endometriosis tends toward natural remission associated with estrogen deprivation.

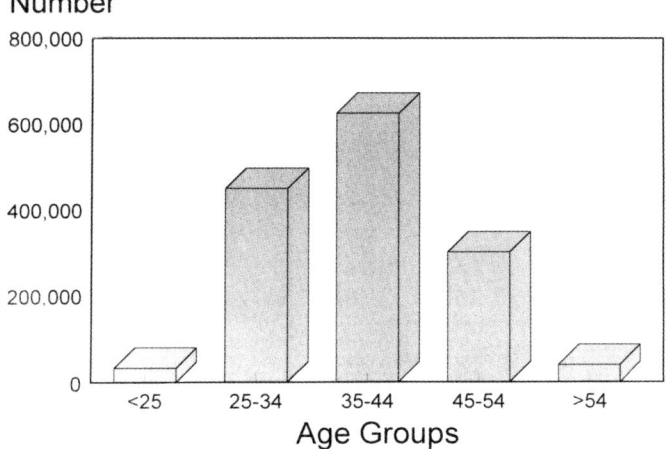

Figure 1.1. Hysterectomies performed for endometriosis in the U.S., 1965–1984: age distribution.

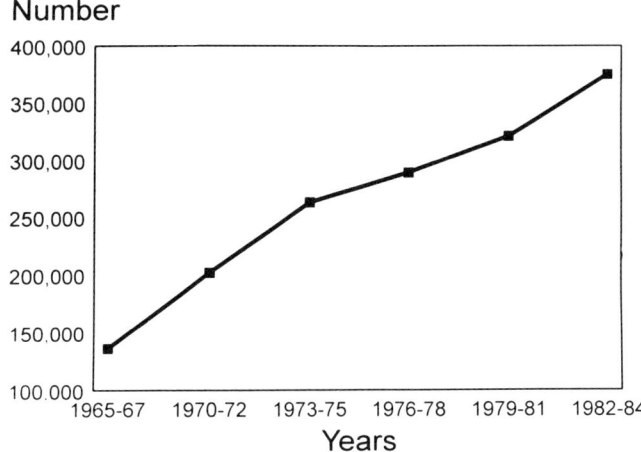

Figure 1.2. Number of hysterectomies performed in the U.S. for endometriosis.

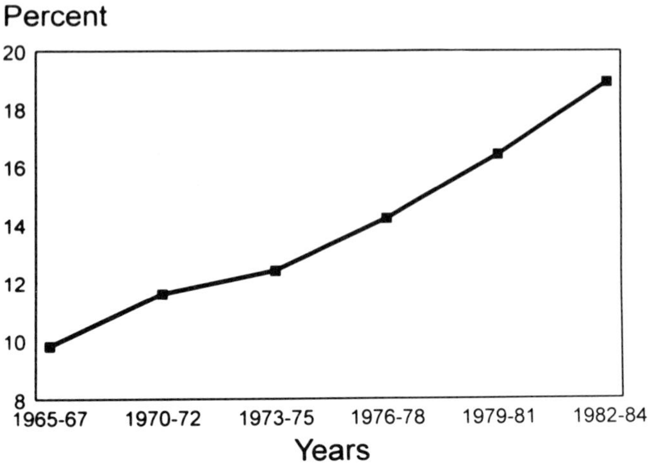

Percent

Figure 1.3. Percent of all hysterectomies performed in the U.S. for endometriosis.

Figure 1.4 shows the changes that occurred in hysterectomy rates, calculated as percentage increases or decreases at the end of the 20-year period as compared with the beginning, for different diagnoses among women of all age groups combined. By far the largest increase was for endometriosis (121%). All other diagnoses were associated with relatively smaller percentage increases or even decreases in hysterectomy rates. Since the occurrence of endometriosis and other diagnoses that lead to hysterectomy is age-related, age-specific changes in hysterectomy rates were examined for the different diagnosis groups. For women of all ages, the relative increase in hysterectomy rates was significantly greater for endometriosis than for all other diagnoses, except for endometrial hyperplasia among women 45 to 54 years of age.[15]

The authors of the NCHS study suggested that changes in medical practices, such as increasing awareness of endometriosis from laparoscopy and/or increasing use of hysterectomy to treat endometriosis, may have accounted for the rising hysterectomy rate associated with endometriosis. It seems unlikely, however, that during the 2 decades studied gynecologists would have performed hysterectomies more frequently *only* for women with endometriosis and not also for women with other conditions considered to be clear indications for hysterectomy. It is improbable that gynecologists would have been performing hysterectomies more frequently only for women with endometriosis during the very time when operative laparoscopy was becoming used for conservative surgical treatment. Also, during those years, several new medical forms of treatment for endometriosis became available.

Another explanation for the rising hysterectomy rates for endometriosis given in the NCHS study report was that demographic changes may have accounted for the results observed (delayed childbearing and/or declining use of oral contraceptives). These explanations may account, in part, for the observed changes. They are also consistent with the hypothesis that the disease was increasing in frequency and/or severity.

Conclusion

Despite thousands of scientific reports in the literature about endometriosis, the true extent of this disease in the general female population is unknown. Since definitive diagnosis requires surgery, our knowledge is limited to selected groups of women who have undergone pelvic surgery for a variety of indications. All existing studies suffer from methodologic limitations that make it difficult to extrapolate their results to the population at large. Until a noninvasive test for endometriosis can be developed, the incidence and prevalence rates of endometriosis in the general population will remain a matter of speculation. Given the significant debility and apparent widespread nature of endometriosis, an accurate enumeration system on a national level needs to developed. This would contribute immensely to our knowledge of the epidemiology of this disease.

References

1. Ballweg ML. Public testimony to the U.S. Senate Committee on Labor and Human Resources, Subcommittee on Aging, May 5, 1993.
2. Wheeler JM. Epidemiology and prevalence of endometriosis. Infertility and Reproductive Medicine Clinics of North America 1992;3(3):545–549.
3. Hasson HM. Incidence of endometriosis in diagnostic laparoscopy. J Reprod Med 1976;16:135–138.
4. Drake TS, Grunert GM. The unsuspected pelvic factor in the infertility evaluation. Fertil Steril 1980;34:27–31.

% Increase or Decrease

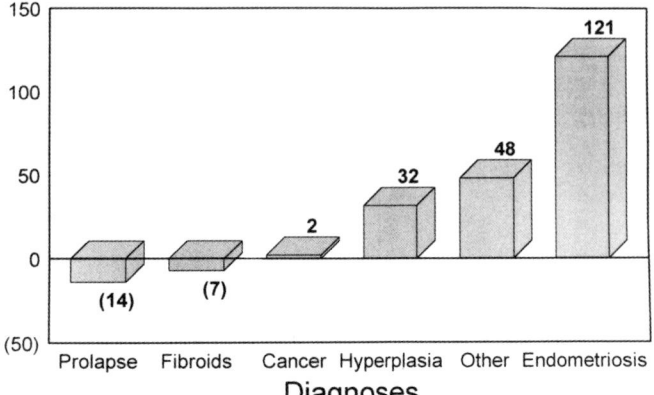

Figure 1.4. Changes in hysterectomy rates in the U.S. between 1965 and 1984.

5. Strathy JH, Molgoard CA, Coulam CB, et al. Endometriosis and infertility: a laparoscopic study of endometriosis among fertile and infertile women. Fertil Steril 1982;38:667–672.
6. Verkauf BS. The incidence, symptoms, and signs of endometriosis in fertile and infertile women. J Fla Med Assoc 1987;74:671–675.
7. Candiani GB, Vercellini P, Fedele L, Colombo A, Candiani M. Mild endometriosis and infertility: a critical review of epidemiologic data, diagnostic pitfalls, and classification limits. Obstet Gynecol Survey 1991;46(6): 374–382.
8. Boling RO, Abbasi R, Ackerman G, Shipul AH Jr, Chaney SA. Disability from endometriosis in the United States Army. J Reprod Med 1988;33:49–52.
9. Haupt BJ, Grave E. Detailed diagnoses and procedures for patients discharged from short-stay hospitals: United States 1979. Hyattsville, MD. National Center for Health Statistics, 1982; DHHS Publication No. (PHS) 82-1274-1.
10. Houston DE, Noller KL, Melton J III, Selwyn BJ. The epidemiology of pelvic endometriosis. Clin Obstet Gynecol 1988;31(4):787–800.
11. Statistical abstracts of the United States. U.S. Bureau of Census Current Population Reports. Series P-25. U.S. Government Printing Office.
12. Vessey MP, Villard-Mackintosh L, Painter R. Epidemiology of endometriosis in women attending family planning clinics. Brit Med J 1993;306:182–184.
13. Prentice A. Epidemiology of endometriosis. Brit Med J 1993;306:585.
14. National Center for Health Statistics. Hysterectomies in the United States, 1965–84. Hyattsville, MD. National Center for Health Statistics, 1987 (Vital and Health Statistics, Series 13, Data from the National Health Survey, No. 92, DHHS Publ No. (PHS) 88-1753).
15. Berger GS. Endometriosis: How many women are affected? Endometriosis Association Newsletter 1993; 14(4):4–6.

2
Pathogenesis of Endometriosis

Ivo Brosens, Gloria Vasquez, Jan Deprest, and Patrick Puttemans

Although the pathogenesis of endometriosis is still under study, much progress has been made recently in identifying the disease. This advance may help us understand its evolution.

History of Surgical Pathology

We believe the surgical pathology of endometriosis offers a rational basis for understanding the pathogenesis and evolution of the disease.

Adenomyoma

What is now universally called endometriosis has a long history. Recognition started with the gross pathology of nodular lesions found at pelvic surgery which appeared to be causing major complaints of pelvic pain and bowel obstruction. The histologic identification of these lesions was consistent with adenomyoma. Such lesions were found outside the uterus in pelvic supportive structures such as the rectovaginal septum, uterosacral ligaments, round ligament, and utero-ovarian ligament, and sometimes extended into the rectum, ovary, and sigmoid colon. In a 1920 report, the pathological lesion was described as "a matrix of non-striped muscle and fibrous tissue. . . . Scattered throughout this matrix or ground-work are isolated glands or groups of glands sometimes lying in direct contact with the muscle, but usually in a characteristic stroma."[1] Much of the nodule, composed of fibromuscular tissue, has finger-like extensions of endometrial tissue suggesting a process of metaplasia, proliferation, and fibrosis rather than one of invasion and destruction. The location of this nodular lesion is typically in the pelvic supportive structures (Fig. 2.1).

Ovarian Endometrial Cyst

It took several decades before the ovarian endometrial cyst was identified as part of the same disease. In 1899, one investigator, on microscopic examination, was "astonished to find areas which were an exact prototype of the uterine glands and interglandular connective tissue."[2] In 1919, another described a case where "the entire cyst, or ovarian cavity as it really is, is lined throughout by a single layer of tall columnar epithelium of the uterine type."[3] The presence of mucosa-type endometriosis and adhesions has become recognized as the characteristic feature of the endometrial cyst.

On large sections of ovaries containing an endometrial cyst, in more than 90% of cases the wall of the cyst was the inverted ovarian cortex (Fig. 2.2).[4] Characteristic features of the ovarian pseudocyst are that it is located on the frontal side of the ovary, is adherent to the surrounding peritoneum or ligaments, and produces an eccentric distension in the ovary. [15]The content of the cyst is frequently drained when the ovary is mobilized during the process of adhesiolysis without any incision of the cortex. The frequent association with lutein cysts is explained by the fact that the pseudo-wall is formed by ovarian cortex in which primordial and developing follicles can be identified.[5]

Peritoneal Endometriosis

It is customary to consider Sampson the discoverer of endometriosis.[6,7] His observations on peritoneal lesions and hemorrhagic cysts of the ovary led him to theorize that during menstruation particles of endometrium might flow in retrograde fashion through the fallopian tubes to be implanted on the peritoneum or into the ovaries. Sampson's theory so impressed the scientific community that the disease has continued to be defined

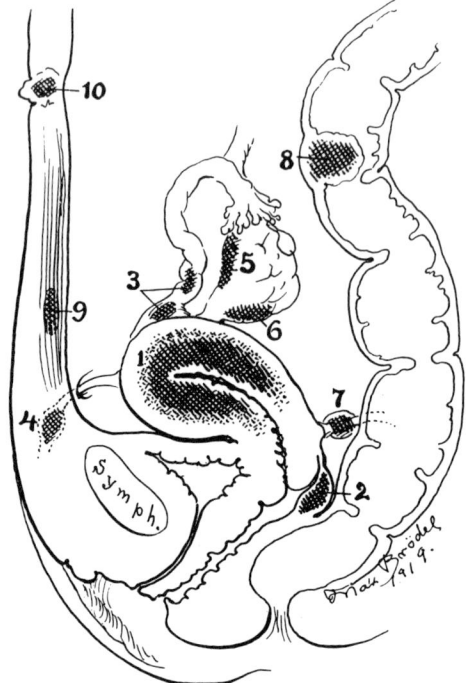

Figure 2.1. Localization of so-called adenomyoma in the pelvic supportive structures and wall of pelvic organs. (Reproduced with permission from *Archives of Surgery*, 1920;1: 215–283. Copyright 1920, American Medical Association.)

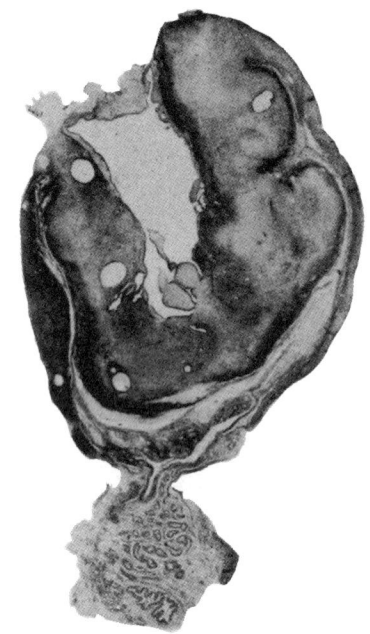

Figure 2.2. Section of ovary cut at right angles to long axis. Illustration shows adhesions above the cavity, which is surrounded successively by thickened invaginated cortex, U-shaped medulla, and remainder of cortex, with broad ligament below (×5, H&E). (Reproduced with permission of *Journal of Obstetrics and Gynaecology of the British Empire*, 1957;64:481–487.)

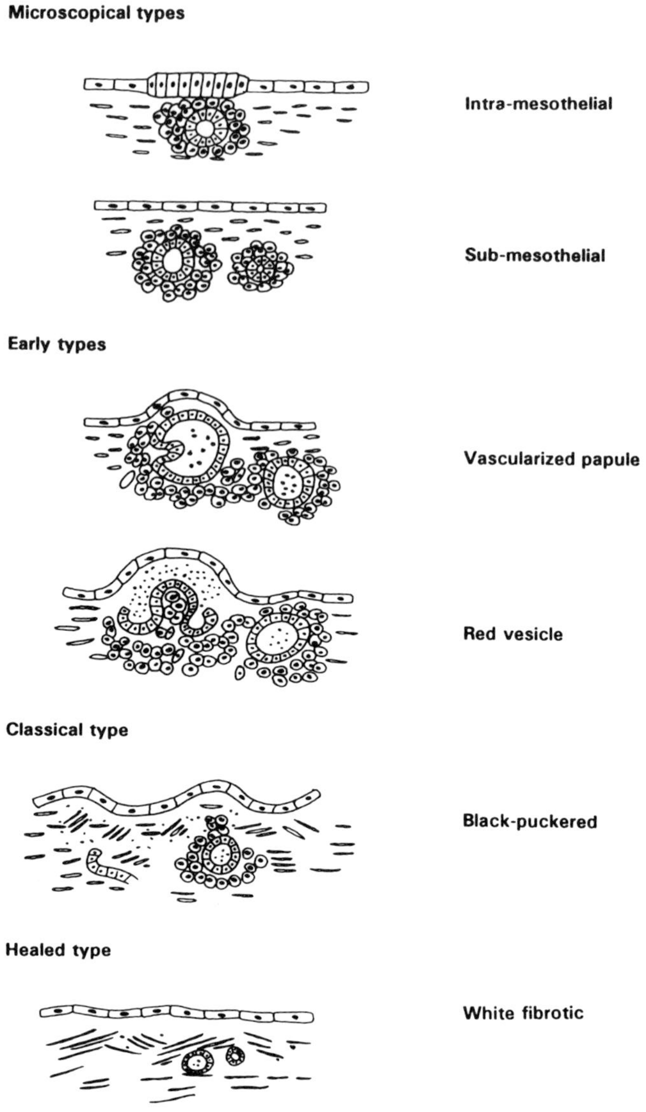

Microscopical types

Intra-mesothelial

Sub-mesothelial

Early types

Vascularized papule

Red vesicle

Classical type

Black-puckered

Healed type

White fibrotic

Figure 2.3. Evolution of peritoneal endometriosis.

by the histologic identification outside the uterine cavity of glands and stroma. During the past decade, microscopic and subtle types of endometrial implants have been described.[8–14] Differences in appearance and color have led investigators to describe more than 20 types of lesions. In addition, terms such as superficial and deep, infiltration and invasion, and intra-, sub-, and retroperitoneal, have been used to describe the varying locations of these lesions.

Pathogenesis of Peritoneal Endometriosis

Four stages can be distinguished in the development of peritoneal endometriosis: microscopic, early active, advanced active (classical), and healed (Fig. 2.3).

Microscopic Lesions

Recent scanning electron microscopic and histologic studies have revealed two types of microscopic lesions

Figure 2.4. Scanning electron microscopy of biopsy taken at laparoscopy from the pouch of Douglas. **A**. General view of the biopsy shows endometrial lining surface (arrows) and underlying endometrial glandular space (asterisk) (×110). **B**. Enlargement of an area of glandular space depicts mainly nonciliated cells and few ciliated cells (small arrows). The endometrial surface epithelium with cuboidal to columnar cells can be appreciated at the cut surface (large arrows) (×550). **C**. Enlargement of the endometrial surface epithelium at the cut surface shows columnar cupuloid secretory cells with numerous microvilli and underlying connective tissue stroma (asterisk) (×2200). **D**. Enlargement is of a neighboring area from the columnar epithelium shown in C. Two cupuloid secretory cells (SC) display microvilli and two neighboring cells, cilia and microvilli (CC). At asterisk note the connective tissue stroma (×5500).

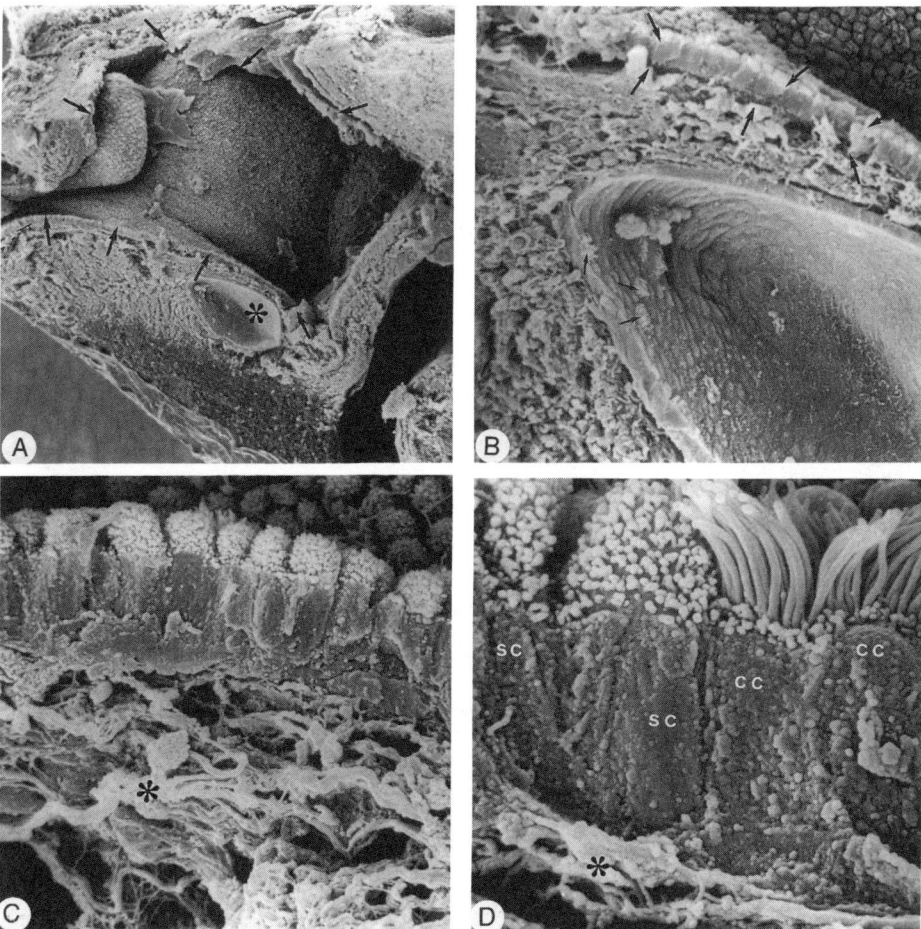

in macroscopically normal-appearing peritoneum.[15] The intraperitoneal lesion, an area where tall epithelium and ciliated cells are replacing the mesothelium (Fig. 2.4), has been found in patients with and without visible endometriosis. The second microscopic lesion, composed of glands and stroma covered by normal mesothelium, has been detected in random biopsies from normal-appearing peritoneum.[13] It is unclear whether or not these lesions develop from implantation or metaplasia. Foci of endometrial tissue growing on the peritoneum have not been detected by scanning electron microscopy.

Retrograde menstruation may have a direct role in establishing endometriosis, but we should also consider the role of growth-stimulating factors that could be carried along by the same process of retrograde menstruation. The cases of "leiomyomatosis peritonealis disseminata" indicate that there may be an individual sensitivity of submesothelial mesenchymal cells to ovarian steroids.

Recent research on the metaplastic potentiality of the secondary Müllerian system into Müllerian structures has been suggested as a factor in the pathogenesis of the early lesion.[16] Studies combining scanning electron microscopy and immunohistochemistry, as well as experimental studies in primates, may help elucidate whether these microscopic lesions develop by implantation, metaplasia, or perhaps by both mechanisms.

Early Active Lesions

We detect early active peritoneal endometriosis when the glandular tissue emerges under the mesothelium as cystic glands (papular excrescences) or as polyps (vesicles) (Fig. 2.5 and color plates 2.5A and B). The glandular papule is a raised, apparently solid lesion with a fine vascularization in continuity with the surrounding peritoneum. It represents one or more proliferating glands distended by secretion. The endometriotic vesicle presents as a blister or a cluster of blisters of the mesothelium. It appears filled with serous, pink or hemorrhagic fluid and is surrounded by marked centripetal vascularization. In these lesions, polypoidal endometrial tissue arising from underlying ruptured glands has been identified. In the early stage, both papular and vesicular lesions are highly vascularized but not fibrotic. The glands are usually in a state of proliferation or secretion (Table 2.1). Approximately one third of these lesions are in phase with the eutopic endometrium (Fig. 2.6 and Table 2.2).

In vivo studies have shown that the red hemorrhagic lesions are very active in prostaglandin production.[11]

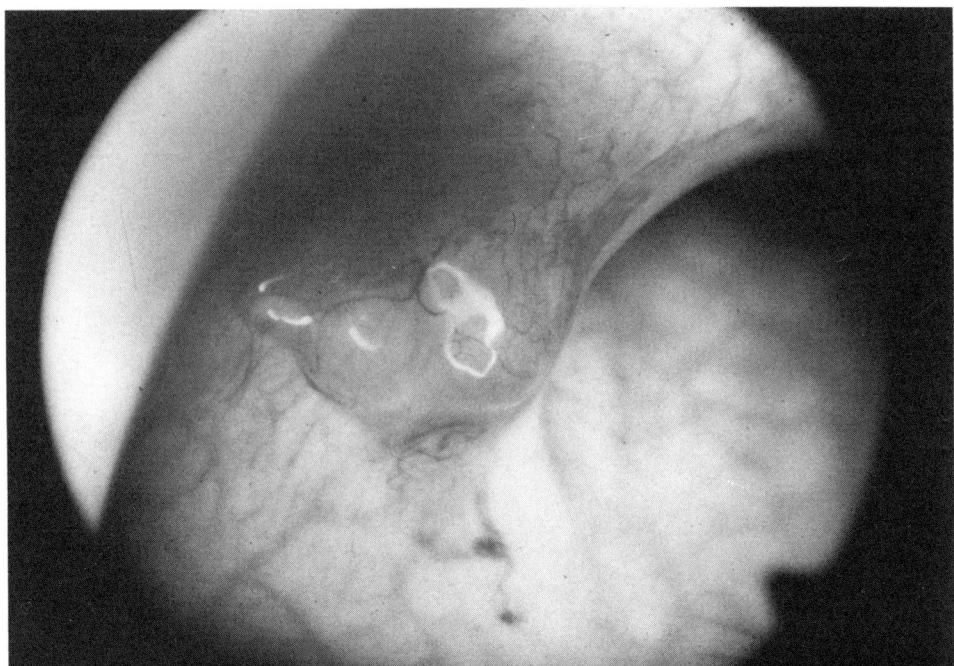

A

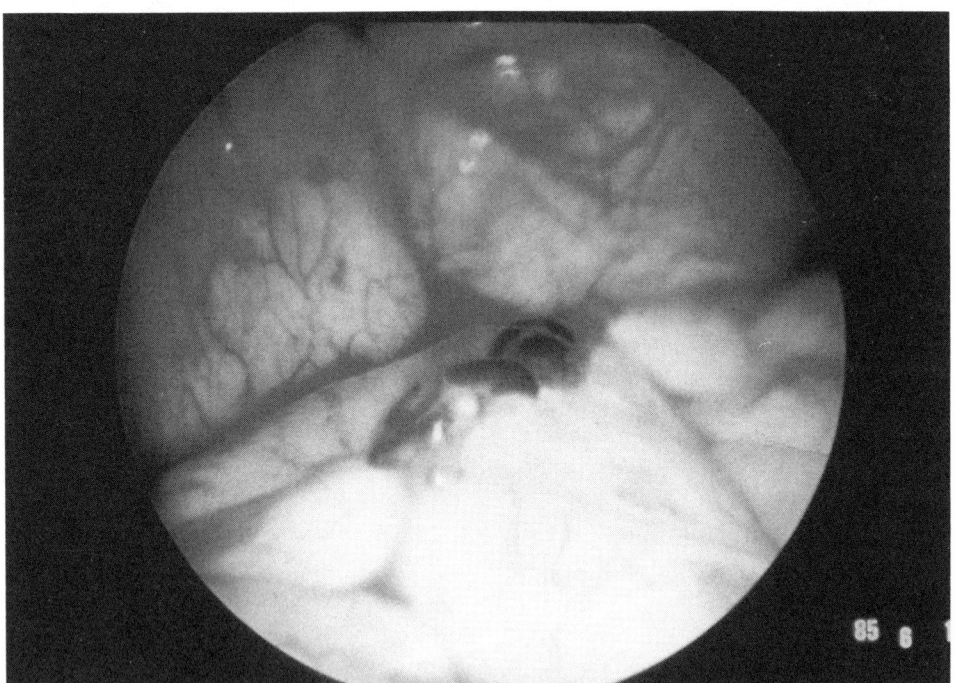

B

Figure 2.5. A. Early peritoneal lesion: papular type. (Lesion represents distended endometrial gland. Note pattern of fine vascularization and absence of bleeding and fibrosis.). **B**. Early peritoneal lesion: sero-hemorrhagic type. (Lesion represents an active implant. Note absence of fibrosis.) See also color plates.

Table 2.1. Correlation between laparoscopic appearance and histologic characteristics of endometriotic peritoneal lesions.

			Glands	
Laparoscopic appearance	Number	Endometriosis not confirmed	At rest	Proliferative or secretory
Pink-red (vesicular, glandular)	25	2 (8%)	8 (32%)	15 (60%)
Black-blue (plaque)	24	12 (50%)	8 (33%)	4 (17%)
White-brown (macula)	19	12 (63%)	7 (37%)	0 (0%)

Source: Vernon et al.[11]

Recent three-dimensional, computerized reconstructions show that the ectopic glands have an interconnecting ramified structure.[14] It is likely that, as the early lesions develop, the tip of one or more glandular ramifications emerges under the mesothelium and becomes visible because of secretion, hemorrhage, or desquamation of active endometrial tissue that bulges and eventually disrupts the thin mesothelial lining. On postscanning sections of electron microscopic-scanned biopsies (Fig. 2.7A and B), it can be seen that these lesions represent the top of larger underlying glandular complexes.[8]

Figure 2.6. Scanning electron microscopy of biopsy taken at laparoscopy from peritoneal surface. **A**. In this polypoid endometrial tissue, note polyps of different size (arrows) arising on the peritoneal surface (×100). **B**. Enlargement is of lower left corner of A. The limits of the endometrial polypoid tissue are shown at arrows (×210). **C**. Enlargement is of area delimited by the three upper arrows in A. Note typical endometrial surface epithelium with both secretory and ciliated cells. No gland openings are observed (×500). **D**. The endometrial surface shows active secretory cells with microvilli and secretory blebs (asterisks), and several ciliated cells (×2100).

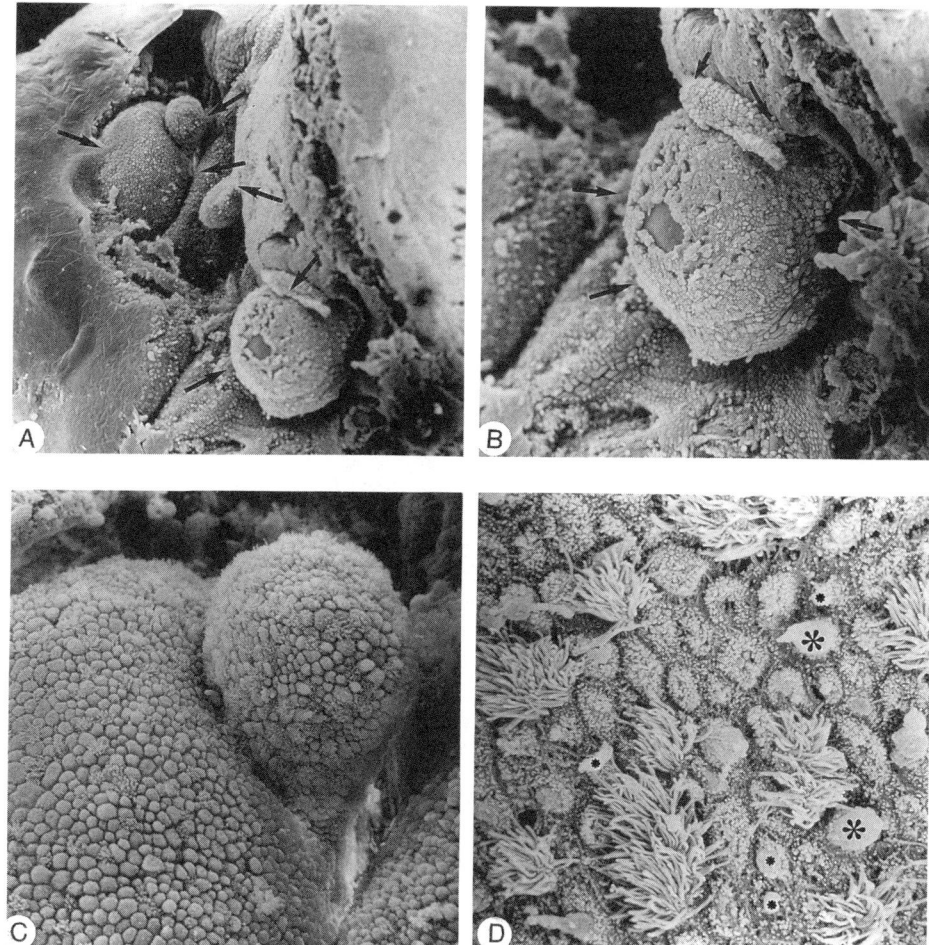

Recently, these papular or vesicular (red) lesions were found to appear and disappear like mushrooms on the peritoneal surface. This finding suggests a fluctuating activation of peritoneal endometriosis.[17] The visual disappearance of endometriosis upon laparoscopic observation after months of hormonal therapy is no guarantee the implant has been truly eliminated. Long-term hormonal therapy masks rather than eliminates peritoneal implants.[18]

Advanced Active Lesions

The advanced active lesions, made prominent because of inflammation, fibrosis, hemorrhage, and pigmentation, form the so-called classic lesions. These lesions are the most easily identified as endometriosis. With increasing fibrosis, the hormonal response during the menstrual cycle apparently decreases and becomes more variable. This implant is known to be very much "out of phase" with the eutopic endometrium. Redwine found that the papular and red vesicular lesions appear at an earlier age than the classic dark or black lesions (Fig. 2.8).[19] During many years of reproductive life, the nonfibrotic and fibrotic lesions coexist, but the fibrotic lesions persist after the glandular or red lesions disappear from the peritoneum. This pattern would suggest that the activation and appearance of early endometriosis is a feature of the initial decades of reproductive life rather than an ongoing process. The seeding process of endometriosis could be limited to the initial phase of reproductive life, thus accounting for the fact that the visible lesions develop intermittently over time. Early active peritoneal lesions can disappear spontaneously or develop into fibrotic active lesions that, with increasing fibrosis, become less and less hormonally responsive. For most of the peritoneal implants, the evolution is apparently a self-limiting disease.

Healed Lesions

Healed lesions have been described as white, and sometimes calcified scars representing remnants of glands embedded in fibrotic tissue. Without the aid of histologic examination, however, it is impossible to exclude the possibility of endometrial activity in these lesions.

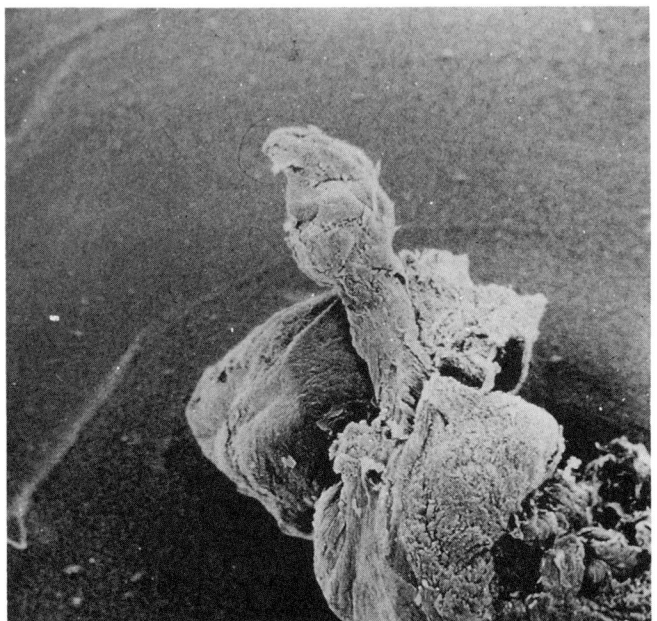

A

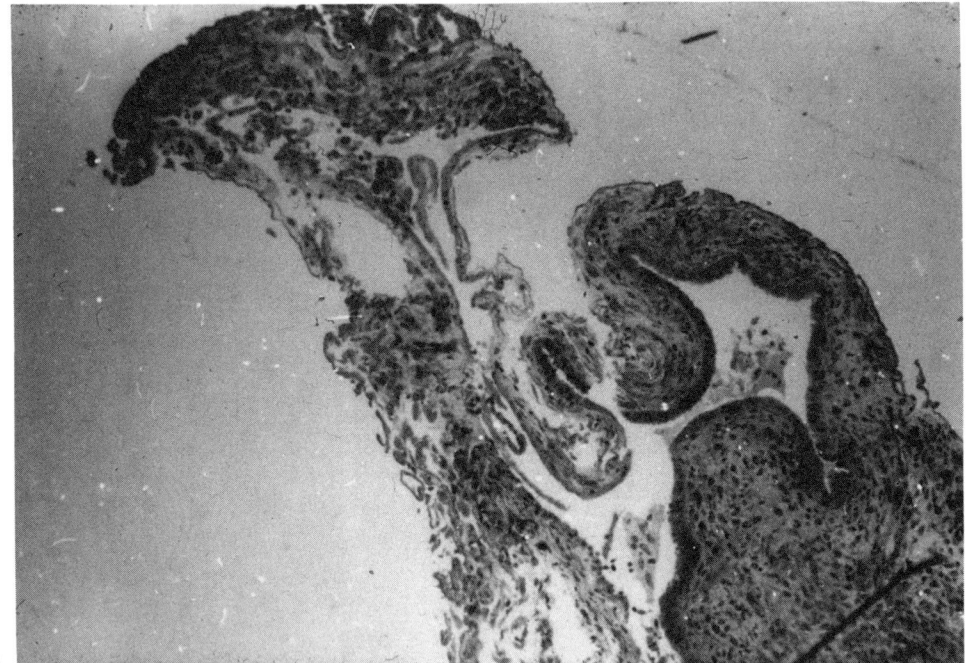

B

Figure 2.7. **A**. Scanning electron microscopy showing polypoid endometrial implants. (The overlying mesothelium forming a hemorrhagic vesicle is ruptured [probably when taking the biopsy]). **B**. Postscanning section of Figure 2.6A. Shown is the underlying glandular complex from which the polyp arises.

Pathogenesis of the Ovarian Endometrial Cyst

Careful histologic studies using step serial sections have demonstrated that, in the vast majority of ovarian endometriomas, the wall is formed by the inverted ovarian cortex.[4] The frontal surface in proximity to the hilus of the ovary is the most frequent site where the folding-in process occurs. Using the technique of ovarian cystoscopy, the site of retraction and inversion can be identified (Fig. 2.9 and color plate 2.9).[20] In early stages, the ovarian cortex can still be recognized by its pearl-white appearance. Endometrial implants are seen as red, vascularized, or hemorrhagic islands at the site of retraction as well as scattered over the ovarian cortex (Fig. 2.10 and color plate 2.10). On histologic examination, the implant frequently has a mucosa-like ap-

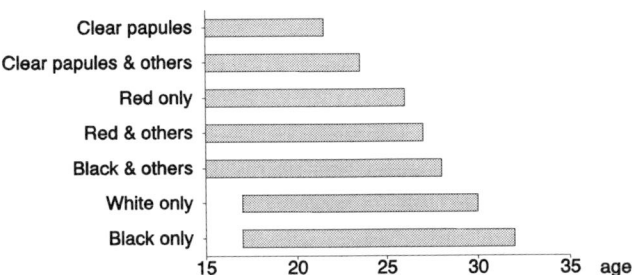

Figure 2.8. Evolution of types of endometriotic lesions with age according to Redwine[19].

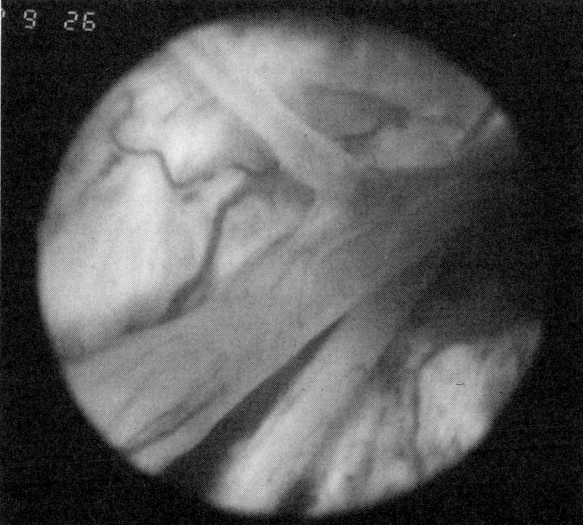

Figure 2.9. Ovarioscopy of endometrial cyst. Note the area of adhesion and retraction of the inverted ovarian cortex at the site of hemorrhagic endometrial implant. See also color plate. (From Brosens IA, Puttemans PJ, Deprest J. The endoscopic localization of endometrial implants in the ovarian chocolate cyst. Fertil Steril 1994;61:1034–8. Reproduced with permission of publisher. The American Fertility Society.)

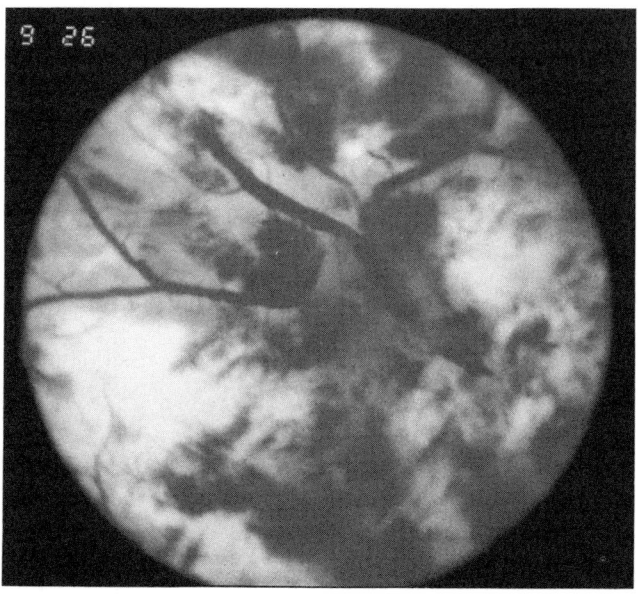

Figure 2.10. Ovarioscopy of endometrial cyst. The implants are scattered over surface of inverted cortex. See also color plate.

pearance (Fig. 2.11 and color plate 2.11). Nieminen was the first to observe the difference in hormonal response between free superficial and enclosed implants.[21] The free mucosa-type lesion can undergo secretory changes during the luteal phase of the cycle, and vascular necrosis and shedding at the time of menstruation (Table 2.2). In many respects, the ovarian endometrioma can be compared with hematometra, an entrapment of blood secondary to obstruction by adhesions.

The pathogenesis of ovarian endometriomas is ap-

parently by a sequence of superficial implants, adhesion formation, invagination of the cortex, and mucosa-like outgrowths on the surface of the inverted cortex; the spilling of the content at dissection; and the frequent combination, particularly in large cysts, with hemorrhagic functional cysts.[5] Progressive distension of the cyst and fibrosis of the wall obscure the original structure and produce a darkly pigmented, fibrotic, and poorly vascularized surface. However, the eccentric localization and the flattening of the wall on the medial

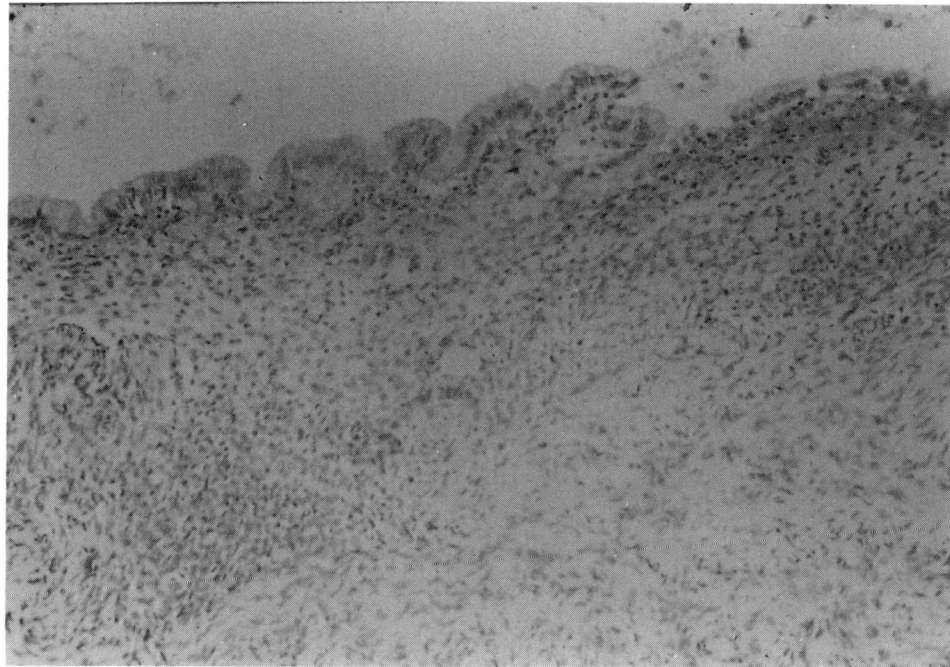

Figure 2.11. Biopsy of endometrial cyst. Specimen shows superficial endometrial tissue growing on the ovarian cortex. See also color plate.

Table 2.2. Type of endometriosis and hormonal response during menstrual cycle.

	Type of lesion	
	Free-growing	Enclosed
Corresponding with endometrium	27/34 (79%)	7/20 (35%)
Corresponding with		
late secretory phase;	7/12 (58%)	0/4 (0%)
menstruation (bleeding)	4/4 (100%)	0/4 (0%)

Source: Nieminen.[21]

side with much of the normal ovarian tissue on the posterior and lateral side remain suggestive of its pathogenesis.

The terminology of deep endometriosis for the ovarian endometrioma is misleading. First, the pathogenesis of the endometriomas is, in most cases, related to superficial and superficially spreading endometriosis and subsequent adhesion formation. Second, the mucosa-type of implant responds to ovarian steroids much as does eutopic superficial endometrium.

A different pathogenesis for some endometriomas is possible. Approximately 10% of ovarian endometrial cysts do not display these external characteristics. It has been suggested that such endometriomas originate from local Müllerian tissue or from colonization of a ruptured follicle by endometrial cells.

Pathogenesis of Nodular Endometriosis

Deep endometriosis presents as a nodular lesion. Histologically, it is characterized by dense tissue composed of fibrous and smooth muscle cells with strands of glands and stroma. It is not surprising that, on descriptive grounds, the lesion had been initially called an adenomyoma. Although the terminology was dropped after Sampson's 1921 publication, there are several reasons for reappraising the terminology.

The major component of the nodular lesion is not endometrial tissue but fibromuscular tissue with sparse, fingerlike extensions of glandular and stromal tissue (Fig. 2.12 and color plate 2.12). The locale characteristically involves pelvic supportive structures such as the uterosacral ligament, the retrocervical fascia, and the rectovaginal septum or the ovarian ligament. The lesion is proliferative and shows poor or absent secretory changes during the luteal phase of the menstrual cycle and vasodilatation, rather than necrosis and bleeding, at the time of menstruation.[21] Also, the well-known resistance to current hormonal therapy makes the lesion morphologically and functionally similar to adenomyosis of the uterus. This fibromyosis type of endometriosis is likely to develop from subperitoneal implants that extend into the underlying pelvic supportive tissue as lesions and usually have some superficial extension. Approximately 25% of superficial lesions of the uterosacral ligament show a component of

Table 2.3. Distribution of type of endometriosis by site.

Site	Number	Fibromyosis type	Classical	Negative
Rectovaginal	11	10 (91%)	0 (0%)	1 (9%)
Uterosacral	28	7 (25%)	15 (54%)	6 (21%)

Source: Nieminen.[21]

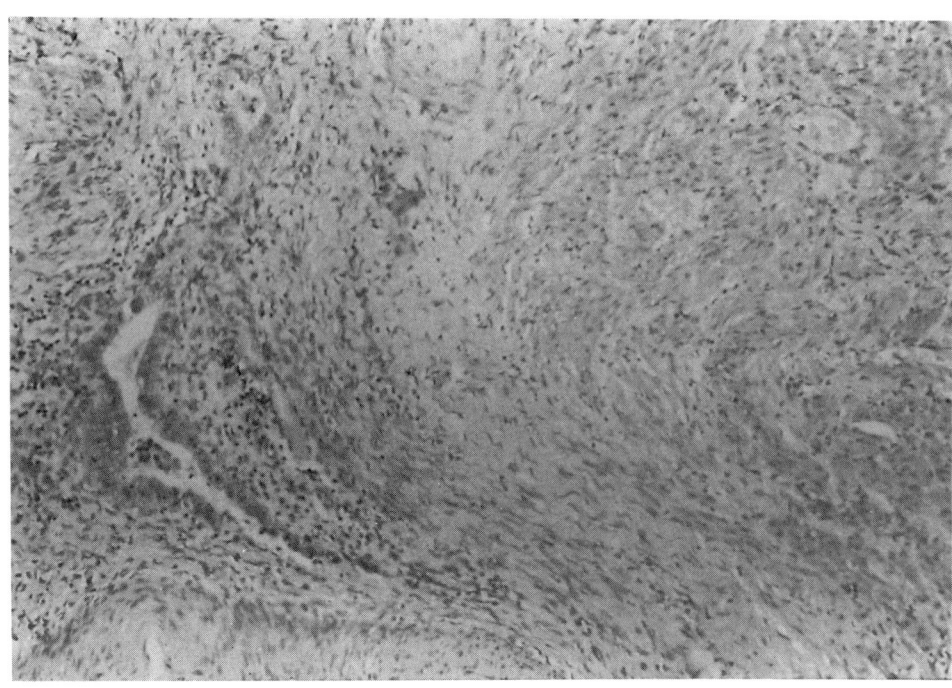

Figure 2.12. Endometriosis of rectovaginal septum. Lesion is characterized by a fibromuscular nodule with fingerlike extensions of endometrial tissue (adenofibromyosis). See also color plate.

fibromyosis (Table 2.3). In contrast with the free mucosa-type implant of the ovary, this lesion develops as an enclosed, fibromuscular nodule with different pathophysiologic characteristics. It is well known that deep endometriotic lesions are frequently associated with pelvic pain, dysmenorrhea, and dyspareunia. Resistance to medical therapy makes surgical excision the treatment of choice. Needle biopsy is useful for identifying the morphologic characteristics of the lesion.

Conclusion

In the pathogenesis of pelvic endometriosis, microscopic mesothelial and submesothelial implants can be considered as the reservoir from which three types of endometriosis arise: the cystic ovarian lesion, the nodular lesion of the pelvic supportive structures, and the visible peritoneal lesion. The three types have different histologic characteristics and pathophysiology.

The ovarian endometrial cyst is a hemorrhagic lesion with mucosa-type implants extending on the inverted cortex. It is associated with the formation of adhesions and fibroreactive tissue. The nodular type is a proliferative lesion of the pelvic supportive fibromuscular tissue in which the endometrial component varies considerably. Peritoneal endometriosis is, except for the microscopic intramesothelial type, a superficial but not free implant because it is covered by mesothelium. Early visible lesions likely originate from microscopic implants and appear and disappear on the peritoneal surface. Advanced peritoneal lesions form after recurrent bleeding; fibroreactive tissue develops into classical, scarred lesions. Superficial endometriosis appears to have a self-limiting evolution and terminates in healed lesions when the stroma is replaced by fibrosis. Progression of the disease may be determined by the localization and the development of the endometrial implant into either a mucosa-type lesion, when it extends into a cystic or open structure, or into a fibromyosis type of lesion, when it extends into the pelvic supportive structures.

References

1. Cullen TS. The distribution of adenomyoma containing uterine mucosa. Arch of Surg 1920;1:215–283.
2. Russel WW. Aberrant portions of the Müllerian duct found in an ovary. Johns Hopkins Hospital Bulletin 1899; 10:8–10.
3. Casler DB. A unique, diffuse uterine tumor, really an adenomyoma, with stroma, but no glands. Menstruation after complete hysterectomy due to uterine mucosa remaining in the ovary. Trans Am Gynecol Soc 1919;44: 69–84.
4. Hughesdon PE. The structure of endometrial cysts of the ovary. J Obstet Gynec Brit Emp 1957;44:481–487.
5. Nezhat F, Nezhat C, Allan CJ, et al. Clinical and histologic classification of endometriomas: Implications for a mechanism of pathogenesis. J Reprod Med 1992;37:771–776.
6. Sampson JA. Perforating hemorrhagic (chocolate) cysts of the ovary. Arch Surg 1921;3:245–323.
7. Sampson JA. Peritoneal endometriosis due to the menstrual dissemination of endometrial tissue into the peritoneal cavity. Am J Ob Gyn 1927;14:422–469.
8. Vasquez G, Cornillie F, Brosens IA. Peritoneal endometriosis: scanning electron microscopy and histology of minimal pelvic endometriotic lesion. Fertil Steril 42:696–703.
9. Jansen RPS, Russell P. Non-pigmented endometriosis: clinical laparoscopic and pathologic definition. Am J Ob Gyn 1986;155:1154–1159.
10. Murphy A, Green W, Bobbie D, et al. Unsuspected endometriosis documented by scanning electron microscopy in visually normal peritoneum. Fertil Steril 1986;46: 522–524.
11. Vernon MW, Beard JS, Graves K, et al. Classification of endometriotic implants by morphologic appearance and capacity to synthesize prostaglandin F. Fertil Steril 1986; 46:801–806.
12. Stripling MC, Martin DC, Chatman DL, et al. Subtle appearances of endometriosis. Fertil Steril 1988;49:427–431.
13. Nisolle M, Paindaveine B, Bourdon A, et al. Histologic study of peritoneal endometriosis in infertile women. Fertil Steril 1990;53:984–988.
14. Donnez J, Nisolle M, Casanas-Roux F. Three-dimensional architectures of peritoneal endometriosis. Fertil Steril 1992;57(5):980–983.
15. Brosens IA, Vasquez G, Gordts S. Scanning electron microscopic study of the pelvic peritoneum in unexplained infertility and endometriosis. Fertil Steril 1984;41(Suppl): S21.
16. Fujii S. Metaplasia: secondary Müllerian system and endometriosis. In Brosens I, Donnez J, eds. The Current Status of Endometriosis, Camforth, UK, The Parthenon Publishing Group, p 19, 1993.
17. Wiegerinck MAHM, Van Dop PA, Brosens IA. The staging of peritoneal endometriosis by the type of active lesion in addition to the revised American Fertility Society Classification. Fertil Steril 1993 (in press).
18. Evers J. The second look laparoscopy for the evaluation of the results of medical treatment of endometriosis should not be performed during ovarian suppression. Fertil Steril 1987;47:502–504.
19. Redwine DB. Age-related evolution in color appearance of endometriosis. Fertil Steril 1987;48:1062–1063.
20. Brosens IA, Puttemans P. Double-optic laparoscopy. Salpingoscopy, ovarian cystoscopy and endo-ovarian surgery with the argon laser. Bailliere's Clin Ob Gyn 1989;3: 595–608.
21. Nieminen U. Studies on the vascular pattern of ectopic endometrium with special reference to cyclic changes. Acta Obstet et Gynecol Scand 1962;41(Suppl. 3):9–81.

3

Histogenesis of Peritoneal Endometriosis

Michelle Nisolle, Françoise Casanas-Roux, and Jacques Donnez

Endometriosis most commonly affects areas of the pelvic peritoneum close to the ovaries: the uterosacral ligaments, the ovarian fossa peritoneum, and the peritoneum of the cul-de-sac. The diagnosis of peritoneal endometriosis at the time of laparoscopy is often made by observation of typically puckered black or bluish lesions, but there are also numerous subtle appearances of peritoneal endometriosis.[1-4] These subtle lesions, frequently nonpigmented, were first diagnosed as endometriosis following confirmation by biopsy in 1986.[1] Experience has led to more frequent identification of subtle lesions, which increased in various reports from 15% in 1986 to 65% in 1988.[1-6]

Lesion Appearance

The typical black peritoneal endometriotic lesion results from tissue bleeding and retention of blood pigment which produce the brown discolored tissue. Puckered black lesions are composed of glands, stroma, scars, and intraluminal debris (Fig. 3.1 and color plates 3.1A, B, and C).

Sometimes, subtle endometriotic lesions are the only lesions seen at laparoscopy. These forms are actually more common and tend to be more active physiologically than the puckered black lesions. The nonpigmented peritoneal endometriotic lesions may be classified, as shown in Table 3.1, as black; red (flame-like, glandular excrescences, petechial peritoneum, hypervascularization areas); and white (white opacification, subovarian adhesions, yellow-brown patches, circular peritoneal defect).[7,8]

Red flamelike lesions of the peritoneum or red vesicular excrescences most often affect the broad liga-ment and the uterosacral ligaments (Fig. 3.2 and color plate 3.2). Histologically, these are due to the presence of active endometriosis surrounded by stroma. In color, translucency, and consistency, glandular excrescences closely resemble the mucosal surface of the endometrium seen at hysteroscopy. Biopsy reveals the presence of numerous endometrial glands. Areas of petechial peritoneum or areas with hypervascularization have been diagnosed as endometriosis in one of our recent studies.[6] These lesions resemble the petechial lesions that result from manipulation of the peritoneum or from hypervascularization of the peritoneum. Generally, they affect the bladder and the broad ligament; histologically, red blood cells are numerous and endometrial glands very rare.

White opacification of the peritoneum, which appears as peritoneal scarring or as circumscribed patches, is often thickened and sometimes raised (Fig. 3.3 and color plate 3.3). Histologically, white opacified peritoneum results from the presence of an occasional retroperitoneal glandular structure and scanty stroma surrounded by fibrotic tissue or connective tissue.

Subovarian adhesions or those between the ovary and peritoneum of the ovarian fossa differ from adhesions characteristic of previous salpingitis or peritonitis. Histologically, connective tissue with sparse endometrial glands is found.

Yellow-brown peritoneal patches resemble "café au lait" patches. The histological characteristics are similar to those observed in white opacification, but blood pigment (hemosiderin) among the stroma cells produces the "café au lait" color.

Circular peritoneal defects have also been described.[2] Serial sections demonstrate the presence of endometrial glands in more than 50% of cases.[7]

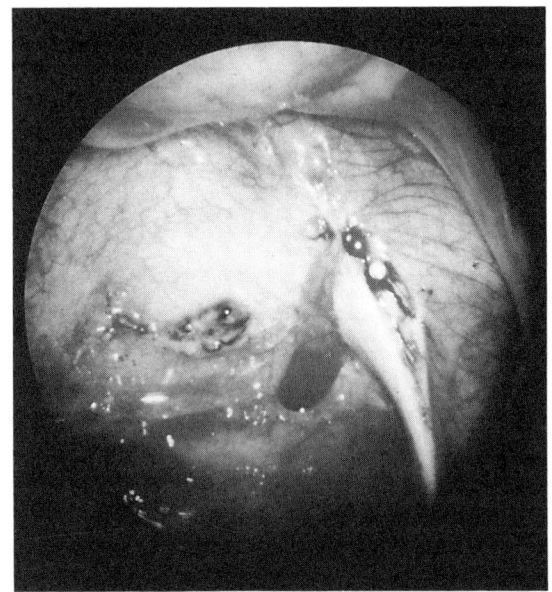

A

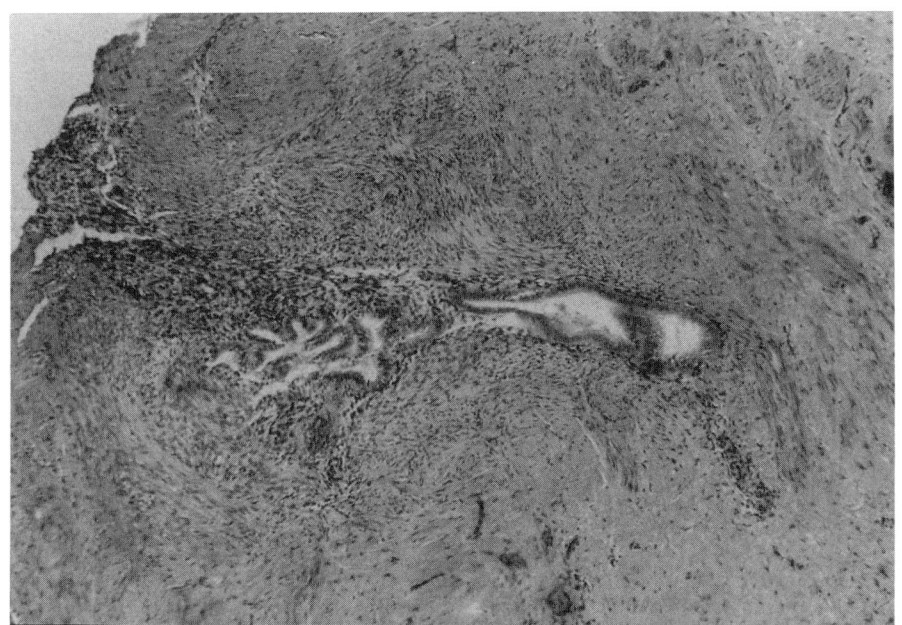

B

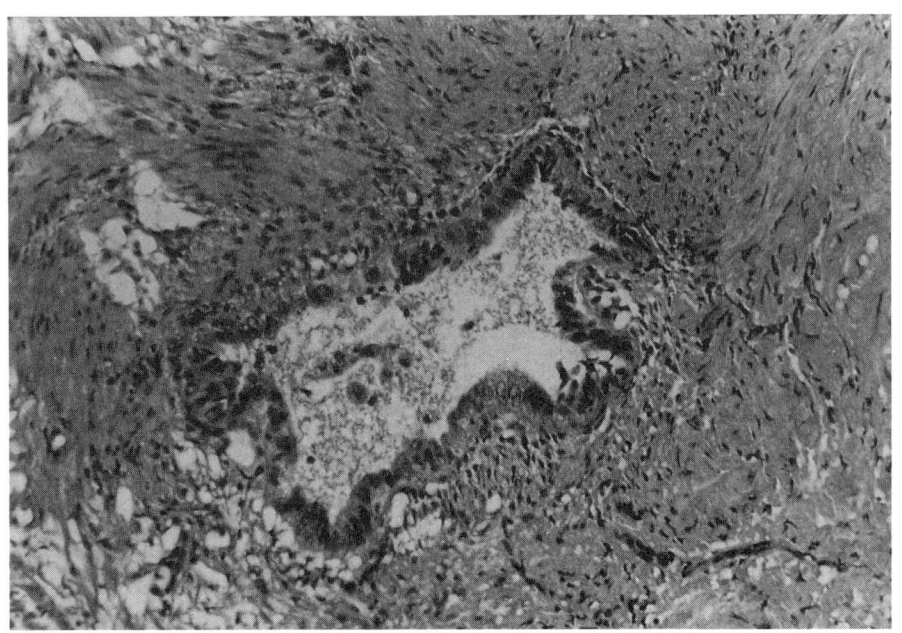

C

Figure 3.1. Typical puckered black lesion. **A**. Laparoscopic appearance: close to the black lesion, other types (red) are seen. **B**. Gomori's Trichrome at ×25 magnification shows combination of endometrial glands and typical stroma. **C**. Higher magnification (×56) of lesion shows intraluminal debris. See also color plates.

Table 3.1. Different appearances of peritoneal endometriosis.

Black:	— Typical puckered, black lesion[a]
Red:	— Red flamelike lesions[a]
	— Glandular excrescences[c]
	— Petechial peritoneum[c]
	— Hypervascularization areas[c]
White:	— White opacification[a]
	— Subovarian adhesions[a]
	— Yellow-brown peritoneal patches[a]
	— Circular peritoneal defects[b]

[a] Jansen and Russell.[1]
[b] Chatman.[2]
[c] Donnez et al.[7]

Histology of Peritoneal Endometriosis

The morphologic characteristics of peritoneal endometriosis were studied in 109 biopsies with histologically confirmed endometriosis (Table 3.2).[6] Endometriotic lesions were considered "active" when typical glandular epithelium appeared as either proliferative or completely unresponsive to hormones, with typical stroma. Such lesions were found in 76% of cases. Areas of oviduct-like epithelium with ciliated cells were demonstrated in 55% of peritoneal endometriotic foci. Epithelial height and mitotic index were calculated in typical glandular epithelium. Epithelial height was measured with a micrometer and the mitotic index was calculated by counting mitotic figures per 2,000 epithelial cells.[9] Their values were $14.8 \pm 3.2\,\mu m$ and 0.6%, respectively.

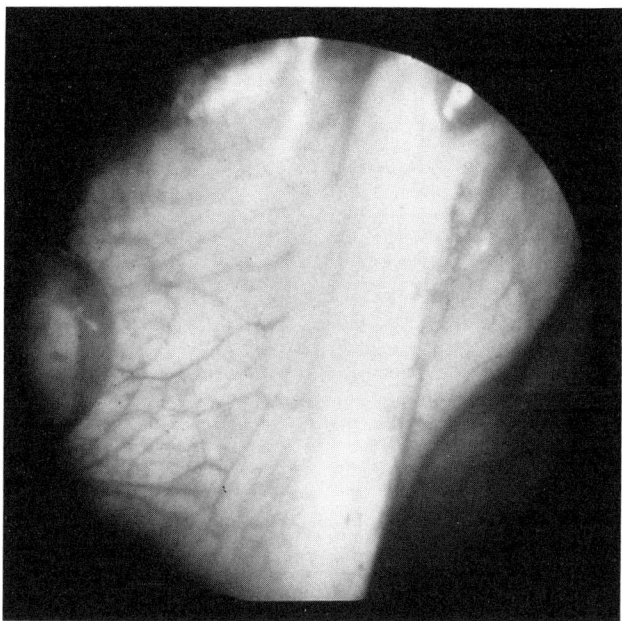

Figure 3.3. Laparoscopic appearance of white opacification of the peritoneum. See also color plate.

Confirmation of endometriosis in subtle lesions was reported by Jansen and Russell.[1] Endometriosis was confirmed in 81% of white opacified lesions, 81% of red flame-like lesions, 67% of glandular lesions, 50% of subovarian adhesions, 47% of yellow-brown patches, and 45% of circular peritoneal defects. Later, Stripling and colleagues confirmed endometriosis in 91% of white lesions, 75% of red lesions, 33% of hemosiderin lesions, and 85% of other lesions.[4] We confirmed the presence of endometriotic lesions in nonpigmented lesions of the peritoneum in more than 50% of cases.[6]

In a recent study, biopsies were taken from normal appearing peritoneum of the uterosacral ligaments among 52 women with visual endometriosis, and from 32 women undergoing laparoscopy for infertility without visually apparent endometriosis. Histologic examination revealed the presence of endometriotic tissue in two cases (6%) in the 32 infertile women without visible endometriosis. This rate was less than one half the rate (13%) observed in biopsies of visually nomal peritoneum taken from patients with visible endometri-

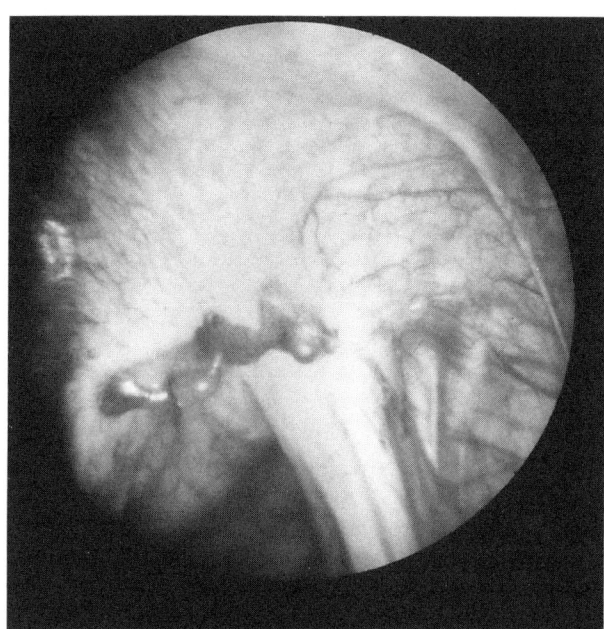

Figure 3.2. Laparoscopic appearance of red flamelike lesion. See also color plate.

Table 3.2. Morphologic characteristics of biopsied peritoneal endometriosis.

Biopsies ($n = 109$)	Number
Typical glandular epithelium and stroma	109 (100%)
Active endometriosis	83 (76%)
Oviductlike epithlium	46 (55%)
Epithelial height (μm)	14.8 ± 3.2
Mitotic index (%)	0.6

Table 3.3. Histologic vs laparoscopic diagnosis of peritoneal endometriosis among infertility patients.

	Endometriosis visible at laparoscopy	Endometriosis not visible at laparoscopy
Biopsy		
Site (+)	86	—
Site (−)	52	32
Histologically proven endometriosis		
Site (+)	80/86 (93%)	—
Site (−)	7/52 (13%)	2/32 (6%)

Site (+) was macroscopically visible endometriotic lesion.
Site (−) was macroscopically normal peritoneum.
Source: Nisolle et al.[6]

osis (Table 3.3). Unsuspected peritoneal endometriosis can thus be found in visually normal peritoneum of infertile women, with or without laparoscopically identifiable endometriosis. The microscopic size of the endometriotic lesions ($313 \pm 185\,\mu m$) explains why the peritoneum had a normal appearance at laparoscopy and why the lesion was not visible even though meticulous inspection was carried out to identify small and nonhemorrhagic lesions.

Hormonal Independence

Using qualitative histochemistry, the microscopic changes present in endometrium have been observed in ectopic implants.[10] Endometrial implants, however, do not demonstrate the characteristic ultrastructural changes of normal endometrium.[11] The fact that endometrial implants can undergo cyclic changes similar histologically to those found in normal endometrium demonstrates that ectopic endometrium responds to gonadal hormones. But the majority of implants do not display histologic changes synchronous with the comparable uterine endometrium.[12] Possible reasons for these differences in ectopic endometrium include a deficiency in steroid receptors; the influence of the surrounding scarification process; pressure atrophy; or hormonal independence of ectopic endometrial glands.

Evaluation of steroid receptors in ectopic endometrial implants is often difficult because of the small number of glandular and stromal cells within the implant and because of the heterogeneity of the tissue. While most implants can be shown to possess progesterone receptors, only 30% have estrogen receptors.[13] In the ovary, implants have far fewer estrogen and progesterone receptors than normal endometrium.[14-15]

Castration, menopause, pregnancy, or therapeutic suppression of gonadal function can dramatically alter the pattern of disease. Hormonal treatment, however, does not eradicate endometriosis. We have shown in both peritoneal endometriosis and ovarian endometriosis, microscopic examination of specimens taken after 6 months of therapy revealed a high incidence of active endometriosis without signs of degeneration. Mitotic activity suggested the presence of hormonally independent glands in endometriotic foci.[14]

New Histologic Aspects

We applied stereometric analysis to study the precise vascularization of peritoneal endometriotic foci.[8] Such vascularization is probably one of the most important factors in the growth and invasion of endometrial glands into other tissue.

In 265 women who were undergoing laparoscopy for infertility, biopsies were taken from areas of the pelvic peritoneum bearing foci of endometriosis (Table 3.4). Among 220 patients who were not given any hormonal therapy, biopsies were taken from typical (puckered black) endometriotic implants ($n = 135$), and from sites of subtle appearances of endometriosis: red lesions ($n = 35$) and white lesions ($n = 50$). Among 45 patients who were given a gonadotropin-releasing hormone agonist (GnRH-a) therapy (Zoladex) for 12 weeks before laparoscopy, biopsies were taken from typical endometriotic implants. A two-dimensional (2-D) computer image analysis was performed by interactive counting of 262,144 points.[8] All endometriotic lesions were examined at 40X magnification. The histologic features were displayed on a television monitor and stored in memory for processing by the measuring program. Histologic structures of interest such as stroma, glandular epithelium and lumen, capillaries, and lymphocytes were examined. Each different structure was discriminated and gray-level images were transferred to

Table 3.4. Morphometric study of stromal vascularization.

	Typical lesions (black) ($n = 135$)	Red ($n = 35$)	White ($n = 50$)	Treated typical lesions ($n = 45$)
Mean number of capillaries per mm² stroma	243	147	206	225
Capillaries mean surface area (μ^2)	118 ± 84	234 ± 192	78 ± 43	71 ± 40
Capillaries/stroma relative surface area ratio	2.4	3.2	1.5	1.4

binary images. Interactive measurements of the selected parameters (number of structures, area and perimeter of the structures per field) were included in the database. In all cases, the mitotic index was calculated.[6,16]

All biopsies showed typical epithelium and stroma of the endometrial type. The results concerning vascularization are shown in Table 3.4. Vascularization (capillaries mean surface area) of the stroma of red lesions was found to be significantly greater than in black or white lesions. After a 12-week GnRH-a regimen, the mean capillary surface area of typical black lesions decreased to $71 \pm 40 \mu^2$, which was significantly lower ($P < 0.001$) than the mean capillary surface areas found in typical black or red lesions but not from that found in white lesions. Treatment did not affect the mean number of capillaries per mm^2 of stroma, but did reduce the ratio of capillaries/stroma surface area, which was significantly different from the untreated typical and red lesions but not from the white lesions.

These results indicated a significant decrease in vascularization of the endometriotic foci after GnRH-agonist therapy. This change was due not to a reduction in the number of capillaries in the lesion, but to a decrease in the surface area of the vessels. In the treated patients, a predominance of smaller vessels was observed when compared with the untreated patients. This reduction in vascularization observed histologically is in accordance with laparoscopic observations after hormonal therapy.

Three-Dimensional Architecture of Endometriosis

To elucidate biologic characteristics of peritoneal endometriotic lesions (for example, how their stereologic development in vivo and how their glandular epithelium and stroma are related to the surrounding tissue), we have recently applied advanced stereographic computer technology to investigate the three-dimensional (3-D) architecture of implants.[7]

Specimens were taken from typical (puckered black) endometriotic implants in 42 women. Group I consisted of 26 women with peritoneal endometriosis who had not previously received any hormonal therapy. Group II consisted of 16 women who had received GnRH-a therapy (Zoladex) for 12 weeks before biopsy (Table 3.5).

Table 3.5. Stereometry of typical endometriotic implants.

Ratio*	Without hormonal treatment ($n = 26$)	With hormonal treatment ($n = 16$)
Epithelium/lesion	20%	15%
Stroma/lesion	62%	52%
Lumen/lesion	13%	25%

*Percentages of the volume of implants attributed to the epithelium, stroma, or lumen.

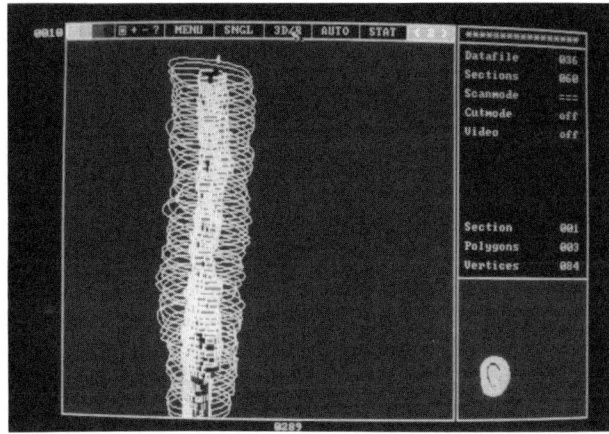

Figure 3.4. 3-D image models displayed as a transparent structure shows cylinder like gland and regular distribution of the glandular epithelium in the stroma. See also color plate.

Histologically, all the biopsy specimens showed typical epithelium and stroma of the endometrial type. The histologic features of the sections were displayed on a monitor on which 2-D figures drawn with a digitizer were superimposed. A computer-assisted reconstruction of 3-D models was developed to generate a complete multicolored model of a complex structure that could be rotated and viewed from any angle or orientation and to calculate the volumes and surfaces within the 3-D model automatically.[7] Lumen volumes were also calculated. Ratios of lumen volume/epithelial volume/stromal volume were determined for each specimen.

The reconstructed 3-D image models of the structures in the peritoneal endometriotic lesion were displayed in color as solid structures. However, models could also be displayed as a transparent structure, when they were simultaneously shown with their stromal and epithelial structures. Stereographically, two types were identified. The first type was composed of cylinder-like glands without ramifications (Fig. 3.4 and color plate 3.4). This lesion showed a regular distribution of the glandular epithelium in the stromal structure, which also was regular. The second type was composed of glands with ramifications (Fig. 3.5 and color plate 3.5). Luminal structures were interconnected with one other. Epithelial structures appeared like fingers and seemed to invade the stroma. The distribution of glandular structures in the stroma was not regular. Many glandular structures formed inside luminal structures whose diameter varied from 22 to 185 μm.

In all groups, the external stromal surface was regular. Like normal uterine epithelial structures, the glandular epithelium had a markedly regular luminal surface. In

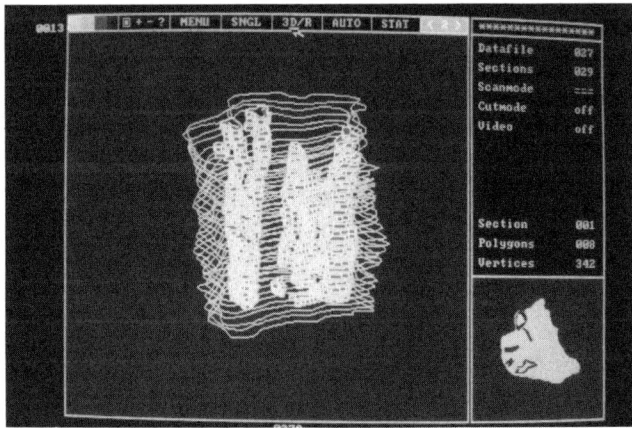

Figure 3.5. 3-D image models displayed as a transparent structure shows glands with ramifications and interconnection of structures. See also color plate.

some cases, the lumens were dilated; in other cases, especially when the ramifications were numerous, the lumens were narrow. The occurrence of cylinderlike glands, and the occurrence of glands with ramifications was similar in the treated and untreated patients. Endometriotic lesion shapes, however, after GnRH-agonist treatment differed significantly ($p < .05$) from the nontreated lesions. Volumes of epithelial, stromal, and luminal structures were measured separately by computer stereometry. The differences observed between the two groups are summarized in Table 3.5.

Stromal Vascularization and Three-Dimensional Evaluation

The typical (puckered black or bluish) peritoneal endometriotic lesion is characterized histologically by both epithelium and stroma of the endometrial type. Subtle appearances have been described and classified as red lesions (vesicular, red flamelike, and glandular excrescences) and white lesions (white opacification, yellow-brown patches, circular peritoneal defects).

When compared with typical lesions, the vascularization of red lesions is greater, and in white lesions and GnRH-agonist treated lesions, reduced. These differences were due to changes in the volume occupied by the vessels as indicated by both the mean capillary surface area and the surface area ratio of capillaries/stroma. Reduction in vascularization can thus be proved following GnRH-a therapy and in white lesions. The significant decrease in the vascularization of the endometriotic foci after GnRH-agonist therapy could account for the diminished inflammatory reaction observed around the endometriotic foci at the time of second-look laparoscopy. Moreover, the mitotic index was also

significantly different in the three groups.[8] Mitotic processes permit the maintenance and growth of peritoneal endometriosis. The absence of mitosis in white lesions proves their low activity.

Our stereographic study showed that two different types of peritoneal endometriotic lesions can be differentiated: (1) a first type without ramification of the glands; (2) a second type in which glands are ramified and connected.[14] Further studies are needed to determine if the two types correlate with the different degree of "aggressiveness" or the different appearances of peritoneal endometriosis.

The apparently multifocal occurrence (in 2-D) of glandular epithelium in one lesion is not confirmed by the 3-D study. Indeed, in each peritoneal lesion, epithelial glands are interconnected by luminal structures. It is probable that in each peritoneal lesion, epithelial structures occur in a single focus of the stroma and may then gradually develop, elongate, and swell to form luminal structures, occasionally with endometrial debris inside. During the expansion, all the glands are connected.

Conclusion

Our stereographic and stereometric studies have shown some new characteristics of peritoneal endometriosis. According to our data there are probably different types of peritoneal endometriotic lesions at different stages of development.[7,8]

Red flamelike lesions and glandular excrescences probably reflect an early stage of implantation of endometrial glands and stroma. In red lesions, a higher incidence of glands with ramifications was observed when compared with typical and white lesions. The increased stromal vascularization could be responsible for the invasion of the ectopic sites by glands and stroma.

Later, menstrual shedding from viable endometrial implants could begin an inflammatory reaction that, in turn, provokes a scarification process that encloses the implant. Intraluminal debris is responsible for the typical black color of the lesion. That scarring is responsible for the vascularization reduction is proven by the marked decrease in the capillaries/stroma relative surface area. Then, the inflammatory process devascularizes the endometriotic foci, and white plaques of old collagen are all that remain of the ectopic implant.

It appears that white opacification and yellow-brown lesions, exhibiting a poor vascularization without mitosis, are latent stages of endometriosis. They are probably inactive lesions that could be quiescent for a long time. We consider typical, red, and white lesions to be different stages of peritoneal endometriosis. Probably, their relative relation to infertility also differs.

References

1. Jansen RPS, Russell P. Nonpigmented endometriosis: clinical laparoscopic and pathologic definition. Am J Obstet Gynecol 1986;155:1154.
2. Chatman DL. Pelvic peritoneal defects and endometriosis; Allen-Masters syndrome revisited. Fertil Steril 1981;36:751.
3. Martin DC, Hubert GD, Vander Zwaag R, El-Zeky F. Laparoscopic appearances of peritoneal endometriosis. Fertil Steril 1989;51:63.
4. Stripling MC, Martin DC, Chatman DL, Vander Zwaag R, Poston WM. Subtle appearances of pelvic endometriosis. Fertil Steril 1988;49:427.
5. Redwine DB. The distribution of endometriosis in the pelvis by age groups and fertility. Fertil Steril 1987;47:173–175.
6. Nisolle M, Paindaveine B, Bourdon A, Berlière M, Casanas-Roux F, Donnez J. Histologic study of peritoneal endometriosis in infertile women. Fertil Steril 1990;53:984.
7. Donnez J, Nisolle M, Casanas-Roux F. Three-dimensional architectures of peritoneal endometriosis. Fertil Steril 1991;57:980.
8. Nisolle M, Casanas-Roux F, Anaf V, Mine JM, Donnez J. Morphometric study of the stromal vascularization in peritoneal endometriosis. Fertil Steril 1993;59:681.
9. Donnez J, Casanas-Roux F, Caprasse J, Ferin J, Thomas K. Cyclic changes in ciliation, cell height, and mitotic activity in human tubal epithelium during reproductive life. Fertil Steril 1985;43:554.
10. Brosens I, Vasquez G, Gordts S. Scanning electron microscopic study of the pelvic peritoneum in unexplained infertility and endometriosis. Fertil Steril 1984;41:215.
11. Lox CD, Word L, Heine MW. Ultrastructural evaluation of endometriosis. Fertil Steril 1984;41:755.
12. Roddick JW, Conkey G, Jacobs EJ. The hormonal response of endometriotic implants and its relationship to symptomatology. Am J Obstet Gynecol 1960;79:1173–1177.
13. Janne O, Kauppila A, Kokko E. Estrogen and progestin receptors in endometriosis lesions: comparison with endometrial tissue. Am J Obstet Gynecol 1981;141:562–566.
14. Bergqvist A, Rannevik G, Thorell J. Estrogen and progesterone cytosol receptor concentration in endometriotic tissue and intrauterine endometrium. Acta Obstet Gynecol Scand 1981;101:53–58.
15. Tamaya T, Motoyaha T, Ohono Y. Steroid receptor levels and histology of endometriosis and adenomyosis. Fertil Steril 1979;31:394–400.
16. Nisolle M, Casanas-Roux F, Donnez J. Histologic study of ovarian endometriosis after hormonal therapy. Fertil Steril 1988;49:423.

4

Classification and Staging of Endometriosis

Mark A. Damario and John A. Rock

A multiplicity of classification schemes for endometriosis has evolved since clinical recognition of the disorder. Such systems, which have taken various forms, have been mostly descriptive based on the morphologic appearance of the disease. From these descriptions, investigators have made inferences regarding the pathogenesis and clinical consequences of this disorder. Attempts to group patients into categories were made with the presumption that certain outcomes with and without treatment could be predicted.

Despite the voluminous literature on the subject, the pathogenesis of endometriosis is not completely understood. Although endometriosis is frequently cited as a cause of pelvic pain and infertility, the mechanisms involved have not been fully elucidated. Clinically, some women with advanced disease have few if any symptoms, whereas others with even small implants have incapacitating pain. The relative place of medical or surgical therapy for infertility associated with early stages of endometriosis remains controversial. Some studies have failed to identify the value of any therapy. Even the diagnosis of endometriosis remains a major challenge, with the discovery of subtle nonpigmented lesions along with the now well-documented phenomenon of microscopic endometriosis. Attempts to classify endometriosis have been hampered by these factors and by our incomplete understanding of the disorder.

In this chapter, we trace the evolution of classification systems for endometriosis. Then, we present the limitations of the present system. Finally, we discuss potential future directions regarding revisions or improvements in the current classification scheme.

Early Classification Systems

In 1921, Sampson became the first to classify endometriosis by describing hemorrhagic cysts of the ovary and their associated adhesion formation.[1] He placed "ovarian hematomas" into four subgroups: follicular, corpus luteal, stromal, and endometrial; and he subdivided the last group into three types: (1) glands without stroma, (2) glands with stroma resembling normal endometrium, and (3) a combination of the first two types. He appreciated the capability of endometriotic cysts to form adjacent adhesions, ranging from minimal filmy strands to extensive obliteration of the cul-de-sac. Although he would consider conservative surgery for minimal disease in women desiring to preserve fertility, Sampson believed that cure of the disease and maximum relief of the pain required removal of the uterus, fallopian tubes, ovaries, and all endometriotic tissue.

Wicks and Larsen in 1949 also categorized endometriosis on the basis of histologic characteristics of resected lesions.[2] Their classification system was similar to those in use for grading malignancy. Grade 1 lesions contained phagocytic cells, blood pigment, and debris with little activity. Grade 4 lesions demonstrated glands and stroma typical of active endometrial tissue and were presumed responsive to normal cyclic stimulation from the ovary. Wicks and Larsen did not correlate symptoms or clinical findings with their histologic grading scheme, but urged the collection of such data.

In the early part of the century, it was felt that endometriosis was a progressive, often invasive and

Table 4.1. Huffman's classification of endometriosis.

Stage I
  a. Limited to uterosacral ligaments and/or
  b. Limited to one ovary and/or
  c. Superficial peritoneal implants.

Stage II
  a. Extensive involvement of one ovary, with lesser involvement of
     second ovary and/or
  b. Superficial implants both ovaries and/or
  c. Superficial bowel implants and/or
  d. Infiltrating lesions of uterus or uterosacral ligaments.

Stage III
  a. Extensively infiltrating both ovaries and/or
  b. Bilateral ovarian endometriotic cysts and/or
  c. Deeply invading rectovaginal lesions and/or
  d. Infiltrating nonobstructing bowel implants.

Stage IV
  a. Vesical invasion and/or
  b. Intestinal invasion, obstructive and/or
  c. Ureteral involvement.

From Huffman[6] by permission of *American Journal of Obstetrics-Gynecology.*

incapacitating disease. Its presence was often felt to be justification for castration. When reports of successful pregnancies after conservative surgery began to appear, interest in conservatism increased.[3,4]

In 1950, Ware published a report on 13 women with endometriosis who had become pregnant; 12 had previously undergone a conservative surgical procedure.[5] Ware advised that "conservative surgical treatment, with preservation of childbearing function in young women and those without children, be recommended whenever possible in cases of endometriosis."

In 1951, Huffman offered a classification scheme based on the anatomic presentation of endometriosis and its similarity to malignancy (Table 4.1).[6] He was the first to recommend treatment based on the stage of disease. Using his system to classify 300 of his patients, he studied the relationship between the stage of endometriosis and the pregnancy rate after conservative operations. He noted that in patients with stages I and II disease, the subsequent pregnancy rate was 47%. This led to his recommendation that childbearing potential be conserved in women with stages I and II disease as well as selected cases of stage III disease.

In 1954, Sturgis and Call correlated the presence of pelvic pain with histopathologic stages of endometriosis.[7] They divided the diseases into three stages: (1) early development, (2) active stage, and (3) endometrial inactivity (postmenopause). They believed that the deep fibrotic encapsulation of long-standing pelvic endometriosis was responsible for chronic dysmenorrhea and pelvic pain. They also identified microscopic foci of glands or stroma within peritoneal scar tissue. This led to their recommendation that both endometriotic implants and their associated adhesions be excised to ensure relief of pain.

It is apparent that current knowledge of the disease's process and available diagnostic methods influence classification systems. Before diagnostic endoscopy became available, a patient would have had to have severe symptoms or clinical findings to receive treatment for endometriosis.

In 1958, Kistner examined the use of progestins in the treatment of endometriosis. Patients for such therapy were selected by symptoms and clinical findings.[8] Criteria were (1) acquired, progressive dysmenorrhea; (2) cul-de-sac and uterosacral nodularity and tenderness; (3) fixed retroversion of the uterus; and (4) tender adnexal masses. Most patients met at least three of these criteria. Kistner realized the limitations of failing to have a histologic diagnosis and suggested culdoscopy or other modes of visualization of the pelvis would be useful.

In 1962, Riva and associates reported their experience with norethynodrel.[9] The diagnosis of endometriosis was confirmed by visualization at culdoscopy, colpotomy, or laparotomy. Riva's group was the first to attempt to use scalar criteria to develop a classification scheme. They grouped patients according to a cumulative count of pelvic structures involved, but found that their scheme's results correlated poorly with treatment outcome.

Four years later, Beecham stated that a painstaking effort to detail endometriotic lesions would "serve no useful purpose."[10] He offered a simplified classification scheme with four stages based on physical examination or operative findings (Table 4.2). His system was designed solely to facilitate recordkeeping, and he did not support it with clinical data.

In 1974, Mitchell and Farber proposed a surgical staging system based on the similarity of endometriosis to malignant disease (Table 4.3).[11] In fact, their stage V included endometriotic lesions giving rise to adenocarcinoma. They used their system to determine whether to apply medical or surgical treatment plans. In stages I and II, progestin therapy was recommended for pain relief; lysis of adhesions and resection of implants were

Table 4.2. Beecham's classification of endometriosis.

Stage I	Scattered, small (1–2 mm) spots anywhere in the pelvis at laparotomy.
Stage II	Uterosacral ligaments, broad ligaments, cervix, and ovaries are, collectively or individually, fixed, tender, nodular, and slightly enlarged.
Stage III	The same as stage 2, with ovaries at least twice normal size; uterosacral ligaments, rectum, and adnexa are confluent and the cul-de-sac is obliterated.
Stage IV	Massive involvement; internal pelvic viscera cannot be clearly distinguished by palpation.

Stages II, III, and IV may be used to describe either the palpable finding on physical examination or the palpable-visual findings at operation.

From Beecham[10] with permission from The American College of Obstetricians and Gynecologists (*Obstetrics and Gynecology*, 1966; 28:437.)

Table 4.3. Mitchell and Farber's classification of endometriosis.

Stage I	One or more small superficial implants (less than 5 mm) on the pelvic peritoneum.
Stage II	Larger superficial implants involving uterosacral ligaments, rectovaginal septum, and/or ovaries.
Stage III	Endometriomas of the ovary greater than 5 cm in diameter with or without superficial involvement of broad ligament and adjacent organs.
Stage IV	Penetration of vagina, bowel, or urinary tract and distant metastases (lymph nodes, umbilicus, surgical wounds, and so forth).
Stage V	Endometriomas giving rise to adenocarcinoma.

Source: Mitchell & Farber[11] with permission.

recommended in cases of infertility. The pregnancy rate following conservative surgery was reported to be 32%. Mitchell and Farber felt that surgical exploration to rule out ovarian malignancy was necessary in advanced stages. Total abdominal hysterectomy and bilateral salpingo-oophorectomy were recommended for those with extensive disease.

Modern Classification Systems

Prior to 1973, numerous reports discussed the value of conservative operations in promoting fertility in women with endometriosis. Because of the lack of means to group patients and compare treatment outcomes objectively, a clinician could not confidently counsel a couple regarding their prognosis for future fertility. The reported pregnancy rates after conservative operations varied widely and were difficult to interpret.

In 1973, diagnostic laparoscopy provided a simpler way of documenting pelvic endometriosis. Because this method improved diagnosis, there was an increase in classifications systems that more accurately predicted outcomes.

Acosta and coauthors promptly outlined a new classification system (Table 4.4) based on the premise that success of surgery in the infertile woman depended primarily on the severity of disease at the time of initial diagnosis.[12] They performed a retrospective analysis of 107 patients who underwent conservative surgery and assigned cases to three categories (mild, moderate, and severe) according to the site and distribution of lesions, scarring, and adhesions. Pregnancy had resulted in 75%, 50%, and 33% of women with mild, moderate, and severe disease, respectively. Although the assignment to stages was admittedly arbitrary, this system was the most concise and complete yet devised. Furthermore, a direct relationship had been established between the initial stage of disease and subsequent pregnancy rates.

Several factors influenced the 1973 Acosta classification. The presence of periovarian or peritubal

adhesions separated mild from moderate disease. At that time, many would use those findings at laparoscopy as a reason to proceed with conservative surgery rather than hormonal therapy. Petersohn had suggested in 1970 that the finding of pelvic adhesions was important in predicting reproductive outcome.[13] In his trial of 111 women, those with endometriosis alone had an 80% pregnancy rate, whereas those with both endometriosis and adhesions had a 40% pregnancy rate. The vulnerability of the ovary to adhesions was also becoming apparent from several subsequent reports concerning adhesion formation following wedge resection for polycystic ovarian disease.[14,15] Therefore, in devising their system, Acosta and co-workers treated the extent of ovarian involvement as a major factor, because of the risk of adhesions after removal of an endometrioma. But the shortcomings of this system eventually became apparent for its arbitrariness and failure to distinguish between unilateral and bilateral disease.

Ingersoll expanded the Acosta staging system by adding stage 0 and stage IV (involvement of extragenital sites).[16] Unfortunately, he presented no data supporting his system.

In 1977, Kistner and colleagues described another system with sharply delineated stages (Table 4.5).[17] This approach was based on their perceived impression of the natural history of the disease: from peritoneal

Table 4.4. Acosta's classification of pelvic endometriosis.

Mild	1. Scattered, fresh lesions (i.e., implants not associated with scarring or retraction of the peritoneum) in the anterior or posterior cul-de-sac or pelvic peritoneum. 2. Rare surface implant on ovary, with no endometrioma, without surface scarring and retraction and without periovarian adhesions. 3. No peritubular adhesions.
Moderate	1. Endometriosis involving one or both ovaries, with several surface lesions, with scarring and retraction, or small endometriomata. 2. Minimal periovarian adhesions associated with ovarian lesions described. 3. Minimal peritubular adhesions associated with ovarian lesions described. 4. Superficial implants in the anterior and/or posterior cul-de-sac with scarring and retraction. Some adhesions, but not sigmoid invasion.
Severe	1. Endometriosis involving one or both ovaries with endometrioma >2 × 2 cm (usually both). 2. One or both ovaries bound down by adhesions associated with endometriosis, with or without tubal adhesions to ovaries. 3. One or both tubes bound down or obstructed by endometriosis; associated adhesions or lesions. 4. Obliteration of the cul-de-sac from adhesions or lesions associated with endometriosis. 5. Thickening of the uterosacral ligaments and cul-de-sac lesions from invasive endometriosis with obliteration of the cul-de-sac. 6. Significant bowel or urinary tract involvement.

From Acosta et al[12] with permission from The American College of Obstetricians and Gynecologists (Obstetrics and Gynecology, 1973; 42:19–25).

Table 4.5. Kistner's classification of endometriosis.

Stage I	Areas of endometriosis are present on the posterior pelvic peritoneum (cul-de-sac, uterosacral ligaments) or on the surface of the broad ligaments, but do not exceed 5 mm in diameter. Avascular adhesions may involve the tubes, but the fimbriae are free. The ovaries may show a few avascular adhesions but there is no ovarian fixation. The surfaces of the bowel and the appendix are normal.
Stage IIA	Areas of endometriosis are present on the posterior pelvic peritoneum (cul-de-sac, uterosacral ligaments) and the broad ligaments, but do not exceed 5 mm in diameter. Avascular adhesions may involve the tubes, but the fimbriae are free. Ovarian involvement by endometriosis has been subclassified as follows: IIA-1: Endometrial cyst or surface is 5 cm or less IIA-2: Endometrial cyst or surface is over 5 cm IIA-3: Ruptured endometrioma; the bowel and the appendix are normal.
Stage IIB	The posterior leaf of the broad ligament is covered by adherent ovarian tissue. The tubes present adhesions not removable by endoscopic procedures. The fimbriae are free. The ovaries are fixed to the broad ligament and show areas of endometriosis over 5 mm in diameter. The cul-de-sac presents multiple implants but there is no adherent bowel nor is the uterus in fixed position. The bowel and the appendix are normal.
Stage III	The posterior leaf of the broad ligament may be covered by adherent tube or ovary. The tubal fimbriae are covered by adhesions. The ovaries are adherent to the broad ligament and tube and may or may not show surface endometriosis or endometriomas. The cul-de-sac shows multiple areas of endometriosis, but there is no evidence of adherent bowel or uterine fixation. The bowel and the appendix are normal.
Stage IV	Endometriosis involves the bladder serosa, and the uterus is in fixed, third-degree retroversion. The cul-de-sac is covered by adherent bowel or is obliterated by the fixed uterus. The bowel is adherent to the cul-de-sac, uterosacral ligaments, or uterine corpus. The appendix may be involved by the endometriotic process.

From Kistner et al.[17] Reproduced with permission of the publisher, The American Fertility Society.

implants to ovarian involvement, then tubo-ovarian disease, and finally extensive spread throughout the pelvis. For the first time in any staging system, adhesions were described according to their amenability to lysis by the operative laparoscope. Extrapelvic endometriosis was not considered because it was not thought to have an impact on fertility.

In 1978, Buttram proposed an expanded classification of endometriosis by revising the stages in the Acosta system (Table 4.6).[18] This new system, more detailed and precise than any previous one, considered unilateral disease as well as bilateral disease. Buttram also provided a table to revert from the new classification system to Acosta's original categorization.

Cohen proposed yet another classification the following year (Table 4.7).[19] This scheme, based on laparoscopic findings, included a category for distant sites. An original addition was the inclusion of adenomyosis as a class of severe endometriosis.

Table 4.6. Buttram's expanded classification of endometriosis.

Stage I (Peritoneal)
A. No peritoneal involvement.
B. Scattered superficial surface endometrial implants on the pelvic peritoneum (anterior or posterior cul-de-sac, uterosacral ligaments, or the broad ligaments) which do not exceed 5 mm in diameter. Neither tubal nor ovarian involvement.
C. Same as under B, but invasive endometriosis or plaques of endometrial implants >5 mm in diameter. Fine, filmy adhesions may be present which may be lysed without great danger of resultant adhesions.

Stage II (Ovarian): 1, Right; 2, Left; 3, Bilateral
A. No ovarian involvement.
B. Superficial surface endometrial implants of ovary <5 mm in diameter which can be removed by scraping or fulguration without great danger of resultant adhesions. Fine, filmy adhesions may be present and lysed without great danger of resultant adhesions.
C. Invasive endometriosis (plaque or endometrioma) >5 mm but <2 cm and requiring surgical removal. Fine, filmy adhesions may be present and lysed without great danger of resultant adhesions.
D. Invasive endometriosis >2 cm requiring surgical removal or a ruptured endometrioma of any size. Fine, filmy adhesions may be present and lysed without great danger of resultant adhesions.
E. B, C, or D with sufficient dense adhesions to fix ovary to adjacent tissue (usually posterior leaf of broad ligament).

Stage III (Tubal): 1, Right; 2, Left; 3, Bilateral
A. No tubal involvement.
B. Superficial endometrial implants on tube which do not exceed 5 mm in diameter and which can be removed by scraping or fulguration without great danger of resultant adhesions. Fine, filmy adhesions may be present and lysed without great danger of resultant adhesions.
C. Invasive endometriosis (plaque or endometrioma) requiring surgical removal. Fine, filmy adhesions may be present and lysed without great danger of resultant adhesions.
D. Tube involved with adhesions which distort tubal anatomy and/or limit tubal movement. Fimbriae are free and tube is patent. B or C may be present.
E. Fimbriae are covered by adhesions or distal end of tube is occluded. B, C, or D may be present.

Stage IV (Cul-de-sac)
A. Neither B nor C is present.
B. Invasive endometriosis of bladder or colon.
C. Posterior cul-de-sac obliterated and/or uterus fixed and retroverted. Bowel or adnexa may be adherent to cul-de-sac area. B is usually present.

From Buttram.[18] Reproduced with permission of the publisher, The American Fertility Society.

Table 4.7. Cohen's classification of endometriosis.

Mild endometriosis
  I.   Superficial implants at one site
  II. Superficial implants at two or more sites

Moderate endometriosis
  III. Implants with puckering and fibrosis; mild adhesions
  IV. Ovaries moderately adherent to endometrial implants
  V.   Multiple implants of ovaries, bladder peritoneum, ligaments with adhesions

Severe endometriosis
  VI. Endometrial cyst, unilateral or bilateral, without tubal involvement
  VII. Endometrial cyst, unilateral or bilateral, with tubal involvement
  VIII. Adenomyomata
  IX. Severe endometriosis and pelvic inflammatory disease
  X.   Severe endometriosis and/or extragenital, bowel, urinary tract, distant organ involvement

From Cohen.[19] Reproduced with permission from *The Journal of Reproductive Medicine.*

Patient's name_____

Stage I (Mild) —1–5
Stage II (Moderate) —6–15
Stage III (Severe) —16–30
Stage IV (Extensive) —31–54

Total _____

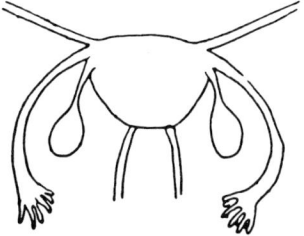

PERITONEUM	ENDOMETRIOSIS		<1 cm	1–3 cm	>3 cm
			1	2	3
	ADHESIONS		Filmy	Dense w/partial culdesac obliteration	Dense w/complete culdesac obliteration
			1	2	3
OVARY	ENDOMETRIOSIS		< 1 cm	1–3 cm	>3 cm or ruptured endometrioma
		R	2	4	6
		L	2	4	6
	ADHESIONS		Filmy	Dense w/partial ovarian enclosure	Dense w/complete ovarian enclosure
		R	2	4	6
		L	2	4	6
TUBE	ENDOMETRIOSIS		<1 cm	>1 cm	Tubal occlusion
		R	2	4	6
		L	2	4	6
	ADHESIONS		Filmy	Dense w/tubal distortion	Dense w/tubal enclosure
		R	2	4	6
		L	2	4	6

Figure 4.1. American Fertility Society classification of endometriosis. (Reproduced with permission of the publisher, The American Fertility Society.)

The AFS Classification System

None of these schemes received universal acceptance. Therefore, a panel was formed by the American Fertility Society (AFS) to devise a system of classification that would promote uniform reporting of results. The Society's 1979 report proposed a unique and innovative approach (Fig. 4.1).[20] A weighted value system was used to document involvement of the peritoneum, fallopian tubes, and ovaries. The stage of endometriosis was then derived from the cumulative score. An anatomic drawing was also provided to document the surgical findings.

Soon, however, critics pointed out shortcomings. Hasson emphasized that pain as well as infertility should be considered.[21] He offered his modification, which increased the point scoring of uterosacral ligament involvement and deep lesions. Brosens and colleagues pointed out that the system seemed to be designed to assess the efficacy of surgical, but not medical, therapy.[22] In 1981, Rock, Guzick, and co-workers presented the first comparative evaluation of the classification systems of Buttram, Kistner, and the AFS by retrospectively classifying 214 patients who had previously undergone conservative surgery for endometriosis.[23] They reported an overall pregnancy rate of 54%. Although the trend was the same in all three

Table 4.8. Pregnancy rates after conservative surgery for endometriosis: A comparison of different classification systems.

Classification and stage	No. of patients	Pregnant Number	Rate	Patient-months of follow-up	Monthly fecundity rate (%)
Buttram*					
Mild	43	29	67%	1,063	2.7
Moderate	71	35	49%	2,024	1.7
Severe	100	51	51%	3,246	1.6
Kistner et al*					
I	45	31	69%	1,110	2.8
IIA	81	44	54%	2,157	2.0
IIB	38	20	53%	1,179	1.7
III	29	11	38%	1,198	0.9
IV	21	9	43%	689	1.3
American Fertility Society**					
Mild	45	28	62%	1,261	2.2
Moderate	88	48	55%	2,424	2.0
Severe	66	33	50%	2,236	1.5
Extensive	15	6	40%	412	1.5
Total	214	115	54%	6,333	1.8

*Differences among monthly fecundity rates significant at $P < .01$.
**If, in the American Fertility Society Classification, mild and moderate are compared with severe and extensive, the difference is significant at $P < .05$.

From Rock et al.[23] Reproduced with permission of the publisher, The American Fertility Society.

Patient's Name _____   Date _____

Stage I   (Minimal) - 1-5
Stage II (Mild)   - 6-15   Laparoscopy _____ Laparotomy _____ Photography _____
Stage III (Moderate) - 16-40   Recommended Treatment _____
Stage IV (Severe)   - >40
Total _____   Prognosis _____

PERITONEUM	ENDOMETRIOSIS	<1cm	1-3cm	>3cm
	Superficial	1	2	4
	Deep	2	4	6
OVARY	R Superficial	1	2	4
	Deep	4	16	20
	L Superficial	1	2	4
	Deep	4	16	20

	POSTERIOR CULDESAC OBLITERATION	Partial		Complete	
		4		40	

	ADHESIONS	<1/3 Enclosure	1/3-2/3 Enclosure	>2/3 Enclosure
OVARY	R Filmy	1	2	4
	Dense	4	8	16
	L Filmy	1	2	4
	Dense	4	8	16
TUBE	R Filmy	1	2	4
	Dense	4*	8*	16
	L Filmy	1	2	4
	Dense	4*	8*	16

*If the fimbriated end of the fallopian tube is completely enclosed, change the point assignment to 16.

Additional Endometriosis: _____   Associated Pathology: _____

_____   _____
_____   _____
_____   _____

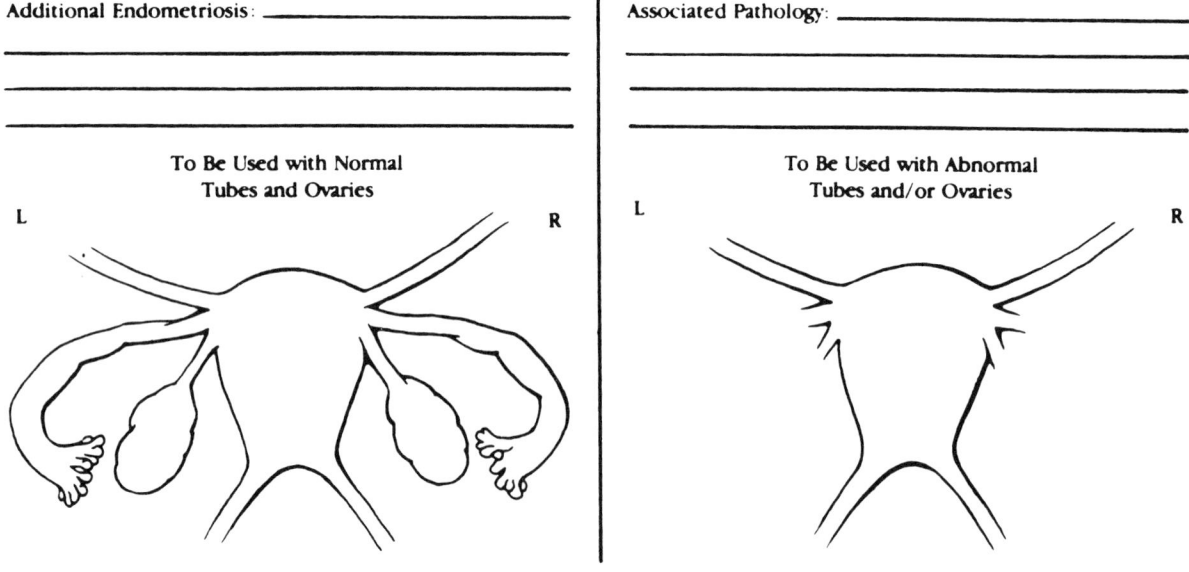

To Be Used with Normal   To Be Used with Abnormal
Tubes and Ovaries   Tubes and/or Ovaries

Figure 4.2. Revised American Fertility Society classification of endometriosis. (Reproduced with permission of the publisher, The American Fertility Society.)

classifications (diminishing pregnancy rates with advancing stage of disease) the rates were not statistically different in the AFS classification unless the mild plus moderate categories were combined and compared with the severe plus extensive categories (Table 4.8). Guzick and co-workers reviewed the point-scoring system by dose-response methodology.[24] They confirmed that the arbitrary point scores and divisions between stages failed to correlate the severity of endometriosis with pregnancy rates after surgery. They recommended that empirically derived scores be used in place of arbitrary scores.

The Revised AFS Classification

Because of the problems encountered in the original AFS classification, a revised and even more detailed scheme (AFS-r) was designed and approved in 1985.[25] This system (Fig. 4.2) eliminated the extensive disease stage, removed tubal endometriosis as a separate category, and created a category for minimal disease. It also provided a means of differentiating between superficial and deep lesions of the peritoneum and ovaries, gave a more detailed quantification of adnexal adhesions, and distinguished filmy from dense adhesions. As before, the system did not include extragenital sites, but provided space to record additional pathology and less frequently involved sites. Complete cul-de-sac obliteration was automatically classified as severe disease. Buttram supported this notion by reporting in his own 1985 series a 68% pregnancy rate associated with partial obliteration of the cul-de-sac in contrast with a 36% pregnancy rate following complete obliteration.[26]

It was apparent that the new AFS-r classification system still suffered from some of the methodologic flaws that characterized earlier systems. It still was derived arbitrarily and unsupported by clinical data, and as understanding of the disease process continued to evolve, relative weights of disease sites shifted and emphasis on adhesions grew. The designers hoped that the new classification scheme would prove useful as a clinical tool to aid in the documentation and study of the disease. They anticipated that, as more knowledge is obtained and the classification system is evaluated, future revisions would prove useful.

Flaws in Revised AFS Classification

There is growing evidence that the current American Fertility Society system (AFS-r) for classifying endometriosis may be inadequate. The scoring system, although derived from expert clinical opinion, is based on arbitrary information and not empiric data. The statistical applicability of the scalar system and the cutoff points between stages have been questioned.

There also appears to be a significant potential for observational error and interobserver variability in light of the now recognized varied and subtle appearances of endometriosis. The usefulness of the system for all outcome variables, particularly pelvic pain as well as infertility, has also been debated.

The use of the scalar system with arbitrary weighted groupings has limited the overall effectiveness of the AFS classification. Several reports have failed to demonstrate a significant difference in cumulative pregnancy rates as a function of AFS-r score or between AFS-r stages.[23,24] Guzick, as early as 1982, had pointed out two problems associated with the AFS-r scoring system.[24] First, the point scores applying to individual categories do not reflect empirically derived relative weights. For example, the point score is 20 for an unruptured solitary endometrioma of 4 cm, whereas the point score is 4 for widely scattered deep peritoneal implants totaling 3 cm. But is the one really five times worse than the other, with respect to pain or fertility impairment? The second problem he pointed out is that demarcations between stages of endometriosis were equally arbitrary. Guzick described a method to determine optimal cutoff points that would improve the discriminatory power of the AFS-r classification system. A large multicenter collaborative effort, however, would be required to verify this approach.

As we learn more about endometriosis, we are increasingly aware of the problems of observational error in attempts to stage the disease precisely. The accuracy of reports using the AFS-r classification system is hard to assess and has not been evaluated for reliability or reproducibility.

There is growing appreciation that endometriosis has many appearances. Jansen and Russell in 1986 described several distinctive appearances of nonpigmented endometriotic lesions.[27] These include (1) white opacification of the peritoneum with or without thickening; (2) red, flamelike lesions of the peritoneum often raised above the peritoneal surface; (3) glandular excrescences on the peritoneal surface; (4) isolated or otherwise unexplained lesions between the undersurface of the ovary and the peritoneum of the ovarian fossa; (5) yellow-brown patches; and (6) circular peritoneal defects. Biopsies confirmed endometriosis in 81% of white opacified lesions, 81% of red, flamelike lesions, 67% of glandular lesions, 50% of subovarian adhesions, 47% of yellow-brown patches, and 45% of circular peritoneal defects. Other authors have also found an association between nonpigmented lesions and endometriosis.[28–31]

Nonpigmented endometriotic lesions are frequently subtle in appearance. Stripling and coauthors noted that increased documentation of subtle, nonpigmented lesions was related to the surgeon's experience and awareness and anticipation of such lesions.[31] In their 1988 series, subtle lesions were documented at laparoscopy in 32% of patients in the first five months and in 72% of patients in the last five months of their study. Martin and co-workers reported an increase in the diagnosis of endometriosis at laparoscopy from 42% in 1982 to 72% in 1988, which they largely attributed to increased awareness of subtle lesions.[28]

Age-related evolution and color appearance of endometriosis was suggested by Redwine.[32] An evolution in appearance with age was noted, that is, non-hemorrhagic lesions were usually seen in younger women, whereas black lesions were seen in older women. Vernon and associates related the gross and histologic appearance of endometriotic implants with their capacity to produce prostaglandin F.[33] As judged by prostaglandin F production, younger, reddish, petechial implants were more biochemically active than intermediate, brownish implants, which in turn were more active than older, powder-burn black implants. This relationship probably reflects the extent to which endometrial glands present in each class of implant are functioning. Thus, dark-pigmented lesions, which are the typical visual criteria for the diagnosis of endometriosis, are late consequences of this cycle and are likely to be inactive in terms of prostaglandin F production. Thus, scoring of endometriotic implants perhaps should take into account their appearance as well as their size and location.

Even more elusive than the identification of nonpigmented lesions is the now well-documented phenomenon of microscopic endometriosis.[34] Vasquez and colleagues described characteristics of minimal peritoneal endometriotic lesions using scanning electron microscopy techniques.[35] Also using scanning electron microscopy, Murphy and co-workers were able to identify microscopic endometriosis in 25% of random biopsies of visually normal appearing peritoneum in patients with endometriosis.[36] In addition, Brosens and co-workers documented microscopic implants by scanning electron microscopy in patients with unexplained infertility in whom no visible endometriosis was seen at laparoscopy.[37]

It is clear that the documentation of the extent of disease by visually inspecting the peritoneum is difficult. Atypical nonpigmented lesions and microscopic implants have further complicated identifying or tabulating the cumulative size of the lesions.

There are other flaws in the present AFS-r classification system. The system does not take into account endometriosis involving extrapelvic sites. A classification and staging system for extrapelvic endometriosis has been proposed by Markham and associates.[38]

Finally, the revised AFS system is of limited use in predicting pelvic pain, with or without treatment. Traditional teaching stresses the lack of correlation between pelvic pain and the extent of the disease. Fedele et al., for example, found no relationship between the revised AFS classification system and the types (dysmenorrhea, pelvic pain, and deep dyspareunia) or severity (scale of 1 to 10) of pain in 160 women studied.[39]

Recent information strongly links pelvic pain with deeply invasive endometriotic implants. Cornillie and associates studied the histologic and clinical importance of deeply infiltrating endometriotic lesions.[40] They evaluated 53 patients using a CO_2 laser excisional technique at laparoscopy. They noted deeply infiltrating implants in the cul-de-sac and uterosacral ligaments, but not in the ovarian fossae. They found that lesions penetrating deeper than 5 mm were more likely to be histologically active, to be in phase with the endometrium, and to be associated with pelvic pain. Superficial implants, in contrast, were found mostly in patients complaining of infertility. Koninckx and co-workers also have recently found that the degree of pelvic pain was not related to the total surface area of endometriosis or type of lesions, but that pain was correlated most strongly with the depth of penetration of the deepest lesion.[41] There appears, therefore, to be a dichotomy between measures associated with pelvic pain and those associated with infertility. The revised AFS classification system does not adequately address this issue.

Future Directions

The revised AFS classification system has provided an objective and widely applied method for staging the severity of endometriosis visualized at laparotomy and laparoscopy. It appears to have many shortcomings, however, and there is interest in revising the current system.

Many believe that endometriosis staging and evaluation should differ for infertility and pelvic pain. There seem to be different anatomic and pathophysiologic factors associated with each. Because the present AFS-r system is admittedly arbitrary, some investigators are interested in evaluating empiric data to determine point values and cutoff scores, an undertaking that would require a large, multicenter collaboration. They hope that empirically derived weighted point values and scores will increase the predictive value of the system. Some have suggested using computerized pelvic mapping to store and accumulate descriptive data in extensive detail.[42] Compilations of these mappings and other important variables could then be analyzed for their relative predictive values. It is possible that appropriate multivariate analysis of the data accumulated could provide physicians with information regarding fertility potential, relief of pain, or risk of disease recurrence for a particular patient.

Intensive research continues regarding the peritoneal environment in endometriosis. Perhaps a physiologic factor will be identified that could be incorporated into a staging system to increase the sensitivity and specificity of the system.

Conclusions

Classification of any disease into statistically valid groupings is a vital step in advancing its treatment. None of the existing classification schemes for endometriosis meet this test but as our knowledge and understanding of this disease improve, we can expect better, more useful means of staging endometriosis to follow.

References

1. Sampson JA. Perforating hemorrhagic (chocolate) cysts of the ovary. Arch Surg 1921;3:245–323.
2. Wicks MJ, Larson CP. Histologic criteria for evaluating endometriosis. Northwest Med 1949;48:611–613.
3. Holmes WR. Endometriosis. Am J Obstet Gynecol 1942; 43:255–266.
4. Beecham CT. Surgical treatment of endometriosis. JAMA 1949;139:971–976.
5. Ware HH. Endometriosis and pregnancy. Am J Obstet Gynecol 1950;59:715–728.
6. Huffman JW. External endometriosis. Am J Obstet Gynecol 1951;62:1243–1252.
7. Sturgis SH, Call BJ. Endometriosis peritonei—relationship of pain to functional activity. Am J Obstet Gynecol 1954; 68:1421–1431.
8. Kistner RW. The use of newer progestins in the treatment of endometriosis. Am J Obstet Gynecol 1958;75:264–278.
9. Riva HL, Kawasaki DM, Messinger AJ. Further experience with norethynodrel in treatment of endometriosis. Obstet Gynecol 1962;19:111–117.
10. Beecham CT. Classification of endometriosis [editorial]. Obstet Gynecol 1966;28:437.
11. Mitchell GW, Farber M. Medical versus surgical management of endometriosis. In Reid DE, Christian CD, eds. Controversy in Obstetrics and Gynecology, volume 2. Philadelphia, WB Saunders, 1974, pp 631–636.
12. Acosta AA, Buttram VC, Besch PK, et al. A proposed classification of pelvic endometriosis. Obstet Gynecol 1973;42:19–25.
13. Petersohn L. Fertility in patients with ovarian endometriosis before and after treatment. Acta Obstet Gynecol Scand 1970;49:331–333.
14. Toaff R, Toaff ME, Peyser MR. Infertility following wedge resection of the ovaries. Am J Obstet Gynecol 1976;124:92–96.
15. Buttram VC, Vaquero C. Post-ovarian wedge resection adhesive disease. Fertil Steril 1975;26:874–876.
16. Ingersoll FM. Selection of medical or surgical treatment of endometriosis. Clin Obstet Gynecol 1977;20:849–864.
17. Kistner RW, Siegler AM, Behrman SJ. Suggested classification for endometriosis: relationship to infertility. Fertil Steril 1977;28:1008–1010.
18. Buttram VC. An expanded classification of endometriosis. Fertil Steril 1978;30:240–242.
19. Cohen MR. Laparoscopy and the management of endometriosis. J Reprod Med 1979;23:81–84.
20. American Fertility Society. Classification of endometriosis. Fertil Steril 1979;32:633–634.
21. Hasson HM. Classification for endometriosis [letter]. Fertil Steril 1981;35:368–369.
22. Brosens IA, Cornillie F, Koninckx P, et al. Evolution of the revised American Fertility Society classification of endometriosis. Fertil Steril 1981;35:368–369.
23. Rock JA, Guzick DS, Senger C, et al. The conservative surgical treatment of endometriosis: Evaluation of pregnancy success with respect to the extent of disease as categorized using contemporary classification systems. Fertil Steril 1981;35:131–137.
24. Guzick DS, Bross DS, Rock JA. Assessing the efficacy of the American Fertility Society's classification of endometriosis: Application of a dose-response methodology. Fertil Steril 1982;38:171–176.
25. American Fertility Society: Revised classification of endometriosis. Fertil Steril 1985; 43:351–352.
26. Buttram VC. Evolution of the revised American Fertility Society classification of endometriosis. Fertil Steril 1985; 43:347–350.
27. Jansen RPS, Russel P. Nonpigmented endometriosis: clinical, laparoscopic, and pathologic definition. Am J Obstet Gynecol 1986;155:1154–1159.
28. Martin DC, Hubert GD, Vander Zwaag R, et al. Laparoscopic appearances of peritoneal endometriosis. Fertil Steril 1989;51:63–67.
29. Nisolle M, Paindaveine B, Bourdon A, et al. Histologic study of peritoneal endometriosis in infertile women. Fertil Steril 1990;53:984–988.
30. Chatman DL, Zbella EA. Pelvic peritoneal defects and endometriosis: Further observations. Fertil Steril 1986; 46:711–714.
31. Stripling MC, Martin DC, Chatman DL, et al. Subtle appearance of pelvic endometriosis. Fertil Steril 1988;49: 427–431.
32. Redwine DB. Age-related evolution in color appearance of endometriosis. Fertil Steril 1987;48:1062–1063.
33. Vernon MW, Beard JS, Graves K, et al. Classification of endometriotic implants by morphologic appearance and capacity to synthesize prostaglandin F. Fertil Steril 1986; 46:801–806.
34. Schenken RS. Microscopic endometriosis. Contr Gynecol Obst 1987;16:7–12.
35. Vasquez G, Cornillie F, Brosens IA. Peritoneal endometriosis: scanning electron microscopy and histology of minimal pelvic endometriotic lesions. Fertil Steril 1984; 42:696–702.
36. Murphy A, Green W, Bobbie D, et al. Unsuspected endometriosis documented by scanning electron microscopy in visually normal peritoneum. Fertil Steril 1986; 46:522–524.
37. Brosens I, Vasquez G, Gordis S. Scanning electron microscopy study of the pelvic peritoneum in unexplained infertility and endometriosis. (Abstr) Presented at the 40th Annual Meeting of the American Fertility Society, New Orleans, April 1984, A# 48.
38. Markham SM, Carpenter SE, Rock JA. Extrapelvic endometriosis. Obstet Gynecol Clin NA 1989;16: 193–219.
39. Fedele L, Parazzini F, Bianchi S, et al. Stage and localization of pelvic endometriosis and pain. Fertil Steril 1990; 53:155–158.
40. Cornillie FJ, Oosterlynck D, Lauweryns JM, et al.

Deeply infiltrating pelvic endometriosis: Histology and clinical significance. Fertil Steril 1990;53:978–982.

41. Koninckx PR, Meuleman C, Demeyere S, et al. Suggestive evidence that pelvic endometriosis is a progressive disease whereas deeply infiltrating endometriosis is associated with pelvic pain. Fertil Steril 1991;55:759–765.

42. Wheeler JM, Malinak LR. Application of computerized pelvic mapping to the conservative surgical treatment of endometriosis: Analysis of anatomic areas in relations to prognosis for postoperative pregnancy. (Abstr) Presented at the 41st Annual Meeting of the American Fertility Society, Chicago, September 1985, A# 12.

5
Pathogenesis of Pelvic Pain in Endometriosis

Alan B. Copperman and David Olive

Endometriosis is associated with a variety of pain symptoms. Despite the strong clinical correlation, however, the pathophysiology of this association is not well understood. Appearance, location, depth of invasion, and other factors may all influence symptoms.

Advances in laparoscopic technology and growth in its popularity have contributed to the increased attention paid to pelvic endometriosis in recent years. Discovery of diverse and subtle forms of the disease shows that endometriosis is a heterogeneous entity.[1-3] As these morphologically distinctive forms are correlated with clinical presentations, our understanding of the pathophysiology of endometriosis improves. Improved delineation of the relationship between endometriosis and pain is essential, both for understanding the disease process and for establishing direction for future scientific analysis. Furthermore, such an understanding will allow more precise therapeutic strategies to ameliorate and eliminate endometriosis-associated pain.

Anatomy and Physiology of Pain

The perception of pain arises via an integration of various stimuli through a multitude of neuronal pathways. The cerebral cortex processes the nociceptive impulses and brings them to conscious awareness. There are established cortical projections for somatic structures, with specific body areas localized to well-defined parts of the cortex. Visceral pain is more diffuse than pain of somatic origin, because there is no specific identification in the sensory cortex. A variety of mechanisms can induce visceral pain: distension or abnormal muscular contraction; sudden stretching of the capsule of solid organs; hypoxia or necrosis of viscera; production of an algesic substance, for example, prostanoids; chemical irritation of visceral nerve endings; and inflammation.[4]

The pelvic organs receive their innervation solely from the autonomic nervous system, which is composed of sympathetic and parasympathetic fibers (Figs. 5.1 and 5.2). Most afferent stimuli are transmitted via sympathetic nerves through cell bodies that lie in a thoracolumbar distribution. The parasympathetic nerve fibers, which also transmit stimuli, have cell bodies in the sacral dorsal ganglia.

Sensory innervation of pelvic organs is a function of their embryologic origin. Organs which are Müllerian in embryonic origin, such as the uterus, fallopian tubes, and upper vagina, transmit impulses via sympathetic fibers into the spinal cord at the level of T-10, T-11, T-12, and L-1.[5] Impulses from the uterus travel through the uterosacral ligaments to the uterine plexus.[6] Other uterine afferents penetrate the cervix and lower uterine body and accompany the uterine arteries between layers of the broad ligament.[7] From the uterus, they join other pelvic afferents to form the pelvic plexus (also known as the inferior hypogastric plexus) which sits at the level of the rectum and vagina. Each pelvic plexus is composed of interlacing nerve fibers and numerous minute ganglia, spread over an area of 2 or 3 cm. They receive branches from the sacral ganglia of the sympathetic trunk and parasympathetic fibers, as well.

The parasympathetic component of the pelvic plexus is provided by the pelvic splanchnic nerves ("nervi erigentes"), which leave the spinal cord in the second, third, and fourth sacral nerves. These fibers ascend into the abdomen in the hypogastric plexus and are distributed with the branches of the inferior mesenteric artery. Impulses from the upper vagina, cervix, and lower uterine segment travel through the parasympa-

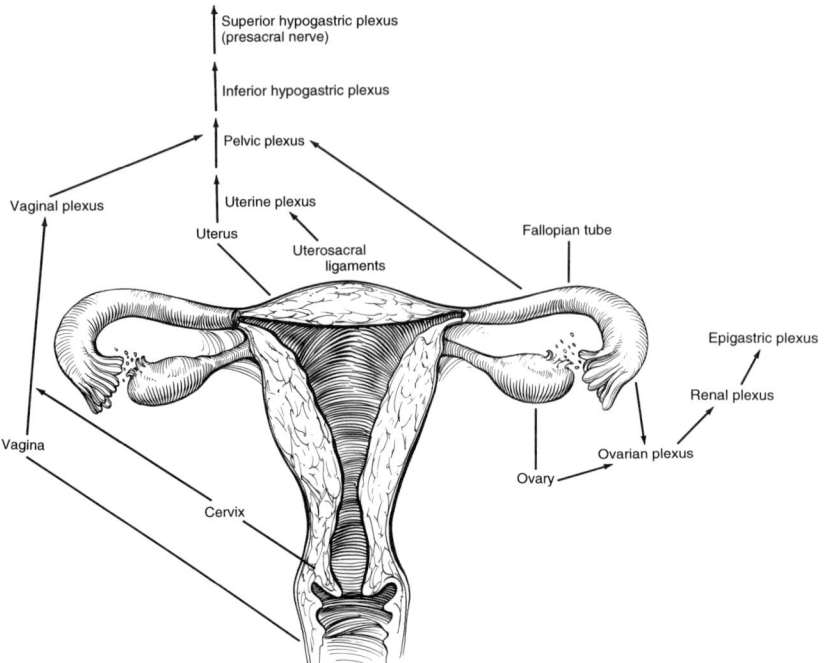

Figure 5.1. The neural supply to the pelvic viscera.

thetic system via the nervi erigentes to the sacral nerve roots (S_2-S_4).[4] Their ganglia (termed Frankenhauser's ganglia) are located lateral to the cervix.

The ovaries and distal fallopian tubes derive their nerve supply independently. The afferent supply from the adnexa travels with the ovarian vascular supply through the ovarian plexus to the inferior mesenteric plexus and ascends with the sympathetic chain to enter the spinal cord at T-9 and T-10.

The bladder, rectum, perineum, and anus are derived from the urogenital sinus, and are innervated by both sympathetic and parasympathetic systems. Afferents from the perineum and anus combine to form branches of the pudendal nerve, eventually leading to the second

and fourth sacral root ganglia (S_2 and S_4). All the sacral and coccygeal nerves receive gray rami communicantes from the sympathetic trunk.

Converging fibers from the sympathetic and parasympathetic networks pass through the superior hypogastric plexus, in front of the fifth lumbar vertebrum, between the common iliac arteries. The superior hypogastric or interiliac plexus sits at the level of the bifurcation of the aorta, where the intermesenteric nerves join with branches from the second, third, and fourth sacral nerves, and with a few filaments from the first two sacral ganglia. The plexus is commonly referred to as the presacral nerve, although there is complete fusion to form a single nerve in only 24% of individuals.[8]

The physiology of pain conduction is similarly complex. Current pain theory suggests that stimulation of specific pain fibers activates direct connections to the cerebral cortex. The viscera are innervated by small diameter a-delta and C primary afferent nerves that terminate in mechanoreceptors. The receptors provide a graded response depending on the intensity of the stimulus. A noxious stimulus is then coded by the intensity of neural discharge and subjected to further modification in the spinal cord and central nervous system. Bidirectional transmission of information occurs from periphery to brain, and from brain to spinal cord. Finally, modulation of peripheral nociceptive signals is affected by motivational and affective states.[9]

Endometriosis and Pain

Pelvic pain associated with endometriosis can present in a variety of ways as dysmenorrhea, dyspareunia, or chronic noncyclic pelvic pain. While endometriosis and

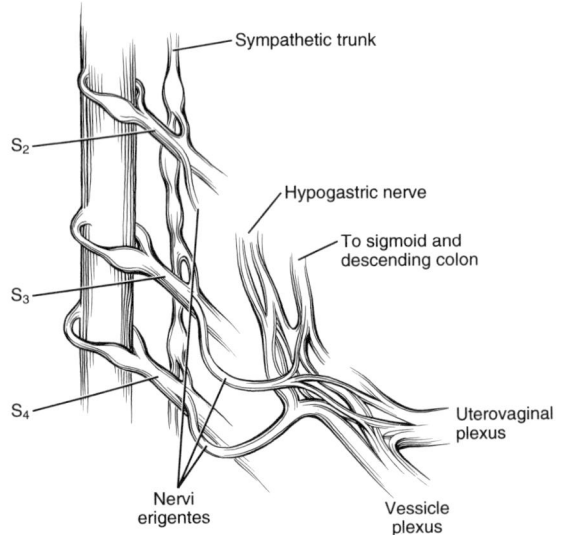

Figure 5.2. Sympathethic and parasympathetic innervation of the uterovaginal and vesicle plexes.

its painful sequelae are often confined to the pelvis, such symptoms have also been reported in the gastrointestinal, urinary, and pulmonary systems.[10-12]

It is difficult to make an accurate estimate of the prevalence of endometriosis in patients with pelvic pain. Reported series of cases have differed with respect to surgical indications, operator experience in disease diagnosis, and presence of multiple morphologic forms of disease. In general, grossly evident endometriosis is diagnosed in approximately 30% to 50% of women undergoing laparoscopy for pelvic pain.[13,15] Prevalence of microscopic lesions, however, may be higher. In one series of pelvic pain patients without obvious pathology, biopsies taken from the broad ligament, uterosacral ligaments, and posterior cul-de-sac revealed microscopic foci of endometriosis in 50%.[16] This is in contrast with the prevalence of visible endometriosis in the general population, which is estimated to be 7% to 15% in studies of asymptomatic multiparous women undergoing laparoscopic tubal sterilization, and 6% to 10% in women undergoing all abdominal surgical procedures.[17-20]

Symptoms of endometriosis may vary with location, stage of disease, type of lesion, and depth of invasion. A thorough preoperative history and physical examination with specific attention to the nature of the pain, its relationship to the menstrual cycle, and evidence of dyspareunia, dyschezia, or dysuria may aid in diagnosis. Pelvic pain reported to be in the same location for 6 months or longer is usually associated with organic pathology.[18] Also, focal tenderness on preoperative pelvic examination is associated with some pathology in 97% of patients, and with endometriosis in 66%.[21] Not all investigators have found pain symptoms to depend on implant location.[22] In fact, some have found no relation between the prevalence and severity of pain symptoms and the stage of endometriosis or site of lesions.[23] Overall, however, it appears that pelvic pain is more severe in advanced stages of endometriosis than in earlier stages.[24]

Dysmenorrhea is the most commonly reported symptom in endometriosis sufferers.[25] Overall, 50% to 91% of patients with endometriosis report dysmenorrhea.[23,24,26-30] The association, however, is neither well understood nor universal. Evaluation of patients undergoing laparoscopic sterilization revealed no increase in prevalence of dysmenorrhea in one study of 32 women with stage I endometriosis.[22] In another study of infertile patients, there was also no increase in incidence of dysmenorrhea in patients with endometriosis.[24] Though not entirely reliable as predictors of disease, however, menstrual symptoms should raise your suspicion for the presence of endometriosis.

Another symptom commonly associated with endometriosis is dyspareunia, generally described as pain deep in the pelvis. A strong association between ad-

vanced stages of endometriosis and deep dyspareunia has been shown by several authors.[24,25,31] The pain is most severe before menstruation and is often associated with specific coital positions.[32] Proposed mechanisms of dyspareunia include immobilization of the pelvic organs during coital activity and direct pressure on areas of endometriosis in the uterosacral ligaments in the cul-de-sac. Even in early endometriosis, there may be extensive involvement of the pelvic peritoneum, which is particularly sensitive to the traction and stretching that occurs during coitus.[33] It is also possible that, upon deep penetration, fibrotic areas or endometriosis-associated adhesions stretch.

Chronic pelvic pain is defined as pain which has been present for at least 6 months.[34] Such pain, frequently associated with advanced stages of endometriosis, can be episodic or continuous.[24] The patient who has episodic pain may have severe discomfort interrupted by pain-free intervals. Three patterns of intermittent pain are often described to the gynecologist: dyspareunia, midcycle pain, and dysmenorrhea. The patient with continuous pain is rarely free from her complaint, although certain factors may lessen or exacerbate the pain.

Study of the relationship between endometriosis and pelvic pain has been limited by current classification schemes. The methods of classification devised by the American Fertility Society were designed to estimate fertility prognosis, not pain severity or response to treatment. To create a scale that reflects pain, anatomic disease must be accurately correlated with initial pain intensity or the degree of pain relief with treatment. To do this, however, requires an accurate and precise method of quantifying pelvic pain. While many pain scales have been validated for both acute or chronic pain, none have been specifically validated for pain of pelvic origin.[35-38]

Pathogenesis of Pain

Numerous investigators have attempted to explain the pathogenesis of endometriosis-associated pain. The heterogeneity of the disease process, however, suggests that a range of pathophysiologic processes are involved. Mechanisms theorized to be responsible for pain include inflammation, pressure, adhesions, neuronal involvement, increased prostaglandin production, and psychologic factors.

Different types of lesions may cause pain via different routes. Atypical papular lesions may produce more prostaglandins than older lesions. These lesions may be responsible for functional pain symptoms, such as dysmenorrhea.[31] Classic lesions are thought to be older or burnt out endometriosis.[39] These might be more likely to provoke organic-type pain from mechanical pressure of cystic nodules and from stimulation of pain fibers by scars and stretching of areas of fibrotic infiltration, as could occur during intercourse upon deep penetration.[31]

Recently, the depth of infiltration of endometriosis has been recognized to correlate with pelvic pain.[39,40] Since depth cannot be easily assessed by inspection alone, surgical excision is required to make an accurate evaluation. Very deep implants appear to be more active and may be found exclusively in patients with pain. Cornillie and co-workers found that nearly all women with lesions deeper than 1 cm suffer from severe pain.[41] In this study, women with superficial (<1 mm), intermediate (2 to 4 mm), or deep (5 to 10 mm) infiltration had pain in 17%, 53%, and 37% of cases, respectively. Total lesion volume, however, has not been found to be directly related to patient symptoms.[39,41]

Peritoneal fluid inflammatory cells, especially macrophages, are increased in number in patients with endometriosis as in other inflammatory conditions.[42,43] This accumulation of white blood cells may release lysosomal enzymes and induce tissue damage and pain. Tissue damage due to acute and chronic inflammation may leave a marked degree of fibrosis and adhesions.

Adhesion formation is common in patients with endometriosis, and may be related to the degree of pain. Adhesions may cause pain by direct nerve damage, from tissue destruction and scar formation, or by devitalization and ischemia of parts of the internal pelvic organs, secondary to damage to the blood supply. Organs such as bowel or adnexa may also be adherent

in abnormal areas and cause any movement to place traction on their nerve supply. Over time, scarring of the posterior uterine surface may become extensive enough to produce a fixed retroflexion possibly resulting in sacral pain because of direct pressure. Pain may be referred to the back, lower abdomen, rectum, and thighs due to the proximity of lumbar and sacral nerves.

Sturgis and Call have suggested that endometriotic lesions surrounded by a fibrotic capsule are likely to cause pain.[44] In support of this theory, Ripps and co-workers found 96% of lesions associated with focal tenderness to be fibrotic.[21] Menstrual pain may be related to a buildup of pressure within the fibrotic lesion prior to or during menstruation. This pressure may be enough to stimulate pain fibers in the capsular tissue. Alternatively, the cyclic menstrual pain may be related to sequential swelling with extravasation of blood and menstrual debris from endometrial glands into surrounding tissue.[45]

Perineural involvement with endometriosis or with its subsequent adhesion formation may also play a role in pain syndromes. The presence of perineural inflammatory reaction, particularly in deep endometriosis, has been demonstrated.[41] An association between pain syndromes and uterosacral ligament involvement has also been described.[46] Additional evidence of endometriosis directly irritating nerve fibers stems from reports of painful syndromes involving the obturator nerve in the obturator fossa or the femoral nerve in the inguinal canal.[47]

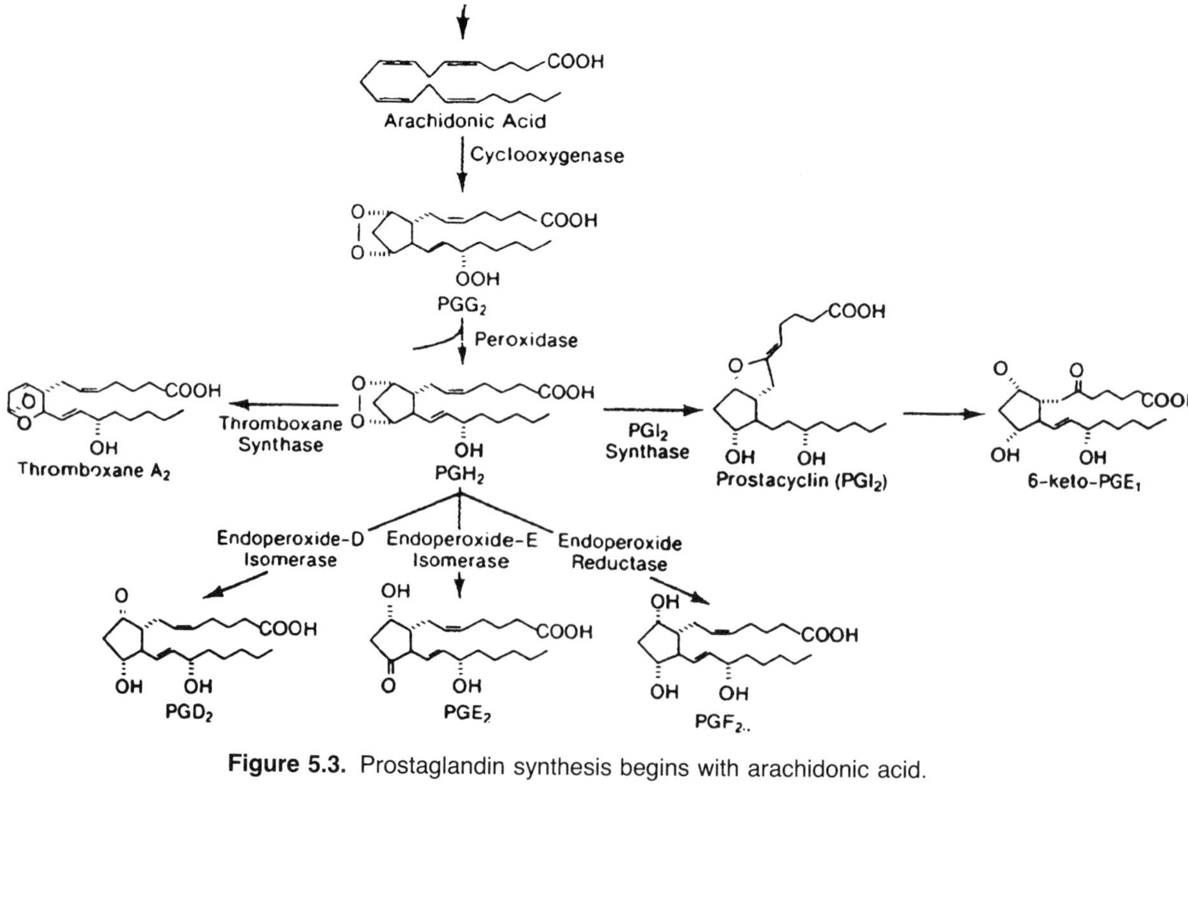

Figure 5.3. Prostaglandin synthesis begins with arachidonic acid.

Several investigators have examined the relationship between endometriosis and prostaglandin production in an attempt to elaborate the role of these compounds in the pathogenesis of pelvic pain.[42,48,49,54] Peritoneal fluid inflammatory cells, such as macrophages, are known to produce prostaglandins.[43] The peritoneum itself, ovary, and retrograde menstrual debris may all contribute to the peritoneal pool of prostaglandins.[49]

In an attempt to delineate this mechanism, a number of prostanoids have been postulated as mediating the painful effects in endometriosis (Fig. 5.3). Eicosanoid products of the cyclooxygenase pathway such as prostacyclin (PGI_2) and prostaglandin E_2 (PGE_2) have been shown to sensitize pain receptors to chemical mediators and mechanical stimuli.[55] Leukotriene B_4 (LTB_4), a product of the lipoxygenase pathway, is a known chemotactic agent, and may initiate an influx of leukocytes.[56] These leukocytes can potentially release lysosomal enzymes, and lead to tissue destruction and adhesion formation. Other prostaglandins possibly involved include prostaglandin $F2\alpha$ ($PGF2\alpha$), thromboxanes A_2 and B_2 (TxA_2, TxB_2), and 6-keto-prostaglandin $F1\alpha$ (6-KF).

Numerous experimental animal models for endometriosis have been evaluated.[57] Autotransplantation in rats of uterine squares to the peritoneal cavity shows that viable endometrial implants produce $PGF2\alpha$ at concentrations similar to those measured in uterine tissue.[58] In rabbits with artificially induced peritoneal endometriosis, peritoneal fluid $PGF2\alpha$ levels are significantly elevated over controls.[53]

A number of investigators have attempted to determine peritoneal prostaglandin levels in women with endometriosis. Badaway found that women with endometriosis, regardless of pelvic pain, show significantly elevated levels of $PFG2\alpha$ in the peritoneal fluid.[48] Drake's team reported an elevated concentration of TxB_2 and 6-KF, the stable metabolites of TxA_2 and prostacyclin, in a group of patients with pelvic pain.[50] Rock and co-workers, however, found normal levels of peritoneal fluid TxB_2 and 6-KF in women between days 8 and 12 of their menstrual cycle.[52]

Dawood and others investigated patients with chronic pelvic pain and found that, except for an increase in 6-KF, the peritoneal fluid prostaglandins measured in patients with endometriosis did not differ from normal women, women with chronic PID, and other women with chronic pelvic pain.[49] Rapkin and Bhattacherjee also examined the relationship between peritoneal fluid eicosanoids and chronic pelvic pain and found no correlation between the symptoms, underlying diagnosis, and concentration of eicosanoids PGE_2, PGI_2, and LTB_4.[51]

While these studies present conflicting data, it appears that at least a subgroup of patients with pelvic pain may suffer from increased prostglandin exposure.[50,54] It is unclear whether this is primarily a result of the activity of the lesions or the degree of inflammatory response.[59] The wide varieties in lesion activity, inflammatory response, the relative insensitivity of pain quantification methods, and the transient nature of prostaglandin action further complicate investigation into this association.

Psychological factors may also play a role in the pathogenesis and persistence of chronic pelvic pain. Patients with chronic pelvic pain frequently have abnormal psychological profiles, including a history of depression and/or dysfunctional family backgrounds. These findings seem to be unrelated to the presence or absence of underlying pelvic pathology.[60] Sexual and physical abuse may promote the chronicity of pelvic pain.[61] Such findings support the importance of obtaining a history of physical abuse, both current and from childhood, when evaluating these patients. The implementation of a multidisciplinary pain management approach often seems indicated.[62] The involvement of a psychologist may be successful in ameliorating feelings of helplessness that promote passive "illness" behavior and depressed mood.

Conclusion

While much has been learned about the diagnosis and treatment of endometriosis over the past century, a full understanding of the pathogenesis of pelvic pain in endometriosis remains to be uncovered. Numerous theories abound, with little data to support them. Tools currently available to study this issue are substandard, and the degree of investigative interest minimal. Nevertheless, pelvic pain remains the preeminent consequence of endometriosis, affecting the vast majority of symptomatic women. A precise understanding of the mechanisms generating pelvic pain are an absolute requirement if therapeutic maneuvers are to attack this process directly. If researchers are to make any important strides in this direction, a change in focus from description to delineation of mechanisms will be required. Only then, when the scientific method has been applied to these questions, can time-honored theories of endometriosis-associated pain be validated and extended.

References

1. Stripling M, Martin D, Chatman D, et al. Subtle appearance of pelvic endometriosis. Fertil Steril 1988;49:427–431.
2. Martin D, Hubert G, Vander Zwaag R, et al. Laparoscopic appearances of peritoneal endometriosis. Fertil Steril 1989;51:63–67.
3. Jansen R, Russell P. Nonpigmented endometriosis: clinical, laparoscopic, and pathologic definition. Am J Obstet Gynecol 1986;155:1154–1159.

4. Rapkin A. Neuroanatomy, neurophysiology, and neuropharmacology of pelvic pain. Clin Obstet Gynecol 1990; 33:119–129.

5. Pomeranz B, Wall P, Wever W. Cord cells responding to fine myelinated afferents from visceral, muscle and skin. J Physiol 1968;199:511–532.

6. Counsellor V. The treatment of dysmenorrhea by resection of the presacral nerves: evaluation of end results. Am J Obstet Gynecol 1934;28:161–167.

7. Gray H. Anatomy: Descriptive and surgical. In Pick T, Howden R, eds. (XV ed.) New York, Bounty Books, 1977, 1257.

8. Fliegner J, Umstad M. Presacral Neurectomy—A reappraisal. Aust NZ J Obstet Gynecol 1991;31:76–79.

9. Melzack R. Neurophysiological foundations of pain. In Sternbach R, ed. The psychology of pain. 2nd ed. New York, Raven Press, 1986, 1–24.

10. Badaway S, Freedman L, Numann P, Bonaventura M, Kim, S. Diagnosis and management of intestinal endometriosis: A report of five cases. J of Reprod Med 1988; 33:851–855.

11. Kerr WJ. Endometriosis involving the urinary tract. Clin Obstet Gynecol 1966;9:331–357.

12. Horsfield K. Catamenial pleural pain. Eur Respir J 1989; 2:1013–1014.

13. Vercillini P, Fedele L, Molteni P, Arcaini L, Bianchi S, Candiani G. Laparoscopy in the diagnosis of gynecologic chronic pelvic pain. Int J Gynaecol Obstet 1990;32:261–265.

14. Chatman D, Zbella E. Pelvic peritoneal defects and endometriosis: Further observations. Fertil Steril 1986;46:711–714.

15. Goldstein D, deCholnoky C, Emans S, et al. Laparoscopy in the diagnosis and management of pelvic pain adolescents. J Reprod Med 1980;24:251–256.

16. DeBrux J, Bret J, Demay C, Bardiaux M. Recurring pelvic peritonitis. Amer J Obstet Gynecol 1968;102:501–505.

17. Barbieri R. Etiology and epidemiology of endometriosis. Am J Obstet Gynecol 1990;162:565–567.

18. Kresch A, Seifer D, Sachs L, Barrese I. Laparoscopy in 100 women with chronic pelvic pain. Obstet Gynecol 1984;64:672–674.

19. Wheeler J, Malinak L. Epidemiology of endometriosisassociated infertility. J Reprod Med 1989;34:41–46.

20. Boling R, Abbasi R, Ackerman G, et al. Disability from endometriosis in the United States Army. J Reprod Med 1988;33:49–52.

21. Ripps B, Martin D. Focal pelvic tenderness, pelvic pain and dysmenorrhea in endometriosis. J Reprod Med 1991; 36:470–472.

22. Liu D, Hitchcock A. Endometriosis: Its association with retrograde menstruation, dysmenorrhea and tubal pathology. Br J Obstet Gynaecol 1986;93:859–862.

23. Fedele L, Parazzini F, Bianchi S, et al. Stage and localization of pelvic endometriosis and pain. Fertil Steril 1990; 53:155–158.

24. Fedele L, Bianchi S, Bocciolone L, et al. Pain symptoms associated with endometriosis. Obstet Gynecol 1992;79: 767–769.

25. Mahmood T, Templeton A, Thomason L, et al. Menstrual symptoms in women with pelvic endometriosis. Br J Obstet Gynecol 1991;98:558–563.

26. Shaw R. Nafarelin in the treatment of pelvic pain caused by endometriosis. Am J Obstet Gynecol 1990;162:574–576.

27. Buttram VJ. Conservative surgery for endometriosis in the infertile female: A study of 206 patients with implications for both medical and surgical therapy. Fertil Steril 1979;31:117–121.

28. Garcia C, David S. Pelvic endometriosis: infertility and pelvic pain. Am J Obstet Gynecol 1977;129:740–747.

29. Ranney B. Endometriosis: Conservative operations. Am J Obstet Gynecol 1970;107:743–750.

30. Williams T, Pratt J. Endometriosis in 1000 consecutive celiotomies: Incidence and management. Am J Obstet Gynecol 1977;129:245–250.

31. Vercellini P, Bocciolone L, Vendola N, et al. Peritoneal endometriosis. Morphologic appearance in women with chronic pelvic pain. J Reprod Med 1991;36:533–536.

32. Galle P. Clinical presentation and diagnosis of endometriosis. In: Obstet Gynecol Clin North Am 1989;16:29–42.

33. Fedele L, Marchini M, Acaia B, et al. Dynamics and significance of placebo response in primary dysmenorrhea. Pain 1989;36:43–47.

34. Slocumb J. Operative management of chronic abdominal pelvic pain. Clin Obstet Gynecol 1990;33:196–204.

35. Flandry F, Hunt J, Terry G, et al. Analysis of subjective knee complaints using visual analog scales. Am J Sports Med 1991;19:112–118.

36. Jensen M, Karoly P, Braver S. The measurement of clinical pain intensity: a comparison of six methods. Pain 1986;27:117–126.

37. Tait R, Pollard C, Margolis R, et al. The Pain Disability Index: psychometric and validity data. Arch Phys Med Rehabil 1987;68:438–441.

38. Wilkie D, Savedra M, Holzemer W, et al. Use of the McGill pain questionnaire to measure pain: a meta-analysis. Nurs Res 1990;39:36–41.

39. Koninckx P, Meuleman C, Demeyere S, et al. Suggestive evidence that pelvic endometriosis is a progressive disease, whereas deeply infiltrating endometriosis is associated with pelvic pain. Fertil Steril 1991;55:759–765.

40. Martin D, Hubert G, Vander Zwaag R, et al. Depth of infiltration of endometriosis. J Gynecol Surg 1989;5:55.

41. Cornillie F, Oosterlynck D, Lauweryns J, et al. Deeply infiltrating pelvic endometriosis: histology and clinical significance. Fertil Steril 1990;53:978–983.

42. Halme J, Becker S, Wing R. Accentuated cyclic activation of peritoneal macrophages in patients with endometriosis. Am J Obstet Gynecol 1983;148:85–90.

43. Piper P. Pharmacology of leukotriene. Br Med Bull 1983; 39:255.

44. Sturgis S, Call B. Endometriosis peritonei. Relation of pain to functional activity. Amer J of Obstet Gynecol 1954;68:1421–1431.

45. Droegemueller W, Herbst A, Mishell D, et al. Comprehensive Gynecology. Missouri: The C.V. Mosby Company, 1987, 1149.

46. Nesbitt R, Rizk P. Uterosacral ligament syndrome. Obstet Gynecol 1971;37:730–733.

47. Redwine D, Sharp D. Endometriosis of the obturator nerve. A case report. J Reprod Med 1990;35:434–435.

48. Badaway S, Marshall L, Gabal A, et al. The concentration of 13, 14-dihydro-15-keto-prostaglandin F_2alpha and prostaglandin E_2 in peritoneal fluid of infertile patients with and without endometriosis. Fertil Steril 1982;38:166–170.

49. Dawood M, Khan-Dawood F, Wilson L. Peritoneal fluid prostaglandins and prostanoids in women with endometriosis, chronic pelvic inflammatory disease, and pelvic pain. Am J Obstet Gynecol 1984;148:391–395.

50. Drake T, O'Brien W, Ramwell P, et al. Peritoneal fluid thromoxane B_2 and 6-keto prostaglandin F1α in endometriosis. Am J Obstet Gynecol 1981;140:401–422.
51. Rapkin A, Bhattacherjee P. Peritoneal fluid eiscosanoids in chronic pelvic pain. Prostaglandins 1989;38:447–452.
52. Rock J, Dubin N, Ghodgaonkar R, et al. Cul-de-sac fluid in women with endometriosis: Fluid volume and prostanoid concentration during the proliferative phase of the cycle—days 8 to 12. Fertil Steril 1982;37:747–750.
53. Schenken R, Asch R. Surgical induction of endometriosis in the rabbit: Effect on fertility and concentrations of peritoneal fluid prostaglandins. Fertil Steril 1980;34:581–587.
54. Ylikorkala O, Vlinikka L. Prostaglandins and endometriosis. Acta Obstet Gynecol Scand 1983;113(Suppl):105–107.
55. Ferreira S, Nakamura M, Salete De Abreu Castro M. The hyperalgesic effects of prostacyclin and prostaglandin E_2. Prostaglandins 1978;16:31–37.
56. Bray M. The pharmacology and pathophysiology of leukotriene B_4. Br Med Bull 1983;39:249.
57. Vernon M. Experimental endometriosis in laboratory animals as a research model. Prog Clin Biol Res 1990;323:49–60.
58. Vernon M, Wilson E. Studies on the surgical induction of endometriosis in the rat. Fertil Steril 1985;44:684–694.
59. Vernon M, Beard J, Graves K, et al. Classification of endometriotic implants by morphologic appearance and capacity to synthesize prostaglandin F. Fertil Steril 1986;46.
60. Harrop-Griffiths J, Katon W, Walker E, et al. The association between chronic pelvic pain, psychiatric diagnoses, and childhood sexual abuse. Obstet Gynecol 1988;71:589–594.
61. Rapkin A, Kames L, Darke L, et al. History of physical and sexual abuse on women with chronic pelvic pain. Obstet Gynecol 1990;76:92–96.
62. Rapkin A, Kames L. The pain management approach to chronic pelvic pain. J Reprod Med 1987;32:323–327.

6

Pathogenesis of Infertility in Endometriosis

George M. Grunert and Robert R. Franklin

There is no single, unifying explanation for the infertility of all patients with endometriosis. By understanding the possible multiple relationships, clinicians can provide the rationale for treatment of endometriosis in the infertile couple. Our present knowledge stems from clinical experience, clinical and epidemiological studies, and basic scientific studies in animals with endometriosis.

Does Endometriosis Cause Infertility?

A critical appraisal of the literature shows that an undisputed relationship between endometriosis and infertility may not be established. To prove a causal relationship, researchers must establish that fertility is present before the occurrence of endometriosis, that infertility follows the development of endometriosis, and that the removal of the endometriosis restores fertility. Since we cannot prospectively perform laparoscopies on fertile women, induce or document infertility, and then treat the disease, such a cause-and-effect relationship may never be proven definitively. Indeed, the link between endometriosis and infertility is based largely on population studies comparing the prevalence of endometriosis in fertile and infertile women and on reports of enhancement of fertility after the treatment of endometriosis. The results of experimental introduction of endometriosis into fertile animals have been used to extrapolate its effect on humans. Even here, though, the conclusion that endometriosis causes infertility may not be valid, because experimentally introduced endometriosis may not parallel the course of the disease in humans.

"Classic" reports relate that 6% to 58% of women with infertility have endometriosis and 30% to 50% of women with endometriosis are infertile.[1-3] The wide variation in prevalence rates of endometriosis reported in infertility patients may be due to referral patterns to infertility surgeons as well as the diligence of investigators in searching for endometriosis. The data on the rate of infertility in women with endometriosis are not contemporary, but came from studies done in the 1930s and 1940s. Therefore, they reflect a population of patients referred to large centers for major surgical management of severe endometriosis.[4-6] The fact that many studies predate the advent of laparoscopy, and are based on patients who underwent laparotomy for symptoms other than infertility, means that the association may not be extrapolated to today's infertility population.

In studies comparing findings at laparoscopy for infertility with the findings at the time of tubal sterilization, there is general agreement that endometriosis is more prevalent in infertile women. The reported rates of endometriosis in the infertile group range from 21% to 48% compared with 1% to 5% in fertile women undergoing laparoscopic tubal ligation.[7-9]

There is little disagreement that women with endometriosis and mechanical distortion of the pelvis have a clear cause for diminished fertility. Adhesions, distal tubal sacculation, distal tubal occlusion, and proximal tubal obstruction can all occur in patients with moderate or severe endometriosis.[10] Inoue and colleagues reported on 2,080 infertile women, 1,263 of whom had minimal or mild endometriosis. There was no difference in the rate of conception when expectant management, medical therapy, or surgical treatment of the endometriosis were compared.[11] Currently, a debate about the relationship of endometriosis and infertility centers on the role of minimal and mild degrees of endometriosis in infertility.

In an attempt to address the relationship of minimal and mild endometriosis and infertility, Jansen prospectively evaluated a group of women who were to undergo therapeutic donor insemination.[12] He found that 7 (8%) of 91 women had minimal or mild endometriosis at laparoscopy before insemination. The group with endometriosis had a lower pregnancy rate per cycle (fecundity rate) (2/56, 4%) than the normal group (46/380, 12%). In a retrospective review of donor insemination patients, Yeh and Seibel also found that patients with endometriosis had both a lower fecundity rate and a lower overall pregnancy rate when compared with patients free of endometriosis.[13] In contrast, in a retrospective study without controls, Portuondo and co-workers reported nine conceptions in ten patients with untreated, laparoscopically documented mild endometriosis who underwent donor insemination.[14] No data on cycle fecundity was given. Toma and colleagues, in another donor insemination study, confirmed the decreased fecundity rate, but found that neither laparoscopic ablation nor danazol therapy of patients with minimal or mild endometriosis increased the fecundity rate to that of non-endometriosis patients.[15] Additional prospective studies of the effect of medical or surgical therapy on fertility in women with minimal or mild degrees of endometriosis have not demonstrated an improvement in the chances of pregnancy per cycle compared with controls.[16–19]

Although experimental transplantation of endometriosis in animals may not represent a true model of endometriosis in humans, it has been used to test the hypothesis that endometriosis can cause infertility. In rats, rabbits, and primates, successful peritoneal transplantation has resulted in decreased fertility.[20–22] In none of these studies was the extent of endometriosis described sufficiently to provide stage-for-stage comparison with observations in humans. However, Schenken and Asch noted decreased fertility only in animals with ovarian adhesions.[22]

Evidence linking endometriosis and infertility is inferred from the fact that endometriosis is more prevalent in infertility patients, that endometriosis decreases the fecundity rate in donor insemination patients, and that the induction of experimental endometriosis in animals results in decreased fecundity. A number of hypotheses attempt to explain the link (Table 6.1).

Table 6.1. Possible mechanisms of infertilty associated with endometriosis.

Mechanical pelvic factors
Peritoneal fluid abnormalities
   Embryo/gamete toxicity
   Macrophages
   Prostaglandins
Ovulatory/endocrine abnormalities
   Abnormal follicular dynamics
   Anovulation
   Hyperprolactinemia
   Luteal phase defect
   Luteinized unruptured follicle
Spontaneous abortion
Immunologic abnormalities

Evidence pertaining to each of these possible mechanisms is reviewed in the following sections.

Mechanical Pelvic Factors

Pelvic endometriosis and the body's inflammatory response to it can produce massive, dense, cohesive adhesions. These adhesions distort the pelvic architecture and may directly interfere with oocyte release from the ovaries or hinder tubal pickup of oocytes. Fimbrial distortion or destruction, the formation of fimbrial bridges, and even distal occlusion with formation of a hydrosalpinx can result. Fimbrial or intraluminal implants or serosal implants with tubal constriction are additional causes of tubal occlusion or distortion. Progressive involvement, with the resulting fibrosis and adhesion formation, can lead to frank obstruction and hydrosalpinx. In a mouse system, distal tubal endometriosis without physical occlusion has been shown to interfere with fimbrial function and ovum capture.[23]

Haney and Fortier, in examining pathologic findings in a group of patients undergoing proximal tubal resection and anastomosis for occlusion, found endometriosis to be the etiologic factor in 14% of cases.[24] Marana and Quagliarello confirmed such a finding.[25] Although not proven histologically, further support for endometriosis as a cause for proximal obstruction is given by the reports of resolution following treatment with danazol.[26,27] Resolution of proximal obstruction was seen both with and without concurrent pelvic endometriosis. Similarly, Urman and co-workers found endometriosis to be the cause of midtubal occlusion in 13% of women undergoing resection and anastomosis.[28]

Ovarian endometriosis and endometriomas have been associated with ovarian dysfunction and anovulation. In extreme cases, destruction of the ovarian stroma can occur. Fixation of the ovary or sacculation of the ovary in adhesions may prevent mechanical release of the oocyte into the abdomen at ovulation.

Transcervical falloposcopy now allows detailed observation of the endosalpinx and tubal lumen. Although endometriosis has not been reported as an endosalpingeal lesion, except in patients with occlusion, Kerin and colleagues reported intratubal adhesions in 25% of patients with pelvic endometriosis.[29] Marana and co-workers, however, were unable to confirm this finding.[30]

Pregnancy rates following conservative surgery for moderate or severe endometriosis are reported to be 37% to 75% and 29% to 48%, respectively.[2] This compared with 7% in patients followed with observation only.[31] Thus, there appears to be an undisputed association between moderate and severe degrees of endometriosis, anatomic distortion of the pelvis, and infertility. Treatment of these patients clearly has a beneficial effect on fertility.

Peritoneal Fluid Abnormalities

Because the fallopian tubes and ovaries are constantly bathed in fluid, investigators have sought peritoneal abnormalities that might explain endometriosis-associated infertility. The search for a constituent of peritoneal fluid in patients with endometriosis that would have an effect on fertility has focused on the areas of direct embryo or gamete toxicity, prostaglandins, peritoneal macrophage function, and free radical formation. Drake and colleagues reported that the volume of peritoneal fluid in women with pelvic endometriosis was increased.[32] Subsequently, Syrop and Halme observed that endometriosis patients who conceived had a lower volume of intraperitoneal fluid than those who remained infertile.[33] However, even this observation is inconsistent. Peritoneal fluid volume varies throughout the menstrual cycle, peaking at mid-cycle. Rezai and co-workers measured peritoneal fluid volume only in the mid-follicular phase, and found no significant increase in volume in endometriosis patients.[34,35]

Embryo Gamete Toxicity

Oak and colleagues examined the effect on sperm motility of peritoneal fluid from women with unexplained infertility, women with infertility due to endometriosis, and fertile controls on sperm motility.[36] They found a significant reduction in sperm motility in both the unexplained infertility and endometriosis groups, compared with the fertile control group. The degree of reduction of sperm motility in the endometriosis group correlated with the volume of peritoneal fluid. Burke, in a similar study, found that adding peritoneal washings from women with endometriosis depressed sperm velocity, motility percentage, and motility index, when compared with washings from nonendometriosis patients.[37] Coddington and co-workers took this one step further and demonstrated that, in addition to decreasing sperm motion, peritoneal fluid from women with endometriosis inhibited sperm binding to the zona pellucida in a hemizona assay.[38]

If there is an inhibitory effect of peritoneal fluid from endometriosis patients on sperm function, we would expect to see fertilization inhibited. While this has not been directly demonstrated in humans, a filterable and partially heat-labile component of peritoneal fluid from endometriosis patients decreased fertilization in vitro in a murine model.[39] Intraperitoneal injection of peritoneal fluid from endometriosis patients also significantly impaired fertility in vivo in superovulated hamsters.[40] Dodds and colleagues, in an in vitro murine model, demonstrated a progressive decrease in fertilization rate with increasing concentrations of peritoneal fluid from endometriosis patients, but found no decrease in fertility with intraperitoneal injections of fluid in an in vivo experiment.[41]

Postfertilization detrimental effects of peritoneal fluid from endometriosis patients have been demonstrated. Morcos and co-workers compared Hams F-10 media with and without added cell-free, heat inactivated peritoneal fluid from patients with endometriosis in a two-cell mouse embryo culture system.[42] There was significant reduction in the percentage of embryos that reached the blastocyst and hatching stages in the endometriosis group. This effect has been confirmed by Prough and colleagues who fractionated cell-free peritoneal fluid and found that the greatest reduction in embryo growth was in the fraction greater than 100,000 daltons.[43] Taketani and colleagues reported that levels of interleukin-1 (IL-1, a product of activated macrophages) and tumor necrosis factor (TNF, a product of both activated macrophages and B-lymphocytes) were elevated in peritoneal fluid from women with endometriosis.[44] The levels were significantly higher than in nonendometriosis controls and higher than in patients with endometriosis who were treated with danazol or buserelin. In a mouse two-cell system, co-cultured with oviducts and peritoneal fluid, embryo toxicity was demonstrated only in the untreated endometriosis group, whereas the treated and control groups showed no toxicity. Kuo and co-workers used a co-culture system with oviductal epithelial cells and demonstrated that the detrimental effect on embryo growth from peritoneal fluid from endometriosis patients was similar to that seen when IL-1, without peritoneal fluid, was added.[45] They were also able to abolish the inhibitory effect of both peritoneal fluid extract and IL-1 with indomethacin, which suggests that the toxicity may be due to stimulation of oviductal production of prostaglandin-E2. This indirect, prostaglandin-mediated effect on IL-1 is supported by the finding that the addition of recombinant IL-1 itself, or in combination with recombinant interleukin 2 (IL-2, a product of activated T cells) did not inhibit murine embryonic development.[46]

This series of studies provides a scientific basis for the hypothesis that there is a factor (or factors) in the peritoneal fluid of endometriosis patients that inhibits sperm motility and function, oocyte fertilization, and embryonic growth. It appears that this action may depend on a large molecular weight substance, such as IL-1, IL-2, or TNF, perhaps acting in concert with other pelvic factors, such as tubal epithelium or peritoneal epithelium, and possibly modulated by prostaglandins.

Prostaglandins

Prostaglandins (PGs), thromboxanes (TXs), and leukotrienes (LTs), oxidant derivatives of dietary essential fatty acids, share arachidonic acid as a common precursor. Together, these substances comprise a group of compounds known as eicosanoids, which serve as both paracrine and autocrine regulators of cellular function.

Conversion to begin synthesis of this family is controlled by phospholipase A_2, the activity of which is increased by trauma, thrombi, toxins, catecholamines, bradykinins, angiotensin, and sex steroids. Eicosanoids are essential for the maintenance of many cellular functions. Absolute deprivation of precursor essential fatty acids causes loss of fertility, failure of growth, and death. Because they are intended to serve only local functions, they have characteristically short half-lives that range from seconds to several minutes. This brevity makes detection difficult. Studies, therefore, commonly measure metabolic end-products such as 6-keto-prostaglandins and thromboxane-B_2.[47]

PG-$F_{2\alpha}$ and PG-E_2 are secreted by almost all tissues, including those of the myometrium, endometrium, tubal endothelium, and peritoneum. PG-E_2 causes relaxation of smooth muscle, including that of the myometrium and tubal muscularis, whereas PG-$F_{2\alpha}$ produces smooth muscle contraction. The degree and location of contraction and relaxation are modulated by estrogen and progesterone levels. Indirect evidence for an essential role for PGs in tubal motility is provided by a variety of studies of interference with tubal function by administration or inhibition of PG activity. 15-methyl-PG-$F_{2\alpha}$, a potent PG analog, accelerates tubal motility and reduces fertility in rabbits and monkeys.[48,49] Although these actions provide an attractive hypothesis for the effect of pelvic endometriosis on fertility, a similar study in humans failed to demonstrate an effect on tubal motility.[50] These two PGs are also important in controlling cornual and myometrial contractions, in dysmenorrhea, and in controlling hemostasis during menstruation.

PGs are essential components of follicular function, ovulation, and corpus luteum function. Ovulation can be inhibited by cyclooxygenase blockage and by intrafollicular injection of antibodies to PG-$F_{2\alpha}$.[51] Disruption of intrafollicular PG activity has also been implicated in the luteinized unruptured follicle syndrome.[52] In contrast, direct injection of PG-$F_{2\alpha}$ into the corpus luteum also produces luetolysis in Rhesus monkeys.[53,54] There is evidence that PG-$F_{2\alpha}$ directly decreases LH-receptor formation and inhibits corpus luteum response to LH by inhibiting LH binding to receptors.[55] In primates, estradiol administration induces luteal regression, an event that can be blocked by indomethacin. This finding supports the hypothesis that this regression is mediated by prostaglandins.[56] These effects have all been reported in primates. To date, there is no conclusive evidence for such a direct role for PGs or PG synthetase inhibitors in the luteinized unruptured follicle syndrome or in leutolysis in humans.

PGI$_2$ (prostacycline) is produced by vascular wall endothelium, the heart, the stomach, and, to a lesser degree, by the endometrium and corpus luteum. PGI$_2$ causes smooth muscle relaxation and vasodilation and inhibits platelet aggregation. TXA$_2$ is produced by platelets, the lung, and the spleen and is essentially an antagonist of PGI$_2$, producing platelet aggregation and intense vasoconstriction. The vascular and platelet effects of these two compounds are essential in maintaining vascular permeability, preventing spontaneous platelet aggregation, and promoting and limiting the inflammatory response. They may play a role in corpus luteum formation and in the control of hemostasis at menstruation.

Leukotrienes, a third metabolite of arachidonic acid, are involved in the anaphylactic immune response, and produce vascular permeability and bronchoconstriction. They serve as chemotactic agents, attracting leukocytes to the site of inflammation. No important role for LTs in reproduction has been described.

For there to be a true role for PGs in infertility associated with endometriosis, an increased concentration or production of PGs must be documented. Several studies have demonstrated elevations of stable metabolites of PGs in peritoneal fluid from endometriosis patients compared to controls.[57-60] Although direct measurement of the active compounds PG-$F_{2\alpha}$ and PG-E_2 is difficult, many investigators have reported no significant increase in these substances in patients with endometriosis, while others have reported elevated levels.[61-65]

Increased PG levels in peritoneal fluid in patients with endometriosis would appear to offer an attractive explanation for infertility. Effects on tubal motility, oocyte capture, follicular rupture, luteinized unruptured follicle syndrome, corpus luteum formation, and leuteolysis have all been demonstrated in animal models. None of these effects, however, has been consistently seen in humans. The evidence for the presence of increased levels of PGs in peritoneal fluid is also inconsistent. Although PGs may play a role in some endometriosis patients, they cannot be universally accountable for infertility in these patients.

Peritoneal Macrophages

In bone marrow, colony-forming unit-granulocyte-macrophage (CFU-GM) cells are the progenitors of the myeloid and monocytic cell lines. CFU-GM cells differentiate into monocytes under the influence of macrophage colony stimulating factor (M-CSF). Monocytes circulate in the peripheral blood for up to 3 days, and then migrate into peripheral tissues to become macrophages, dermal Langerhans' cells, and Kupffer cells. As a result of this process, normal peritoneal fluid contains 0.5 to 1.5 × 10^5 macrophages per milliliter.[66] Macrophages identify and process antigens for presentation to lymphocytes in the initiation, coordination, and propagation of both cellular and, to a lesser degree, humoral immune responses. They also directly phagocytize organisms, foreign bodies, and, to a limited degree, cells and they remove debris. Macrophages undergo activation in response to a number of stimuli including lymphokines (interluekin-3 and interleukin-4), granulocyte-macrophage colony stimulating factor (GM-CSF), interferon-gamma, macrophage activating factor (MAF), and migration inhibitory factor (MIF). Activated macrophages phagocytize foreign bodies and microorganisms, process the antigens from these bodies, and present them to helper T cells, initiating the cellular immune response. Macrophages produce a wide variety of substances of importance in the immune response, including interleukin-1 (IL-1) and tumor necrosis factor (TNF), which amplify lymphocyte reactions. These normal, physiologic functions could, in the proper circumstances, also be directed against the normal reproductive processes and decrease fertility.

Studies of peritoneal fluid macrophages are nearly unanimous in agreement that the total number of peritoneal fluid macrophages is increased in women with endometriosis.[67–70] It has been argued that the increased number of macrophages results from an increase in peritoneal fluid volume, with the concentration kept constant. Haney and co-workers and Halme and colleagues reported an increase in the concentration of macrophages in peritoneal fluid from women with endometriosis compared with controls.[71,72] This finding has not consistently been supported by other investigators. The control groups for these studies were either fertile women or women with pelvic adhesions not related to endometriosis. Because macrophage concentration is higher in women with patent tubes than in women with tubal occlusion, and varies with phase of the menstrual cycle, control groups should be matched for these factors. One series, which compared patients with endometriosis with those with unexplained infertility and patent tubes, at comparable times in the menstrual cycle, noted no increase in total number or concentration.[73] Induction of endometriosis in a rabbit model did not increase peritoneal fluid volume, total macrophage numbers, or concentration.[74]

To support the hypothesis that macrophages may play a role in infertility in patients with endometriosis, one must demonstrate not only increased macrophage numbers but also increased macrophage activation. Macrophage activation can be confirmed by detecting changes in cell size or morphology, or cellular capping (segregation of specific cell membrane receptors). Increases in the activity or concentration of intracellular enzymes such as acid phosphatase, myeloperoxidase, or leucine aminopeptidase are consistent with activation. Others have used measurement of the ability to generate peroxides, superoxides, and oxygen-free radicals by chemoluminescence as biochemical evidence of activation. Activation can also be confirmed in vitro by demonstrating phagocytosis or by demonstration of the production of IL-1 or TNF.[75] Halme and co-workers

have confirmed activation of macrophages from peritoneal fluid of endometriosis patients by showing increased staining for myeloperoxidase, increased concentrations of acid phosphatase and leucine aminopeptidase, increased macrophage size, and cellular capping.[61,67,70] Other authors have also shown increased phagocytic activity.[63,70,76]

Since the predominant function of macrophages is phagocytosis of foreign organisms and cells, it is not surprising that Muscato and colleagues were able to show phagocytosis of sperm in vivo.[77] Incubation of sperm in peritoneal fluid results in a decrease in sperm motility and survival and, using peritoneal fluid from endometriosis patients, in percent motility and straight line velocity.[36,78] Chaco and co-workers used culture media that had been incubated with peritoneal macrophages and showed a significant decrease in sperm penetration of zona-free hamster oocytes (SPA assay).[79] They further showed the same decrease in penetration with media incubated with killed macrophages and with media heat-inactivated after exposure to macrophages. Similar studies using cell-free preparations of peritoneal fluid showed no such effect.[80,81] Sueldo and colleagues, assessing the effect of cell-free peritoneal fluid on fertilization in a mouse system, confirmed a decrease in fertilization rate.[39]

Besides the cellular response of macrophages to foreign cells and organisms, activated peritoneal fluid macrophages from endometriosis patients produce increased amounts of prostaglandins, IL-1 and TNF.[82] The peritoneal fluid concentrations of IL-1 and TNF are increased in endometriosis patients.[44] Macrophages removed from the fluid produced these factors spontaneously.[83] Sueldo and co-workers found that the addition of IL-1 to culture media significantly decreased zona-free hamster oocyte sperm penetration assay results, interfered with human zona pellucida binding of sperm, and inhibited mouse embryo development.[84] They hypothesized that IL-1 secretion by peritoneal macrophages may be responsible for the detrimental effects on mouse embryo growth reported by others. In an in vivo murine system, Uda and Umesaki found a decreased conception rate and decreased litter number when peritoneal macrophages were stimulated by intraperitoneal injection.[85] The effect of macrophage stimulation was reversed by concurrent administration of steroids. Uda also studied the effect of intraperitoneal injection of IL-1 and found a similar decrease in conception rate. Histologic study showed decreased intracellular glycogen in the endometrium, which the author felt could impair implantation.[86] In this same study, a decreased rate of mouse embryo growth and blastulation was evident when IL-1 was added to culture media.

Peritoneal macrophages from endometriosis patients are also associated with an increased production of reactive oxygen products (peroxides, superoxides, and oxygen-free radicals), as demonstrated by increased chemoluminescence of peritoneal cells from endometriosis patients. Murphy and colleagues described the presence of oxidized LDL (OX-LDL) in peritoneal fluid from endometriosis patients and found a dose-dependent decrease in sperm motility with increasing concentration of OX-LDL, in the range observed in endometriosis patients.[87] They speculated that OX-LDL disrupted cellular membranes and interfered with the activity of cell membrane-bound enzymes. OX-LDL is also a potent stimulator of TXA_2, producing platelet aggregation and vasospasm.

Thus, there is evidence of both an increased number of macrophages in the peritoneal fluid of endometriosis patients and increased activation of these macrophages. The activated macrophages can directly phagocytize sperm and may indirectly affect sperm motility, velocity, and the ability of sperm to bind to the zona pellucida and to fertilize oocytes. IL-1, a primary product of macrophages, impairs fertilization and embryo growth rates and may have an additional adverse effect on endometrial receptivity. Reactive oxygen products, produced by activated macrophages, may also disrupt sperm activity, and can trigger vasospasm and platelet aggregation. While theoretically attractive, a direct effect of macrophage activity on human reproduction and a beneficial effect of inhibition of macrophage proliferation or function on fertility, remain to be documented.

Endocrine Abnormalities

Because prostaglandins are important regulators of ovarian follicular development, ovulation, and corpus luteum function, a relationship between endometriosis and the occurrence of endocrine abnormalities has been hypothesized. If such a relationship exists, we would expect to see this manifested by anovulation or other qualitative abnormalities of ovarian function.

Anovulation

Acosta and co-workers described a possible relationship between endometriosis and anovulation.[88] In a series of 107 patients with endometriosis, 29 (27%) were anovulatory. Induction of ovulation in this group resulted in 11 patients (38%) becoming pregnant. In a similar study, Soules and colleagues found 58 (17%) of 350 infertile women with endometriosis were anovulatory or oligo-ovulatory.[89] Concurrent treatment of endometriosis and ovulatory abnormalities resulted in a 43% pregnancy rate. Badawy and co-workers found 28 of 103 women with endometriosis and infertility had ovulatory dysfunction (anovulation, oligo-ovulation, or luteal phase defect).[90] Dmowski and colleagues described a group of patients with mild endometriosis and ovulatory dysfunction. Patients treated concurrently with danazol and ovulation induction had a 70% preg-

nancy rate, whereas induction of ovulation alone resulted in only a 28% pregnancy rate.[91] Combining results of these studies, an overall rate of ovulatory dysfunction of 21% has been reported in women with endometriosis, with a 41% pregnancy rate following ovulation induction.

The finding that rabbits with experimentally induced endometriosis have decreased numbers of ovulation sites lends support for an association between endometriosis and anovulation. This effect, however, appears to be related to periovarian adhesion formation rather than directly to the presence of endometriosis.[92]

Looking at a population of infertility patients as a whole, 18% were anovulatory.[1] Treatment of the ovulation problems resulted in a pregnancy rate of 65%. Thus, while anovulation certainly exists in women with endometriosis, the rate does not appear to be increased over the general population of infertility patients. Anovulation may well be a concurrent problem unrelated to endometriosis except, perhaps, in those with ovarian adhesions.

Hyperprolactinemia

Prolactin is necessary for normal reproductive function, but abnormal elevations of the hormone are associated with disorders of ovulation and corpus luteum function. This may occur at a hypothalamic, pituitary, or ovarian level. Hirschowitz and colleagues described an association between galactorrhea and endometriosis in nine patients, eight with galactorrhea and two with hyperprolactinemia.[93] They felt that the conditions were associated, but not necessarily causally related. Hargrove and Abraham, in a similar study, reported that seven of 14 patients with endometriosis and luteal phase defects had galactorrhea, and three had hyperprolactinemia. Brosens and co-workers and Balasch and Vanrell were unable to confirm an increased incidence of hyperprolactinemia in endometriosis patients.[94,95] Other investigators have reported increased nocturnal levels of prolactin in women with endometriosis and an increased prolactin response to thyrotropin releasing hormone (TRH) infusion in endometriosis patients.[96,97] Gendron and colleagues were unable to confirm this and, in fact, found a higher prolactin response to TRH stimulation in normal controls, compared with infertile women with and without mild endometriosis.[98]

Because prolactin can be produced locally by secretory endometrium, Haney and co-workers examined peritoneal fluid concentrations of prolactin, thinking there might be a prolactin effect which would not be found on sampling peripheral blood.[99] They found no difference among three groups: fertile women, and infertile women with and without endometriosis. Chew and colleagues repeated this study and found an elevation of peritoneal fluid prolactin only in the luteal phase in endometriosis patients compared with controls.[100]

As with other factors described, hyperprolactinemia or hyperprolactinemia in response to TRH infusion has been seen in a small number of women with endometriosis. While the two conditions do coexist in some patients, there is insufficient information to define a cause and effect relationship.

Abnormal Follicular Dynamics

An emerging area of investigation concerns the pattern of follicular growth seen on serial ultrasound examination. The relatively recent development of transvaginal ultrasound technology allows precise monitoring of follicular growth. Thomas and co-workers found only 12 of 18 cycles (67%) in women with minor endometriosis were sonographically normal.[101] Abnormalities seen were absent, inadequate, or abnormal folliculogenesis; premature follicular rupture; and luteinized unruptured follicles. A more precise study of follicular growth was performed by Doody and colleagues who compared patterns in 46 endometriosis patients with 18 controls.[102] Significant differences were seen in the rate of follicular growth and the duration of follicular growth before ovulation. The clinical and physiologic consequences of these observations are unknown.

Luteal Phase Defect

Luteal phase defect (LPD) is manifested by endometrial development chronologically out of phase with endometrium from a luteal phase of normal length, or dyssynchronous development of endometrial glands and stroma.[103] This defect may result from abnormal follicular development, inadequate production of progesterone by the corpus luteum, or diminished responsiveness of the endometrium to hormonal stimulation. Classically, the diagnosis is made by a late luteal phase endometrial biopsy, comparing the histologic dating with the subsequent menses. Because LPDs can occur in normal women, the diagnosis is substantiated by demonstration of an out-of-phase biopsy in consecutive cycles.[104]

While a variety of studies have used nonclassical techniques for diagnosing LPD (basal body temperature charts, measurements of serum progesterone, biopsies in the midluteal phase, or biopsies in only a single cycle without second cycle confirmation), only three investigations have used late luteal phase endometrial biopsies for diagnosis. Badawy and co-workers confirmed LPD in 12% of women with endometriosis, Pittaway and colleagues in 9%, and Balasch and Vanrell in 19%.[90,95,105] These findings are not different from the reports of a 3% to 20% incidence of LPD in an unselected infertility population.[106]

Other subtle luteal endocrine abnormalities have also been described. Hargrove and Abraham as well as Cheesman and colleagues reported subnormal midluteal phase progesterone levels, a finding not substantiated, however, by Dmowski and co-workers who measured daily serum progesterone levels throughout the luteal phase.[107–109] Brosens and colleagues and Cheesman and colleagues, measuring urinary estradiol metabolites, found a delay in the preovulatory decline of estradiol in patients with endometriosis.[94,110] Cheesman and colleagues also found a biphasic pattern of urinary excretion of LH prior to ovulation. Thomas and co-workers, measuring daily serum LH, estradiol, and progesterone levels, failed to find any significant difference between women with and without endometriosis.[101] While in some women with endometriosis there may be subtle differences in LH, estradiol, and progesterone secretory patterns, this does not appear to be a common mechanism for infertility. Similarly, the incidence of LPD does not appear greater than in infertility patients in general.

Luteinized Unruptured Follicle Syndrome

The luteinized unruptured follicle (LUF) syndrome has been described as a condition characterized by regular menses; normal estradiol, progesterone, and LH excretion patterns; and a failure of physical follicular rupture and oocyte release. Initially, this condition was diagnosed by an absence of ovarian stigma at laparoscopy and by decreased levels of progesterone and estradiol in peritoneal fluid. The latter finding presumably resulted from failure of the follicle to release its hormone-containing fluid. In animal studies, LUF has also been diagnosed by the histologic find of a persistent, luteinized simple cyst. More recently, serial ultrasound determinations have been used to follow follicular development, diagnosing LUF when there was evidence of progesterone production and luteinization without follicular rupture.

Schenken and colleagues reported LUF to be a significant factor in infertility in monkeys with surgically induced endometriosis who had periovarian adhesions.[22] Theoretically, this entity could be related to a decrease in LH receptors in granulosa cells in patients with endometriosis, as reported by Ronnberg and colleagues.[111] If the follicles of patients with endometriosis are incapable of responding to an LH surge, only partial luteinization with inadequate production and failure of rupture could occur.

Brosens and colleagues reported that only 21% of women with endometriosis undergoing laparoscopy in the luteal phase had stigma of ovulation, compared with 94% of controls with infertility due to male factor or tubal disease without endometriosis.[92] Other studies, using the same criteria, including two subsequent studies from the same group of investigators, failed to confirm these findings.[112,113] A potential source of error in the first study, which was not controlled for the stage of disease, is the possibility that periovarian adhesions may have hidden the stigma from laparoscopic view.

Ultrasound offers a noninvasive method of documenting follicular rupture; it has been used in three studies of endometriosis patients in which investigators found LUF in less than 20% of cycles in infertile women with and without endometriosis.[101,114,115] In a study of 183 cycles in normal, fertile women, Kerin and co-workers found LUF in 5% of cycles; they concluded that LUF was a random event occurring in both fertile and infertile patients and was not a reproducible cause of infertility.[116] Based on serial ultrasound monitoring of follicular growth and rupture, LUF appears to be a sporadic phenomenon and not a true syndrome associated with endometriosis. As with other infertility mechanisms, patients with endometriosis may occasionally also have LUF, but LUF does not appear to play a major role in the causation of infertility in endometriosis patients.

Spontaneous Abortion

A variety of retrospective reports have noted an increased incidence of spontaneous abortion in women with endometriosis, along with a decrease in spontaneous abortion rates after treatment of the disease.[117–124] Potential mechanisms for an increased incidence of spontaneous abortion in endometriosis patients include abnormalities of luteal phase progesterone production, alterations in prostaglandin dynamics leading to increased uterine irritability and contractions, implantation failure due to immunologic rejection or endometrial abnormality, and the association of endometriosis with uterine anomalies and leiomyomata.

Metzger and colleagues studied 139 infertile women with endometriosis, 63% of whom reported having a previous spontaneous abortion.[125] Of this group, 99 underwent conservative surgery, and 44 elected observation only. Of the 99 patients in the surgery group, 32 (32%) conceived, while 32 of the 44 (73%) in the observation group conceived. None of the surgery patients aborted (0%), whereas six (19%) of the control pregnancies aborted. Since the selection for treatment was nonrandom, it is likely that the patients with more severe disease and symptoms may have elected surgery. Although an association is plausible, the link between endometriosis and spontaneous abortion is unclear.

Immunologic Abnormalities

Sampson's theory of the histogenesis of endometriosis is that it results from repeated deposit of endometrium in the pelvis as a result of retrograde menstruation.[126] If true, then every menstruating woman with patent tubes has the potential to develop endometriosis.[127] Reasons for the failure of all women to develop endometriosis include: there may be varying degrees of the ability of endometrium from different individuals to implant in the peritoneal cavity; there may be a required volume of tissue inoculum for the development of endometrio-

sis; the peritoneum of some women may be more susceptible to implantation; or women who do not develop endometriosis may have the immunologic ability to reject endometrial implantation. In fertile women without endometriosis, the number and activity of macrophages varies throughout the menstrual cycle, being most numerous and active at the time of menses. In women without endometriosis, retrograde menses may activate the cellular immune system resulting in the rejection of what is, in effect, a monthly autologous tissue transplant. This possibility is supported by the observation in animals that the transfer of endometrium to the peritoneal cavity does not produce endometriosis, whereas transfer to an immunologically privileged site (such as the eye), transfer to an abraded or irritated peritoneal site, or transfer in immunocompromised animals does result in endometriosis.

The cellular immune response is initiated by antigen processing by macrophages, dendritic cells, and Langerhans' cells. The processed antigen is presented to T-lymphocytes (70% to 75% of circulating lymphocytes) in the form of an antigen-MHC protein complex. After differentiation and growth, this results in a population of cytolytic lymphocytes capable of directly attacking and killing foreign cells. This reaction is amplified by the production of a variety of local inflammatory factors: prostaglandins, interleukins, leukotrienes, and other factors designed to increase the body's response. Alternatively, large granular lymphocytes (natural killer cells or NK cells) comprise about 10% of peripheral lymphocytes and have the ability to directly kill certain tumor cells or virally infected cells without the need for antigenic recognition and processing.

In the humoral immune response, new antigens are captured and processed by B-lymphocytes, which account for 10% to 15% of peripheral circulating lymphocytes. The activated B-lymphocytes, under the necessary influence of helper T-lymphocytes, form a clone of specific antibody-producing plasma cells. The plasma cells then produce antigen-specific antibodies that attach to and assist in the control of foreign antigens. If the B-lymphocytes have previously recognized antigens, precursor B-lymphocytes with antigen-specific antibody are already present and can act more rapidly, without the need for primary antigen processing.

Humoral Immune Response

Antibody formation and complement function has been investigated in endometrium, serum, and peritoneal fluid of patients with endometriosis. Weed and Arquembourg theorized that women with endometriosis may produce antibodies to endometrial antigens, either as a reaction to retrograde menstruation or to peritoneal implants.[128] They found fibrosis and lymphocytic and plasma cell infiltration in the endometrium of women with endometriosis. Three groups have found increased levels of IgG and/or IgA in the endometrium of endometriosis patients; these findings suggest an immune response to endometrial antigens results in the antibody response to endometrium.[129–132]

Immunodiffusion, hemagglutination, indirect immunofluorescence, and immunohistochemical techniques have all been used to confirm the presence of serum antiendometrial antibodies in women with endometriosis.[129,133–137] A similar pattern was not seen in women without endometriosis. A wide variety of serum antibodies to cellular elements (antinuclear antibodies) and to cellular proteins (anti-DNA, anticardiolipin, antiphospholipid antibodies), and other nonspecific antigens have been reported in endometriosis patients similar to the reports of such antibodies in women with repeated abortion.[138–140] This pattern raises the possibility that endometriosis may represent a form of autoimmune disease.

Antibodies by themselves are not capable of destroying cells. Antibody-coated cells activate the complement system, which then causes agglutination and lysis of cells. Weed and Arquembourg, in their study of endometrium from endometriosis patients found complement in endometrium, not seen in nonendometriosis controls.[128] Bartosik and colleagues also found complement in the endometrium of endometriosis patients.[141] Peripheral serum complement levels have been found by different investigators to be decreased, increased, or not different from controls.[128,132,142]

Peritoneal fluid findings also have been conflicting. Halme and Mathur found no increase in antibodies in peritoneal fluid from endometriosis patients.[143] Badawy and co-workers found increased levels of complement in peritoneal fluid, whereas Meek and colleagues found decreased peritoneal fluid IgA and complement levels in endometriosis patients.[132,144]

Because the humoral response is produced by B-lymphocytes and modulated by helper T-lymphocytes, two studies have looked at B-cell and T-cell activity. Startseva described increased B-cell and reduced T-cell activity in a group of women with adenomyosis and endometriosis, consistent with activation of the humoral immune system.[145] Cunningham and colleagues found a difference in B-cell and T-cell responses depending on the stage of endometriosis.[146] Women with minimal and mild endometriosis showed increased antibody response to challenge with antigens, along with normal levels of helper T cells and decreased levels of suppressor T cells. In contrast, women with moderate and severe degrees of endometriosis had no increase in antibody response compared with controls, but had increased levels of helper T-cell activity and decreased levels of suppressor T cells. The antibody response could be restored to normal by adding T cells to the B-cell preparation. The authors hypothesized that women with mild disease, by mounting an increased humoral response to endometriosis, limited its progression. Women with severe disease either had an ineffective response because of the overwhelming volume of antigen presented to the immune system which resulted in a decreased number of suppressor T cells, or, perhaps, developed severe disease because of a preexisting defect in the T-cell system.

Similar antibody studies of women with pelvic inflammatory disease have revealed the presence of antiendometrial antibodies.[131,136,140] It may be that antiendometrial antibody formation and complement activation and deposition are nonspecific results of inflammation involving endometrium or endometriosis.

There is a substantial body of evidence demonstrating activation of the humoral immune system in women with endometriosis. This humoral response appears to decrease as the disease progresses, either as a result of the volume of antigen overcoming the body's ability to respond or because a subset of patients with deficient response cannot limit the growth of endometriosis. If antiendometrial antibodies, endometrial inflammation, or deposition of complement in the endometrium are related to infertility in these patients, one would expect to see a decrease in embryo implantation as a result of the endometrial abnormalities. However, in IVF procedures in women with endometriosis as the primary diagnosis, this has not been reported.[147–149] If implantation is impaired, one might expect an increase in the spontaneous abortion rate, but this has not been confirmed.

Cellular Immune Response

The primary immune response to foreign cells (tissue transplants, cancer cells, virus-infected cells) is the cellular immune system. If the immune response to endometrial cells parallels the response to other foreign cells, one would expect to see activation or abnormality of the cellular immune system. Techniques to evaluate the competence and function of the cellular immune system include skin testing with cellular antigens, in vitro testing of proliferation of elements of the cellular system in response to antigen, and evaluation of the number and state of activation of macrophages and T-lymphocytes, cytotoxic T-lymphocytes, and natural killer cells.

Dmowski and co-workers found cutaneous response to injected endometrial antigens to be diminished in rhesus monkeys with spontaneous endometriosis. This finding confirms the acquisition of a degree of tolerance to the ectopic endometrial tissue.[150] In the same animals, they reported decreased lymphocyte proliferation in response to autologous endometrial antigens in vitro. Similar findings of decreased peripheral lymphocyte reaction to endometrial cells were reported in women with moderate and severe endometriosis.[142] Tests of nonendometriosis antigenic response were similar between endometriosis and control groups, suggesting that the observations were limited to endometriosis and were not the result of a more generalized immunosuppression.

Most investigators have found increases in either the number or concentration of macrophages as well as in macrophage activity in peritoneal fluid from endometriosis patients. Looking at other components of the cellular immune system in peritoneal fluid, Badawy and colleagues reported an increase in the overall number of T- and B-lymphocytes as well as in the helper T-cell to suppressor T-cell ratio in both peripheral blood and peritoneal fluid from women with endometriosis.[151] These findings were confirmed by Hill and associates who also demonstrated increased numbers of peritoneal fluid lymphocytes, macrophages, and helper T-lymphocytes in women with unexplained infertility when compared with fertile controls.[152] They suggested that some women with an anatomically normal pelvis and unexplained infertility may actually have a marked immunologic response to transplanted endometrial tissue with resulting infertility but no histologic endometriosis.

More recent investigations have focused on the activity of natural killer (NK) lymphocytes. These cells are responsible for directly attacking and destroying intact foreign cells, such as tumor and tissue transplantation cells. Oosterlynck and co-workers noted decreased peripheral NK cell cytotoxicity in peripheral lymphocytes from women with endometriosis.[153] These same investigators also demonstrated NK activity in peritoneal fluid from normal controls, and a decrease in peritoneal fluid NK activity in endometriosis patients. The decrease correlated with the severity of the endometriosis.[154] These findings were confirmed by Garzetti and colleagues.[155] Seeking an explanation for the decrease in NK activity, Kanzaki and colleagues found that incubation of NK cells from healthy volunteers with sera from endometriosis patients inhibited NK activity, with the degree of inhibition proportional to the time of incubation.[156] They postulated the existence of a substance in the serum of endometriosis patients that suppressed NK cell activity, perhaps intended to allow the continued growth of ectopic endometrial cells, much in the same fashion as occurs with cancer patients. That this inhibition is a result of endometriosis, and not vice versa, was demonstrated by the work of Kikuchi and co-workers who confirmed both a decrease in the absolute number and percentage of NK cells in peripheral blood from endometriosis patients.[157] After treatment of endometriosis, there was an increase in both the number and percentage of NK cells to normal.

The second subset of lymphocytes capable of destroying foreign cells are the cytolytic lymphocytes (CL), products of T-lymphocyte differentiation. Vigano and co-workers described a deficiency in this group of cells in their response to stromal cell antigens in women with endometriosis compared with controls.[158] No difference

was seen in the reaction to a leukemic cell line, confirming that this reduction was specific for endometrial stromal cells. Braun and colleagues examined peritoneal fluid cellular cytotoxicity and found increased cytotoxicity in women with stages I and II endometriosis, but a decrease in cytotoxicity in stages III and IV disease.[159] That this decrease could be reversed by adding indomethacin suggests the decrease is mediated by prostaglandin effects. No effect of indomethacin on cytotoxicity in fertile women or stage I or II endometriosis patients was seen. Cytoxicity was also increased in patients treated with either danazol or GnRH agonists, when compared with untreated women with the same stage of disease.

It appears there is a decrease in the number and activity of peripheral and peritoneal NK cells in endometriosis patients, this decrease is mediated through a humoral substance present in serum from endometriosis patients, and treatment of the endometriosis can return the NK function to normal. In addition, peritoneal fluid cytotoxicity is increased from women with minimal and mild endometriosis and decreased in women with moderate and severe disease, which can be restored either by inhibition of prostaglandin synthesis or by treatment of the disease. The humoral products of the cellular immune response (prostaglandins, thromboxane, leukotrienes, macrophage activating and inhibiting factors, tumor necrosis factor, interleukins) have all been identified in peritoneal fluid from endometriosis patients and, directly or indirectly, have been implicated in the pathophysiology of infertility associated with endometriosis.

Conclusion

How can we reconcile all this information to provide an explanation for infertility in patients with endometriosis? Women with moderate or severe disease who have anatomic distortion of the pelvis, adhesions, or tubal occlusion have an obvious reason for infertility. It is the majority of women with minimal, mild, or moderate disease without apparent physical disruption of oocyte release, capture, or tubal anatomy function who are perplexing to the clinician. There is no consensus that endometriosis produces infertility in this group, but there may well be a subpopulation in whom one or more of the many factors we have reviewed may play a role.

It appears that the scene is set for endometriosis to develop in all women who have retrograde menstruation. There is evidence of a cyclic immune response to this repetitive exposure to transplanted endometrial tissue. The majority of women are able to reject implantation because of immunologic competence, intermittent discontinuation of reflux of active cellular elements (as in pregnancy or other causes of amenorrhea), or because of the low volume of tissue presented, (as in patients taking oral contraceptives). Increases in the amount of reflux (as in women with outflow obstruction) may overwhelm a competent immune system and lead to implantation and growth of endometriosis.

Women with minimal and moderate degrees of endometriosis, and some women with unexplained infertility without visible endometriosis, appear to have increased humoral and cellular immunologic responses to endometrial antigens. This may limit the growth of disease beyond the early stages. Unfortunately, byproducts of this response (macrophage activation, lymphocytic activation, PGs, TXs, LTs, and other factors associated with the immune and inflammatory responses) may also decrease fertility by humoral toxicity to or cellular phagocytosis of gametes, interfering with ovulation, gamete interaction and fertilization, or by deleterious effects on embryo growth, effects on tubal or uterine motility, interference with corpus luteum function, and possibly other endometrial effects. Although many of these effects have not been documented unequivocally, they are all plausible.

Progression of endometriosis to a moderate or severe stage is associated with a diminution of both humoral and cellular immune responses. This may occur because women with decreased immunologic competence cannot adequately protect themselves from progression of endometriosis, or it may represent exhaustion of the immune system from an overwhelming volume of antigenic material. Fibrosis and adhesion formation, as a result of the inflammatory response, adds an anatomic cause for infertility. Immunologic competence can be restored by addition of lymphocytes from nonendometriosis patients, inhibition of prostaglandin synthesis, medical suppression of active growth of disease, or surgical reduction of the volume of endometriosis.

Our understanding of the mechanisms of immunologic disorders observed in endometriosis patients is in its infancy. Further elucidation of the role of the immune system in the genesis of endometriosis may provide a basis for improved therapy of endometriosis and associated infertility in the future.

References

1. Hull MGR, Glazener CMA, Kelly NJ, et al. Population study of causes, treatment, and outcome of infertility. Brit Med J 1985;291:1693–1697.
2. Buttram VC Jr, Reiter RC. Endometriosis. In Buttram VC Jr, Reiter RC, eds. Surgical treatment of the infertile female. Baltimore, Williams & Wilkins, 1985, pp 89–148.
3. Counseller VS. Endometriosis. A clinical and surgical review. Am J Obstet Gynecol 1938;36:877–890.
4. Counseller VS. The clinical significance of endometriosis. Am J Obstet Gynecol 1939;37:788–792.
5. Haydon GB. A study of 569 cases of endometriosis. Am J Obstet Gynecol 1942;43:704–709.
6. Fallon J, Brosnan JT, Moran WG. Endometriosis. Two hundred cases considered from the viewpoint of the practitioner. N Engl J Med 1946;235:669–672.
7. Hasson HM. Incidence of endometriosis in diagnostic laparoscopy. J Reprod Med 1976;16:135–138.
8. Drake TS, Grunert GM. The unsuspected pelvic factor in the infertility investigation. Fertil Steril 1980;34:27–31.
9. Strathy JH, Moulgaard CA, Coulam CB, et al. Endometriosis and infertility: a laparoscopic study of endometriosis among fertile and infertile women. Fertil Steril 1982;38:667–672.
10. Mage G, Chany Y, Bruhat MA. Endometriosis: mechanical factors of infertility. Contr Gynec Obstet 1987;16:144–146.
11. Inoue M, Kobayashi Y, Honda I, Awaji H, Fujii A. The impact of endometriosis on the reproductive outcome of infertile patients. Am J Obstet Gynecol 1992;167:278–282.
12. Jansen RPS. Minimal endometriosis and reduced fecundability: prospective evidence from an artificial insemination by donor program. Fertil Steril 1986;46:141–143.
13. Yeh J, Seibel MM. Artificial insemination with donor sperm: a review of 108 patients. Obstet Gynecol 1987;70:313–316.
14. Portuondo JA, Eschanojauregui AD, Herran C, Alijarte I. Early conception in patients with untreated mild endometriosis. Fertil Steril 1983;39:22–25.
15. Toma SK, Stovall DW, Hammond MG. The effect of laparoscopic ablation or danocrine on pregnancy rates in patients with stage I or II endometriosis undergoing donor insemination. Obstet Gynecol 1992;80:253–256.
16. Schenken RS, Malinak LR. Conservative surgery versus expectant management for the infertile patient with mild endometriosis. Fertil Steril 1982;37:183–186.
17. Seibel MM, Berger MJ, Weinstein FG, et al. The effectiveness of danazol on subsequent fertility in minimal endometriosis. Fertil Steril 1982;38:534–537.
18. Hull ME, Moghissi KS, Magyar DF, et al. Comparison of different treatment modalities of endometriosis in infertile women. Fertil Steril 1987;47:40–44.
19. Bayer SR, Seibel MM, Saffan DS, et al. Efficacy of danazol treatment for minimal endometriosis in infertile women. A prospective, randomized study. J Reprod Med 1988;33:179–183.
20. Vernon MW, Wilson EA. Studies on the surgical induction of endometriosis in the rat. Fertil Steril 1985;44:684–694.
21. Schenken RS, Asch RH. Surgical induction of endometriosis in the rabbit: effects on fertility and concentrations of peritoneal fluid prostaglandins. Fertil Steril 19909;34:581–587.
22. Schenken RS, Asch RH. Etiology of infertility in monkeys with endometriosis: luteinized unruptured follicles, luteal phase defects, pelvic adhesions, and spontaneous abortions. Fertil Steril 1984;41:122–130.
23. Suginami H, Yano K, Nakhashi N, et al. Fallopian tube and fimbrial function in endometriosis: with a special reference to an ovum capture inhibitor. Prog Clin Biol Res 1990;323:81–97.
24. Fortier KJ, Haney AF. The pathologic spectrum of uterotubal junction obstruction. Obstet Gynecol 1985;65:93–98.
25. Marana R, Quagliarello J. Proximal tubal occlusion: microsurgery versus IVF—a review. Int J Fertil 1988;33:338–340.

26. Ayers JW. Hormonal therapy for tubal occlusion: danazol and tubal endometriosis. Fertil Steril 1982;38: 748–750.

27. Claman P, Taymor ML, Berger MJ, et al. Danazol therapy for proximal obstruction of the oviduct. J Reprod Med 1986;31:687–689.

28. Urman B, Gomel V, McComb P, et al. Midtubal occlusion: etiology, management and outcome. Fertil Steril 1992;57:747–750.

29. Kerin J, Daykhovsky L, Grundfest W, et al. Falloposcopy. A micro-endoscopic transvaginal technique for diagnosing and treating endotubal disease incorporating guide wire cannulation and direct balloon tuboplasty. J Reprod Med 1990;35:606–612.

30. Marana R, Muzil L, Rizzi M, et al. Salpingoscopy in patients with endometriosis-associated infertility. Acta Eur Fertil 1990;21:247–249.

31. Garcia CR, David SS. Pelvic endometriosis: infertility and pelvic pain. Am J Obstet Gynecol 1977;129:740–747.

32. Drake TS, Metz SA, Grunert GM, et al. Peritoneal fluid volume in endometriosis. Fertil Steril 1980;34:280–281.

33. Syrop CH, Halme JH. A comparison of peritoneal fluid parameters of infertile patients and the subsequent occurrence of pregnancy. Fertil Steril 1986;46:631–635.

34. Maathuis JB, Van Look PFA, Michie EA. Changes in volume, total protein and ovarian steroid concentrations of peritoneal fluid throughout the human menstrual cycle. J Endocrinol 1978:76:123–133.

35. Rezai H, Ghodgaonkar RB, Zacur HA. Cul-de-sac fluid in women with endometriosis: fluid volume, protein and prostanoid concentration during the periovulatory period—days 13 to 18. Fertil Steril 1987;48:29–32.

36. Chantler EN, Williams CA, Elstein M. Sperm survival studies in peritoneal fluid from infertile women with endometriosis and unexplained infertility. Clin Reprod Fertil 1985;3:297–303.

37. Burke RK. Effect of peritoneal washings from women with endometriosis on sperm velocity. J Reprod Med 1987;32:743–746.

38. Coddington CC, Oehninger S, Cunningham DS, et al. Peritoneal fluid from patients with endometriosis decreases sperm binding to the zona pellucida in the hemizona assay: a preliminary report. Fertil Steril 1992; 57:783–786.

39. Sueldo CE, Lambert H, Steinleitner A, et al. The effect of peritoneal fluid from patients with endometriosis on murine sperm-oocyte interaction. Fertil Steril 1987;48: 697–699.

40. Steinleitner A, Lambert H, Kazensky C. Peritoneal fluid from endometriosis patients affects reproductive outcome in an in vivo model. Fertil Steril 1990;53:966–969.

41. Dodds WG, Miller FA, Friedman CI, et al. The effect of periovulatory peritoneal fluid from cases of endometriosis on murine in vitro fertilization, embryo development, oviduct transport, and implantation. Am J Obstet Gynecol 1992;166:219–224.

42. Morcos RN, Gibbons WE, Findley WE. Effect of peritoneal fluid on in vitro cleavage of 2-cell mouse embryos: possible role in infertility associated with endometriosis. Fertil Steril 1985;44:678–683.

43. Prough SG, Aksel S, Gilmore SM, et al. Peritoneal fluid fractions from patients with endometriosis do not promote two-cell mouse embryo growth. Fertil Steril 1990; 54:927–930.

44. Taketani Y, Kuo TM, Mizuno M. Comparison of cytokine levels and embryo toxicity in peritoneal fluid in infertile women with untreated or treated endometriosis. Am J Obstet Gynecol 1992;167:265–270.

45. Kuo TM, Taketani Y, Ayabe T, et al. Influence of peritoneal fluid with endometriosis on the development of mouse embryos. Nippon Sanka Fujinka Gakkai Zasshi 1990;42:1284–1290.

46. Schneider EG, Armant DR, Kupper TS, et al. Absence of a direct effect of recombinant interleukins and cultured peritoneal macrophages on early embryonic development in the mouse. Biol Reprod 1989;40:825–833.

47. Speroff L, Glass RH, Kase NG. Prostaglandins. In Speroff L, Glass RH, Kase NG, eds. Clinical gynecologic endocrinology and infertility. Baltimore: Williams & Wilkins, 1989;351–378.

48. Spilman CH, Beuving DC, Roseman TJ, et al. Effect of vaginally administered 15(S)-methyl-PGF$_{2\alpha}$ on egg transport and fertility in rabbits. Proc Soc Exp Biol Med 1976;151:575–578.

49. Eddy CA. Ovum transport in the Rhesus monkey following postovulatory intravaginal 15(S)-methyl-prostaglandin-F$_{2\alpha}$ methyl ester administration. Am J Obstet Gynecol 1980;137:966–971.

50. Croxatto HB, Oritz ME, Guiloff E, et al. Effect of 15(S)-methyl-prostaglandin-F$_{2\alpha}$ on human oviductal motility and ovum transport. Fertil Steril 1978;30:408–414.

51. Karim SM, Hillier K. Prostaglandins in the control of animal and human reproduction. Br Med Bull 1979;35: 173–180.

52. Killick S, Elstein M. Pharmacologic production of luteinized unruptured follicles by prostaglandin synthetase inhibitors. Fertil Steril 1987;47:773.

53. Sargent EL, Stouffer RL. An obligatory luteotropic role for prostaglandins in the Rhesus monkey. Presented at the 20th Annual Meeting for the Society of a Study of Reproduction, 1987.

54. Auletta FJ, Kamps DL, Pories S. An intracorpus luteum site for the luteolytic action of prostaglandin F$_{2\alpha}$ in the Rhesus monkey. Prostaglandins 1984;27:285–288.

55. Auletta FJ, Agins H, Scommegna A. Prostaglandin F$_{2\alpha}$ mediation of the inhibitory effect of estrogen on the corpus luteum of the rhesus monkey. Endocrinology 1978;103:1183–1188.

56. Auletta FJ, Caldwell BV, Speroff L. Estrogen-induced luteolysis in the rhesus monkey: reversal with indomethacin. Prostaglandins 1976;11:745–749.

57. Drake TS, O'Brien WF, Ramwell PW. Peritoneal fluid thromboxane B2 and 6-keto-prostaglandin F$_{1\alpha}$ in endometriosis. Am J Obstet Gynecol 1981;140:401–404.

58. Dawood MY, Kahn-Dawood FS, Wilson L Jr. Peritoneal fluid prostaglandins and prostanoids in women with endometriosis, chronic pelvic inflammatory disease, and pelvic pain. Am J Obstet Gynecol 1984;148:391–395.

59. Ylikorkala O, Viinikka L. Prostaglandins and endometriosis. Acta Obstet Gynecol Sand 1983;113:105–107.

60. DeLeon FD, Vijayakumar R, Brown M. Peritoneal fluid volume, estrogen, progesterone, prostaglandin, and epidermal growth factor concentrations in patients with and without endometriosis. Obstet Gynecol 1986;68: 189–194.

61. Halme J, Becker S, Hammond MG, et al. Increased activation of pelvic macrophages in infertile women with mild endometriosis. Am J Obstet Gynecol 1983;145: 333–337.

62. Sgarlata CS, Hertelendy F, Mikhail G. The prostanoid content in peritoneal fluid and plasma of women with endometriosis. Am J Obstet Gynecol 1983;147:563–565.

63. Chacho KJ, Chacho MS, Andresen PY, et al. Peritoneal fluid in patients with and without endometriosis: prostanoids and macrophages and their effects on the spermatozoa penetration assay. Am J Obstet Gynecol 1986; 154:1290–1299.

64. Badawy SZ, Cuenca V, Marshall L, et al. Cellular components in peritoneal fluid in infertile patients with and without endometriosis. Fertil Steril 1984;42:704–708.

65. Badawy SZ, Marshall L, Cuenca V. Peritoneal fluid prostaglandins in various stages of the menstrual cycle: role in infertile patients with endometriosis. Int J Fertil 1985;30:48–52.

66. van Furth R, Raeburn JA, van Zwet TL. Characteristics of human mononuclear phagocytes. Blood 1979;54:485–2500.

67. Halme J, Becker S, Haskill S. Altered maturation and function of peritoneal macrophages: possible role in pathogenesis of endometriosis. Am J Obstet Gynecol 1987;156:783–789.

68. Haney AF, Misukonis MA, Weinberg JB. Macrophages and infertility: oviductal macrophages as potential mediators of infertility. Fertil Steril 1983;39:310–315.

69. Olive DL, Weinberg JB, Haney AF. Peritoneal macrophages and infertility: the association between cell number and pelvic pathology. Fertil Steril 1985;44:772–777.

70. Cao SJ. Relation between macrophages in peritoneal fluid of endometriosis and infertility. Chung Hua Fu Chan Ko Tsa Chih 1992;27:93–95.

71. Haney AF, Muscato JJ, Weinberg JB. Peritoneal fluid cell populations in infertility patients. Fertil Steril 1981; 35:696–698.

72. Halme J, Becker S, Hammond MG, et al. Pelvic macrophages in normal and infertile women: the role of patent tubes. Am J Obstet Gynecol 1982;142:890.

73. Zeller JM, Henig I, Radwanska E, et al. Enhancement of human monocyte and peritoneal macrophage chemoluminescence activities in women with endometriosis. Am J Reprod Immun Microbiol 1987;13:78–82.

74. Johnson JV, Rozek MM, Moreno AC, et al. Surgically induced endometriosis does not alter peritoneal factors in the rabbit model. Fertil Steril 1991;56:343–348.

75. Hurst BS, Rock JA. Endometriosis: pathophysiology, diagnosis, and treatment. Obstet Gynecol Surv 1989;44: 297–304.

76. Dunselman GA, Hendrix MG, Bouckaert PX, et al. Functional aspects of peritoneal macrophages in endometriosis of women. J Reprod Fertil 1988;82:707–710.

77. Muscato JJ, Haney AF, Weinberg JB. Sperm phagocytosis by human peritoneal macrophages: a possible cause of infertility in endometriosis. Am J Obstet Gynecol 1982;144:503–510.

78. Oak MK, Chatler EN, Williams CA, et al. Sperm survival studies in peritoneal fluid from infertile women with endometriosis and unexplained infertility. Clin Reprod Fertil 1985;3:297–303.

79. Chacho KJ, Andreson PG, Scommegna A. The effect of peritoneal macrophage incubates on the spermatozoa assay. Fertil Steril 1987;48:694–696.

80. Halme J, Hall JL. Effect of pelvic fluid from endometriosis patients on human sperm penetration of zona-free hamster ova. Fertil Steril 1982;37:573–576.

81. Muse K, Estes S, Vernon M, et al. Effect of endometriosis on sperm motility in peritoneal fluid in vitro. Fertil Steril 1986;46:99.

82. Buyalos RP, Rutanen EM, Tsui E, et al. Release of tumor necrosis factor alpha by human peritoneal macrophages in response to toxic shock syndrome toxin-1. Obstet Gynecol 1991;78:182–186.

83. Mori H, Sawairi M, Nakagawa M, et al. Peritoneal fluid interleukin-1 and tumor necrosis factor in patients with benign gynecologic disease. Am J Reprod Immunol 1991;26:62–67.

84. Sueldo CE, Kelly E, Montoro L, et al. Effect of interleukin-1 on gamete interaction and mouse embryo development. J Reprod Med 1990;35:868–872.

85. Uda S, Umesaki N. The role of the peritoneal macrophage in infertility associated with endometriosis— animal experiment. Nippon Sanka Fujinka Gakkai Zasshi 1991;43:497–502.

86. Uda S. The role of the peritoneal macrophage on the infertility associated with endometriosis. Osaka City Med J 1992;38:11–26.

87. Murphy AA, Garzo VG, Morales A, et al. Effects of oxidized LDL on human sperm motility: a possible role in endometriosis associated infertility. Presented at the 47th Annual Meeting of the American Fertility Society, 1991.

88. Acosta AA, Buttram VC, Besch PK, et al. A proposed classification of pelvic endometriosis. Obstet Gyencol 1973;42:19–26.

89. Soules MR, Malinak LR, Bury R, et al. Endometriosis and anovulation: a coexisting problem in the infertile female. Am J Obstet Gynecol 1976;125:412–417.

90. Badawy SZ, Nusbaum M, Taymor E, et al. Ovulatory dysfunction in patients with endometriosis. Diag Gynecol Obstet 1981;3:305–307.

91. Dmowski WP, Radwanska E, Binor A, et al. Mild endometriosis and ovulatory dysfunction: effect of danazol treatment on success of ovulation induction. Fertil Steril 1986;46:784–789.

92. Kaplan CR, Eddy CA, Olive DL, et al. Effect of ovarian endometriosis on ovulation in rabbits. Am J Obstet Gynecol 1989;160:40–44.

93. Hirschowitz JS, Soler NG, Wortsman J, et al. The galactorrhea-endometriosis syndrome. Lancet 1978;1: 896–898.

94. Brosens IA, Koninckx PR, Corvelevyn PA. A study of plasma progesterone, oestradiol-17beta, prolactin and LH levels, and of the luteal phase appearance of the ovaries in patients with endometriosis and infertility. Br J Obstet Gynaecol 1978;85:246–250.

95. Balasch J, Vanrell JA. Mild endometriosis and luteal function. Int J Fertil 1985;30:4–6.

96. Radwanska E, Heig I, Rana N, et al. Nocturnal prolactin (PRL) levels in infertile women with and without endometriosis. Presented at the annual meeting of the Society for Gynecologic Investigation, 1985.

97. Muse K, Wilson EA, Jawad MJ. Prolactin hyperstimulation in response to thyrotropin-releasing hormone in patients with endometriosis. Fertil Steril 1982;38:419–422.

98. Gendron R, Ainmelk Y, Belisle S. Prolactin response to thyrotropin-releasing hormone in patients with mild endometriosis. Presented at the annual meeting of the Canadian Fertility and Andrology Society, 1983.

99. Haney AF, Handwerger S, Weinberg JB. Peritoneal fluid prolactin in infertile women with endometriosis: lack of evidence of secretory activity by endometrial implants. Fertil Steril 1984;42:935–938.

100. Chew PC, Peh KL, Loganath A. Elevated peritoneal fluid luteinizing hormone and prolactin concentrations in infertile women with endometriosis. Int J Gynaecol Obstet 1990;33:35–39.

101. Thomas EJ, Lenton EA, Cooke ID. Follicle growth patterns and endocrinologic abnormalities in infertile women with minor degrees of endometriosis. Br J Obstet Gynaecol 1986;93:852–858.
102. Doody MC, Gibbons WE, Buttram VC Jr. Linear regression analysis of ultrasound follicular growth series: evidence for an abnormality of follicular growth in endometriosis patients. Fertil Steril 1988;49:47–51.
103. Jones GS. The luteal phase defect. Fertil Steril 1976;27:351–356.
104. Brodie BL, Wentz AC. An update on the clinical relevance of luteal phase inadequacy. Semin Reprod Endocrinol 1989;7:138–162.
105. Pittaway DE, Maxson W, Daniell J, et al. Luteal-phase defects in infertility patients with endometriosis. Fertil Steril 1983;39:712–713.
106. Strauss JF III, Gurpide E. The endometrium: regulation and dysfunction. In Yen SSC, Jaffe RB, eds. Reproductive Endocrinology. Philadelphia, WB Saunders Co, 1991, 309–356.
107. Hargrove JT, Abraham GE. Abnormal luteal function in endometriosis. Fertil Steril 1980;34:302.
108. Cheesman KL, Cheesman SD, Chatterton RT Jr, et al. Alterations in progesterone metabolism and luteal function in infertile women with endometriosis. Fertil Steril 1983;40:590–595.
109. Dmowski WP, Cohen MR, Wilhelm JL. Endometriosis and ovulatory failure: does it occur? Should ovulatory stimulating agents be used? In Greenblatt RB ed. Recent Advances in Endometriosis. Princeton, NJ, Excerpta Medica Foundation, 1976.
110. Cheesman KL, Ben-Nun I, Chatterton RT Jr, et al. Relationship of luteinizing hormone, pregnanediol-3-glucuronice, and estriol-16-gulcuronide in urine of infertile women with endometriosis. Fertil Steril 1982;38:542–548.
111. Ronnberg L, Kauppila A, Rajaniemi H. Luteinizing hormone receptor disorder in endometriosis. Fertil Steril 1984;42:64–68.
112. Koninckx PR, Brosens IA. The luteinized unruptured follicle. Observations on peritoneal fluid steroid hormones and plasma follicle stimulating hormone concentrations. Fertil Steril 1980;33:242.
113. Koninckx PR, De Moor P, Brosens IA. Diagnosis of the luteinized unruptured follicle syndrome by steroid hormone assays on peritoneal fluid. Br J Obstet Gynaecol 1980;87:929–934.
114. Gibbons WE, Buttram VC Jr, Rossavik IK. The observed incidence of luteinized unruptured follicles in a population of infertile women undergoing ovulation monitoring by ultrasound. Fertil Steril 1984;41:19.
115. Hamilton CJ, Wetzels LC, Evers JL, et al. Follicle growth curves and hormonal patterns in patients with the luteinized unruptured follicle syndrome. Fertil Steril 1985;43:541–548.
116. Kerin JF, Kirby C, Morris D, et al. Incidence of the luteinized unruptured follicle phenomenon in cycling women. Fertil Steril 1983;40:620–626.
117. Norwood GE. Sterility and fertility in women with pelvic endometriosis. Clin Obstet Gynecol 1960;3:456–461.
118. Devereux WP. Endometriosis: long-term observation, with particular reference to incidence of pregnancy. Obstet Gynecol 1963;444–448.
119. Peterson L. Fertility in patients with ovarian endometriosis before and after treatment. Acta Obstet Gynecol Scand 1970;49:331–337.
120. Spangler DB, Jones GS, Jones HW. Infertility due to endometriosis: conservative surgical therapy. Am J Obstet Gynecol 1971;109:850–856.
121. Naples JD, Batt RE, Sadigh H. Spontaneous abortion rate in patients with endometriosis. Obstet Gynecol 1981;57:509–512.
122. Rock JA, Guzick DS, Sengos C. The conservative surgical treatment of endometriosis: evaluation of pregnancy success with respect to the extent of disease as categorized using contemporary classification systems. Fertil Steril 1981;35:131–137.
123. Wheeler JM, Johnston BM, Malinak LR. The relationship of endometriosis to spontaneous abortion. Fertil Steril 1983;39:656–660.
124. Groll M. Endometriosis and spontaneous abortion. Fertil Steril 1984;41:933–935.
125. Metzger DA, Olive D, Stohs GF, et al. Association of endometrios and spontaneous abortion: effect of control group selection. Fertil Steril 1986;45:18–22.
126. Sampson JA. Peritoneal endometriosis due to the menstrual dissemination of endometrial tissue to the peritoneal cavity. Am J Obstet Gynecol 1927;14:422–426.
127. Bartosik D, Jacobs SL, Kelly LJ. Endometrial tissue in peritoneal fluid. Fertil Steril 1986;46:796–800.
128. Weed JC, Arquembourg PC. Endometriosis: can it produce an autoimmune response resulting in infertility? Clin Obstet Gynecol 1980;23:885–893.
129. Mathur S, Peress MR, Williamson HO, et al. Autoimmunity to endometrium and ovary in endometriosis. Clin Esp Immunol 1982;50:259–266.
130. Saifuddin A, Buckley CH, Fos H. Immunoglobulin content of the endometrium in women with endometriosis. Int J Gynecol Pathol 1983;2:255–263.
131. Kreiner D, Fromowitz FB, Richardson DA, et al. Endometrial immunofluorescence associated with endoemtriosis and pelvic inflammatory disease. Fertil Steril 1986;46:243–245.
132. Badawy SZ, Cuenca V, Stitzel A, et al. Autoimmune phenomena in infertile patients with endometriosis. 1984;63:271–275.
133. Chihal JH, Mathur S, Holtz GL, et al. An endometrial antibody assay in the clinical diagnosis and management of endometriosis. Fertil Steril 1986;46:408–411.
134. Badawy SZ, Cuenca V, Freliech H, Stefanu C. Endometrial antibodies in serum and peritoneal fluid of infertile patients with and without endometriosis. Fertil Steril 1990;53:930–932.
135. Garza D, Mathur S, Dowd MM, et al. Antigenic differences between the endometrium of women with and without endometriosis. J Reprod Med 1991;36:17–82.
136. Wild RA, Shivers CA. Antiendometrial antibodies in patients with endometriosis. Am J Reprod Immunol Microbiol 1985;8:84–86.
137. Fernandez-Shaw S, Hicks BR, Yudkin PL. Anti-endometrial and anti-endothelial auto-antibodies in women with endometriosis. Hum Reprod 1993;8:310–315.
138. Cowchock S, Smith JB, Gocia B. Autoantibodies to phospholipids and nuclear antigens in patients with repeated abortions. Am J Obstet Gynecol 1986;155:1002–1010.
139. Gleicher N, El-Roeiy A, Confino E, et al. Autoantibodies in patients with unexplained infertility and recurrent pregnancy loss. Presented at the 34th Annual Meeting of the Society for Gynecologic Investigation, Atlanta, 1987.
140. El-Roeiy A, Dmowski WP, Gleicher N, et al. Danazol but not gonadotropin-releasing hormone agonist sup-

preses autoantibodies in endometriosis. Fertil Steril 1988;0:864–871.

141. Bartosik D, Damjanov I, Viscarello RR. Immunoproteins in the endometrium: clinical correlates of the presence of complement fractions C3 and C4. Am J Obstet Gynecol 1987;156:11–15.

142. Steele RW, Dmowski WP, Marmer DJ. Immunologic aspects of human endometriosis. Am J Reprod Immunol 1984;6:33–36.

143. Halme J, Mathur S. Lack of local autoimmunity in mild endometriosis. Fertil Steril 1984;43:541.

144. Meek SC, Hodge Dd, Muisch JR. Autoimmunity in infertile patients with endometriosis. Am J Obstet Gynecol 1988;158:1365–1373.

145. Startseva NV. Clinico-immunological aspects of genital endometriosis. Akush Ginekol (Mosk) 1980;3:23–26.

146. Cunningham DS, Hansen KA, Coddington CC. Changes in T-cell regulation of responses to self antigens in women with pelvic endometriosis. Fertil Steril 1992;58:114–119.

147. Mahadevan MM, Trounson AO, Leeton JF. The relationship of tubal blockage, infertility of unknown cause, suspected male infertility, and endometriosis to success of in vitro fertilization and embryo transfer. Fertil Steril 1983;40:755–762.

148. Jones HW Jr, Acosta AA, Andrews MC, et al. Three years of in vitro fertilization at Norfolk. Fertil Steril 1984;42:826–834.

149. Oehinger S, Acosta AA, Kreiner D, et al. In vitro fertilization and embryo transfer (IVF/ET): an established and successful therapy for endometriosis. J In Vitro Fert Embryo Transf 1988;5:249–256.

150. Dmowski WP, Steele RW, Baker GF. Deficient cellular immunity in endometriosis. Am J Obstet Gynecol 1981; 141:377–383.

151. Badawy SZ, Cuenca V, Stitzel A. Immune rosettes of T and B lymphocytes in infertile women with endometriosis. J Reprod Med 1987;32:194–197.

152. Hill JA, Faris HM, Schiff I, et al. Characterization of leukocyte subpopulations in the peritoneal fluid of women with endometriosis. Fertil Steril 1988;50:216–222.

153. Oosterlynck DJ, Cornille FJ, Waer M, et al. Women with endometriosis show a defect in natural killer activity resulting in a decreased cytotoxicity to autologous endometrium. Fertil Steril 1991;56:45–51.

154. Oosterlynck DJ, Meuleman C, Waer C, et al. The natural killer activity of peritoneal fluid lymphocytes is decreased in women with endometriosis. Fertil Steril 1992;58:290–295.

155. Garzetti GG, Ciavattini A, Provinciali M, et al. Natural killer cell activity in endometriosis: correlation between serum estradiol levels and cytotoxicity. Obstet Gynecol 1993;81:665–668.

156. Kanzaki H, Wang HS, Kariya M, et al. Suppression of natural killer cell activity by sera from patients with endometriosis. Am J Obstet Gynecol 1992;167:257–261.

157. Kikuchi Y, Ishikawa N, Hirata J, et al. Changes of peripheral blood lymphocyte subsets before and after operation of patients with endometriosis. Acta Obstet Gynecol Scand 1993;72:157–161.

158. Vigano P, Vercellini P, DiBlasio AM, et al. Deficient antiendometrium lymphocyte-mediated cytotoxicity in patients with endometriosis. Fertil Steril 1991;56:894–899.

159. Braun DP, Gebel H, Rotman C, et al. The development of cytotoxicity in peritoneal macrophages from women with endometriosis. Fertil Steril 1992;57:1203–1210.

7

Approach to the Patient With Suspected Endometriosis

Kamran Moghissi

Endometriosis is defined by the presence of tissue that is biologically and morphologically similar to normal endometrium in locations other than the endometrial cavity and myometrium. Although the cause of endometriosis has not been clearly established, clinical and experimental observations indicate that retrograde menstruation, vascular or lymphatic dissemination, direct implantation, and metaplasia – alone or in concert – may be responsible. Other factors, such as genetic predisposition and immunologic disturbances, may also play a role.

Risk factors include late marriage, delayed fertility, low parity, high socioeconomic status, and short menstrual cycle (27 days or less). In young girls, there appears to be an association with obstructive and congenital anomalies of the genital tract.[1]

Prevalence

It is impossible to assess accurately the prevalence in the general population. Estimates are based on examination of pelvic or abdominal structures by laparoscopy or laparotomy in women who have symptoms. Thus, the observed frequency varies with the indications for these procedures as well as the diagnostic accuracy of the operating surgeon. In a composite of nine studies involving 33,598 women, the mean prevalence rate was 1% (range 0.1% to 9.0%).[2] In another series of eight reports encompassing 860 laparoscopies performed for pelvic pain, the mean was 19% (range 5% to 32%).[2] Among infertility patients, the prevalence of endometriosis has been reported to be as high as 30% to 60%, whereas in the general population the prevalence has been estimated to be 7% to 10%.

Contrary to earlier reports, black women, particularly those in higher socioeconomic classes, may be as frequently affected as white women.[3] In a series of 260 diagnostic laparoscopies in black women, 21% were found to have endometriosis.[4] Similarly, the disease was diagnosed in 30% of black women examined by laparoscopy for pelvic pain.[4]

Endometriosis does not occur in premenarchal girls but is frequently diagnosed in teenagers.[5] In postmenopausal women, the growth of endometriosis is arrested; implants atrophy and are resolved. However, symptoms of the disease may persist or reappear, particularly in women who receive estrogen replacement therapy.[6]

Clinical Presentation

The most common sites of pelvic endometriosis are the ovaries, pelvic peritoneum, cul-de-sac, uterosacral ligaments, posterior surface of the uterus, sigmoid colon, and bladder. Other affected structures in the abdomen include the appendix, ileum, and diaphragm. Endometriosis may also affect the vulva, vagina, cervix, rectovaginal septum, abdominal wall, umbilicus, bronchi, lungs, kidneys, and inguinal regions.

Since most implants are confined to the pelvic cavity, the clinical manifestations of the disease predominantly relate to pelvic pain, menstrual disorders, and infertility. Other symptoms may appear when endometriosis affects abdominal viscera or extraabdominal sites. However, endometriosis may be present but produce no symptoms. Extensive endometriosis may cause little or no pain in some women, whereas mild disease may be associated with severe pain. Pain is usually more intense when uterosacral ligaments are involved.

Pain

Pelvic pain, the most common symptom of endometriosis, usually appears in the third or fourth decade of life and occurs in the form of dysmenorrhea. The pain typically starts 1 or 2 days before the onset of menses and lasts for the duration of the flow. Pelvic pain may be associated with rectal pressure and backache radiating to the thighs. The pain resulting from extraabdominal endometriosis depends on the location of the implants.

Some patients complain of dyspareunia, particularly with deep coital penetration. This symptom is more likely when the rectovaginal septum or uterosacral ligaments are affected. It is also observed when the cul-de-sac is obliterated or ovaries adhere to the cul-de-sac. Some women may experience constant dull aches or pain, usually exacerbated during menstruation. Occasionally, a woman has a history of pain with defecation (dyschezia).

The pathophysiology of pain in endometriosis is not entirely clear. It may be that minimal bleeding from the implants causes an inflammatory reaction of the surrounding tissues and compression of nerve endings. Another contributing factor may be the synthesis and release of prostaglandins from the ectopic endometrial tissue.

Menstrual Abnormalities

Abnormal menstrual bleeding is another important symptom of pelvic endometriosis. These disturbances may manifest as premenstrual spotting, hypermenorrhea, or metrorrhagia. Ovulatory dysfunction, reported by many investigators, may cause these abnormalities.

Infertility

Frequently associated with infertility, endometriosis is diagnosed in 30% to 60% of patients with otherwise unexplained infertility who undergo laparoscopy.[2] When there are adhesions or anatomic distortion of pelvic organs, the infertility can be readily explained. However, it is not clear why minimal or mild disease is associated with infertility. Several hypotheses have been advanced to explain this relationship: ovulatory disorders, abnormalities of peritoneal fluid, adverse effects of prostaglandins and other toxic substances released from ectopic endometrial implants, disturbance of the immune system, and increased rate of spontaneous abortion.

Ovulatory Disorders

Numerous investigators have attempted to demonstrate a link between ovulatory dysfunction and endometriosis. Abnormalities reported in these studies cover the entire spectrum of ovulatory disorders, anovulation, luteal phase defects, subtle anomalies of follicular phase or luteinizing hormone (LH) surge, and luteinized

unruptured follicle syndrome (LUFS). These dysfunctions are also observed in infertile women who do not have endometriosis. Contradictory results have been reported. For example, some studies indicate that patients with endometriosis have abnormal follicular growth patterns, as documented by ultrasonic monitoring, but other studies do not confirm these findings.[7,8] Some data also indicate no statistically significant difference in overall pregnancy rates of patients with minimal to mild endometriosis (stage I or II AFS-r), who are treated either medically or by surgical excision, compared with controls.[9-11,28] However, other evidence suggests that patients with minimal endometriosis have a lower monthly fecundity rate when compared with controls.[12] Information derived from reports of women undergoing in vitro fertilization (IVF) indicates a decreased rate of follicular development and retrieval, and decreased rate of oocyte fertilization and pregnancy compared with controls.[13,14] Thus, it appears that even minimal pelvic endometriosis may be associated with, as yet, undefined factors that lead to a decline in fecundity.

Other groups have implicated LUFS as both a cause and a result of endometriosis. LUFS is characterized by a menstrual cycle that appears to be ovulatory by usual clinical and hormonal criteria. However, the oocyte is trapped within the follicle. The condition may be diagnosed by laparoscopy (absence of ovulatory stigma), ultrasonography (absence of follicular collapse), or examination of peritoneal fluid (failure of progesterone levels to rise). In one study, LUFS was diagnosed in 79% of patients with endometriosis but in only 6% of the controls.[15] Other investigators, however, have not confirmed these findings.[16,17]

The relationship of endometriosis to luteal phase deficiency has been extensively investigated. Some studies have demonstrated a link between these conditions, whereas others have not (Table 7.1).

The evidence to support an association between luteal phase deficiency (LPD) and endometriosis is based on three types of studies: luteal phase endometrial biopsies, mid-luteal phase progesterone levels or its metabolites, and such hormonal changes as abnormalities of LH surge or estradiol secretion. A review of these contradictory studies indicates that the rate of occurrence

Table 7.1. Association of luteal phase deficiency and endometriosis.

Study	Endometriosis cases (Number)	Proportion with luteal phase deficiency
Grant[18]	96	45%
Groll[19]	80	56%
Pittaway et al[20]	75	5%
	68 (controls)	9%
Balasch & Vanrell[21]	27	19%
	50 (controls)	22%

of LPDs in patients with endometriosis is approximately 10% to 20%, which is not statistically significantly different from other infertile patients. Thus, an increased incidence of luteal phase defect is not a likely cause of infertility in patients with endometriosis.

Hyperprolactinemia has also been proposed as a possible mechanism by which patients with minimal endometriosis are rendered infertile. Several studies have shown the presence of galactorrhea, elevated basal and thyrotropin-releasing hormone (TRH)-stimulated prolactin and nocturnal hyperprolactinemia in patients with endometriosis.

A high frequency of spontaneous abortion in infertile women with endometriosis has been observed in several studies.[19] However, most of these studies have not included a control population. Furthermore, suppression of endometriosis with medication does not appear to lower the spontaneous abortion rate. Therefore, it is possible that high spontaneous abortion rates are characteristic of women with infertility and not just of women with endometriosis. The majority of spontaneous abortions associated with endometriosis are not thought to be caused by the disease.[22,23]

Physical Examination

You should suspect endometriosis when there are the typical symptoms of pain, menstrual disorders, and infertility. Physical examination may confirm your clinical suspicion. Physical exam findings in patients with endometriosis vary and depend, to a large extent, on the location and stage of the disease. In mild to moderate stages, the physical and pelvic examination findings may be entirely normal.[24]

On pelvic examination, a common finding in mild disease is tender nodularity of the posterior cul-de-sac and uterosacral ligaments. With more advanced disease, in addition to thickening and nodularity of these structures, fixed tender retroversion of the uterus and thickening or masses of the rectovaginal septum may be palpable.

Adnexal involvement is characterized by ovarian enlargement, with or without tenderness. Speculum examination may reveal lesions on the surface of the cervix or in the vagina. Umbilical lesions are usually visible and tender on palpation. Pain or bleeding from any site coinciding with menses should raise the index of suspicion and lead to careful evaluation of the specific anatomic areas involved such as lungs, inguinal canal, umbilicus or previous incisions.

Diagnosis

Laparoscopy is the most reliable procedure for detecting pelvic or abdominal endometriosis. The best time to perform this procedure during the menstrual cycle depends on the type of abnormalities being investigated.

Laparoscopy Techniques

In infertile women, valuable information is obtained when laparoscopy is performed in the luteal phase. You will be able to visualize ovulatory stigma, detect corpus hemorrhagicum, and diagnose luteal phase deficiency if a simultaneous endometrial biopsy is performed. In patients with suspected endometriosis without associated infertility, laparoscopy may be performed at any time during the menstrual cycle.

Diagnostic laparoscopy should be performed with the "two-puncture technique." This approach allows introduction of a suprapubic probe or atraumatic grasping instrument to examine pelvic and abdominal structures thoroughly. The availability of video equipment is a distinct advantage. It enables the operator to visualize various organs on a large screen and to document the presence of endometrial lesions or other pathologic entities by photography or video recording.

Diagnostic laparoscopy must be thorough and systematic. On entering the abdomen, note the color, character and amount of peritoneal fluid. Sanguinous fluid often indicates endometriosis. Starting from one side of the pelvis, the ovary, fallopian tube, anterior uterine surface, broad ligaments, and bladder area are carefully inspected progressing to the opposite side. If ovaries are fixed, they should be mobilized and the ovarian surface and fossa examined. Endometriosis of the ovarian fossa is relatively common and may be completely missed if this manuever is omitted. The uterus should be raised and the posterior surface of the uterus examined. Cul-de-sac fluid should then be aspirated to allow careful inspection of the cul-de-sac, uterosacral ligaments, sigmoid colon and ureters.

Next, direct attention to the abdominal viscera, small and large bowels, and appendix. Similarly inspect liver, spleen, and diaphragm. In the course of this evaluation, note the presence, size, color, and other characteristics of endometriosis. Endometriosis of the diaphragm may lead to unusual complaints of pain in the shoulder during menses. Adhesions between diaphragm to liver (Curtis-Fitz-Hugh syndrome) are usually associated with pelvic inflammatory disease rather than endometriosis.

Besides the black, bluish, red, and brown lesions classically reported as being consistent with endometriosis, several other types have recently been described. These include nonpigmented peritoneal lesions that may be whitish or light gray and fibrotic.[25] When in doubt, perform biopsies to establish the diagnosis. Even in lesions having the typical visual appearance of endometriosis, histologic examination may reveal non-endometriotic conditions such as hemangiomas, carbon particles, old suture materials, trophoblastic proliferation, and old ectopic pregnancies.[25] Table 7.2 shows the reported rates of histologic confirmation of different

Table 7.2. Histologic confirmation of endometriosis by lesion type.

Lesion type	Histologic confirmation (%)
Black	94–98
White	78–91
Red	75–92
Glandular	66–67
Yellow-brown	22–47
Subovarian adhesions	39–50
Peritoneal pockets	39–47

Source: Pittaway[25] with permission.

lesion types. Several reports have documented endometriosis in biopsy material obtained from normal appearing peritoneal surfaces.[26,27] Old corpus luteum cysts of the ovary may be mistaken for endometrial (chocolate) cysts. Thus, to make accurate diagnoses, you must be familiar with the vagaries of endometrial lesions. Even for expert laparoscopists, endometriosis may be missed. Whenever laparoscopy is done for endometriosis associated with infertility, chromotubations should be performed. Other endoscopic techniques such as sigmoidoscopy, colonoscopy, and cystoscopy may be useful to diagnose extragenital endometriosis.

At the completion of laparoscopy, it is important to carefully document the extent and staging of endometriosis. During the last 20 years, several classifications have been proposed. Among those most commonly utilized is the American Fertility Society Revised Classification.[28] Regardless of the system used, it is essential to stage the disease. Only in this way can you properly assess the severity of endometriosis and monitor the course of any treatment.

Imaging Technique

Imaging techniques used for the diagnosis of endometriosis consist of radiography, ultrasonography, computed tomography (CT), and magnetic resonance imaging (MRI). In general, these techniques are of limited value. Radiographic procedures include hysterosalpingography (which may reveal cornual tubal obstruction due to endosalpingiosis), gynecography, and occasionally barium enema. None of these procedures is sufficiently specific to aid in the diagnosis of endometriosis.

Ultrasonography, highly accurate for assessing pelvic and adnexal masses, may help you differentiate between solid and cystic lesions and identify their exact location. This information is particularly useful in formulating preoperative decisions regarding a laparoscopic approach versus laparotomy for diagnosis and management of pelvic tumors. CT scanning, a more expensive technique requiring radiation exposure, does not offer much additional information. MRI does not expose the patient to radiation, but is very expensive and not readily available in all institutions. Although reliable in determining the size and location of ovarian cysts and possibly large endometriomas, MRI cannot establish a specific diagnosis of endometriosis. It should be reserved for unusual cases and those with diagnostic problems. MRI has been found to be of value for the diagnosis of adenomyosis.

Serum Markers

CA-125 is an antigen associated with a high molecular weight glycoprotein that is expressed on a number of tissues derived from human celomic epithelium. It was originally found to be expressed in many epithelial ovarian cancers. A monoclonal antibody to CA-125 has been produced by immunizing mice with human ovarian carcinoma antigens. Using this monoclonal antibody, CA-125 may be detected in the serum of patients with ovarian cancer as well as endometriosis, leiomyoma, pelvic inflammatory disease, and ovarian hyperstimulation syndrome.

CA-125 levels may also be elevated during pregnancy and with diseases such as appendicitis, chronic liver disease, and peritonitis. Numerous investigators have examined the value of CA-125 for endometriosis. These studies indicate that the serum CA-125 level is elevated in most women with endometriosis. However, the serum test has low sensitivity and is not appropriate for general screening purposes.[25,29] But, in clinical situations that have a high prevalence of endometriosis, CA-125 may be used as an additional diagnostic tool. The concentration of CA-125 seems to correlate with both the severity and the clinical course of endometriosis. The response of endometriosis to medical or surgical therapy may be monitored by serial determination of CA-125 levels. It has been suggested that persistent or recurrent elevations of CA-125 after surgical treatment may indicate a poor prognosis for pregnancy.[25]

Two other substances are being investigated as markers for endometriosis. Antiendometrial antibodies have been detected in the serum of women with endometriosis using a variety of immunologic assays.[25,30] Preliminary studies have demonstrated a high sensitivity (74% to 83%) with a fairly low false–positive rate (0% to 21%). The level of endometrial antibodies does not appear to correlate with the stage of disease. These assays are not, as yet, generally available and are at present used mostly as research tools.

Another protein marker, "endometrial secretory protein PP14," has been found to have a sensitivity of 74% for all stages of endometriosis. Its level seems to decrease in women receiving medical treatment for endometriosis.[31] However, there is a significant overlay with normal values in mild disease.

Conclusion

Endometriosis affects pelvic structures primarily, but it may also be found at a variety of other sites. The presence of typical clinical symptoms and physical findings should alert you to proper diagnostic procedures and, ultimately, laparoscopy. Laparoscopy should be thorough and performed by an expert intimately familiar with the pathologic presentation of this disease and its vagaries. Confirmatory biopsies should be obtained whenever possible and when the diagnosis is in doubt.

References

1. Schifrin BS, Erez S, Moore JG. Teen-age endometriosis. Am J Obstet Gynecol 1973;116:973–980.
2. Pauerstein CJ. Clinical presentation and diagnosis in endometriosis. In Schenken RS, ed. Contemporary concepts in clinical management. Philadelphia, JB Lippincott Co., 1989, pp 127–144.
3. Chatman DL. Endometriosis in the black woman. Am J Obstet Gynecol 1976;125:987–989.
4. Chatman DL. Endometriosis and the black woman. J Reprod Med 1976;16:303–306.
5. Huffman JW. Endometriosis in young teen-age girls. Pediatr Ann 1981;10:44–49.
6. Djursing H, Petersen K, Weberg E. Symptomatic postmenopausal endometriosis. Acta Obstet Gynaecol Scand 1981;60:529–530.
7. Doody MC, Rossavik IK, Gibbons WE. Women with endometriosis have significantly abnormal ultrasonographic follicular growth parameters. Fertil Steril 1986;46(Suppl):91.
8. Thomas EJ, Lenton EA, Cooke IO. Follicle growth patterns and endocrinological abnormalities in infertile women with minor degrees of endometriosis. Br J Obstet Gynaecol 1986;93:852–858.
9. Bayer SR, Seibel MM, Saffan DS, et al. Efficacy of danazol treatment for minimal endometriosis in infertile women. J Reprod Med 1988;33:179–183.
10. Hull ME, Moghissi KS, Magyar DF, et al. Comparison of different treatment modalities of endometriosis-associated infertility. Fertil Steril 1987;47:40–44.
11. Schenken RS, Neolinak LR. Conservative surgery versus expectant management for infertile patients with mild endometriosis. Fertil Steril 1982;37:183–186.
12. Jansen RPS. Minimal endometriosis and reduced fecundability. Prospective evidence from an artificial insemination by donor program. Fertil Steril 1986;46:141–143.
13. O'Shea RT, Chen C, Weiss T, et al. Endometriosis and in vitro fertilization. Lancet 1985;2:723.
14. Wardle PG, McLaughlin EA, McDermott A, et al. Endometriosis and ovulatory disorder: reduced fertilization in vitro compared with tubal and unexplained infertility. Lancet 1985;2:236–239.
15. Brosens IA, Koninckx PR, Corveleyn PA. A study of plasma progesterone, oestradiol-17, prolactin, and LH levels, and of the luteal-phase appearance of the ovaries in patientswith endometriosis and infertility. Br J Obstet Gynaecol 1978;85:246–250.
16. Dmowski WP, Rao R, Scammegna A. The luteinized unruptured follicle syndrome and endometriosis. Fertil Steril 1980;33:30–34.
17. Kerin JF, Kirby C, Morris D, et al. Incidence of the luteinized unruptured follicle phemonenon in cyclingwomen. Fertil Steril 1983;40:620–626.
18. Grant A. Additional sterility factors in endometriosis. Fertil Steril 1966;17:514–519.
19. Groll M. Endometriosis and spontaneous abortion. Fertil Steril 1984;41:933–935.
20. Pittaway DE, Maxson W, Daniell J, et al. Luteal-phase defects in infertility patients with endometriosis. Fertil Steril 1983;39:712–713.
21. Balasch J, Vanrell JA. Mild endometriosis and luteal function. Int J Fertil 1985;30:4.
22. Pittaway DE, Ellington CP, Klimek M. Preclinical abortion and endometriosis. Fertil Steril 1988;49:221–233.
23. Metzger DA, Olive DL, Stoho GF, et al. Association of endometriosis and spontaneous abortion effect of control group selection. Fertil Steril 1986;45:18–22.
24. Rawson JMR. Prevalence of endometriosis in asymptomatic women. J Reprod Med 1991;36:513–515.
25. Pittaway DE. Diagnosis of endometriosis. Infertil Reprod Med Clin North Am 1992;3:619–631.
26. Nisolle M, Paindaveine B, Bourdon A, et al. Histologic study of peritoneal endometriosis in infertile women. Fertil Steril 1990;53:984–988.
27. Jansen RPS, Russell P. Nonpigmented endometriosis: clinical, laparoscopic, and pathologic definition. Am J Obstet Gynecol 1986;155:1154–9.
28. American Fertility Society. Revised classification of endometriosis. Fertil Steril 1985;43:351–352.
29. Pittaway DE. CA-125 in women with endometriosis. Obstet Gynecol Clin North Am 1989;16:237–51.
30. Kennedy SH, Starky PM, Sargent IL, et al. Antiendometrial antibodies in endometriosis measured by an enzyme-linked immunoabsorbant assay before and after treatment with danazol and nafarelin. Obstet Gynecol 1990;75:914–918.
31. Telima S, Kanppila A, Ronnbert L, et al. Elevated serum levels of endometrial secretory protein PP14 in patient with advanced endometriosis. Amer J Obstet Gyencol 1989;161:866–871.

Part 2
Surgical Management Techniques

8

Rationale for Surgical Treatment of Endometriosis

Dan Martin

Do All Patients With Endometriosis Need Treatment?

Rawson found that 50% of patients undergoing sterilization and 61% of patients having surgery for myomata had asymptomatic endometriosis.[1] My own group found a similar occurrence of 25% in patients having tubal sterilization reversals.[2] Such findings suggest that some women who have endometriosis may not need treatment.

However, we do not know who will have progression of their disease and who may need subsequent treatment. Moen and Muss found that 16% of patients undergoing sterilization at pregnancy termination and 22% of women undergoing interval sterilization have endometriosis.[3] When this rate was analyzed for the number of years since the last delivery, the odds ratio increased to 4.5 at ten years when compared with the first five years after delivery.[4] This suggests that even though these women were symptom-free, the prevalence, or perhaps recognition, of the disease was increasing as the interval from the last pregnancy increased. With longer followup some women may become symptomatic as their disease progresses.[5]

Cycle of Progression and Regression

Sampson noted a change from a red raspberry appearance to a blueberry appearance as lesions aged.[6] Karnaky stated that it required four to ten years for water blister lesions to progress to scarred blue-domed cysts.[7] Redwine quantitated these changes and demonstrated a change in the observed appearance from clear to red to scarred black lesions over seven to ten years.[8] Such changes were also noted by Koninckx and co-workers in documenting an increase from 23% to 63%

in the occurrence of scarred black lesions over a 20-year age interval. Koninckx and I also found a decreased occurrence of red and polypoid lesions and an increased occurrence of deep infiltration over the same time span.[5]

Jansen and Russell also observed a progressive change to pigmented lesions within 6 to 24 months in six patients having second-look laparoscopy.[9] Davis and co-workers found red lesions in 86% of adolescents with an average age of 17 as opposed to 20% of patients undergoing laparoscopic-assisted vaginal hysterectomy with an average of 37 years. Of interest, red lesions were significantly associated with symptoms such as diarrhea and vomiting.[10]

D'Hooghe's team reported similar changes in baboons.[11] They demonstrated that 91% of baboons had additional lesions at second-look laparoscopy whereas 52% had regression at the sites of original lesions. In the control group, none of which had endometriosis at first look, 70% had developed endometriosis by second-look laparoscopy. All endometriosis was stage I. The investigators also documented specific changes in lesion color. White vesicles changed to white plaques; red vesicles to black spots; organ zones to white plaques; and black spots to white plaques. The medical modification of these changes was documented by Thomas and Cooke. They found no progression while patients were on suppressive therapy, whereas there was a 47% progression without therapy.[12]

Mahmood's team confirmed this work and showed progression of endometriosis in 64% of women who had no therapy, 33% of danazol-treated patients, 22% of diathermy-treated patients, and 20% of those treated with surgery and danazol with 9 to 18 months of follow-up.[13] The spontaneous regression rate was 27%; the rate of regression increased with both medical and surgical treatment. These authors concluded the natural course of the disease is unpredictable, and that endometriosis should be treated even if asymptomatic. Mahmood and Templeton's progression rates for diathermy and combined diathermy and danazol are greater than Redwine's recurrence rate of 7% at one to two years following laparoscopic excision or Wheeler's recurrence rate of 7% at one to two years following laparotomy. Redwine reported a 19% recurrence at five years and Wheeler a 20% recurrence.[14,15]

Expectant Management

Expectant management is based on the theory that some patients with endometriosis may have regressing rather than progressing or stable endometriosis. Asymptomatic endometriosis and spontaneous resolution of symptoms are not uncommon. Pregnancy frequently occurs without treatment.

This approach may be useful when there is asymptomatic involvement of the bowel, periureter, and rectovaginal septum. If there is no pain and no compromise of the lumen of the ureter or bowel, surgery may be avoidable. Medical suppression may not be needed. When pain is present, it often can be controlled with medical suppression, and the morbidity and expense of pelvic surgery can be avoided.

Nontender masses in the rectovaginal septum that are biopsy-proven endometriosis need to be observed for their proximity to the anal verge. A distance of 1.5 cm or more may be necessary for placement of the circular gastrointestinal anastomotic device (GIA). If a rectovaginal septal mass is growing and extending down toward the anal verge, surgery may be indicated to avoid a permanent colostomy. Permanent colostomy, however, may be necessary when a deep anastomosis cannot be performed.

Medical Management

In certain patients, medical suppression may break the cycle of pain. It may be short term, with GnRH analogs or danazol, or long term, with medications such as combined estrogen/progestin preparations or pure progestins. Table 8.1 lists various indications proposed by different physicians.

There is some suggestion that medical suppression may be helpful by allowing the body to provide its own form of treatment for the disease. In theory, this approach would encourage the regression of disease in a number of patients.

Surgical Management

Pain is the most common indication for surgical treatment, particularly when a pelvic mass is present. This treatment also appears reasonable when focal tenderness is present.

As a pragmatic decision, surgery is avoided on teenagers with no palpable masses until after a trial of oral contraceptive suppression and nonsteroidal anti-inflammatory drugs (NSAIDs). Teenagers who have pain so severe that it interferes with their activities but which does not respond to oral contraceptive suppression and NSAIDs frequently benefit from therapeutic laparoscopy.

Focal tenderness and a possible mass may be the first findings that suggest deep retroperitoneal involvement. These patients frequently need early therapy because delay only increases the depth of infiltration and the extent of dissection needed.

Moore and co-workers reported on five patients seen over ten years with deep retroperitoneal involvement.[16] These patients had little or no peritoneal disease; four had AFS-r stage 0–score 0 and the fifth had stage 1–score 1.[17] Three of these patients had either complete ureteral obstruction, hydronephrosis, or full-thickness involvement of the rectum. The disease produced severe symptoms, was difficult to diagnose, and offered challenges at surgery. This deep retroperitoneal disease may be recognized only during menses.[5]

Exposure

The surgical exposure needed for the treatment of endometriosis is determined, in part, by the goals of surgery. When a tissue diagnosis is needed, biopsy or excisional technique is used. When fertility is to be preserved, the techniques require a balance that removes as much diseased tissue as possible but causes as little residual trauma as feasible. An overly aggressive excisional approach may result in subsequent adhesions that may be more a factor in infertility than the endometriosis itself. Pain secondary to fibrotic endometriosis, however, particularly in the bowel, requires resection of all palpable and visual abnormalities.

Recognition of lesions may be difficult. Near-contact laparoscopy has been used to identify lesions as small as $180\,\mu$ to $200\,\mu$.[2,18,19] However, not all lesions are recognized at laparoscopy or laparotomy. Small lesions can be missed because of their size, whereas larger lesions may be missed because of their position.[16,20–23] These deep lesions may be more evident on palpation.[5,24,26]

Table 8.1. Indications for medical suppression.

Cornual occlusion
Myomectomy
Persistent infertility or pain following surgical excision
Preoperative preparation to decrease ovarian size and functional cysts
Recurrent miscarriages

Laparotomy

Laparotomy has been the standard for surgical therapy of endometriosis. Palpation, examination of retroperitoneal spaces, examination of bowel, and delicate handling of deep lesions are easier at laparotomy than at laparoscopy. Laparoscopic excision of deep bowel lesions has been associated with a high persistence.[24] Open surgery is used when circumstances indicate a need for laparotomy.[27,28] Laparotomy is most useful in patients who continue to have persistent pelvic pain after an initial laparoscopic approach and in those with bulky tumors.

Laparoscopy

Laparoscopy can be used to identify, remove, and confirm lesions as small as $180\,\mu$.[2] Video monitoring provides magnification and high resolution.[29] This monitoring technique increases the ability of the assistants and other personnel to assist at surgery. However, relying on video can decrease detection, resolution, depth of field, and field of vision.

Although coagulation and vaporization are adequate for most cases, excision has been used to resect lesions as deep as 14 mm and to dissect the ureter and bowel away from endometriosis and adhesions.[24,30,32] The CO_2 laser can be used for deep and delicate dissections with excellent visualization. Scissors, bipolar coagulation, thermal coagulation, and unipolar knives are more commonly available pieces of equipment.[14,33–35] The use of scissors and bipolar or thermal coagulation must be mastered before learning laser or advanced unipolar knife techniques. Although laparoscopy is generally equal to or better than other treatments in all groups studied, the learning curve for extensive disease can be so long that few physicians will decide to work through the complications associated with this change in technique.[29,36–38]

Extent of Surgery

The extent of surgery depends on the patient's history, physical findings, and goals of surgery. A primary approach is generally used on patients whose problem is infertility or focal pelvic tenderness, but who have no palpable nodules and who are having their first operation. The secondary approach is generally used when nodules are present or when pain and focal tenderness are the main problems. The tertiary approach is one in which the surgeon and patient are prepared for bowel surgery, ureteral anastomosis or implantation, and laparotomy. These patients have generally had the diagnosis made at a previous laparoscopy or laparotomy.

For all patients undergoing laparoscopy, the surgeon must be prepared to coagulate any recognized lesions and to lyse adhesions. These steps can be performed with bipolar or thermal coagulation and mechanical scissors. Monopolar equipment is not necessary for this level of care.

The secondary level of care is used in those patients who have previously had laparoscopy or who have a clinical history or physical findings suggesting the need for deep tissue techniques. Those techniques include vaporization with laser or monopolar electrosurgery or dissection and excisional techniques using any form of dissecting and excisional equipment.

The tertiary approach is for those patients who have large palpable nodules or who have failed to respond to other forms of therapy. These patients frequently have had intravenous pyelograms, barium enemas, colonoscopies, sonographies, and other diagnostic testing. In addition, these patients are bowel prepped and frequently have self-banked blood. Preoperative permission for exploratory laparotomy, bowel resection and anastomosis, and the possibility of ureteral resection and implantation is discussed and clarified. This type of approach is generally used for those complaining of chronic pain and is not commonly used for infertility patients.

Peritoneum and Soft Tissue

Small implants ($\leq 2\,$mm) may be treated with many energy sources. These are sampled by biopsy or excision prior to treatment. Coagulation can distort tissue because of the thermal transfer and heating. This distortion may interfere with recognition and dissection. Vaporization or excision is more useful for larger lesions. These techniques are carried down to the level of healthy tissue (Fig. 8.1).

Deep lesions are more accurately excised than vaporized.[5,24,32,39] Excision is started by cutting through the peritoneum and into the loose connective tissue with scissors, knife, or laser.[40] A probe, irrigating solution, knife, or laser is then used to dissect these layers. Once the tissue is excised, it is removed. Specimens too large to be removed through the trocar can be cut or morcellated into smaller areas or bagged to be removed through the trocar incision, a minilaparotomy, or a colpotomy.[31]

If carbon accumulates, the field is obscured both at the time of surgery and at subsequent laparoscopy. Carbon can be confused with or can hide endometriosis.[25,41] High-power density electrosurgical or superpulse laser techniques decrease carbonization by facilitating rapid vaporization and thus decreasing the amount of lateral tissue desiccated or coagulated.[42]

Ovary

Ovarian endometriomas are managed according to their size. Those of less than 5 mm are biopsied and coagulated, vaporized, or excised. The infiltration of these

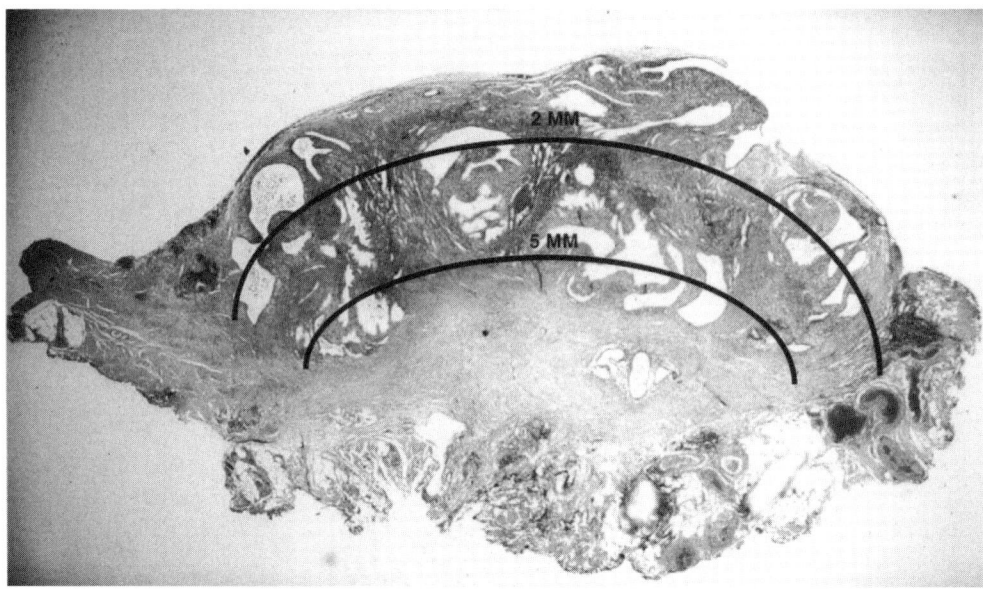

Figure 8.1. This micrograph of a histologic slide demonstrates the depth of expected efficacy for various techniques. The most superficial line is at 2 mm. Bipolar electrosurgery, thermal cautery, and argon or KTP coagulation are effective at this 2 mm depth. The second line is at 5 mm. This is at or beyond the limits of a Nd:YAG laser coagulation. Either vaporization or excision is necessary for lesions at this depth. The full depth of the lesion is 7 mm. Vaporization to this depth is tedious and creates excess smoke. Excision is generally needed.

small lesions can be very irregular and vaporization is taken 2 to 4 mm into healthy appearing stroma.

When endometriomas are 2 to 5 cm in size, the ovary is opened and drained and the inner wall inspected. A modification of Semm's technique for stripping is used.[43] The opening of the ovary for this stripping can be performed with any type of equipment but should be at the dependent portion or on the lateral (broad ligament) side to avoid bowel adhesions. A relaxing incision to facilitate definition of the plane of the pseudocapsule may be useful, both in developing the dissection plane and in determining the histology.[25] Surface implants and endometriosis infiltrating into a corpus luteum have

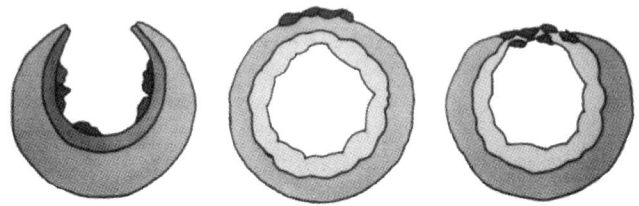

Figure 8.2. Chocolate cysts can be endometriomas, corpora lutea, other hemorrhagic cysts, or combinations of any of these. In order to distinguish endometriosis overlying or invading a corpus luteum, excision of the surface of the ovary and the most superficial level of the chocolate cyst is performed first. Then, the deep lining is resected or a biopsy performed separately.

different scores from an ovarian endometrioma (Fig. 8.2).[44-46] When the capsule is adherent to the hilar vessels, coagulation is used instead of stripping to avoid tearing these vessels.

For endometriomas that exceed 5 cm, stripping techniques may require two to five hours at laparoscopy and then require a laparotomy.[25] Removing these large cysts rather than performing a staged procedure may also increase the chance of sacrificing the ovary.[27,43,47,48] A staged procedure involves draining, biopsy, and coagulating the inner lining of large cysts at an initial laparoscopy. These steps are followed by serial sonography with or without medical suppression. A subsequent laparoscopy is performed if the cyst recurs.

Limiting the amount of surgery, using laparoscopy, avoiding sutures, and early ambulation have all been associated with decreased need for repeat operations.[25,27,29,50,51]

Bowel

Bowel involvement is suggested by palpable tumor near the organ, rectovaginal tenderness, a rectovaginal shelf, rectal bleeding at the time of menses, or persistent pain after laparoscopic removal of recognized lesions.

Lesions smaller than 1 cm are easier to feel than see. Most of them may push into the lumen; a superficial manifestation may represent only the tip of an iceberg.[26,27] Approximately 50% of appendiceal lesions are more readily recognized by palpation than visualization. In addition, few lesions are found by barium enema, colonoscopy, sonography, CT scan, or MRI scan. The main advantage to colonoscopy in the presence of a bowel mass is to rule out adenocarcinoma of the bowel.

Dealing with tumor in the rectovaginal septum generally requires a gynecologist or general surgeon familiar with bowel surgery in this area. Deep rectosigmoid resection and anastomosis is a distinct possibility at this level and laparotomy may be indicated.[26,28,43,53] Furthermore, the uterosacral ligaments can be infiltrated, with extension toward the sacrum or pelvic floor. This level of the uterosacrals or perirectal tissue is more palpable through the rectosigmoid than through the vagina. If the infiltration is not noted preoperatively, it is easy to miss at surgery. If the mucosa is fixed, full thickness penetration is often present. With any concern regarding bowel muscularis involvement, a preoperative general surgery consult, barium enema, sigmoidoscopy, and colonoscopy are advisable to rule out bowel cancer.

Laparoscopic dissection and excision in this area can be superficial or deep. The CO_2 laser is focused in repeat pulse or superpulse to avoid distortion and damage associated with coagulation and vaporization. Laparoscopic vaporization will generally be adequate for 50% to 90% of bowel lesions and adhesions. Bowel surgery is generally avoided in infertility patients who do not have symptoms attributable to bowel infiltration.

In one study of five patients with bowel distortion associated with pain and tenderness an initial partial-thickness resection was attempted at laparoscopy.[24] Immediate laparotomy was performed for bowel resection in two of these. Although the other three had apparent resection of their endometriosis, persistent pain and tenderness resulted in delayed laparotomy. All five had deep muscularis involvement. Those patients who have persistent pain may require medical suppression and/or laparotomy.[24,26,28,43,53–55]

Patients scheduled for laparotomy are bowel prepped whenever bowel involvement is suspected. In addition, self bloodbanking should be discussed with these patients because these procedures, frequently lasting three to five hours, can be associated with marked blood loss and subsequent transfusion.

Bladder

Bladder implants of up to 5 mm are handled much as the peritoneal lesions are. Larger lesions approach and may invade the bladder muscularis. Deep muscularis penetration should be anticipated as the lesions get larger. Lesions of 2 cm and greater often require resection of the bladder dome at laparotomy.

Ureter

When endometriosis lies over the ureter, two techniques are useful. Solution can be injected to push the ureter away and to provide a barrier between the ureter and the surgical destruction.[33,56] An alternate technique is to make an incision in the peritoneum above and away from the ureter. The peritoneum is then grasped and pulled toward the midline. A blunt probe is used to push the ureter away as the laser is used to incise into loose connective tissue. The laser is not aimed at the ureter. The lesion is resected in its entirety using this technique.

When the ureter does not push away from the peritoneum, the chance of infiltration in the ureter is great. The periureteral vessels can also bleed and techniques for hemostasis may harm the ureter. If the ureter is transected or damaged in the process of resecting endometriosis, some urologists feel that anastomosis in a diseased area should not be performed and that an implantation is indicated. If you are not prepared for ureteral implantation avoid cutting near the ureter, especially when it is adherent to endometriosis.

Staged Procedures

Staging of surgery for endometriosis has been described by Semm and Donnez.[47,48] This involves removing as much endometriosis as reasonable at first surgery, and then placing the patient on three to nine months of hormonal suppression. Asymptomatic patients are observed. For others, repeating the pelviscopy to remove any remnant endometriosis and to treat both adhesions and tubal disease may be necessary.

A staged procedure for ovarian endometriomas that involves drainage, irrigation, examination, biopsy, and coagulation of the inner lining of large cysts at an initial laparoscopy may be useful. This decreases the extent of removal of healthy ovary.[57] Serial sonography, with or without medical suppression, is used to monitor persistence or recurrence. A subsequent laparoscopy is performed if the cyst recurs.

Other surgeons suggest that endometriosis, particularly around the ureter, bowel, or major blood vessels, be left behind intentionally.[54,55] Observation may prove that partial treatment provides sufficient relief and that laparotomy or medical therapy is not necessary. When pain is persistent, medical therapy, a second laparoscopy, and laparotomy are considered. When there is marked endometriosis, a second laparoscopy may remove additional lesions or recurrent lesions. Repeat laparoscopy for recurrent endometriosis is particularly useful in younger patients.

Laparotomy may reveal palpable lesions that are not seen at laparoscopy.[5,16,24] Because of the increased incidence of palpable bowel disease in this group, bowel prep is routinely performed on all patients who are prepared for laparotomy.

Pregnancy

Life-table analyses of pregnancy rates in four separate studies suggest that laparoscopic techniques are equal to medication or laparotomy in mild or moderate cases and equal to or better than laparotomy in severe cases.[29,36-38] The outcome in these series may be related to limiting the amount of surgery, limiting the trauma from retraction, avoiding sutures, and/or early ambulation.[25,27,29,50-52] Nezhat and co-workers demonstrated a 60% to 79% resolution of adhesions and no new adhesion formation following laparoscopic lysis.[58] As adhesions may influence the outcome, ongoing use and development of agents to decrease adhesions appear useful.[59,60]

When pregnancy rates are analyzed by years of infertility and presence of other factors, younger women and patients who have short-term infertility have the best chance of having children. The prognosis is poorer for older patients and those with long-term infertility particularly when other factors are present.[61-64]

Pain

Focal tenderness associated with scarred lesions resolves when these lesions are resected.[5,16,24,25,65] Pain relief is much harder to quantitate than pregnancy rates or resolution of focal tenderness. Pain may be due to endometriosis, endometriosis and other factors combined, or only to other factors with endometriosis as a coincidental finding. Pain relief after laparoscopic surgery has been reported to be similar to that occurring after laparotomy.[66-68]

Conclusion

General guidelines for surgical management of endometriosis are given, but the treatment of any patient must be individualized. Although coagulation and medical suppression can be a good first-line approach to symptomatic diseaes, observation, deep dissection, or supportive care may be needed for comprehensive care.

References

1. Rawson JMR. Prevalence of endometriosis in asymptomatic women. J Reprod Med 1991;36:513–515.
2. Martin DC, Hubert GD, Vander Zwaag R, et al. Laparoscopic appearances of peritoneal endometriosis. Fertil Steril 1989;51:63–67.
3. Moen MH, Muus KM. Endometriosis in pregnant and nonpregnant women at tubal sterilization. Hum Reprod 1991;6(5):699–702.
4. Moen MH. Is a long period without childbirth a risk factor for developing endometriosis. Hum Reprod 1991; 6(10):1404–1407.
5. Koninckx PR, Martin DC. Deep endometriosis: a consequence of infiltration or retraction or possibly adenomyosis externa? Fertil Steril 1992;58:924–928.
6. Sampson JA. Benign and malignant endometrial implants in the peritoneal cavity, and their relation to certain ovarian tumors. Surg Gynecol Obstet 1924;38:287–311.
7. Karnaky KJ. Theories and known observations about hormonal treatment of endometriosis in-situ and endometriosis at the enzyme level. Arizona Medicine, 1969, January:37–41.
8. Redwine DB. Age-related evolution in color appearance of endometriosis. Fertil Steril 1987;48:1062–1063.
9. Jansen RPS, Russell P. Nonpigmented endometriosis: clinical, laparoscopic, and pathologic definition. Am J Obstet Gynecol 1986;155:1154–1159.
10. Davis GD, Thillet E, Lindemann J. Clinical characteristics of adolescent endometriosis. Presented at The Modern Surgical Management of Endometriosis, Phoenix, March 8, 1993.
11. D'Hooghe TM, Bambra CS, Isahakia M, et al. Evolution of spontaneous endometriosis in the baboon (*Papio anubis, Papio cynocephalus*) over a 12-month period. Fertil Steril 1992;58:409–412.
12. Thomas EJ, Cooke ID. Impact of gestrinone on the course of asymptomatic endometriosis. Brit Med J 1987; 294:272–274.
13. Mahmood TA, Templeton A. The impact of treatment on the natural history of endometriosis. Hum Reprod 1990;5: 965–970.
14. Redwine DR. Conservative laparoscopic excision of endometriosis by sharp dissection: life table analysis of reoperation and persistent or recurrent disease. Fertil Steril 1991;56:628–634.
15. Wheeler JM, Malinak LR. Recurrent endometriosis. Contr Gynecol Obstet 1987;16:13–21.
16. Moore JG, Binstock MA, Growdon WA. The clinical implications of retroperitoneal endometriosis. Am J Obstet Gynecol 1988;158:1291–1298.
17. American Fertility Society. Revised American Fertility Society classification of endometriosis: 1985. Fertil Steril 1985;43:351–353.
18. Redwine DB. The distribution of endometriosis in the pelvis by age groups and fertility. Fertil Steril 1987;47: 173–175.
19. Stripling MC, Martin DC, Poston WM. Does endometriosis have a typical appearance. J Reprod Med 1988;33: 879–884.
20. Brosens IA, Vasquez G, Gordts S. Scanning electron microscopic study of the pelvic peritoneum in unexplained infertility and endometriosis. (abstract) Fertil Steril 1984; 41:21S.
21. Nisolle M, Paindaveine B, Bourdon A, et al. Histologic study of peritoneal endometriosis in infertile women. Fertil Steril 1990;53:984–988.
22. Vasquez G, Cornillie F, Brosens IA. Peritoneal endometriosis: scanning electron microscopy and histology of minimal pelvic endometriotic lesions. Fertil Steril 1983; 42:696–703.
23. Cornillie FJ, Brosens IA, Vasquez G, et al. Histologic and ultrastructural changes in human endometriotic implants treated with the antiprogesterone steroid ethylnorgestrienone (Gestrinone) during 2 months. Int J Gynecol Pathol 1986;5:95–109.

24. Martin DC, Hubert GD, Levy BS. Depth of infiltration of endometriosis. J Gynecol Surg 1989;5:55–60.
25. Martin DC, Diamond MP. Operative laparoscopy: comparison of lasers with other techniques. Curr Probl Obstet Gynecol Fertil 1986;9:563–601.
26. Weed JC, Ray JE. Endometriosis of the bowel. Obstet Gynecol 1987;69:727–730.
27. Martin DC. Therapeutic laparoscopy. In Martin DC, ed. Laparoscopic appearance of endometriosis, 2nd ed, volume I. Memphis; Resurge Press, 1990, pp 21–29.
28. Coronado C, Franklin RR, Lotze EC, et al. Surgical treatment of symptomatic colorectal endometriosis. Fertil Steril 1990;53:411–416.
29. Nezhat C, Crowgey SR, Nezhat F. Videolaseroscopy for the treatment of endometriosis associated with infertility. Fertil Steril 1989;51:237–240.
30. Martin DC, Vander Zwaag R. Excisional techniques for endometriosis with the CO_2 laser laparoscope. J Reprod Med 1987;32:753–758.
31. Martin DC. Laparoscopic and vaginal colpotomy for the exicision of infiltrating cul-de-sac endometriosis. J Reprod Med 1988;33:806–808.
32. Davis GD, Brooks RA. Excision of pelvic endometriosis with the carbon dioxide laser laparoscope. Obstet Gynecol 1988;72:816–819.
33. Reich H. Laparoscopic treatment of extensive pelvic adhesions, including hydrosalpinx. J Reprod Med 1987; 32:736–742.
34. Murphy AA. Operative laparoscopy. Fertil Steril 1987;47: 1–18.
35. Gomel V. Operative laparoscopy: time for acceptance. Fertil Steril 1989;52:1–11.
36. Adamson GD, Hurd SJ, Pasta DJ, et al. Laparoscopic endometriosis treatment: is it better? Fertil Steril 1993;59: 35–44.
37. Adamson GD, Lu J, Subak LL. Laparoscopic CO_2 laser vaporization of endometriosis compared with traditional treatments. Fertil Steril 1988;50:704–710.
38. Olive DL, Martin DC. Treatment of endometriosis-associated infertility with CO_2 laser laparoscopy: the use of one- and two-parameter exponential models. Fertil Steril 1987;48:18–23.
39. Cornillie FJ, Oosterlynck D, Lauweryns JM, et al. Deeply infiltrating pelvic endometriosis: histology and clinical significance. Fertil Steril 19990;53:978–983.
40. Martin DC, ed. Laparoscopic Appearance of Endometriosis. Color Atlas. Memphis, Resurge Press, 1993, p 22.
41. Stripling MC, Martin DC, Chatman DL, et al. Subtle appearance of pelvic endometriosis. Fertil Steril 1988;49: 427–431.
42. Taylor MV, Martin DC, Poston W, et al. Effect of power density and carbonization on residual tissue coagulation using the continuous wave carbon dioxide laser. Colposc Gynecol Laser Surg 1986;2:169–175.
43. Semm K. Course of endoscopic abdominal surgery. In Semm K, Friedrick ER, eds. Operative manual for endoscopic abdominal surgery. Chicago, Year Book Med Publ, 1987, pp 130–213.
44. Martin DC. Chocolate cysts. Memphis: Media Services (videotape), Baptist Memorial Hospital, 1993.
45. Sampson JA. Perforating hemorrhagic (chocolate) cysts of the ovary. Their importance and especially their relation to pelvic adenomas of the endometrial type ("adenomyoma" of the uterus, rectovaginal septum, sigmoid, etc.). Arch Surg 1921;3:245–323.
46. Nezhat F, Nezhat C, Allan DJ, et al. Clinical and histologic classification of endometriomas. Implications for a mechanism of pathogenesis. J Reprod Med 1992;37:771–776.
47. Semm K. Postoperative care after endoscopic abdominal surgery. In Semm K, Friedrick ER, eds. Operative manual for endoscopic abdominal surgery. Chicago, Year Book Med Publ, 1987, pp 228–238.
48. Donnez J, Nisolle M, Karaman Y, et al. CO_2 laser laparoscopy in peritoneal endometriosis and in ovarian endometrial cyst. J Gynecol Surg 1989;5:361–366.
49. Fallon J, Brosnan JT, Moran WG. Endometriosis. Two hundred cases considered from the viewpoint of the practitioner. N Engl J Med 1946;235:669–673.
50. Brumsted JR, Deaton J, Lavigne E, et al. Postoperative adhesion formation after ovarian wedge resection with and without ovarian reconstruction in the rabbit. Fertil Steri 1990;53:723–726.
51. DeLeon FD, Edwards M, Heine MW. A comparison of microsurgery and laser surgery for ovarian wedge resection. Int J Fertil 1990;35:177–179.
52. Das K, Penney LL, Critser JK. Effects of passive motion and early vs delayed ambulation on adhesion formation in rat uterine surgery. Int J Fertil 1990;35:245–248.
53. Grunert GM, Franklin RR. Management of recurrent endometriosis. In Wilson EA, ed. Endometriosis. New York: Alan R. Liss, 1987:173–184.
54. Buttram VC, Reiter RC. Endometriosis. In Buttram VC, Reiter RC, eds. Surgical treatment of the infertile female. Baltimore: Williams & Wilkins, 1985:89–147.
55. Martin DC. Laparoscopy. In Nichols DH, ed. Gynecologic and Obstetrics Surgery. St. Louis, Mosby-Year Book, 1993, pp 735–749.
56. Nezhat C, Nezhat FR. Safe laser endoscopic excision or vaporization of peritoneal endometriosis. Fertil Steril 1989;52:149–151.
57. Martin DC, Berry JD. Histology of chocolate cysts. J Gynecol Surg 1990;6:43–46.
58. Nezhat CR, Nezhat FR, Metzger DA, et al. Adhesion reformation after reproductive surgery by videolaseroscopy. Fertil Steril 1990;53:1008–1011.
59. Diamond MP, Cunningham T, Linsky CB, et al. Laparoscopic application of Interceed (TC7) in the pig. J Gynecol Surg 1989;5:145–148.
60. INTERCEED (TC7) Adhesion Barrier Study Group. Prevention of postsurgical adhesions by INTERCEED (TC7), an absorbable adhesion barrier: a prospective, randomized multicenter clinical study. Fertil Steril 1989; 51:933–938.
61. Martin DC. CO_2 laser laparoscopy for endometriosis associated with infertility. J Reprod Med 1986;31:1089–1094.
62. Hull MGR. Infertility treatment: Relative effectiveness of conventional and assisted conception methods. Hum Reprod 1992;7(6):785–796.
63. Keye WR, Hansen LW, Astin M, et al. Argon laser therapy of endometriosis: a review of 92 consecutive patients. Fertil Steril 1987;47:208–212.
64. Kojima E, Yanagibori A, Yuda K, et al. Nd:YAG laser endoscopy. J Reprod Med 1988;33:907–911.
65. Ripps BA, Martin DC. Focal pelvic tenderness, pelvic pain and dysmenorrhea in endometriosis. J Reprod Med 1991;36:470–472.
66. Davis GD. Management of endometriosis and its associated adhesions with the CO_2 laser laparoscope. Obstet Gynecol 1986;68:422–425.

67. Keye WR, McArthur GR. Laser laparoscopy: argon. In
    Keye WR, ed. Laser surgery in gyneoclogy and obstetrics,
    2nd ed. Chicago, Year Book Med Publ, 1990, pp 208–
    221.

68. Nezhat C, Winer WK, Crowgey SR. Videolaseroscopy for
    the treatment of endometriosis and other diseases of
    the reproductive organs. Obstet Gynecol Forum 1987;
    1:1–4.

9

The History of Surgical Treatment of Endometriosis

Jan Deprest and Ivo Brosens

Introduction

Some sources refer to Rokitansky, in 1860, as being the first to describe a case he called adenomyoma.[1] But an earlier case that clearly showed all characteristics of endometriosis was described by Diesterweg in 1883.[2] He reported on a woman who had been operated on twice within two years for "polyps" on the posterior uterine wall. The tumors contained "cysts lined with ciliated epithelium" and were "filled with blood." It was Cullen's work that forced scientists to recognize that these tumors contain heterotopic uterine epithelium, stroma, and glands.[3] Sampson in the 1920s is, however, usually credited with describing the clinical entity of endometriosis and suggesting menstrual regurgitation as the cause.[4,5]

The disease, although benign, was generally considered to have the potential for invading adjacent organs and distorting normal anatomy. At that time, it was diagnosed only in what we now consider "advanced" stages. For years, the only cure was surgery that removed en bloc all foci of disease and the involved organs. Treatment consisted of *radical surgery* because the uterus and ovaries were presumed to be causative. It was not until the 1960s that *conservative surgery* was considered to be a valid alternative.[6] Medical treatment was also welcomed as a promising, less mutilating alternative that preserved endocrine and reproductive functions.

Wheeler and Malinak recently suggested that there is a cyclicity in the popularity of medical versus surgical treatment of endometriosis over the years.[7] Today, it seems both medical and surgical therapy, often combined, are simultaneously developed. Each treatment modality was enhanced from time to time by new developments.

Medical therapy, which is essentially suppressive in nature, benefited from three new major advances. In 1958 combined estrogen-progestogen (pseudopregnancy) treatment was proposed by Kistner.[8] In 1976, the FDA approved danazol, and in the late 1980s GnRH-agonists were introduced. Medical treatment, however, continues to fail to eradicate implants. Furthermore, metabolic, symptomatic, and contraceptive side effects are limiting.

Surgical therapy also has evolved. In the 1960s, conservative surgery was introduced; in the 1980s there was the development of endoscopic instrumentation and lasers. In 1985, Decherney even predicted somewhat prematurely the death of laparotomy.[9,10] More recently, the laparoscopic approach for radical surgery has become a fact.

As treatments have changed, so has terminology. In the early days, any surgery for endometriosis was considered *conservative* if the ovaries were preserved. Today, surgery is considered conservative only when functional reproductive organs are preserved. Initially, *radical* surgery included en bloc resection of uterus, ovaries, and all endometriotic implants; but today, in some selected cases, the ovaries are preserved.

In the past, authors often did not refer to the approach or route through which surgery was accomplished (laparotomy or laparoscopy). Neither did they use magnification loupes. Today, the terminology and techniques of microsurgery are extended to endoscopic surgery because of the magnification provided by the endoscope and new instrumentation.[11] It is well to remember that the use of the endoscope does not ensure atraumatic surgery. Endoscopy is only a method of access. When comparing results of various approaches, it is important to check carefully what each term meant at a particular time and in the hands of a specific author or group.

Surgical Diagnosis

Today, noninvasive techniques cannot diagnose or stage endometriosis correctly. The surgical approach remains the gold standard to confirm the presence and extension of disease. Previously, diagnosis was confirmed during laparotomy; today, laparoscopy is the route of choice to describe accurately the type, extent, and activity of lesions, to obtain biopsies and, ultimately to stage disease.[12-15] Diagnostic laparoscopy originated in the beginning of this century, but clinical applications began 50 years ago with the introduction of cold light illumination by Fourestière and the rod lens-system by Hopkins.[16,17] In Europe, gynecologic laparoscopy became accepted in the 1930s because of the pioneering work of Raoul Palmer in France, Hans Fraugenhein in Germany, and Patrick Steptoe in England. Later laparoscopy revived in North America under Jordan M. Phillips, who founded the American Association of Gynecologic Laparoscopists in 1971. Increased use of laparoscopy as a diagnostic tool and greater awareness of endometriosis, especially in infertility patients, prompted the diagnosis of the disease at earlier stages.[18] The introduction of cutting and coagulation instruments, such as monopolar or bipolar electrocoagulators and thermocoagulation devices, made surgical sampling possible.[19-21] Diagnostic accuracy has continued to improve since the introduction of ovarioscopy and microlaparoscopy.[22]

Surgical Treatment for Infertility

The management of endometriosis depends on the stage of the disease, the symptoms, and on the desire for future fertility.

Conservative Surgery

In 1929, Wharton published the first report on conservative surgery for endometriosis.[23] Over the next 50 years, numerous investigators have described refined operative techniques. Four objectives of conservative surgery were formulated by Buttram in 1979: (1) removal of all visible endometriosis and adhesions; (2) where possible, restoration of normal anatomy; (3) complete hemostasis; (4) and application of the rules of atraumatic and reconstructive surgery.[24] These objectives, although initially formulated for open surgery, continue to apply to any surgical treatment whether microsurgical or macrosurgical, and whether open or laparoscopic. Conservative surgery, as we know it today, became popular in the late 1960s. Initially, it was used for patients with advanced stages and/or previous surgery. Later, indications were extended to patients with less advanced stages. However, the benefits of surgical treatment of minimal or mild stages have not yet been proven.[18,25,26]

Surgical techniques have been described in detail by Buttram and by Malinak and Wheeler.[24,27] Superficial endometriosis is eradicated by coagulation or vaporization. As vital structures are present in the lateral pelvic sidewall, excisional techniques or thermal destruction with collateral protection is mandatory. Nodular lesions, particularly those involving the posterior cul-de-sac and uterosacral ligaments are excised. Reperitonealization is recommended for large denuded areas. Large ovarian endometriomas are enucleated rather than thermally treated, and subcapsulary closure of the ovary is performed. Reapproximation of uterosacral ligaments is advocated, pulling the cervix into the posterior fornix of the vagina and supporting the ovaries. Uterosuspension has been recommended to prevent adnexal structures from becoming adherent. Although adjuvants for the prevention of adhesions might be helpful, Buttram has stressed that surgical technique and skills are more important.

The use of magnification for infertility surgery in the female was introduced by Swolin.[28] It was performed with the use of binocular lenses or an operative microscope.[27,29] Microsurgical instruments such as glass hooks (rather than traumatic clamps), microscissors, microforceps, electromicrosurgical needles of 0.1 mm and bipolar microsurgical forceps of 0.2 mm are used. The operating field is continuously irrigated with isotonic balanced electrolyte solution. Gordts and coworkers described microsurgical techniques for ovarian endometrioma.[29] Using an elliptical incision along the axis of the ovary, the capsule is enucleated, following the plane of cleavage. After careful hemostasis, the ovary is repaired with inverted 5/0 nonabsorbable surgical suture (Prolene) stitches in the stroma and an 8/0 running suture on the cortex. In selected cases, free peritoneal grafts are applied over the denuded peritoneum.

Table 9.1 provides an overview by Candiani of the results of open conservative surgery for (advanced) endometriosis.[30] Extreme caution must be taken when comparing the results of these studies. They are not of similar design, are usually case series, and do not all include the same stages of disease.[10] There is no clear evidence that any technique is superior.

Laparoscopic Surgery

Today, laparoscopy can be extended into an operative procedure that provides treatment at the same time of the diagnosis. Simultaneous diagnosis and treatment reduce delay in treatment, number of procedures, and costs. However, there is no scientific proof that the laparoscopic approach benefits the patient more than

Table 9.1. Conservative laparotomy surgery for severe endometriosis.

Study	Classifiation	Number of patients	Pregnancy rate	MFR*
Acosta et al[92]	Acosta	39	33%	
Hammond et al[93]	Acosta	2	0%	
Sadigh et al[94]	Acosta	42	48%	
Garcia & David[95]	Acosta	49	29%	
Schenken & Malinak[62]	Acosta	21	29%	
Buttram[96]	Acosta/ Buttram	68	47%	
Rock et al[97]	AFS**	81	48%	1.5
Weeler & Malinak[98]	Acosta	119	30%	
Rantala et al[99]	Acosta	46	39%	
Chong & Baggish[100]	AFS**	10	30%	
Gordts et al[29]	AFS**	57	35%	
Olive & Lee[101]	Acosta	34	29%	1.4
Candiani et al[102]	AFS	8	38%	1.2
Donnez et al[103]	AFS	15	47%	2.6
Total		591	38%	

* Monthly Fecundity Rate per 100 women.
** Includes stage III (severe) and IV (extensive).

Source: Candiani.[30]

open surgery (Table 9.2). Correct indications, surgical experience and techniques, the completeness of the procedure, and the prevention of adhesion formation remain of utmost importance for the final result. Not only the goals of laparoscopic surgery but also the principles of gentle tissue handling and microsurgical techniques should remain the same as in open surgery.

Operative laparoscopic removal of endometriosis was first introduced by Semm in 1974.[32] In the United States, diagnostic laparoscopy began its revival in the early 1970s, but reports of laparoscopic surgery for endometriosis were first published in the late 1970s.[33–36]

Operative laparoscopy requires a two- to four-puncture technique and the use of some basic instruments: atraumatic probe, atraumatic forceps, and excisional (scissors or electrosurgical or laser knife) and hemostatic devices (monopolar, bipolar, or endo-coagulators). The loss of depth perception and the inability to palpate the involved tissues directly present major problems in identifying the extent of disease. But other advantages of laparoscopy offset these limitations.

Mechanical excision with laparoscopic scissors is an accepted treatment modality, but it may cause bleeding and subsequent adhesions.[37] The first electrosurgical high-frequency alternating current generator was designed in the 1920s by Cushing and Bovie; since then the principles have not changed.[38] Unipolar high-frequency electrosurgical removal is an established procedure but carries the risk of burning vital structures.[39] Bipolar coagulation was introduced as a safer alternative because tissue necrosis is more limited, and hazards by the unpredictable route of monopolar current are avoided.[20] Semm has argued for the use of an endocoagulator whose heat is generated by a resistance element at the top of a Teflon-coated probe.[21,32] Although very safe, coagulation with this device does not go deeper than 1 to 2 mm, making treatment of deeper implants incomplete.[40]

The vaporization of endometriotic implants has become popular since the introduction of the CO_2 laser in 1979 by Bruhat.[41] Successively other lasers were developed and used such as Nd:Yag by Lomano, Argon laser by Keye, and more recently KTP/532 by Daniell, and diode laser by Lower.[42–45] An interesting applica-

Table 9.2. Conservative laparoscopic surgery for severe endometriosis.

Author	Classification and stage	Modality	Number of patients	Pregnancy rate	MFR*
Hasson[36]	Hasson	Unipolar	5	75%	
Feste[84]	AFS III	CO_2	5	40%	
Martin[104]	AFS III	CO_2	4	25%	
Ingersoll[105]	Acosta	Excision/unipolar bipolar	20	60%	
Davis[106]	AFS-r III + IV	CO_2	33	52%	
Nezhat et al[107]	AFS III + IV	CO_2	27	44%	2.5
Martin[108]	AFS III + IV	CO_2	14	64%	
Keye et al[109]	AFS III	ARgon	5	20%	2.5
Olive & Martin[110]	AFS III	CO_2	20	50%	4.5
Donnez[111]	AFS III	CO_2	7	43%	2.4
Gast et al[112]	AFS-r III	CO_2	19	47%	2.6
Damewood & Rock[113]	AFS-r III + IV	Excision/bipolar	14	21%	2.1
Corson etr al[114]	AFS-r IV	ND:YAG	7	57%	
Canis et al[115]	AFS-r IV	Excision/CO_2	24	38%	3.3
Sutton & Hill[116]	AFS-r IV	CO_2	2	100%	
Total			206	48%	

* Monthly Fecundity Rate per 100 women.

Source: Candiani.[30]

tion of endo-ovarian argon fiber laser to destroy endometrial implants was developed by Brosens, which is not absorbed by the distending saline solution but interacts with the pigmented endometriotic lesions.[22]

Surgery for Pelvic Pain

Open Surgery

Pelvic pain, the most common symptom in endometriosis, is present in almost one third of patients. Presacral neurectomy (PSN) or interruption of the presacral nerve originating from the intermediate and superior hypogastric plexus, was introduced in 1898 by Jaboulay.[46] In 1949, Cotte reported on about 1500 cases with a success rate of 98%. In a later compilation, the success rate was 86%; in cases of secondary dysmenorrhea, 72%.[49]

Although division of the uterosacral ligaments was first described in 1899 by Ruggi, it was proposed only in 1954 by Doyle as an alternative to PSN.[50,51] The rationale was that the nerve supply to the cervix is not necessarily completely interrupted by PSN.[52] The procedure could be done either by the vaginal or abdominal route. The latter was recommended for cases of endometriosis. Initially, a peritoneal fold was interposed after division. Later, both ligaments were sutured together to the midline of the posterior face of the isthmus, about 1 cm higher than the original insertion, and using stainless steel sutures. Impressive results of 86% pain relief were noted; in cases of secondary dysmenorrhea, with concomitant treatment of pelvic pathology, even a 87% success rate was reported.[53] With the arrival of medical therapy and because of the lack of controlled studies both procedures were largely abandoned.

Laparoscopic Surgery

There has been a renewed interest in surgery for pelvic pain as these procedures are now feasible through the laparoscope. The procedure originally described by Doyle has been revived as laparoscopic uterine nerve ablation (LUNA). First suggested in 1974 by Frangenheim and Kleindienst, some later series reported the use of laser instrumentation (Table 9.3).[54,55] The technique varies among surgeons. Next to division and/or removal of part of the uterosacral ligaments, Sutton and Donnez vaporize the posterior aspect of the uterine isthmus to interrupt crossing fibers.[56,57] Although it appears easy, at first view, it must be stressed that complications such as hemorrhage, even with fatal outcome, and damage to the ureter have been reported.[58] Failures were explained by alternative pathways of pain fibers accompanying the vessels, incompleteness of the procedure, and inappropriate selection of patients for the procedure.[59] The true

Table 9.3. Laparoscopic uterine nerve ablation.

Author	Energy source	Total No./ No. with secondary dysmenorrhea	Failure rate (primary/ secondary) dysmenorrhea)
Feste[84]	CO_2	186/NS	13%/NS
Daniell[85]	KTP	100/80	28%/25%
Lichten & Bombard[55]	Mechanical & electrosurgery	11/NS	<20%/NS
Sutton & Nisolle[56]	CO_2	126/100	16%/13%
Donnez & Nisolle[57]	CO_2	100/NS	9%/NS
Perry & Azziz[86]	Not stated	NS/200	NS/50%
Gürgan et al.[59]	CO_2	23/3	30%/NS
Stutts et al[87]	Mixed	91/NS	22%/NS

NS Not stated.

efficiency of the procedure for pain associated with endometriosis has not been established in prospective, placebo-controlled studies. The long-term effect appears to be limited.

More recently, presacral neurectomy came within reach of the laparoscopic surgeon (Table 9.4). It requires intimate knowledge of anatomy of the retroperitoneal space and advanced surgical skills. The time needed to acquire the ability to perform such advanced laparoscopic procedures exceeds that of laparotomy.[60] The success rates of laparoscopically performed procedures appear to be the same as those through the open approach. But both approaches need rigorous evaluation. Meanwhile, patient selection should be restricted to those with centrally located dysmenorrhea which fail to respond to medication.

Radical Surgery

In the early days of treating endometriosis, radical surgery was the sole treatment. Now, it is seldom indicated prior to attempted conception, but rather reserved for patients with intractable pain who have completed their family or for cases of previously failed conservative surgery. About 12% of all endometriosis patients require radical surgery, but this could be an underestimate.[61] Such surgery usually includes the removal of ovaries. Whether this step is necessary, however, is still debated. But there is strong evidence

Table 9.4. Laparoscopic presacral neurectomy.

Author	Energy source	Number of patients	Failure rate
Perez[88]	—	25	8%
Nezhat et al.[60]	CO_2	86	10%
Perry & Azziz[86]	Nd:YAG	50	8%
Perez & Redwine[89]	Electrosurgery and Nd:YAG	58	4%

that the only realistic therapy for a permanent cure is removal of both uterus and ovaries.[62,63] Montgomery and Studd showed that when ovarian tissue is preserved, the reoperation rate can be as high as 45%.[64]

Total abdominal hysterectomy and/or bilateral salpingo-oophorectomy is normally performed by a low transverse incision (Pfannenstiel, Cherney, Maylard), but some cases might benefit from a vertical incision. Whatever the incision selected, the goal is to obtain proper access to the lateral pelvic walls, because the disease is usually extensively spread. If the ovaries are normal and to be preserved, some authors advocate the fixation of these structures away from the vaginal vault, in order to prevent subsequent pain during intercourse.[8]

The most recent change in radical surgery is that these operations can be performed endoscopically. In 1989, Reich described the first case of laparoscopic hysterectomy.[65] For severe endometriosis requiring radical surgery, and where the vaginal route is obviously more difficult, laparoscopic assisted hysterectomy seems a realistic alternative: the completeness of the laparoscopic removal of endometriotic implants and/or adhesions is enhanced by the good visualization of the peritoneum and all lesions. Then, the procedure can be completed totally via laparoscope or with a combined vaginal and laparoscopic approach still offering the patient all advantages of vaginal hysterectomy.

Laparoscopic hysterectomy appears to be not only a feasible, but also a safe procedure with acceptable complication rates and improved recovery rate.[66,67] In a Belgian multicentric register of 182 cases, 34% of laparoscopic hysterectomies were performed because of endometriosis (all stages).[66] The rate of major complications was 2%. In Liu's series of 215 patients, 44% were operated on because of endometriosis with a complication rate of 9.2%.[67] This technique needs further evaluation, particularly to see what happens if this procedure is performed by less experienced laparoscopic surgeons. We also have to await long-term results and reoperation rates.

Rectovaginal Endometriosis

Cullen described this nodular form of endometriosis in 1920.[3] The relationship between active implants in the posterior pouch of Douglas and deep dyspareunia has been clearly demonstrated.[68] The histology of this longtime neglected entity has been reviewed.[69,70] Although medication may reduce pain caused by these foci, surgical excision is advocated by many authors.[69,71,72] Reich pioneered many of these advanced endoscopic techniques, such as of cul-de-sac desobliteration and resection of nodules in the rectovaginal septum.[73] Others, like Koninckx, Nezhat, Martin using the CO_2 laser, and Redwine, with sharp excision, have reported good success rates.[60,68,72,74] The proximity of

vital structures, and especially the potential for bowel perforation, makes this type of major endoscopic surgery appropriate only for highly experienced laparoscopists. The extent of the disease seems only to be evaluative during excision, but the benefits of CO_2 laser regarding this aspect remain to be proven.[60,68,72]

Extrapelvic Endometriosis

Intestinal Endometriosis

Management is based on localization, extent, and impact on bowel function.[75] After medical pretreatment, surgery may be conservative, such as local resection of individual spots (enterotomy), or, in more extensive cases, partial or segmental resection of involved bowel. Always, the aim is complete removal of all endometriotic lesions.

In cases of intestinal obstruction, immediate intervention is needed; in other cases, preoperative mechanical and/or antibiotic bowel preparation is mandatory. The patient should be informed about the possibility of laparotomy. Colonoscopy, barium enema, IV pyelogram, and general surgery consultation is recommended. At surgery, superficial and intramural lesions are locally excised and reperitonealized. Prepared enterotomy carries few risks and closure is performed transversely in layers to minimize the risk of postoperative bowel stricture.[76] If bowel preparation is performed, segmental resection can be anastomosed primarily.

During the past few years, the feasibility of endoscopic management has been demonstrated (Table 9.5). Nezhat reported a successful endoscopic proctectomy for rectal endometriosis.[77] A worrying observation by Martin was the 100% failure rate in his experience.[78] New technology for bowel reanastomosis, and development of devices such as rectal and vaginal probes will make this surgery more feasible and, perhaps, more successful. Meanwhile, endoscopic surgery for these lesions is restricted to specialized centers. Elsewhere, laparotomy remains the standard.[78,79]

Urinary Tract Endometriosis

Bladder and ureter lesions occur in fewer than 1% of cases. In case of obstruction, immediate intervention is mandatory. If lesions are nonobstructive, medical pretreatment may benefit the patient.[75] Segmental

Table 9.5. Laparoscopic surgery for intra- and transmural bowel endometriosis.

Author	Procedure
Reich et al.[90]	Enterotomy
Redwine & Sharpe[91]	Enterotomy, segmental resection
Nezhat et al.[77]	Enterotomy, proctectomy
Martin[72]	Enterotomy

resection and anastomosis of the ureter or ureteral reimplantation by laparotomy have been the preferred approaches. However, in 1992, Nezhat resected a ureter implant and performed laparoscopic uretero-ureteral anastomosis.[80]

The Future

A number of changes in therapeutic strategies have been predicted in the field of both medical and surgical treatment of endometriosis. Further improvement of the approach of videolaparoscopy is expected: cameras and monitors are improving as resolution increases even up to high definition television (HDTV) level of over 1,200 lines. As smaller fiberoptic endoscopes are developed, diagnostic procedures can be done under local anesthesia as an office procedure.[61] There is already some experience in three-dimensional video technology, which could make advanced endoscopic surgery more accessible to the vast majority of gynecologists. Because of the complexity of the endoscopic approach, formal credentialing and organization of postgraduate training courses is needed.[82]

Energy modalities are changing: safety might be enhanced by the use of bipolar cutting devices. As new lasers with variable wavelengths are introduced, they might offer a combination of cutting and coagulation in a so-called bloodless scalpel.

An exciting new field of photodynamic therapy is under development.[81,83] Theoretically, a photosensitizing drug may be administered and retained by the endometriotic implants. Lesions would then be exposed to light of a certain wavelength, which interacts with the drug, causing destructive oxidation of cellular structures. The vascular and neoproliferative nature and the sensitivity to hormones of endometriotic tissue make it a good model for photodynamic therapy. Although still experimental, this selective treatment at the cellular level may transform the dream of treating microscopic disease to reality.

References

1. Rokitansky C. Zesch Gessellsch Aertze, (Wien) 1860;16: 577.
2. Diesterweg A. Ein fall von Cystadenofibroma Uteri. Z Geburtshilfe 1883;9:191.
3. Cullen TS. Adenomyoma des Uterus. Vorlag von Augustus Hirschwald, Berlin.
4. Sampson JA. Perforating hemorrhagic (chocolate) cysts of the ovary. Arch Surg 1921;3:245.
5. Sampson JA. Peritoneal endometriosis due to the menstrual dissimination of endometrial tissue into the peritoneal cavity. Am J Obstet Gynecol 1927;14:422.
6. Rogers SF, Jacobs WM. Infertility and endometriosis: conservative surgical approach. Fertil Steril 1968;19:529.
7. Wheeler JH, Malinak LR. The surgical management of endometriosis. Obstet Gynecol Clin North Am 1989;16: 147.
8. Kistner RW. The use of newer progestins in the treatment of endometriosis. Am J Obstet Gynecol 1958;75: 264.
9. DeCherney AH. The leader of the band is tired. Fertil Steril 1985;35:521.
10. Gant NF. Infertility and endometriosis: comparison of pregnancy outcomes with laparotomy versus laparoscopic techniques. Am J Obstet Gynecol 1992;166:1072.
11. McComb PF. A new suturing instrument that allows the use of microsuture at laparoscopy. Fertil Steril 1992;57: 936.
12. Janssen RPS, Russell P. Non-pigmented endometriosis. Clinical laparoscopic and pathologic definition. Am J Obstet Gynecol 1986;155:1154.
13. Stripling MC, Martin DC, Chatman DL, Vander Zwaag R and Poston WM. Subtle appearance of pelvic endometriosis. Fertil Steril 1988;49:427.
14. Wiegerinck AHMM, Van Dop PA, Brosens IA. The staging of peritoneal endometriosis by the type of active lesion in addition to the revised American Fertility Society classification. Fertil Steril 1993 (in press).
15. The American Fertility Society. Revised AFS classification of endometriosis. Fertil Steril 1985;43:351.
16. Fourestière M, Gladu A, Vulmière J. La péritonéoscopie. Presse Médicale 1943;5:46.
17. Hopkins HH. On the diffraction theory of optical images. Proceedings of the Royal Society 1953;A217:408.
18. Wheeler JH. The epidemiology of endometriosis-associated infertility. J Reprod Med 1990;34:41.
19. Frangenheim H. Laparoscopy and culdoscopy in gynecology. London, Butterworth, 1972.
20. Rioux JE, Cloutier D. Bipolar cautery for sterilization by laparoscopy. J Reprd Med 1974;13:6.
21. Semm K. Endocoagulation: a new field of endoscopic surgery. J Reprod Med 1976;16:195.
22. Brosens I, Puttemans P. Double-optic laparoscopy: salpingoscopy, ovarian cystoscopy and endo-ovarian surgery with the Argon laser. Ballière's Clin Obstet Gynaecol 1989;3:595.
23. Wharton L. Conservative surgical treatment of pelvic endometriosis. South Med J 1929;22:267.
24. Buttram VC. Principles of conventional conservative surgery. In Chadha DR, Buttram VC, eds. Current Concepts in Endometriosis, New York, Alan R. Liss, Inc., 1990, p 269.
25. Malinak LR, Wheeler JH. Does mild endometriosis cause infertility? Semin Reprod Endocrinol 1988;6:239.
26. Brosens I. Endometriosis related to infertility. Curr Opinions Obstet Gynecol 1991;3:205.
27. Malinak LA, Wheeler JH. Conservative surgery for endometriosis. In Wilson EA, ed. Endometriosis. New York, Alan R Liss, Inc. 1987, p 141.
28. Swolin K. Electromicrosurgery. In Crosiagnani R, ed. Microsurgery in Female Infertility. London, Academic Press, 1980, p 35.
29. Gordts S, Boeckx W, Brosens I. Microsurgery of endometriosis in infertile patients. Fertil Steril 1984;42: 520.
30. Candiani GB, Vercellin P, Fedele L, et al. Conservative surgical treatment for severe endometriosis in infertile women: are we making progress? Obstet Gynecol Surv 1991;46:410.
31. Brosens I, Boeckx W, Page G. Microsurgery of ovarian endometriosis. Hum Reprod 1988;3:365.

32. Semm K. The laparoscopic instrumentation. In Semm K, ed. Atlas of Gynecologic Laparoscopy and Hysteroscopy. Philadelphia, WB Saunders Co., 1977;30.
33. Phillips JM, Keith D, Keiler L, et al. Survey of gynecologic laparoscopy. J Reprod Med 1975;15:45.
34. Eward RD. Cauterization of stage I & II endometriosis and resulting pregnancy rate. In Phillips JM, ed. Endoscopy in Gynaecology. Downey, CA, AAGL, 1978.
35. Cohen MR. Laparoscopy and the management of endometriosis. J Reprod Med 1979;23:81.
36. Hasson HM. Electrocoagulation of pelvic endometriotic lesions with laparoscopic control. Am J Obstet Gynecol 1979;135:115.
37. Redwine D. Conservative laparoscopic excision of endometriosis by sharp dissection: life table analysis of reoperation and recurrent disease. Fertil Steril 1991;56: 628.
38. Cushing H, Bovie WT. Electrosurgery as an aid to the removal of intracranial tumors. Surg Gynecol Obstet 1928;47:731.
39. Chamberlain G, Brown JC. Gynaecological laparoscopy. The Report of the Working Party of the Confidential Enquiry into Gynaecological Laparoscopy. London, Royal College of Obstetricians and Gynaecologists, 1978.
40. Keye WR. Laparoscopic treatment of endometriosis. Obstet Gynecol Clin North Am 1989;16:157.
41. Bruhat MA, Mage C, Manhes M. Use of the carbon-dioxide laser via laparoscopy. In Kaplan I, ed. Laser Surgery III, Proceedings of the Third Congress of International Society for Laser Surgery, Tel Aviv, 1979, p 273.
42. Lomano JM. Nd:YAG laser ablation for early pelvic endometriosis: a report of 61 cases. Laser Surg Med 1987;7:56.
43. Keye WR, Dixon J. Photocoagulation of endometriosis by the Argon laser through the laparoscope. Obstet Gynecol 1983;62:383.
44. Daniell JF, Miller W, Tish R. Initial evaluation of the use of the KTP532 laser in gynaecologic laparoscopy. Fertil Steril 1986;46:373.
45. Lower AM, Coumbe A, Armstrong P, et al. Scandinavian Laser Society, Oslo, March 1993.
46. Jaboulay M. Le traitement de la névralgie pelvienne par la paralyse du sympathique sacre. Lyon Méd 1898;90: 102.
47. Cotte G. La symphathectomie hypogastrique: a-t-elle sa place dans la thérapeutique gynécologique? Presse Méd 1925;33:98.
48. Cotte G. Technique of presacral neurectomy. Am J Surg 1949;78:50.
49. Black WT. Use of presacral sympathectomy in the treatment of dysmenorrhea: a second look after 25 years. Am J Obstet Gynecol 1964;89:16.
50. Ruggi C. La sympatectomia abdominale utero-ovarica come mezzo di cura di alcune lesiani interne degli organi genitali della donna. Bologna, Zanichelli, 1899.
51. Doyle JB. Paracervical uterine denervation for dysmenorrhea. Trans New Engl Obstet Gyne Soc 1954;8: 143.
52. Wente JC. Conduction of visceral pain. N Engl J Med 1952;246:686.
53. Doyle JB, DeRosiers JJ. Paracervical uterine denervation for relief of pelvic pain. Clin Obstet Gynecol 1963; 6:742.
54. Frangenheim H, Kleindienst W. Chronic pelvic disease of unknown origin. In Phillips JM, ed. Gynecologic laparoscopy. New York, Stratton 1974, p 52.
55. Lichten EM, Bombard J. Surgical treatment of dysmenorrhea with laparoscopic uterine nerve ablation. J Reprod Med 1987;32:37.
56. Sutton CD. CO_2 laser laparoscpoy in endometriosis. Ballière's Clin Obstet Gynaecol 1989;3:499.
57. Donnez J, Nisolle M. CO_2 laser laparoscopic surgery. Ballière's Clin Obstet Gynaecol 1989;3:525.
58. Granger DA, Soderstrom RM, Schiff SF, et al. Ureteral injury at laparoscopy. Obstet Gynecol 1990;75:839.
59. Gurgan T, Urman B, Ahm T, et al. Laparoscopic CO_2 LUNA for treatment of drug resistant primary dysmenorrhea. Fertil Steril 1992;58:422.
60. Nezhat C, Silfen S, Nezhat F, et al. Surgery for endometriosis. Curr Op Obstet Gynecol 1991;3:385.
61. Cook AS, Rock JA. The role of laparoscopy in the treatment of endometriosis. Fertil Steril 1991;55:663.
62. Schenken RS, Malinak LR. Reoperation after initial treatment of endometriosis with conservative surgery. Am J Obstet Gynecol 1978;131:416.
63. Wheeler JH, Malinak LR. Recurrent endometriosis: incidents, management and prognosis. Am J Obstet Gynecol 1983;146:247.
64. Montgomery JC, Studd JW. Oestradiol and testosterone implants after hysterectomy for endometriosis. Contrib Gynecol Obstet 1987;16:241.
65. Reich H, DeCaprio J, McGlynn F. Laparoscopic hysterectomy. J Gynecol Surg 1989;5:213.
66. Belcohyst: Deprest J, Cusmano P, Hardy A, et al. Multicentric registration on laparoscopic hysterectomy: A one year's experience. Abstract book of Raoul Palmer Club of Gynaecologic Endoscopy. September 10–11, 1992, Clermont Ferrand, France.
67. Liu CY. Laparoscopic Hysterectomy. Report of 213 cases. Gynaecol Endosc 1992;1:73.
68. Koninckx PR, Meuleman C, Demeyere S, et al. Suggestive evidence that pelvic endometriosis is a progressive disease, whereas deeply infiltrating endometriosis is associated with pelvic pain. Fertil Steril 1991;55:759.
69. Cornillie FH, Oosterlynck O, Lauwereyns J, et al. Deeply infiltrating pelvic endometriosis: histology and clinical significance. Fertil Steril 1990;53:978.
70. Brosens I. Classification of endometriosis revisited. Lancet 1993;341:630.
71. Donnez J, Nisolle M, Casanas-Roux F, et al. Endometriosis: rationale for surgery. In Borsens I, Donnez J, eds. Current Status of Endometriosis: Research and Management. New York, Parthenon Publishers, 1993, p 385.
72. Martin DC. Laparoscopic and vaginal colpotomy for the excision of infiltrating cul-de-sac endometriosis. J Reprod Med 1988;33:806.
73. Reich H. New techniques in advanced laparoscopic surgery. Ballière's Clin Obstet Gynaecol 1989;3:655.
74. Redwine DB, Perez JJ. En bloc resection for treatment of the obliterated cul-de-sac in endometriosis. J Reprod Med 1992;37:695.
75. Markham SM, Carpenter SE, Rock JA. Extrapelvic endometriosis. Obstet Gynecol Clin North Am 1989;16: 193.
76. Grunert GM, Franklin RR, Bailly MR. Surgical management of intestinal endometriosis. In Brosens I, Donnez J, eds. Current Status of Endometriosis: Research and Management. New York, Parthenon Publishers, 1993, p 447.
77. Nezhat C, Nezhat F, Pennington E. Laparoscopic proctectomy for infiltrating endometriosis of the rectum. Fertil Steril 1992;57:1129.

78. Martin DC. Laparoscopic treatment of endometriosis. In Azziz R, Murphy AA, eds. Practical Manual of Operative Laparoscopy and Hysteroscopy. New York, Springer Verlag, 1992, p 101.

79. Corenado C, Franklin RR, Lotze EC, et al. Surgical treatment of symptomatic colerectal endometriosis. Fertil Steril 1990;53:411.

80. Nezhat C, Nezhat F, Green B. Laparoscopic treatment of obstructed ureter due to endometriosis by resection and ureterostomy. J Urol 1992;148:865.

81. Keye WR. The present and future application of lasers to the treatment of endometriosis and infertility. Int J Fertil 1986;31:160.

82. Brosens I. Endoscopic surgery. Eur J Obstet Gynaecol Reprod Biol 1993;48:155.

83. Manyak MJ, Nelson LM, Solomon D, et al. Photodynamic therapy of rabbit endometrial implants. Fertil Steril 1989;52:140.

84. Feste JR. Laser laparoscopy, a new modality. J Reprod Med 1985;30:413.

85. Daniell JF. Fiberoptic laser laparoscopy. Ballière's Clin Obstet Gynaecol 1989;3:545.

86. Perry CP, Azziz R. In Azziz R and Murphy AA, eds. Practical Manual of Operative Laparoscopy and Hysteroscopy. Springer-Verlag, New York, 1992, p 143.

87. Stutts L, Yarbrough R, Perry CP, et al. LUNA: long-term follow-up of 91 patients. In Hunt RB and Martin DC, eds. Endoscopy in Gynecology, AAGL. Baltimore, Port City Press, 1993, p 91.

88. Perez JJ. Laparoscopic Presacral Neurectomy: results in the first 25 cases. J Reprod Med 1990;35:625.

89. Perez JJ, Redwine DB. Laparoscopic presacral neurectomy. In Soderstrom RM, ed. Operative Laparoscopy. New York, Raven Press, 1992, p 157.

90. Reich H, McGlynn F, Budin R. Laparoscopic repair of full thickness bowel injury. J Laparoendosc Surg 1991;1:119.

91. Redwine DB, Sharpe DR. Laparoscopic segmental resection of the sigmoid colon for endometriosis. J Laparoendosc Surg 1991;1:217.

92. Acosta AA, Buttram VC Jr, Besch PK, et al. A proposed classification of pelvic endometriosis. Obstet Gynecol 1973;42:19.

93. Hammond CB, Rock JA, Parker RT. Conservative treatment of endometriosis: The effects of limited surgery and hormonal pseudopregnancy. Fertil Steril 1976;27:756.

94. Sadigh H, Naples JD Jr, Batt RE. Conservative surgery for endometriosis in the infertile couple. Obstet Gynecol 1977;49:562.

95. Garcia CR, David SS. Pelvic endometriosis: infertility and pelvic pain. Am J Obstet Gynecol 1977;129:740.

96. Buttram VC Jr. Conservative surgery for endometriosis in the infertile female: a study of 206 patients with implications for both medical and surgical therapy. Fertil Steril 1979;31:117.

97. Rock JA, Guzick DS, Sengos C, et al. The conservative surgical treatment of endometriosis: evaluation of pregnancy success with respect to the extent of disease as categorized using contemporary classification systems. Fertil Seril 1981;35:131.

98. Wheeler JM, Malinak LR. Postoperative danazol therapy in infertility patients with severe endometriosis. Fertil Steril 1981;36:460.

99. Rantala ML, Kahanpaa KV, Koskimies AI, et al. Fertility prognosis after surgical treatment of pelvic endometriosis. Acta Obstet Gynecol Scand 1983;62:11.

100. Chong AP, Baggish MS. Management of pelvic endometriosis by means of inraabdominal carbon dioxide laser. Fertil Steril 1984;41:14.

101. Olive DL, Lee KL. Analysis of sequential treatment protocols for endometriosis-associated infertility. Am J Obstet Gynecol 1986;154:163.

102. Candiani GB, Fedele L, Vercellini P. Conservative surgical treatment of endometriosis. Acta Eur Fertil 1986;17:173.

103. Donnez J, Lemaire-Rubbers M, Karaman Y, et al. Combined (hormonal and microsurgical) therapy in infertile women with endometriosis. Fertil Steril 1987;48:239.

104. Martin DC. CO_2 laser laparoscopy for the treatment of endometriosis associated with infertility. J Reprod Med 1985;30:409.

105. Ingersoll FM. Selection of medical or surgical treatment of endometriosis. Clin Obstet Gynecol 1977;20:849.

106. Davis GD. Management of endometriosis and its associated adhesions with the CO_2 laser laparoscope. Obstet Gynecol 1986;68:422.

107. Nezhat C, Crowgey SR, Garrison CP. Surgical treatment of endometriosis via laser laparoscopy. Fertil Steril 1986;45:778.

108. Martin DC. CO_2 laser laparoscopy for endometriosis associated with infertility. J Reprod Med 1986;31:1089.

109. Keye WR, Hansen LW, Astin M, et al. Argon laser therapy of endometriosis: a review of 92 consecutive patients. Fertil Steril 1987;47:208.

110. Olive DL, Martin DC. Treatment of endometriosis-associated infertility with CO_2 laser laparoscopy: the use of one and two parameter exponential models. Fertil Steril 1987;48:18–23.

111. Donnez J. CO_2 laser laparoscopy in infertile women with endometriosis and women with adnexal adhesions. Fertil Steril 1987;48:390–94.

112. Gast MJ, Tobler R, Strickler RC, et al. Laser vaporization of endometriosis in an infertile population: the role of complicating infertility factors. Fertil Steril 1988;49:32–6.

113. Damewood MD, Rock JA. Treatment independent pregnancy with operative laparoscopy for endometriosis in an in vitro fertilization program. Fertil Steril 1988;50:463–65.

114. Corson SL, Unger M, Kwa D, et al. Laparoscopic laser treatment of endometriosis with the Nd:YAG sapphire probe. Am J Obstet Gynecol 1989;160:718–23.

115. Canis M, Mage G, Manhes H, et al. Laparoscopic treatment of endometriosis. Acta Obstet Gynecol Scand 1989;150(Suppl):15.

116. Sutton C, Hill D. Laser laparoscopy in the treatment of endometriosis: a 5-year study. Br J Obstet Gynaecol 1990;97:181.

10

Techniques for Ablation and Excision of Endometriosis

Michel Canis, Maurice Antoine Bruhat, Jean Luc Pouly, Michael J.W. Cooper, Arnaud Wattiez, and Hubert Manhes

The goals of surgical treatment of endometriosis are to completely ablate and/or excise active endometriotic tissue and correct anatomic distortions caused by adhesions and cystic lesions.[1] Over the past few years, laparoscopic surgery has become a valuable addition to conventional and microsurgical approaches by laparotomy. The choice of approach (laparotomy or laparoscopy), surgical technique (excision, coagulation, vaporization), and instruments (CO_2 laser, electrocautery, or scissors) is according to the surgeon's preference (see Figs. 10.1 through 10.6 and color plates 10.1 through 10.6). The key issue is to adequately identify and treat the disease. By selecting the most effective surgical modality for each location and each patient, the desired postoperative results can best be achieved. A wide variety of surgical and medical treatments are now available, but it is important to take into account the limits of each approach. For example, medical treatments have no effect on dense pelvic adhesions, whereas surgery is unsuitable for microscopic disease.

Many recent studies have suggested that laparoscopy often offers the best surgical approach. However, many questions have still to be answered: the activity of the implants, postoperative adhesion reformation, and recurrence of disease. Endometriosis remains a poorly understood disease. New treatments seem more likely to be designed in laboratories than in operating theaters.

Operating Room

As for any surgical procedure, adequate preparation and exposure is crucial. The day before surgery at our hospital, each patient is given a bowel prep similar to that used in bowel surgery. When endometriosis is suspected, particularly deep infiltrating disease, the patient is draped to permit access to the vagina. She lies in a modified dorsal lithotomy position with legs slightly flexed (15° to 20°) and abducted to form a 45° angle. This position allows easy manipulation of the uterus, permits intraoperative pelvic examination, provides good access to the vagina and to the rectum, and offers room for proper insertion of ancillary instruments in the suprapubic area. A shoulder brace is placed on the left side and the left arm is fixed alongside the patient's body.

Manipulation of the uterus is performed using a long curette taped to a tenaculum. The Trendelenburg position is routinely used as one of the main laparoscopic retractors. The correct angle, about 10°, pushes the bowel loops and omentum over the superior pelvic brim. A steeper Trendelenburg may be necessary at the beginning of the procedure to achieve initial exposure. The pneumoperitoneum, which serves as a retractor, should be maintained using an automatic insufflator capable of delivering 9L/minute.[2,3] Prophylactic antibiotics are routinely administered to patients with ovarian endometriomas, deep infiltrating peritoneal implants, or a previous history of pelvic inflammatory disease.

Staging Endometriosis

In describing the appearance of peritoneal endometriosis, several authors have reported atypical, subtle, typical, and deeply invasive peritoneal implants.[4-6] One team advocates routine puncture of enlarged ovarian endometriomas.[7] For proper staging, each lesion should be included and each pelvic area routinely assessed and described in the operative report using the AFS-r scoring system. Correct laparoscopic staging includes the following steps:

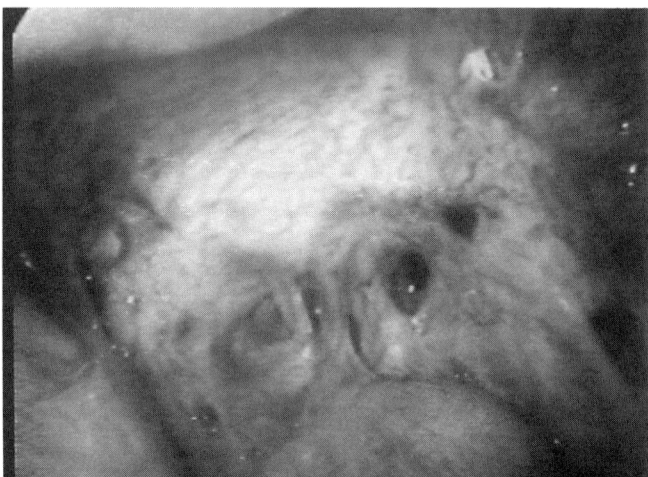

Figure 10.1. Atypical peritoneal implants and partial obliteration of the posterior cul-de-sac. See also color plate.

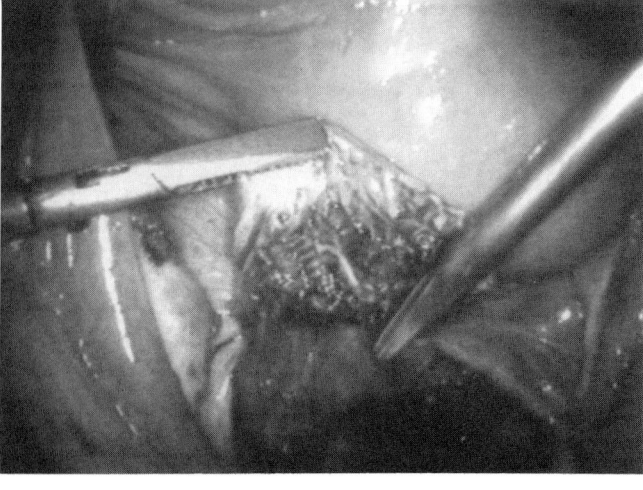

Figure 10.3. Excision of a large nodule (>2cm in diameter) of the rectovaginal septum. See also color plate.

- exposure of pelvis, obtained using laparoscopic retractors and one or two 5mm trocars inserted in suprapubic area;
- removal of adhesions preventing access to the pelvis or holding bowel in the presacral area;
- routine aspiration of peritoneal fluid when managing adnexal masses and inspecting posterior cul-de-sac;
- mobilization of tubes and ovaries when looking for adnexal adhesions;
- complete ovariolysis to detect ovarian endometriomas located on the anterior ovarian surface;
- meticulous inspection of the pelvic peritoneum using magnification provided by the laparoscope when looking for small and/or atypical implants;
- puncture of enlarged ovaries and starlike ovarian scars when looking for small endometriomas;

- intraoperative vaginal and/or rectal examination to assess posterior cul-de-sac and rectum;[8] and
- careful inspection of upper abdomen when looking for bowel or appendicular involvement.

Whenever an ovarian endometrioma has been ruptured or punctured, we copiously irrigate the pelvis, inspect the internal cyst wall, and routinely take biopsies to differentiate endometriomas from functional cysts and to rule out malignancy.[9] Similarly, peritoneal implants should be biopsied to exclude nonendometriotic peritoneal abnormalities such as hemangiomas or Walthard islets. Frozen sections may be useful to help decide on the management of chocolate cysts and to avoid unnecessary ovarian damage when only luteal cysts are present.

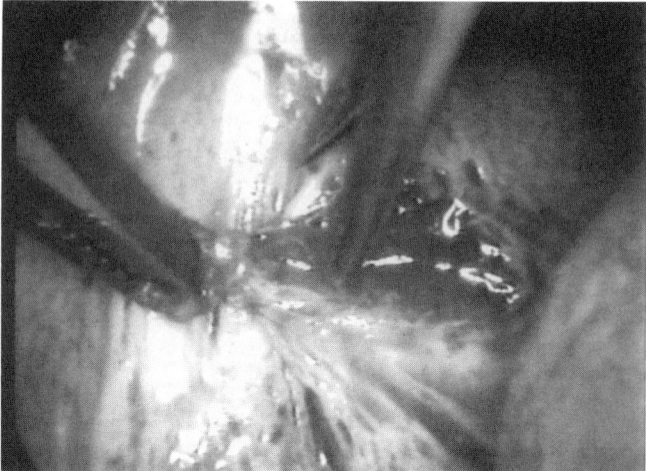

Figure 10.2. Excision of superficial peritoneal implants of the right broad ligament is performed with a grasping forceps and scissors. See also color plate.

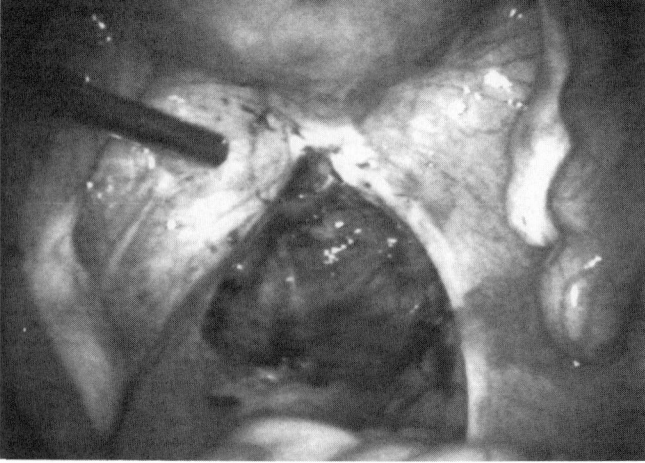

Figure 10.4. Final view after excision of nodule of the rectovaginal septum. See also color plate.

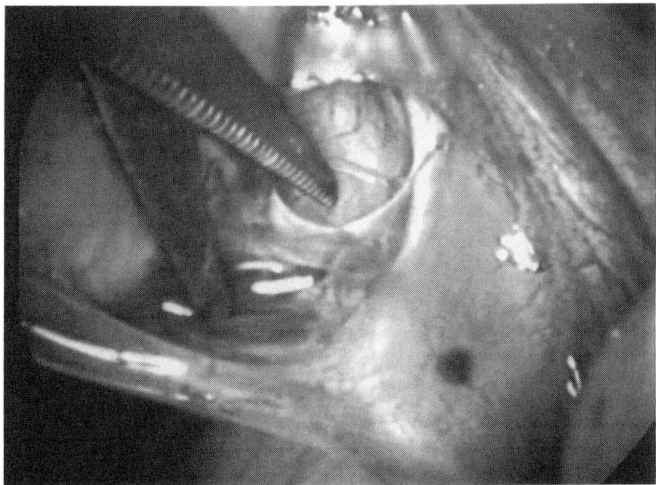

Figure 10.5. Laparoscopic ovariolysis obtained with scissors; subovarian endometriotic adhesions are visible on broad ligament. See also color plate.

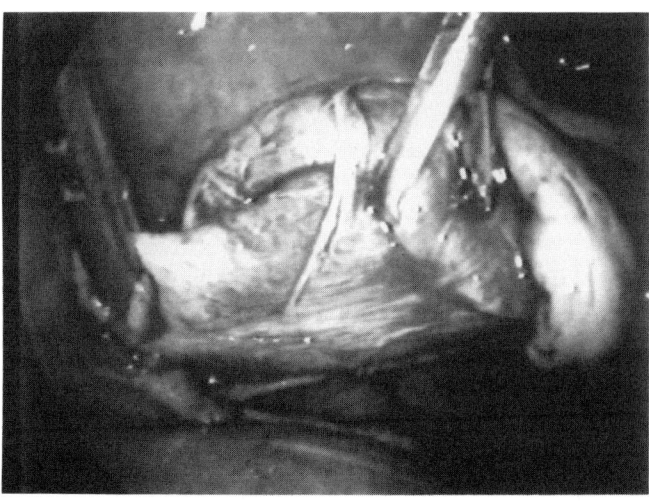

Figure 10.6. Laparoscopic ovarian cystectomy; the red fibrotic tissue on the surface of the cyst wall suggests that one should get closer to the cyst wall to identify the cleavage plane. See also color plate.

General Treatment Principles

Endometriotic implants can be treated using excision or in situ destruction achieved by coagulation or vaporization. Although excision will often include a more extensive dissection of the adjacent structures, coagulation or vaporization are potentially as dangerous to the ureters and rectum and as difficult as excision.

Endometriosis is an invasive disease that traumatizes a very effective healing tissue, the peritoneum. Peritoneal implants are not "intraperitoneal" lesions, but rather superficial or deep retroperitoneal lesions. Therefore, complete treatment includes a retroperitoneal procedure often close to the ureters, the uterine vessels, or the rectum.

The lesions are often surrounded by fibrosis. Active glands and stroma may be identified during histologic examination of tissues that appeared purely fibrotic without any evidence of chocolate cysts. This fibrosis, more abundant around deep infiltrating implants, often produces severe anatomic distortions. For such implants, complete treatment of fibrotic tissue is required.

The key to complete treatment is differentiating normal and abnormal tissues. This ability depends on the surgeon's expertise and on the technique used. Most authorities agree that excisional techniques improve tissue recognition when compared with vaporization and/or coagulation. It may be difficult to distinguish normal coagulated or carbonized tissue from abnormal tissue. Therefore, use only (or mostly) a cutting effect when outlining the limits of lesions to be excised. Similarly, with a CO_2 laser, use a very high-power density to avoid carbonization.

Irrespective of the procedure, identify the tissue before removing it. In simple cases, identification is achieved by inspection; in fibrosis and deep implants, by dissection. In this way, hydrodissection and scissors are actually the best laparoscopic instruments to identify the normal surrounding tissue.

Since permanent visual control is key to safe and complete procedures, careful hemostasis and frequent peritoneal lavages are required. When possible, proceed from the lower to the upper part of the pelvis so that bleeding induced by the first steps will not obscure the operative field. Move from the posterior to the anterior part of the pelvis to allow better visualization.

Conservative laparoscopic surgery should follow all the principles of microsurgery: frequent irrigation of the operative field, minimal and gentle tissue handling, and careful but meticulous hemostasis using fine bipolar forceps to avoid extensive thermal damages. Trauma to the visceral peritoneum and deperitonealized areas, which may cause recurrence of adhesions, should be avoided. Remember that surgical treatment deals only with the visible part of the disease and with sequelae. Surgery has no effect on the causes or on microscopic disease.

Adhesiolysis

Adhesiolysis is the most difficult step and the main limit to laparoscopic treatment of endometriosis. The adhesions should be sectioned or the cleavage plane developed only when put under tension. Proceed from the simple adhesions to the more complex dissections; treatment of filmy adhesions may improve the exposure of dense ones. Since the pouch of Douglas is very useful for rapid aspiration of lavage, the posterior cul-de-sac should be freed as early as possible. Difficult adhesiolysis should be performed using magnification provided by the laparoscope. In most cases, the surgeon uses one hand to hold the laparoscope. A CO_2 laser connected to the laparoscope allows the surgeon to operate with both hands. When cutting with very high-power density, a backstop is mandatory.

Laparoscopic adhesiolysis may be performed using hydrodissection, scissors, atraumatic forceps, or CO_2 laser. First separate the tissues and then cut identified structures. Cutting without prior dissection works well when treating filmy adhesions but not for dense ones. If the dissection is difficult, curved scissors are best. Mechanical dissection does not induce any thermal effects so identification of the tissue is easier than with electrical or laser dissection. Current aspiration-lavage devices can generate pressure high enough to dissect normal tissues but not fibrotic tissue and vessels. Hydrodissection is useful to increase the distance between organs and improve exposure when beginning the cleavage. We use hydrodissection in selected cases, particularly for the treatment of deep infiltrating disease. We do not use medical treatment or intraperitoneal adjuvants to prevent postoperative adhesion formation. However, extensive peritoneal lavage with warm Ringer's lactate solution is performed routinely at the end of the procedure.

Treating Peritoneal Endometriotic Implants

Initially, the lesion margins are identified by close inspection of the peritoneum. The margins are outlined with a cutting instrument, with or without previous coagulation of the adjacent normal peritoneum. The implant is then lifted up with atraumatic forceps, and separated from the normal underlying tissue using dissection and section. Depending on the location, thickness, and size of the implant, excision may be easy or extremely difficult.

Vaporization is achieved using a high-power density beam delivered over a short time. This induces a rapid increase in the temperature of water. As the water changes to vapor, the transformation of thermal energy to mechanical energy tears the cellular membranes and causes tissue separation. This method produces smoke, which should be aspirated. Vaporization is a precise technique if the effect is obtained without carbonization and with minimal thermal damage around the treated area. Since the power density decreases in a Gaussian distribution from the middle of the beam to the periphery, a very high-power density is required to achieve vaporization without carbonization in the periphery of the shot. Most CO_2 lasers are used in the superpulse or ultrapulse mode for this effect. The thermal damage is thus reduced to one third of that observed using the continuous mode. We consider the CO_2 laser the best instrument for vaporizing peritoneal implants. The extinction length of this laser is very short; "what you see is what you get."

Coagulation occurs with lower energies and results in lower temperatures at the tissue level. Between 60°C and 80°C, blanching is obtained with loss of intracellular water and coagulation of proteins. The effect of heat depends on the temperature applied and on the duration of contact. Coagulation is not a precise technique. It is almost impossible to control the depth of the tissue effect. Although the blanching effect may appear limited, thermal damage to adjacent structures may occur, particularly when using large instruments for long periods of contact. Moreover, when treating black endometriotic lesions, the blanching of the surface cannot ensure complete destruction of the lesion. In most cases, when opening the cyst with biopsy forceps, you will see chocolate fluid. This finding indicates that coagulation of the deeper part of the cyst is necessary to achieve complete destruction of this implant. But, when treating superficial peritoneal and/or ovarian implants, if blanching is the desired effect, it can be very effectively achieved using coagulation. Such superficial coagulation is easily obtained using the CO_2 laser with a defocused beam and very low-power densities, a Nd:YAG laser applied with a sapphire tip, or a bipolar forceps (1 mm in diameter) if these instruments are moved fast enough to avoid unnecessary thermal damage. We consider the CO_2 laser the fastest and most convenient choice. The bipolar forceps are as effective but slower and less precise.

Treating Deep Infiltrating Peritoneal Implants

Deep infiltrating endometriotic implants are more common in patients who complain of chronic pelvic pain. Most experts agree that complete excision of endometriotic and fibrotic tissue is required to obtain relief. Complete excision might require rectal resection and/or total abdominal hysterectomy with bilateral salpingo-oophorectomy. However, these invading lesions may be managed intraoperatively using a radical, but still realistic, treatment. Hysterectomy is not a good choice in a young patient, even though it seems necessary to ensure complete excision.

Vaginal and rectal examinations are essential to detect the implants and to conduct the procedure. An assistant trained in operative laparoscopy and in the clinical diagnosis of deep endometriosis should stand between the patient's legs in order to expose the operative field by performing a rectovaginal examination and moving rectal and vaginal probes and the uterine cannula. These laparoscopic retractors should be moved slowly under direct vision to avoid inducing bowel lacerations. It is wise to begin the dissection in an uninvolved area to allow easier and safer identification of adjacent structures. Complete excision of fibrotic tissue can be accomplished, but adhesiolysis is often difficult.

Adhesiolysis is necessary to identify the organs involved in the implant, but it is time-consuming since excision of both margins of the cleavage plane is required. Therefore, whenever it is technically possible, it is faster first to dissect the rectum from the implant. In this way, you know immediately whether or not a rectal procedure will be necessary and, if it is, excision may begin immediately. Once the rectum has been fully dissected, the pelvis is filled with warm Ringer's lactate solution and the rectum with air or methylene blue to identify possible rectal lacerations. Both ureters should be routinely visualized and fully dissected to the uterus whenever the uterosacral ligaments are involved. Excision of lesions should be performed toward the uterus. To allow easier identification of the uterus, the nodule is then outlined anteriorly and excision completed while the assistant checks for complete disappearance of the nodule by palpating the posterior fornix. A vaginal incision is often, but not routinely, required.[10] After a vaginal incision, the procedure is completed either vaginally or laparoscopically depending on the quality of the pneumoperitoneum. The vaginal incision is closed with a transverse suture performed vaginally.

Extensive peritoneal lavage is required to minimize vaginal contamination and to check for bleeding and ureteral peristalsis. Hemostasis is checked again when the uterus is back in its normal situation to identify bleeders hidden by the anteversion.

These extensive procedures will result in large deperitonealized areas that cannot be sutured. We are convinced there is less adhesion reformation in the posterior cul-de-sac when fibrotic tissue is completely excised. Treatment of complete cul-de-sac obliteration is difficult and takes time. It also requires close cooperation and understanding between the surgeon and the assistants.

Excision of uterosacral nodules is easier. The peritoneum is incised laterally to the uterosacral ligament. The ureter is then identified, dissected, and protected using scissors and hydrodissection. The uterosacral ligament is resected beginning posteriorly and working toward the uterus. When the nodule has been freed from the underlying tissue, the anterior part of the ligament is cut and the remaining abnormal peritoneum excised taking care to avoid rectal laceration. Most of these deep uterosacral implants can be treated without vaginal incision. At laparoscopy, uterosacral implants may appear smaller than they really are until their dissection is in progress. Therefore careful palpation of the uterosacral ligaments is required in each patient. Palpation of the uterosacral ligaments should be performed after bilateral ovariolysis, since ovarian endometriomas fixed on the uterosacral ligaments may appear as deep nodules.

In patients complaining of pain, we prescribe postoperative medical treatment for 3 to 6 months. Although laparoscopic treatment of deep infiltrating bowel, rectal, or ureteral endometriosis has been reported, we believe that most of these cases should still be treated by laparotomy.

Treating Ovarian Endometriomas

When treating ovarian endometriomas we have the following four goals:

- to rule out malignancy as when dealing with any ovarian cystic masses;
- to remove all the ovarian ectopic endometrium (in older patients complete excision is required because malignant transformation may occur in ovarian endometriomas);
- to minimize ovarian trauma and preserve follicles; and
- to minimize postoperative adhesion formation or reformation (postoperative adhesions are common after ovarian surgery).[13]

To begin, the peritoneal cavity should be thoroughly scrutinized for signs of malignancy and peritoneal cytology performed.[11] The cyst is then aspirated, irrigated, and opened at laparotomy with scissors on the most dependent part, which is located on the anterior ovarian surface. The internal cyst wall is carefully inspected. An immediate laparotomy is performed if there are signs of malignancy during peritoneal, ovarian, or endocystic examination.

One should also account for the anatomic characteristics of ovarian endometriomas. A 1954 study showed that in more than 90% of ovarian endometriomas the cyst wall represents an inverted anterior ovarian cortex with adhesions and implants on its surface (Fig. 10.7 and color plate 10.7).[14] This finding may explain why most endometriomas are located on the anterior ovarian surface and why the ovary and cyst are generally fixed to the broad ligament.

Anterior ovarian adhesiolysis is essential. The cyst cannot be removed entirely without complete ovariolysis. This anterior ovarian incision is almost unavoid-

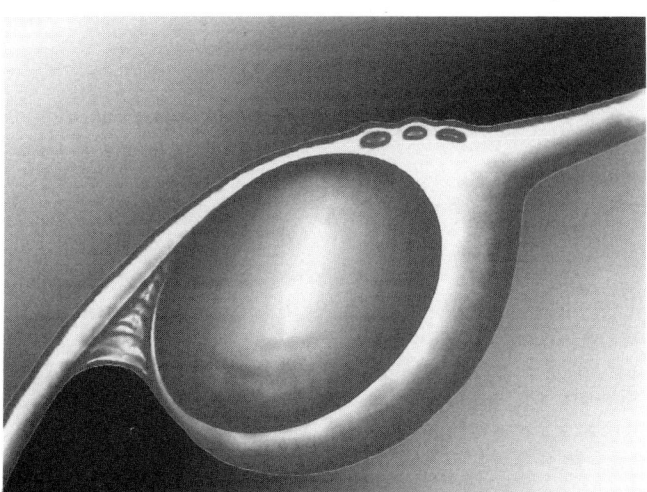

Figure 10.7. Representation of a left ovarian endometrioma fixed to the broad ligament. As suggested by Hughesdon in 1957, the cyst wall is an inverted anterior ovarian cortex fixed to the broad ligament. See also color plate.

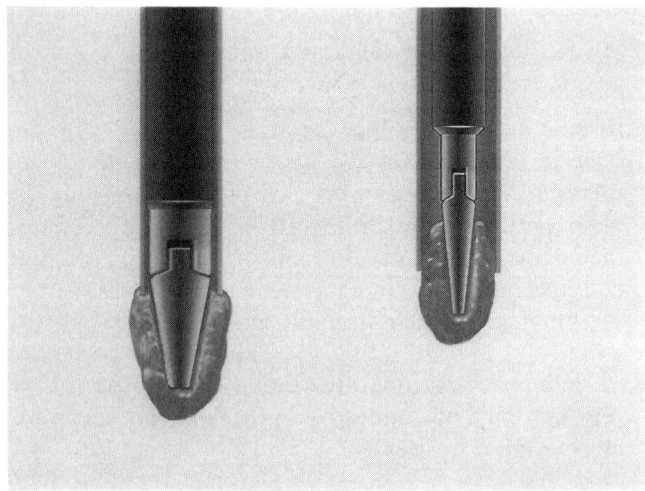

Figure 10.8. On the right, a fragment of the cyst wall is easily removed from the abdomen using a 10 mm trocar and a 5 mm forceps, but it would be cut by the trocar sleeve when removed with a 10 mm forceps, as shown on the left. See also color plate.

able. The ovary should first be freed from all adhesions to allow complete dissection of the cyst. Usually, during the ovariolysis, the endometrioma will be opened spontaneously, as if the cyst were fixed to the broad ligament. In contrast, an incision located on the posterior ovarian aspect does not allow complete treatment, does not avoid rupture on the anterior surface, and may induce sequelae in an area not commonly involved by adhesions.

Several techniques have been described to treat ovarian endometriomas. These include ovarian cystectomy or stripping of the lining, laser vaporization, or excision.[15-18] We have found CO_2 laser vaporization very effective at laparotomy, but too time consuming at laparoscopy. The power densities available at the beginning of our experience were too low to obtain a quick and complete ablation of the cyst lining. Subsequently, we have found that ovarian endometriomas can be treated by intraperitoneal cystectomy.

Incising the cyst is essential to obtain good approximation of the ovary after the dissection. A vertical incision located on the anterior ovarian surface is performed starting from the rupture. This incision, which is only grossly approximated at the end of the procedure, is a site for potential adhesions. The incision should be large enough to avoid a difficult dissection. Unnecessary ovarian lacerations induce bleeding and require extensive coagulation. Furthermore, the edges of ovarian lacerations often require sutures to obtain a satisfactory ovarian shape. On the most dependent part, the ovarian cortex is so thin that the cleavage plane cannot be identified. This problem explains why partial resection of the ovarian cortex may be necessary and why the incision should be enlarged to an area

where the cleavage plane can be identified by inspecting the incision. Since the cyst wall and normal ovarian issue have different elasticities, the edges of these tissues separate spontaneously when the cleavage plane has been incised. The cyst wall and the ovarian cortex are grasped with atraumatic grasping forceps and the dissection plane is developed by pulling these forceps slowly in opposite directions. The forceps are frequently drawn down toward the cleavage plane to permit visual control of the dissection and prevent tearing of tissue and associated bleeding. Continuous visual control is necessary to ensure complete removal of the cyst lining.

In difficult cases, three suprapubic instruments are necessary. Two grasping forceps are used to expose the plane developed with scissors, hydrodissection, bipolar coagulation, or CO_2 laser. Difficulties are often encountered with both small and large endometriomas in patients who have received preoperative medical treatment, and also those who have not. During the dissection, these difficulties should be recognized early enough to avoid unnecessary ovarian damage and the diffuse oozing that prevents effective CO_2 laser ablation which could be used in such difficult cases. The initial steps of the dissection are usually easy. Difficulties are encountered close to the ovarian hilum, particularly near the utero-ovarian ligament. These difficulties are obvious when tension on the instruments increases, and when red fibrotic tissue becomes visible on the dissected part of the cyst wall. In such cases, to identify the dissection plane, it is necessary to get closer to the cyst wall. This time-consuming final step requires a microsurgical technique. Poor dissection may result in laceration of the utero-ovarian ligament and compromise ovarian function. This complication was diagnosed at routine second-look laparoscopies in three of our patients. Once the dissection is completed, additional hemostasis is achieved using bipolar coagulation. Then, the ovary is inspected for remaining parts of the cyst wall. The ovarian shape is evaluated. When it is unsatisfactory, it can be approximated using several techniques including fibrin (Fibrogen); 4/0 sutures, which are kept inside the ovary; or superficial coagulation of the remaining ovarian stroma to retract the ovary, just as

Table 10.1. Laparoscopic treatment of ovarian endometriosis.

	Cases (N)	Partial treatment	Complete treatment	P
Cyst diameter				
<3 cm	54	12 (22%)	42 (78%)	>.05
≥3 cm	118	13 (11%)	105 (89%)	
Adhesion score				
≤50	127	13 (10%)	114 (90%)	<.01
>50	45	12 (27%)	33 (73%)	

Table 10.2. Results of second-look laparoscopy after complete treatment of ovarian endometrioma (AFS ovarian score).

Group	Cases (No.)	First laparoscopy	Second laparoscopy	P
Cyst < 3 cm	13	16	2.3 ± 5.4	<.05
Cyst ≥ 3 cm	61	20	1.7 ± 2.4	<.001
Total	74	19.3 ± 1.5	2.1 ± 5.0	<.001
Severe endometriosis	55	19.2 ± 1.5	2.3 ± 5.1	<.001
Moderate endometriosis	19	19.6 ± 1.3	1.8 ± 4.8	<.001
Ovarian adhesion < 16	58	19.2 ± 1.6	2.0 ± 4.7	<.001
Ovarian adhesion = 16	16	19.8 ± 1.0	2.7 ± 6.1	<.001

Statistical comparison of difference in scores between first and second laparoscopy used the Wilcoxon signed rank test.

coagulation of the serosa is used to obtain eversion of the distal part of the tube.[19,20] The relative effectiveness of these techniques has yet to be established in prospective studies.

When removing the cyst from the abdomen, it is essential to avoid contaminating the abdominal wall. We have found a laparoscopic bag or 10 mm trocar helpful. When using a 10 mm trocar, use a 5 mm external reducer, so that the cyst can be grasped with a 5 mm forceps and easily brought inside the trocar. A 5 mm external reducer is essential because if a 10 mm forceps is inserted in a 10 mm trocar, it is impossible to bring the cyst inside the trocar (Fig. 10.8 and color plate 10.8). Laparoscopic bags are also very useful. We had one patient whose recurrent abdominal wall endometrioma was located at a previous suprapubic trocar site after earlier laparoscopic treatment of an endometrioma.

Excision produces more adhesions and is too traumatic to be used routinely.[18] However, partial excision of the cyst wall previously fixed to the broad ligament is often necessary to ensure complete treatment. We often use laparoscopic laser ablation to treat endometriomas of less than 3 cm or for the remaining part of larger cysts when a complete dissection is not possible. Laser treatment of endometriomas is easier and faster when performed after a 3-month course of medical treatment, which reduces the thickness and activity of the ectopic endometrium.[19] Very high-power densities may be used, because the remaining ovarian tissue is a safe backstop. The CO_2 laser is the best instrument to treat superficial ovarian endometriotic lesions, which may be typical, atypical, or subtle in appearances.

Reviewing the data from 172 ovarian endometriomas, we found that the main limiting factors of complete treatment were the overall adhesion score rather than the cyst diameter (Table 10.1). Complete treatment was achieved in 89% of patients whose cysts were more than 3 cm, but in only 73% in patients with an overall adhesion score of more than 50 (including all the adnexal adhesions and the posterior cul-de-sac obliteration). The efficacy of laparoscopic treatment of ovarian endometriomas, including large ones, has been confirmed from data obtained at second-look laparoscopy (Table 10.2).

In a previous report we showed that adhesion formation affected 21% of the adnexae treated by intraperitoneal cystectomy.[16] Furthermore, complete or partial recurrence of adhesions treated at laparoscopy occurred in 82% of the cases. To study contralateral adhesions, contralateral adnexae without deep ovarian endometriosis were selected, including those with an initial adnexal adhesion score of 4 or less. In this group, the mean adnexal adhesion was slightly, but not significantly, higher at second-look laparoscopy (Table 10.3).

In the AFS-r classification scheme, ovarian adhesions are weighted according to the ovarian surface involved, so that recurrence of initial adhesions may be scored more heavily at second-look because of the decreased ovarian diameter. Nevertheless, several points may be made: (1) Postoperative adhesions can occur after

Table 10.3. Results of second-look laparoscopy after complete treatment of ovarian endometrioma (AFS ovarian plus tubal adhesion scores).

Group	Cases (No.)	First laparoscopy	Second laparoscopy	P
Cyst < 3 cm	13	10.0 ± 8.8	5.6 ± 6.8	>.10
Cyst ≥ 3 cm	61	13.4 ± 10.7	9.9 ± 10.1	<.03
Total	74	12.8 ± 10.4	9.1 ± 9.7	<.01
Severe endometriosis	55	14.9 ± 10.9	10.3 ± 10.3	<.01
Moderate endometriosis	19	6.6 ± 5.4	5.9 ± 6.9	>.50
Ovarian adhesion ≤ 4	24	2.9 ± 2.4	6.0 ± 6.8	>.05
Ovarian adhesion > 4–15	34	13.1 ± 6.9	9.3 ± 10.1	<.05
Ovarian adhesion = 16	16	27.0 ± 6.4	13.5 ± 11.4	<.01
Contralateral adhexa				
All cases	21	3.9 ± 8.6	2.6 ± 4.2	>.50
Adnexal adhesion score ≤4	17	0.5 ± 1.3	1.4 ± 2.7	>.05

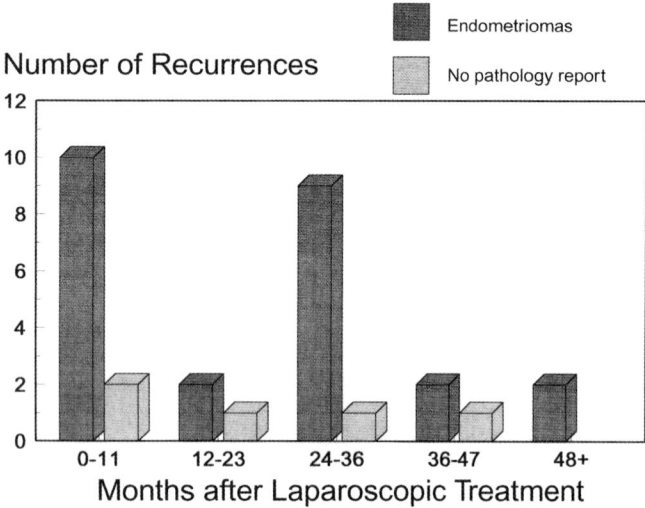

Figure 10.9. Incidence of recurrent ovarian cystic masses is shown after laparoscopic treatment of ovarian endometriomas.

laparoscopic procedures. (2) Although marked improvement of adhesion scores has been reported after laparoscopic adhesiolysis and the dissection of an ovarian endometrioma, the treatment of dense adhesions is disappointing.[21] (3) We should not consider any procedure valuable just because it can be performed laparoscopically. Strict guidelines should be followed to minimize postoperative adhesions.[2,22,23]

We studied endometriosis recurrence rates of 163 patients followed for more than 1 year. The rate of pathologically confirmed recurrences was 16%. Early recurrences were attributed to inadequate or incomplete laparoscopic procedures; late recurrences may simply be consequences of the natural history of the disease (Fig. 10.9).

We felt it was necessary to confirm that ovarian function was not impaired by laparoscopic dissection of ovarian endometriomas, a procedure considered by microsurgeons to be bloody, traumatic, and damaging. We found no significant differences in number of oocytes retrieved for IVF among patients with prior treatment of ovarian endometriomas, patients with tubal infertility, and endometriosis patients without endometriomas (Table 10.4). Marked ovarian damage, however,

Table 10.4. Mean number of oocytes obtained during IVF pickup.

Indication	Cases	Oocytes (mean)
Tubal infertility	253	8.4
Endometriosis		
Without endometrioma	83	8.2
With an endometrioma	67	8.5
Endometrioma treated by		
ovarian cystectomy	34	8.0

can occur during laparoscopic procedures because endometriomas are often located close to the ovarian vessels.

Associated and Radical Procedures

Sectioning of the uterosacral ligaments, presacral neurectomy, and uterine suspension can be performed laparoscopically as well as through laparotomy.[2,24,25] These procedures, often proposed to relieve chronic pain, are more valuable in treating dysmenorrhea and midline pelvic pain than for lateral pain.[26] The efficacy of these techniques in patients treated for endometriosis has not been adequately evaluated and complications can be severe. Damage to the ureter has been reported during laser uterosacral nerve ablation.[17] Presacral neurectomy is a potentially dangerous procedure because it requires dissection of the common iliac veins.[28] We believe laparoscopic uterosacral nerve ablation is indicated only when deep infiltrating implants of the uterosacral ligaments are identified. Presacral neurectomy should be considered only for patients with central pelvic pain, particularly central dysmenorrhea.

Appendectomy is not routinely indicated during laparoscopic treatment of endometriosis. However, macroscopic appendicular endometriotic implants should be removed.

Finally, radical procedures such as oophorectomy, adnexectomy, or hysterectomy also can be performed laparoscopically.[2,29] These radical procedures might be indicated in symptomatic patients over 40 years of age who have undergone several operations. Radical surgical treatment has long been established as a very effective treatment that prevents recurrences even when postoperative hormonal replacement therapy is prescribed.[30] Endometriosis may become in the future one of the indications for laparoscopically assisted vaginal hysterectomy.

Complications

In series of 133 patients who underwent laparoscopic treatment of endometriomas, three required reoperation because of postoperative bleeding.[31] One was reoperated on postoperative day two, one on postoperative day ten, and one three weeks later. All three patients had large cysts. In two cases, the procedure was technically difficult because several endometriomas were removed from one ovary. In the third case late postoperative hemorrhage was attributed to a coagulation disorder induced by nonsteroidal antiinflammatory drugs and low-molecular weight heparin. Two other patients sustained rectal laceration during the excision of a rectovaginal nodule and required immediate laparotomy.

Discussion

Endoscopic surgery has several advantages in comparison with laparotomy surgery. Hospital stay, postoperative recovery, and associated costs are reduced. More important, laparoscopy avoids peritoneal drying. This reduces peritoneal trauma and potential for adhesion formation, which is essential in patients with an inflammatory disease such as endometriosis. However, laparoscopic microsurgical technique is required to ensure complete treatment and optimal results, and this often takes longer than open microsurgical technique.

Provided that treatment is complete, there are no scientific data to demonstrate that any single technique or instrument is better than any other. The surgeon's experience and expertise are much more important than the instrumentation. Each surgeon should use instruments and techniques most familiar to him, taking into account size, location, and thickness of the implant in order to produce the desired postoperative result. In experienced hands, laparoscopic management of ovarian endometriomas is a valuable alternative to the conventional approach by laparotomy. Operative difficulties, however, will often be encountered and persistent endometriomas and postoperative adhesion de novo found at second-look laparoscopy.[32] The three-step medical and surgical treatment, initially proposed a decade ago, and recently reevaluated, may need to be reconsidered in young or infertile patients with endometriomas of more than 8 cm and/or with very active and inflammatory disease.[19,33] Prospective randomized studies are required to compare all the plans of management, including IVF, which can be proposed for patients with severe endometriosis. Only with such information will surgeons of the future be able to manage their patients according to scientific data rather than clinical impressions. In patients with large endometriomas, careful preoperative and laparoscopic examinations are required to rule out malignancy. Consent for a possible laparotomy should be obtained routinely as a safeguard.

Adhesiolysis remains the main limit of the surgical treatment of endometriosis. This limit will obviously differ according to the surgeon's experience and skill. Preoperative and intraoperative patient selection should be managed according to the surgeon's experience, the patient's age, and complaints and physical signs. For example, the management of very severe unilateral adnexal involvement may differ according to the clinical situation. Once the diagnosis of a benign endometrioma has been confirmed, management may be: (1) unilateral adnexectomy using a retroperitoneal approach and a routine dissection of the ureter in a patient over 40; (2) complete adhesiolysis with excision of all active disease in a young patient who complains of severe chronic pelvic pain; or (3) biopsy and laser vaporization of the endometrioma without complete adhesiolysis in an infertile patient who has a normal contralateral adnexa. Other plans of management might also be valuable in differing circumstances. Hence, an individual surgeon may be able to adequately treat the young infertile patient via laparoscopy, but not those with pain or those who are older. Under no circumstances should the surgeon's inexperience or the technical limits of laparoscopic surgery be proposed as valid indications for approximate, incomplete, or unnecessarily radical procedures.

Postoperative adhesions appear to be one of the main limits of laparoscopic surgery. Postoperative adhesions are related to the surgical procedure and to the natural history of the disease. We recently found a 93% intrauterine pregnancy rate in patients who had been treated laparoscopically for nonendometriotic ovarian cysts. We are convinced that adhesion formation is more common following laparoscopic treatment of endometriomas.[15] Since recurrence of dense adhesions is frequent, the value of a second adhesiolysis is doubtful in patients who have extensive dense adhesions at initial laparoscopy (AFS-r score >70). Laparoscopic surgery does not seem to improve the treatment of dense adhesions compared with laparotomy surgery. Since in vitro fertilization pregnancy rates obtained in patients with severe endometriosis and adhesions have been improved by transvaginal ultrasound-guided oocyte retrieval, such patients may best be treated by IVF. We have suggested a stage V be used to classify patients with extensive disease, especially bilateral extensive dense adhesions.[34]

Laparoscopic treatment of severe endometriosis and deep peritoneal implants may be a long procedure (3 hours or more). Appropriate instruments, trained nurses and anesthetists, extensive experience and expertise in endoscopic surgery are prerequisites for this type of

Table 10.5. Pregnancy rates after laparoscopic treatment of endometriosis.

Group	Total cases	Intrauterine pregnancies Number	Rate
All patients	133	49	37%
Stage I	44	16	36%
Stage II	22	7	32%
Stage III	39	13	33%
Stage IV	28	13	46%
Stage IV AFS-r Score			
≤ 70	18	11	61%
Stage IV AFS-r > 70	10	2	20%
Patients previously treated	40	14	35%
Stage I, II, III	24	4	17%
Stage IV	16	10	63%
Patients without previous treatment	93	35	38%
Stage I, II, III	81	32	40%
Stage IV	12	3	25%

surgery. We believe that endoscopic surgery will become the gold standard for treatment of endometriosis in the near future. However, it is only a new surgical approach, not a new treatment based on a better understanding of the disease. Many clinical questions have still to be answered despite the introduction of the so-called "magic" laser beam and endoscopic "wizardry."

References

1. Cook AS, Rock JA. The role of laparoscopy in the treatment of endometriosis. Fertil Steril 1991;55:663–680.
2. Bruhat MA, Mage G, Pouly JL, et al. Operative laparoscopy. New York: McGraw Hill Inc., 1992.
3. Canis M, Mage G, Manhes H, et al. Laparoscopic treatment of endometriosis. Acta Obstet Gynecol Scand 1989; (Suppl. 150):15–20.
4. Janssen RPS, Russel P. Nonpigmented endometriosis: clinical, laparoscopic and pathologic definition. Am J Obstet Gynecol 1986;155:1154–1159.
5. Martin DC, Hubert GD, Vander Zwaag R, et al. Laparoscopic appearances of peritoneal endometriosis. Fertil Steril 1989;51:63–67.
6. Koninckx PR, Meuleman C, Demeyere S, et al. Suggestive evidence that pelvic endometriosis is a progressive disease, whereas deeply infiltrating endometriosis is associated with pelvic pain. Fertil Steril 1991;55:759–765.
7. Candiani GB, Vercellini P, Fedele L. Laparoscopic ovarian puncture for correct staging of endometriosis. Fertil Steril 1990;53:994–997.
8. Reich H, McGlynn F, Salvat J. Laparoscopic treatment of cul-de-sac obliteration secondary to retrocervical deep fibrotic endometriosis. J Reprod Med 1991;36:516–522.
9. Martin DC, Berry JD. Histology of chocolate cysts. J Gynecol Surg 1990;6:43–46.
10. Martin DC. Laparoscopic and vaginal colpotomy for the excision of infiltrating cul-de-sac endometriosis. J Reprod Med 1988;33:806–808.
11. Mage G, Canis M, Manhes H, et al. Laparoscopic management of adnexal cystic masses. J Gynecol Surg 1990;6:7–19.
12. Heaps JM, Nieberg RK, Berek JS. Malignant neoplasms arising in endometriosis. Obstet Gynecol 1990;75:1023–1028.
13. Pittaway DE, Daniell JF, Maxson WL. Ovarian surgery in an infertility patient as an indication for a short-interval second-look laparoscopy: a preliminary study. Fertil Steril 1985;44:611–614.
14. Hughesdon PE. The structure of endometrial cysts of the ovary. J Obstet Gynaecol British Empire 1957;44:481–487.
15. Canis M, Bassil S, Wattiez A, et al. Fertility following laparoscopic management of benign adnexal cysts. Hum Reprod 1992;7:529–531.
16. Canis M, Mage G, Wattiez A, et al. Second-look laparoscopy after laparoscopic cystectomy of large ovarian endometriomas. Fertil Steril 1992;58:617–619.
17. Nezhat C, Crowgey S, Nezhat F. Videolaseroscopy for the treatment of endometriosis associated with infertility. Fertil Steril 1989;51:237–240.
18. Fayez JA, Vogel MF. Comparison of different treatment methods of endometriomas by laparoscopy. Obstet Gynecol 1991;78:660–665.
19. Donnez J, Nisolle M, Karaman Y, et al. CO_2 laser laparoscopy in peritoneal endometriosis and in ovarian endometrial cyst. J Gynecol Surg 1989;5:361–366.
20. Martin DC. Laparoscopic treatment of ovarian endometriomas. Clinical Obstet Gynecol 1991;34:452–459.
21. Operative Laparoscopy Study Group. Postoperative adhesion development after operative laparoscopy: evaluation at early second-look procedures. Fertil Steril 1991;55:700–704.
22. Luciano AA, Maier B, Koch EL, et al. A comparative study of postoperative adhesions following laser surgery by laparoscopy versus laparotomy in the rabbit model. Obstet Gynecol 1990;74:220–224.
23. Nezhat CR, Nezhat FR, Metzger DA, et al. Adhesion reformation after reproductive surgery by videolaseroscopy. Fertil Steril 1990;53:1008–1011.
24. Perez JJ. Laparoscopic presacral neurectomy: results of the first 25 cases. J Reprod Med 1990;35:625–630.
25. Lichten EM, Bombard J. Surgical treatment of primary dysmenorrhea with laparoscopic uterine nerve ablation. J Reprod Med 1987;32:37–41.
26. Tjaden B, Schlaff WD, Kimball A, et al. The efficacy of presacral neurectomy for the relief of midline dysmenorrhea. Obstet Gynecol 1990;76:89–91.
27. Grainger DA, Soderstrom RM, Schiff SF, et al. Ureteral injuries at laparoscopy: Insights into Diagnosis, Management and Prevention. Obstet Gynecol 1990;75:839–843.
28. Nezhat C, Nezhat F. A simplified method of laparoscopic presacral neurectomy for the treatment of central pelvic pain due to endometriosis. Br J Obstet Gynaecol 1992;99:659–663.
29. Canis M, Mage G, Chapron C, et al. Laparoscopic hysterectomy: A preliminary study. Surg Endosc 1993;7:42–45.
30. Montgomery JC, Studd JWW. Oestradiol and testosterone implants after hysterectomy for endometriosis. In Bruhat MA, Canis M, eds. Endometriosis. Karger Basel 1987, Contr Gynec Obstet 16, pp 241–246.
31. Chassagnard F. External endometriosis. Results of laparoscopic treatment of endometriosis in pain and in infertile patients. Indication and results for IVF in endometriosis. These Medicale Clermont Ferrand 1990.
32. Vancaillie T, Schenken RS. Laparoscopic treatment. In Schenken RS, ed. Endometriosis: contemporary concepts in clinical management. Philadelphia, JB Lippincott 1989, 251–266.
33. Mettler L, Semm K. Three step medical and surgical treatment of endometriosis. Ir J Med Sci 1983;152:26–28.
34. Canis M, Pouly JL, Wattiez A, et al. Incidence of bilateral adnexal disease in severe endometriosis (Revised-American Fertility Society, Stage IV). Should a stage V be included in the American Fertility Society Classification? Fertil Steril 1992;57:691–692.

11
Treatment of Ovarian Endometriosis

Camran Nezhat, Farr Nezhat, Ceana Nezhat, and Dahlia Admon

Ovarian involvement occurs in 50% to 70% of all cases of endometriosis.[1] Lesions appear differently at the ovary than at other sites. Superficial ovarian endometriosis, like endometriosis of other parts of the pelvis, can be treated by excision, vaporization or coagulation. Irrigation is performed and all of the charcoal is removed to be sure that the disease is completely treated. Aggressive use of the laser or electrocoagulation should be avoided to decrease the chance of ovarian damage. Ovarian endometriosis may form cystic structures known as endometriomas.

Clinical Presentation and Location

We have seen endometriomas as large as 25 cm, although most are under 10 cm, the average being 4 to 6 cm.[2–4] Their presence is associated with dyspareunia, dysmenorrhea, and infertility. Many, however, are asymptomatic and are found on routine examination or during an evaluation of infertility.

Common sites of small endometriomas (cystic structures filled with chocolate material) are the ovaries, fallopian tubes, uterus, and gastrointestinal tract. They have also been reported in a variety of extrapelvic locations such as the liver surface, perineum, postoperative abdominal incision, and even embedded in the gluteus minimus muscle.[5–9] There have been reports of endometrioma giving rise to an ovarian abscess.[10,11] A single case of endometrioma in an 83-year-old male has been reported.[12]

Large cystic ovarian endometriosis has been reported in pregnancy.[13–16] The differential diagnosis should include dermoid cyst, hemorrhagic corpus luteum, ectopic pregnancy simultaneous with intrauterine gestation, inflammatory tubo-ovarian complex, and colonic pseudomass.

Origin and History of Endometriomas

As with the development of endometriosis, the exact process of endometrioma development has not been clearly elucidated, but several theories may explain its origin. In 1921, Sampson first noted: "The histological findings in these cysts (chocolate cysts) vary in different portions of the same cyst." He also noted that both luteal membrane and ovarian epithelial tissues are frequently present.[17] Sampson believed that in addition to the local spread of endometriosis by salpingeal reflux, some foci may develop from the implantation of endometrioma contents after rupture.[18]

In 1979, Chernobilsky and Morris reported on a variety of epithelial characteristics found in ovarian endometriosis.[19] Since the features included the frequent presence of both endometrial and oviductlike epithelium, such findings may attest to the ovarian tissue as being the common histologic precursor.

Nissole-Pochet and co-workers studied the microscopic characteristics of 113 cases of ovarian endometriosis before and after hormonal therapy.[20] They were able to identify typical endometrial glandular epithelium and stroma. In 18% of the women, the epithelium presented as cyst lining only; in the others, as both the flattened endometrial epithelium and the typical glandular and stromal structures. Also, areas with ciliated cells representing oviductlike epithelium were demonstrated in 47%.

When Martin and Berry examined 41 chocolate cysts they found that 61% were microscopically confirmed

Figures reproduced from *Operative Gynecologic Laporoscopy: Principles and Techniques*, C. Nezhat, Editor, 1995. With permission of McGraw-Hill Publishers.

endometriomas, 27% were corpora lutea, and in no specific histological findings were 12% of cases identified.[21] In evaluating the value of visual diagnosis of endometriomas, Vercellini's team used at least two of the following four microscopic patterns to diagnose endometriosis: the presence of endometrial epithelium, endometrial glands or glandlike structures, endometrial stroma, and hemosiderin-laden macrophages.[22] They confirmed 98% of visually diagnosed endometriomas according to these criteria which are more liberal than the classic histologic criteria which require the presence of both endometrial glands and stroma.[23] Representing the other end of the spectrum are the findings of Fayez and Vogel.[3] They found that none of 66 cysts in 50 patients had endometrial lining. Such findings might be explained by inadequate sampling of the cyst walls for histologic diagnosis.

Authors' Experience

We undertook clinical and pathologic evaluation of 187 consecutive patients with 216 persistent hemorrhagic ovarian cysts (endometriomas).[24] After clinical laparoscopic evaluation to classify the cysts, we removed them for histologic examination. We classified the cysts based on their appearance, cyst content, and ease of removal of the cyst wall from ovarian stroma. We concluded that cysts with an endometrioma appearance can be classified as one of two clinically relevant types. Type I (primary endometriomas) are true endometriomas and

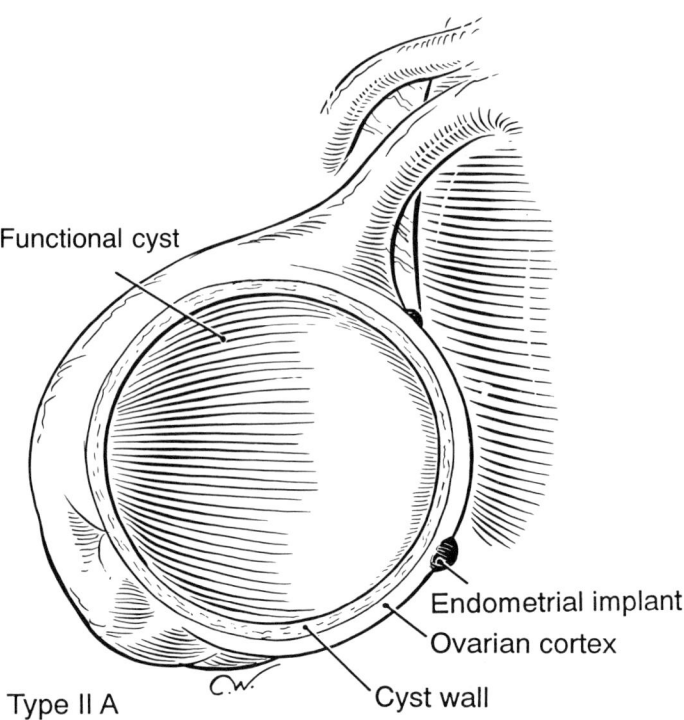

Figure 11.2. Type IIA. The endometrial implant is superficially involved with the ovarian cortex. The implant has not reached the cyst wall.

their origin is the same as that for peritoneal endometriosis. Type II (secondary endometriomas) are follicular or luteal cysts that have been involved or invaded by cortical endometriosis implants or primary endometriomas. Based on the relationship of the cortical endometriosis to the cyst wall, secondary endometriomas are classified into the subtypes IIA, IIB, and IIC. The original presentation of our data included three types, one with two subtypes (types I, II, IIIA, and IIIB).[25] To simplify classification, we made the following modifications.

Type I (Primary Endometriomas)

This variety included 15 small (<2 cm) cysts containing thick, brownish material, which were difficult to remove and often required segmental extraction. Microscopically, all cysts had endometrial lining. Hemosiderin deposition was noted in 11 cysts and five showed fibrosis. The walls were fibrotic, not unlike the fibrosis caused by endometriosis in other pelvic structures. Dense adhesions involved five (33%) of the cysts and three (20%) had filmy adhesions. The growth of these endometriomas appeared to be limited by this fibrosis and scarring (Fig. 11.1).

Type IIA (Secondary Endometriomas)

This group included 57 cysts (2 to 6 cm) containing blood-tinged, yellow fluid, gelatinous clots, or thick,

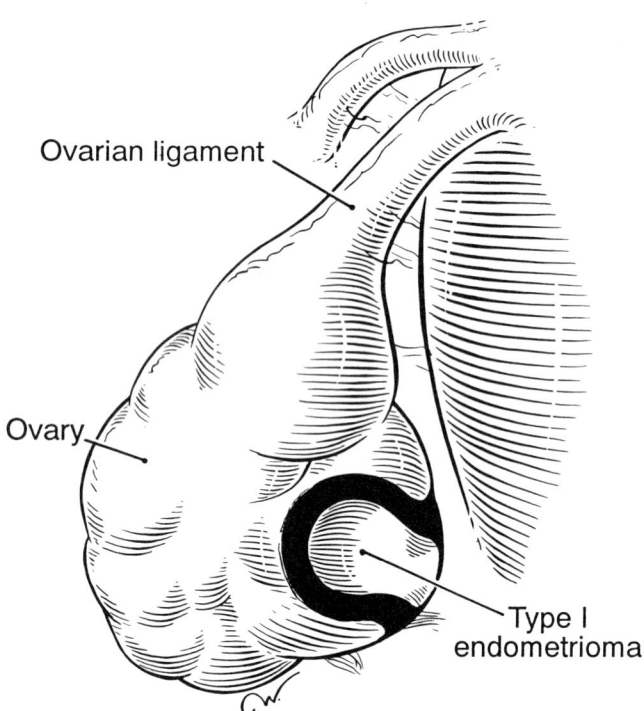

Figure 11.1. Type I. The endometrioma is small and severely attached to the ovary.

brownish material. They appeared to be endometriomas. The capsule separated easily from the ovarian tissue. Endometriosis implants, if present, were superficial and did not penetrate the cyst or the ovarian capsule (Fig. 11.2). Luteinization was found in the lining of 46 cysts, two were hemorrhagic cyst teratomas, and nine were hemorrhagic cysts with unidentifiable lining. No walls had evidence of endometrial tissue. Five (9%) cysts had dense surface adhesions and 11 (19%) had filmy adhesions. It is important to note that while many contained thick, dark, brownish fluid, they could not be called endometriomas at the time of the histologic exam.

Type IIB (Secondary Endometriomas)

We found 46 cysts (3 to 12 cm) containing brownish fluid or degenerating blood clots. The lining of these cysts separated easily from the ovarian capsule and stroma. Adjacent to the areas of endometriosis, however, the ovarian capsule adhered to the cyst wall (Fig. 11.3). Microscopic examination revealed focal endometrial lining in 23 cysts; 14 displayed histologic characteristics of corpora lutea, and nine cysts had an indistinguishable lining. In 35 there was hemosiderin deposition and/or fibrosis. Adhesions between the ovary and pelvic sidewall or uterus and posterior broad ligaments were dense (47%) or filmy (28%).

Type IIC (Secondary Endometriomas)

There were 98 ovarian cysts (3 to 20 cm) that contained dark brownish fluid. Surface endometrial implants were present, penetrating deep into the capsule and the cyst wall and spreading to at least one area of the cyst wall (Fig. 11.4). Thus, the progression of the cyst wall "invasion" formed the basis for differentiating between the IIB and IIC groups. We found it difficult to remove the lining of the cyst wall because of the multiple areas of surface endometriosis invading the cyst through the cyst wall. Surface endometriosis in the presence of dense adhesions was associated with an absence of tissue planes between the capsule and ovarian stroma. In 88 women (90%), the ovary wall was densely adherent to the posterior uterus or lateral pelvic wall.

It is common to observe different types of endometriomas in one ovary. Especially in types IIB and IIC, different stages of cortical endometrial implants to the cyst wall can be seen.

In summary, we identified pure (primary) endometriomas (type I) that were small, developed from surface endometriosis, and difficult to remove. Large type I cysts are almost never present because of the extensive scarring and adhesions. Type IIA endometriomas were usually hemorrhagic luteal, or follicular cysts. The last types (types IIB and IIC) represent endometriomas with features of functional cysts involved

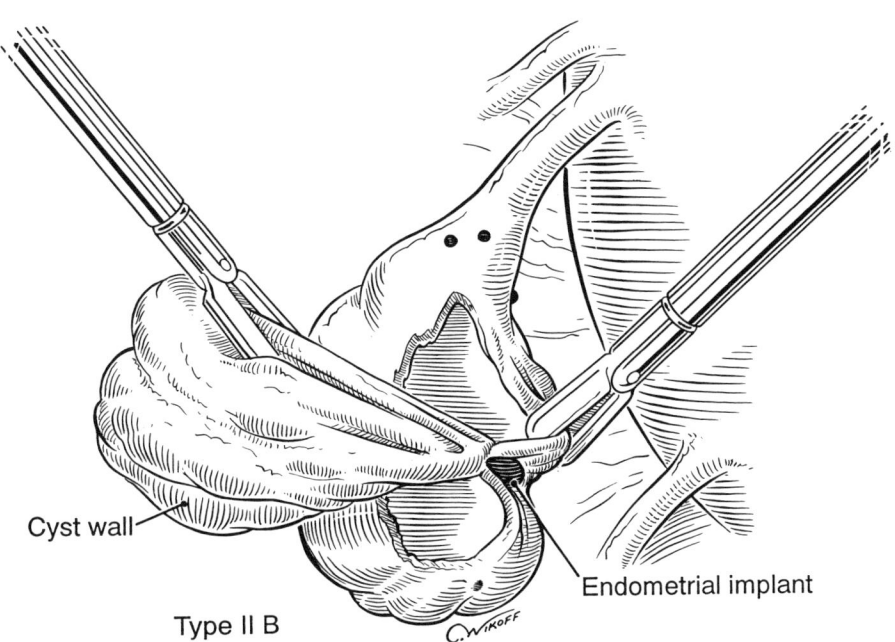

Cyst wall

Endometrial implant

Type II B

Figure 11.3. Type IIB. The endometrial implant has reached the cyst wall, but is not completely invading the cyst wall. The cyst wall can be separated from the ovarian cortex.

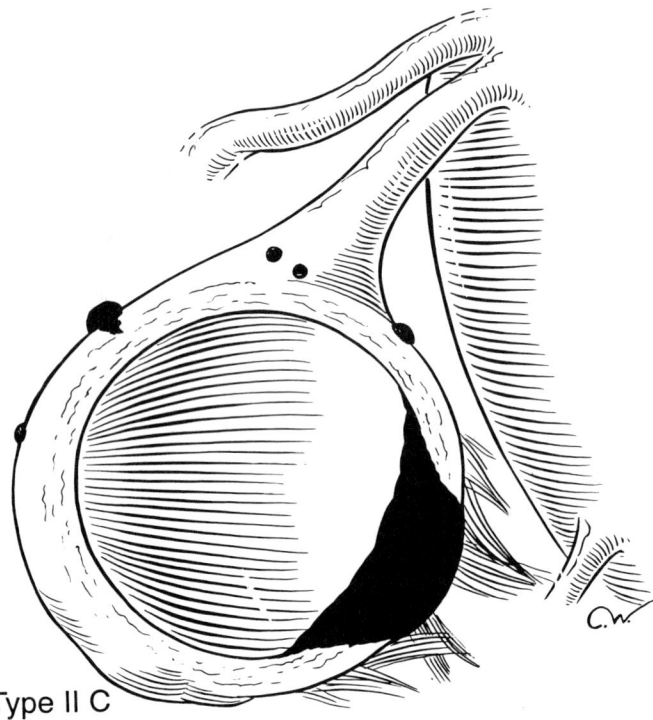

Type II C

Figure 11.4. Type IIC. The endometrial implant has completely reached the cyst wall and has spread. The cyst wall is attached severely to the ovarian cortex with endometriosis and fibrosis. The ovary is attached to the pelvic sidewall with adhesions.

deeply with surface endometriosis. This classification, which accounts for the variation of chocolate cysts, helps to explain the discrepancies among the data of other authors. For example, Vercellini and others observed that the gross characteristics of the examined endometriomas were "ovarian cysts not greater than 12 cm in diameter, adhesions to the pelvic side wall and/or the posterior broad ligaments, powder burns and minute red or blue spots with adjacent puckering on the surface; and tarry, thick, chocolate-colored fluid content."[23] These criteria describe some, but not all, of the ovarian cysts in our types I, IIB, and IIC categories. Using Vercellini's criteria, the false–positive rate is relatively low, but many endometriomas would not be diagnosed.

Stricter classification of endometriomas may aid in future attempts to assess the variety of treatments and postoperative management of adnexal masses. While corpora lutea and follicular cysts may benefit from aspiration and/or hormonal suppressive therapy, definite endometriosis should be completely excised.

Diagnosis and Preoperative Evaluation

The patient typically complains of pelvic pain, infertility, or both. A pelvic mass is frequently detected on physical exam. Other presenting signs are short menstrual cycle, premenstrual spotting, and increased duration and

volume of menses. Endometriosis is known to follow a familial mode of inheritance. Women with a family history of the disorder should be considered at increased risk.

On physical exam, besides the pelvic mass, the uterus is commonly fixed and retroverted. The posterior cul-de-sac and uterosacral ligaments may be tender with manipulation and have palpable nodularity. In one report, diagnostic operations revealed that approximately 10% of pelvic masses resulted from endometriosis.[26] As transvaginal ultrasound becomes more widely used, it may replace the bimanual exam as the modality of choice for screening and diagnosis. Since endometriomas and endometriosis generally involve other organs, it is important to question the patient about possible problems with the bladder, uterus, and bowel. Those with GU involvement will often complain of dysuria, urine frequency, and may have a history of frequent urinary tract infections or recurrent pyelonephritis. Complaints of dyschezia, irregularity of bowel movements, diarrhea, or constipation should alert clinicians to possible rectal or large bowel involvement. When these symptoms are present, an intravenous pyelogram and barium enema may help determine the extent of involvement.

Serum CA-125

The use of serum CA-125 for differentiation among endometriotic and nonendometriotic cysts has been suggested. Pittaway and co-workers studied benign cysts larger than 4 cm.[27] In their investigation, 19 women with endometriomas had a mean serum CA-125 of 53 U/mL compared with 11 U/mL in those with nonendometriotic cysts and 15 U/mL in women with pelvic endometriosis but nonendometriotic benign cysts. Furthermore, all women with endometriomas had serum CA-125 greater or equal to 20 U/mL, whereas all women with nonendometriotic cysts had CA-125 levels below 20 U/mL. These results, however, have not been confirmed by other investigations.

We reviewed the charts of 1,011 women with adnexal masses; 360 patients had endometriomas and 219 had functional cysts which looked pathologic.[28] The mean serum CA-125 appeared or was higher for all endometrioma sizes. However, we observed a sizable overlap in the values. The use of serum CA-125, therefore, is impractical in differentiating among the cyst types, and we do not recommend this test for the diagnosis of endometrioma.

Ultrasound

This modality has long been used to diagnose pelvic endometriosis and ovarian endometriomas. A transabdominal approach is nonspecific in diagnosing endometriosis. In contrast, with the greater resolution of a transvaginal approach, specific features associated with endometriomas have been described.[29]

When we used vaginal probe ultrasonography to evaluate 247 endometriomas, 69% were cystic, 23% were semicystic, and 8% appeared solid.[28] Of the 219 functional cysts, 58% appeared cystic, 25% semisolid, and 4% solid. These characteristics alone do not differentiate endometriomas from other cysts.

For an accurate diagnosis, many findings must be considered simultaneously. These include lesion size, acoustic enhancement, wall thickness, wall contour, presence of fluid-fluid levels, and internal echoes. In a recent study of 38 surgically proven endometriomas, homogeneous internal echoes were found in 82% of all masses and septations in 29%.[4] The wall thickness was 4 mm or less in nearly 90% of all endometriomas.

Transvaginal color Doppler sonography may be of additional use in differentiating malignant adnexal lesions from benign endometriomas. Low pulsatile index of blood vessels associated with lesions can be correlated with an increased probability of malignancy. In a series of 43 surgically proven ovarian masses, Fleischer's group were able to exclude all cases of malignancy with a negative predictive value of 100%.[30] However, a low pulsatile index was found in some benign lesions, resulting in a 73% positive predictive value for this technique. In other words, approximately one quarter of adnexal masses suspected of being malignant by this technique will be benign upon surgical removal and histologic evaluation.

Computed Tomography

While CT scans were the early choice to evaluate a variety of adnexal masses, it failed to differentiate benign ovarian lesions with severe adhesions from malignant disease in repeated trials.[31] It is also difficult with this technique to distinguish many ovarian lesions (including endometriomas) from adjacent loops of bowel. Some findings such as focal hyperdensity inside an ovarian cyst may help distinguish endometriomas from other pelvic masses.[32]

Magnetic Resonance Imaging

MRI appears to be more specific than other imaging techniques in the diagnosis of endometriosis and endometriomas.[33,34] Endometrial implants as small as 3 mm may be accurately diagnosed. Differentiation between endometriomas and loops of small and large bowel is enhanced, though it is still challenging. By examining the cyst in question on both T1 (the time it takes for the nuclei to begin to vibrate out of step with each other) weighted images, an endometrioma is confirmed when the high signal intensity of the cystic component remains unchanged. It has also been suggested that MRI can

distinguish benign from malignant adnexal masses with its ability to differentiate tissue and high resolution.[35]

Diagnostic Laparoscopy

Laparoscopy has the advantage of allowing simultaneous diagnosis, staging, and treatment of ovarian endometriomas. Visual diagnosis of endometriomas at laparotomy and laparoscopy can be highly sensitive and specific. In a study of 245 women who underwent laparotomy for ovarian cysts, Vercellini's team were 96% accurate in their visual diagnosis when compared with the findings of a microscopic exam.[22] Other authors, however, have shown that histologic examination of "chocolate cysts," reveals many to be hemorrhagic corpus luteum or corpus albicans cysts.[21] In our series of 216 presumed endometriomas 46 (21%) were luteal cysts, 2 (1%) were hemorrhagic cystic teratomas, and 9 (4%) were cysts with no residual identifiable lining.[25]

An early promise may lie in determination of CA-125 levels in the fluid obtained from "chocolate cysts."[36] Among 42 women undergoing cystectomy after aspiration of chocolate fluid, 68% had histologically proven endometriomas (the other 27% had corpora lutea and 5% had follicular cysts). When the fluid from these cysts was evaluated, 78% of endometriomas had very high CA-125 concentrations (>10,000 IU/mL). Endometriomas were also found to have low estradiol and progesterone concentrations. This can be contrasted with low CA-125 and elevated estradiol (>2,000 pg/mL) in fluids from corpora lutea.

Medical Therapy

Medical therapy for ovarian suppression may have therapeutic value when used preoperatively. As suggested by Buttram, preoperative treatment with danazol (3 months of 800 mg/day or 6 months of 400 mg/day) may reduce vascularity and result in decreased intraoperative hemorrhage.[37] Ovarian suppression may reduce the size or resolve many follicular and corpus luteum cysts that compose our type II group. The reduction will further decrease manipulation and minimize damage to normal ovarian tissue. It appears that for those women taking preoperative danazol, the overall pregnancy rates were higher than for those who only underwent surgery.[38]

GnRH agonists show promise for treating endometriomas because they lessen the severity of pelvic endometriosis for 6 to 12 months during and after the therapy.[39,40] Their value, however, is questionable when they are used alone, especially with endometriomas >3 cm.[41] Their use following laparoscopic aspiration of an ovarian cyst was without benefit compared with cases with surgery only.[2] We recommend their use for preoperative ovarian suppression in cases of severe and extensive endometriosis.

Surgical Therapy

As medical management of endometriomas has proven ineffective, surgical therapy has become the accepted approach. Laparotomy has long been the conventional modality for treatment of severe endometriosis and endometriomas. However, advances in videoimaging and instrument technology have pushed operative laparoscopy to the forefront of endometriosis surgery.[42,43]

With wider acceptance of operative laparoscopy, numerous authors have proposed different degrees of invasiveness when dealing with endometriomas. The least invasive and the technically simplest approach involves fenestration and removal of chocolate-colored fluid without cystectomy or ablation of the cyst wall.

In 1988, we compared simple aspiration of endometriomas with copious irrigation of the cyst cavity and removal of the entire cyst wall.[44] Fenestration and irrigation were associated with a 50% endometrioma recurrence rate, compared with only 8% in the group with the capsule removed. Fayez and co-workers created a wide opening in the cyst wall to drain its contents completely.[3] This technique created fewer periadnexal adhesions (27%) when compared with complete resec-

tion of endometrioma (100%), stripping of lining (37%), and lining evaporated by CO_2 laser in a continuous mode (30%). Persistence of endometrioma was much higher in all groups in which the cyst wall was not completely removed. All recurrent endometriomas were larger than 4 cm. An even more dramatic finding by Vercellini's team illustrates that simple aspiration and washing of the capsule of endometrioma is not therapeutic.[2] In their series of 33 women, most endometriomas recurred even though many patients took GnRH analogs postoperatively. Hasson found no therapeutic value to simple aspiration.[45] He noted recurrence in eight of nine endometriomas treated by fenestration alone. Our experience parallels these investigations. Therefore, we recommend complete removal of the types I and IIB and C endometriomas.

Surgical Technique

While small, type I endometriomas are difficult to remove intact because of associated fibrosis and adhesions, they can be easily biopsied, drained, and vaporized using laser or electrosurgery or removed in pieces.[25] The larger type I lesions (2 to 3 cm) must be completely removed.

Type IIA lesions (follicular and luteal cysts) are expected to resolve with preoperative ovarian suppression. Patient observation of persistent cysts undergo

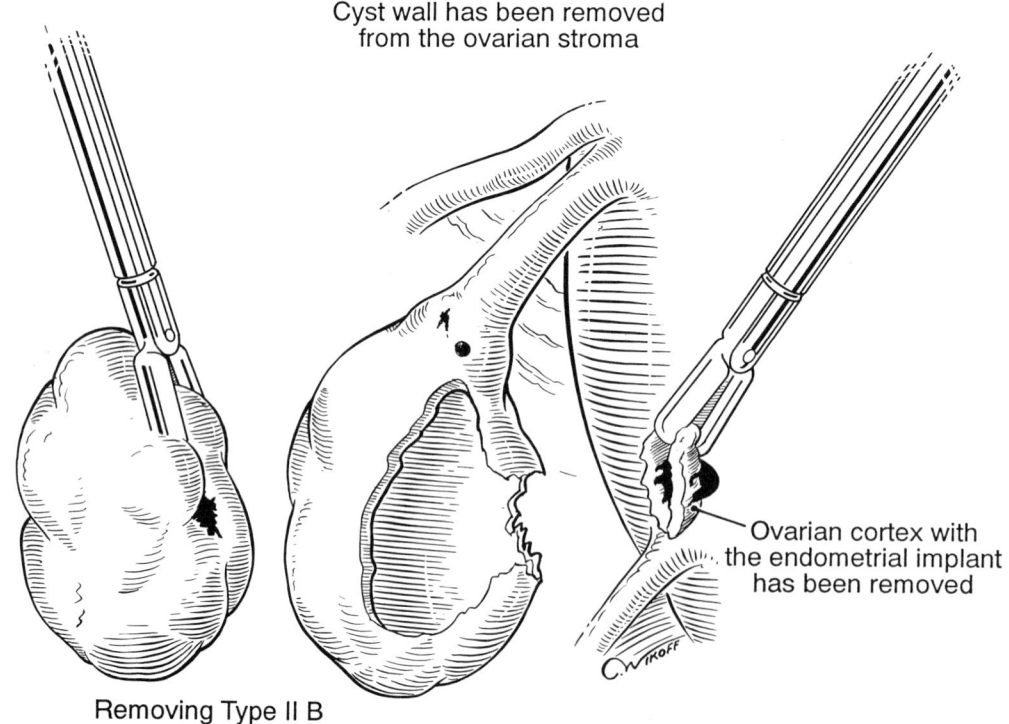

Cyst wall has been removed
from the ovarian stroma

Ovarian cortex with
the endometrial implant
has been removed

Removing Type II B

Figure 11.5. Right: One small portion of ovarian cortex with endometrial material is removed. Left: The main portion of the ovary with endometrial cyst wall; using two grasping forceps and suction-irrigator the cyst wall is separated from the ovarian cortex.

laparoscopy. Periovarian adhesions are lysed and the ovarian cortex is thoroughly evaluated. The cyst is aspirated and deflated. Any superficial ovarian cortex endometriosis is vaporized or excised. The cyst is opened and its interior evaluated for signs of malignancy. The surgeon can usually diagnose this cyst type by its yellowish appearance and ease of removal. A frozen section biopsy is taken to confirm a functional cyst and rule out malignancy. If the operator is not comfortable with the clinical diagnosis, the cyst should be excised. Postoperatively, hormonal suppressive therapy is used for 6 to 8 weeks (danazol 800 mg/day; GnRH analogs or birth control pills) to promote ovarian healing and prevent ovulation.

Types IIB and C are usually larger and associated with more periovarian adhesions. Type IIB lesions are severely attached to the pelvic side wall and the back of the uterus, and will rupture during separation. After dissecting the ovary from the pelvic side wall, the cyst contents are removed with the suction-irrigator probe. The cyst cavity is copiously irrigated. Any spillage is immediately suctioned and irrigated. For type IIB, an opening is made and the suction-irrigator probe introduced inside the cyst cavity. The contents are aspirated. By alternating suction and irrigation, the contents (which may be thick) are removed. The inside of the cyst is evaluated to be sure there are no signs of malignancy (vegetation or excrescences).

For type IIB, that portion of ovarian cortex involved with endometriosis is removed (Fig. 11.5). Using the grasping forceps and the suction-irrigator probe, the cyst wall is grasped and separated from the ovarian stroma by traction and countertraction. Hydrodissection will facilitate complete removal. Small blood vessels from the ovarian bed and more severe bleeding from the ovarian hilum can be controlled by bipolar electrocoagulation.

In type IIC, the ovarian cortex is severely attached to the cyst wall and at the level of opening. This makes it difficult to develop a plane between the cyst wall and ovarian capsule. The portion of the ovary that is attached to the cyst wall is removed until an area is found to develop a plane (Fig. 11.6). The remainder of the procedure is similar to that for type IIB.

The redundant ovarian capsule is approximated by low-power laser, or electrosurgery. If suturing is used to approximate the ovary, all sutures are placed inside the capsule and 4-0 polyglycolic material is used. Fewer sutures will likely result in fewer adhesions.[46]

Low-power continuous laser or bipolar coagulation can be applied to the inside wall of the redundant ovarian capsule, causing the capsule to invert. One must be careful to avoid excessive coagulation of the adjacent ovarian stroma.

Complications of ovarian cystectomy for endometrioma include postoperative adhesion formation,

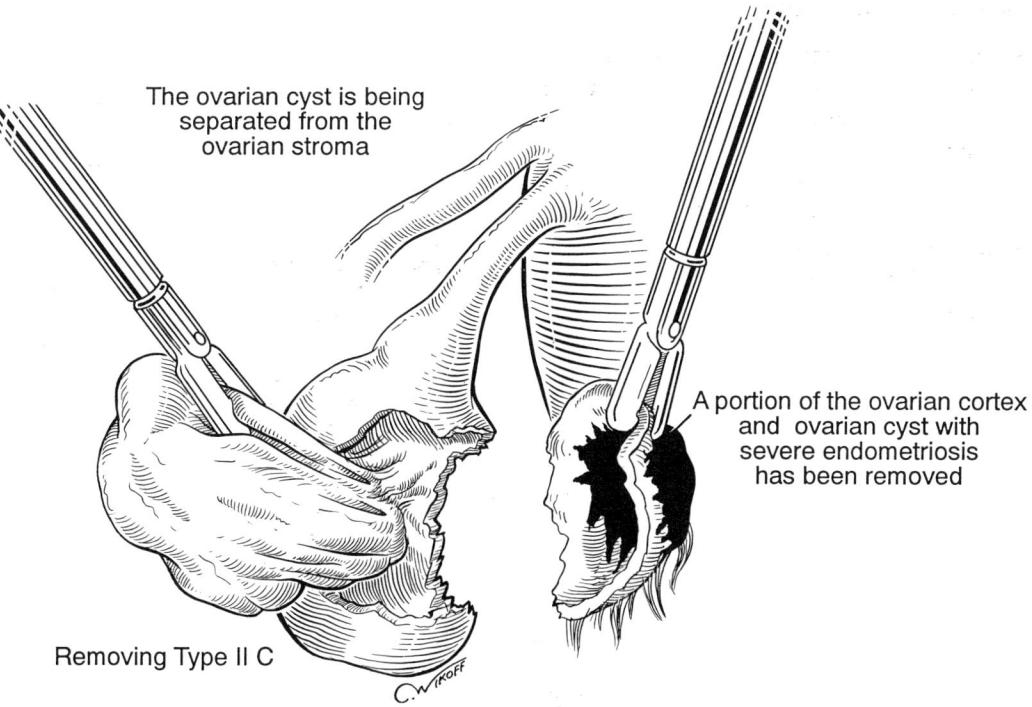

The ovarian cyst is being separated from the ovarian stroma

A portion of the ovarian cortex and ovarian cyst with severe endometriosis has been removed

Removing Type II C

Figure 11.6. Right: Partial oophorectomy is performed to remove the severe involvement of ovarian cortex with endometriosis which is attached to the cyst wall. Left: Main portion of ovary with endometrioma at cyst wall. The remaining cyst wall is stripped out of the ovary.

endometrioma recurrence, and oophorectomy during conservative surgery. Injury to surrounding organs may also occur because of extensive adhesions and surface endometriosis. There is a slight chance of malignancy within the endometrioma.

Second-Look Laparoscopy

This evaluation is important in judging the validity of various surgical approaches, postoperative adhesion formation, and the persistence or recurrence of endometriosis. Canis and others undertook second-look laparoscopy on 42 patients 3 to 6 months following laparoscopic removal of endometriomas >3 cm.[47] In this series, 92% of ovaries had no residual deep ovarian endometriosis. This finding compares with 22% of residual deep ovarian endometriosis found by Fayez and co-workers at second-look laparoscopy after stripping the cystic lining alone.

Second-look laparoscopy has shown that postoperative adhesion formation after surgery for endometriomas is a major problem. However, if dense adhesions were present at initial surgery, ovarian adhesion scores appear to be improved at second look.[48] Our second-look laparoscopy in 67 patients showed that when sutures were used to approximate ovarian cortex following cystectomy, an increased number of adhesions can be expected.

Risk of Malignant Transformation

The risk of malignant transformation in endometriomas is low. Chernobilsky's group reviewed 194 ovarian endometriosis cases and found only seven (4%) with some degree of atypia.[19]

A true malignancy, endometrioid adenocarcinoma of the ovary is seen in 15% to 20% of all epithelial ovarian cancers. In many frank cancers (at least 10% to 20%), adjacent areas of benign endometriosis is seen.[49] This finding suggests that perhaps in some cases, endometriosis is the benign precursor to malignancy. In our series of 1,011 women, four ovarian cancers were found. Intraoperatively, one appeared to be an endometrioma, but was identified as an endometrioid tumor of low malignant potential on pathologic examination.[27]

References

1. Jenkins S, Olive DL, Haney AF. Endometriosis: pathogenic implications of the anatomic distribution. Obstet Gynecol 1986;67:335.
2. Vercellini P, Vandola N, Bocciolone L, et al. Laparoscopic aspiration of ovarian endometriomas. J Reprod Med 1992;37:577.
3. Fayez JA, Vogel MF. Comparison of different treatment methods of endometriomas by laparoscopy. Obstet Gynecol 1991;78:660.
4. Kupfer MC, Schwimer SR, Lebovic J. Transvaginal sonographic appearance of endometrioma: spectrum of findings. J Ultrasound Med 1992;11:129.
5. Grabb A, Carr L, Goodman JD, et al. Hepatic endometrioma. J Clin Ultrasound 1986;14:478.
6. Kennedy SH, Brodribb J, Godfrey AM, et al. Preoperative treatment of an abdominal wall endometrioma with nafarelin acetate: case report. Br J Obstet Gynecol 1988; 95:521.
7. Frydman CP, Schwartz JW, Schwartz IS. Endometrioma of the anterior abdominal wall. Mount Sinai J Medicine 1986;53:160.
8. Punnonen R, Pettersson K, Vanharanta R, et al. Androgen, estrogen and progestin binding in cystosis of benign gynecologic tumors and tumor-like lesions. Hormone and Metabolic Research 1985;7:607.
9. Botha AJ, Halliday AE, Flanagan JP. Endometriosis in gluteus muscle with surgical implantation: a case report. Acta Orthopaedica Scandinavica 1991;62:497.
10. Lipscomb GH, Ling FW, Photopoulos GJ. Ovarian abscess arising within an endometrioma. Obstet Gynecol 1991;78:951.
11. Martino CR, Haaga JR, Bryan PJ. Secondary infection of an endometrioma following fine-needle aspiration. Radiology 1984;151:53.
12. Martin JD, Hauck AE. Endometriosis in the male. Am Surg 1985;51:426.
13. Johnson TR, Woodruff JD. Surgical emergencies of the uterine adnexae during pregnancy. Int J Gynecol Obstet 1986;24:331.
14. Pennes DR, Bowerman RA, Silver TM. Echogenic adnexal masses associated with first-trimester pregnancy: sonographic appearance and clinical significance. J Clin Ultrasound 1985;13:391.
15. Ninia JG. Large endometrioma with intrauterine pregnancy. NY State J Med 1992;92:364.
16. Nezhat F, Nezhat C, Silfen S, et al. Laparoscopic ovarian cystectomy during pregnancy. J Laparoendosc Surg 1991; 1:161–164.
17. Sampson JA. Perforating hemorrhagic (chocolate) cysts of the ovary. Arch Surg 1921;3:245.
18. Sampson JA. The development of the implantation theory for the origin of peritoneal endometriosis. Am J Obstet Gynecol 1940;40:549.
19. Chernobilsky B, Morris WJ. A historic study of ovarian endometriosis with emphasis on hyperplastic and atypical changes. Obstet Gynecol 1979;53:318.
20. Nisolle-Pochet M, Casanas-Roux F, Donnez J. Histologic study of ovarian endometriosis after hormonal therapy. Fertil Steril 1988;49:423.
21. Martin DC, Berry JD. Histology of chocolate cysts. J Gynecol Surg 1990;6:43.
22. Vercellini P, Vendola N, Bocciolone L, et al. Reliability of the visual diagnosis of ovarian endometriosis. Fertil Steril 1991;56:1198.
23. Sternberg SS, ed. Histology for pathologists, 1992, p. 513.
24. Nezhat F, Nezhat C, Allan CJ, et al. Clinical and histologic classification of endometriomas. J Reprod Med 1992; 37:771.
25. Nezhat C, Nezhat F. Letter-to-the-Editor: Comparison of different treatment methods of endometriomas by laparoscopy. Obstet Gynecol 1991;79:315.
26. Killackey M, Neuwirth R. Evaluation and management of pelvic mass: a review of 540 cases. Am J Obstet Gynecol 1988;71:319.
27. Pittaway DE, Fayez JA, Douglas JW. Serum CA-125 in the evaluation of benign adnexal cysts. Am J Ob Gyn 1987;157(6):1426–1428.

28. Nezhat F, Nezhat C, Welander CE, et al. Four ovarian cancers diagnosed during laparoscopic management of 1,011 women with adnexal masses. Am J Obstet Gynecol 1992;167:790.

29. Wood C, Maher P, Hill D. Diagnosis and surgical management of endometriomas. Aust NZ J Obstet Gynecol 1992;32:161.

30. Fleisher AC, Rogers WH, Rao BK, et al. Assessment of ovarian tumor vascularity with transvaginal color Doppler sonography. J Ultrasound Med 1991;10:563.

31. Shields RA, Peel KR, MacDonald HN, et al. A prospective trial of computed tomography in the staging of ovarian malignancy. Br J Obstet Gynecol 1985;92:407.

32. Buy JN, Ghossain MA, Mark AS, et al. Focal hyperdense areas in endometriomas: a characteristic finding on CT. Am J Roentgen 1992;159:769.

33. Arrive L, Hricak H, Martin MC. Pelvic endometriosis: MR imaging. Radiol 1989;171:687.

34. Togashi K, Nishimura K, Kimura I, et al. Endometrial cysts: diagnosis with MR imaging. Radiol 1991;180:73.

35. Mawhinney RR, Powell MC, Worthington BS, et al. Magnetic resonance imaging of benign ovarian masses. Br J Radiol 1988;61:179.

36. Koninckx PR, Muyldermand M, Moerman P, et al. CA 125 concentrations in ovarian "chocolate" cyst fluid can differentiate an endometriotic cyst from a corpus luteum. Hum Reprod 1992;7:1314.

37. Buttram VC. Use of danazol in conservative surgery. J Reprod Med 1990;35:82.

38. Dmowski WP, Kapetanakis E, Scommegna A. Variable effects of danazol on endometriosis at 4 low-dose levels. Obstet Gynecol 1982;59:408.

39. Henzl MR, Corson SL, Moghissi K, et al. Administration of nasal nafarelin as compared with oral danazol for endometriosis: a multicenter double blind comparative clinical trial. N Engl J Med 1988;318:485.

40. Zorn JR, Matheison J, Risquez F, et al. Treatment of endometriosis with a delayed release preparation of the agonist D-Trp^6-luteinizing hormone releasing hormone: long-term follow-up of 50 patients. Fertil Steril 1990;53:401.

41. Schenken RS. Gonadotropin-releasing hormone analogs in the treatment of endometriomas. Am J Obstet Gynecol 1990;162:579.

42. Nezhat C, Crowgery SR, Garrison C. Surgical treatment of endometriosis via laser laparoscopy. Fertil Steril 1986;45:778.

43. Nezhat C, Nezhat F, Pennington E. Laparoscopic treatment of infiltrate rectosigmoid colon and rectovaginal septum endometriosis by the technique of videolaparoscopy and the CO_2 laser. Br J Obstet Gynecol 1992;99:664.

44. Nezhat C, Winder W, Nezhat F. Is endoscopic treatment of endometriosis and endometrioma associated with better results than laparotomy? Am J Gynecol Health 1988;2:10.

45. Hasson HM. Laparoscopic management of ovarian cysts. J Reprod Med 1990;35:863.

46. Nezhat C, Nezhat F. Postoperative adhesion formation after ovarian cystectomy with and without ovarian reconstruction. Presented at the 75th Annual Meeting of the American Fertility Society, Orlando, Florida, October 19–24, 1991.

47. Canis M, Mage G, Wattiez A, et al. Second-look laparoscopy after laparoscopic cystectomy of large ovarian endometriomas. Fertil Steril 1992;58:617.

48. Nezhat C, Nezhat F, Metzger D, et al. Adhesion reformation after reproductive surgery by videolaseroscopy. Fertil Steril 1990;53:1008.

49. Yu J, Grimes DA. Ascites and pleural effusions associated with endometriosis. Obstet Gynecol 1991;78:533.

12

Treatment of Endometriosis of the Cul-de-Sac

David B. Redwine

The cul-de-sac holds special importance in endometriosis treatment. It is the pelvic area most commonly involved by the disease (Table 12.1). Indeed, although Sampson's original publications in the 1920s made it appear that the ovary was the most commonly involved pelvic site, two decades later he realized that peritoneal disease was more common and clinically more important.[1-3] Gynecologic surgeons, therefore, must become proficient in identifying and treating cul-de-sac endometriosis.

The cul-de-sac includes the pouch of Douglas, the uterosacral ligaments, the distal rectosigmoid colon and proximal rectum, and the posterior cervix. Although each of these pelvic areas can be anatomically identified separately, the invasive potential of cul-de-sac endometriosis requires that, for safe and complete surgical treatment, all be considered together.

The high frequency of cul-de-sac involvement is often taken as confirming Sampson's theory: reflux menstruation causing gravitational accumulation, attachment, and implantation of viable endometrial cells preferentially in this area.[4] However, since embryonic organogenesis involves differentiation and migration of cells across the posterior pelvic coelomic epithelium, the high incidence of posterior pelvic involvement could also be taken as evidence supporting embryonic rests or embryologically patterned metaplasia.[5,6]

Endometriosis is frequently encountered when we perform endoscopic evaluation of patients complaining of pain or infertility. However, the endometriosis lesions are not necessarily the sole cause of either of these symptoms. Uncomplicated endometriosis, without pelvic distortion or ovarian endometriomas, is being reevaluated as a cause of infertility. Pain seems to be a more common and more specific symptom of the disease. As a presenting complaint, it is almost three times more frequent than infertility.[7] However, not all pelvic pain is due to endometriosis.

Usually, without realizing it, the clinician treating a patient with endometriosis seeks either relief of symptoms or treatment of disease. Although these endpoints seem separate, the distinction may blur in clinical practice. Even research on the disease is hampered by this lack of focus. Relief of symptoms may result from any of several nonspecific treatments that may have no effect on the disease, whereas completely successful surgical removal of endometriotic implants can occur without any improvement of pain or infertility. It is important to remember that not all pain and not all infertility is caused by endometriosis. You must ask: am I really treating the disease, or just symptoms associated with it (pain and infertility)?

Symptoms and Signs of Cul-de-Sac Endometriosis

Patients with endometriosis of the cul-de-sac report a high frequency of symptoms such as deep dyspareunia, painful bowel movements, and pelvic tenderness. However, endometriosis patients without involvement of the cul-de-sac also frequently have such symptoms (Table 12.2).

Detailed questioning of patients who report painful bowel movements suggests that those with an endometriotic rectal nodule and obliteration of the cul-de-sac frequently suffer throughout the menstrual cycle. They may also have chronic rectal pain, low sacral backache, and painful passage of flatus. Although cyclic rectal bleeding suggests invasion of the bowel wall, 88% of patients with intestinal endometriosis who required full-thickness or segmental resection for treatment of bowel endometriosis did not have this symptom.[8] Some

Table 12.1. Distribution of endometriotic sites among 1,147 patients at a referral center.

Site	Distribution
Cul-de-sac*	801 (70%)
Left broad ligament	591 (52%)
Right broad ligament	496 (43%)
Left uterosacral ligament	459 (40%)
Right uterosacral ligament	418 (36%)
Bladder	354 (31%)
Left ovary	192 (17%)
Fundus	186 (16%)
Right ovary	172 (15%)

*Represented as the pouch of Douglas, excluding the uterosacral ligaments, rectosigmoid colon, and posterior cervix.
All disease was confirmed histologically by the presence of glands and stroma; excludes patients with previous hysterectomy.

Table 12.2. Type and severity of pain* among patients with or without endometriosis of the cul-de-sac.

Symptom* Pain level	Endometriosis of cul-de-sac	
	Disease Present	Disease Absent
Painful bowel movements[a]		
1	114 (24%)	24 (47%)
2	96 (20%)	8 (16%)
3	115 (24%)	11 (22%)
4	107 (22%)	7 (14%)
5	47 (10%)	1 (2%)
Tenderness on exam[b]		
1	25 (5%)	7 (13%)
2	57 (12%)	8 (15%)
3	146 (30%)	13 (25%)
4	184 (38%)	21 (40%)
5	74 (15%)	3 (6%)
Deep dyspareunia[c]		
1	62 (14%)	10 (23%)
2	67 (15%)	4 (9%)
3	115 (25%)	13 (29%)
4	133 (29%)	11 (25%)
5	78 (17%)	6 (14%)
Pelvic pain away from menses[c]		
1	40 (8%)	4 (8%)
2	39 (8%)	10 (19%)
3	127 (27%)	12 (23%)
4	171 (36%)	15 (29%)
5	103 (22%)	11 (21%)
Uterine cramps with menses[d]		
1	62 (14%)	3 (6%)
2	34 (7%)	7 (13%)
3	84 (17%)	7 (13%)
4	144 (30%)	17 (33%)
5	190 (40%)	18 (35%)

*Measured by preoperative 5-point pain scales (1 = not a problem, 5 = debilitating problem).
[a] $p < .01$.
[b] $p = .05$.
[c] $p = >.05$.
[d] $p = >.05$.
Totals within group are not equal since not all patients answered each questionnaire item.

patients with invasive disease may have low-grade fever, malaise, and fatigue. Superficial cul-de-sac disease may be associated with painful bowel movements primarily with menses.

Findings on physical examination can suggest the presence of cul-de-sac endometriosis. Since the external hand cannot be used effectively to palpate the cul-de-sac through the abdominal wall, the internal exam should be performed gently without using external pressure to identify focal tenderness of the cul-de-sac. Reactions of the patient's face and body during examination are important. If light stroking of the cul-de-sac produces a wince or a facial grimace, suspect endometriosis. Arching of the back, movement up the table away from the examiner, or expressions of pain are highly suggestive of cul-de-sac disease. Painful nodularity of the cul-de-sac or uterosacral ligaments is virtually pathognomonic of endometriosis. In one study, 97% of patients with focal tenderness on pelvic exam were found to have pathology, usually endometriosis, at the point of tenderness.[9] If tenderness on exam reproduces the patient's pain, the probability of relief after excision of implants is high. When you encounter marked central cul-de-sac nodularity, check the posterior fornix closely, since invasion into the vagina may have been missed on initial speculum exam (Fig. 12.1 and color plate 12.1). When you find tenderness, resist the temptation to diagnose less common causes of pelvic pain such as pelvic inflammatory disease, ruptured ovarian cysts, or adhesions. Endometriosis should usually lead the list of differential diagnoses in patients with pelvic pain who are between ages 10 and 45, regardless of parity.

Preoperative Imaging Studies

Preoperative ultrasound or radiologic studies are of limited value in the diagnosis of cul-de-sac endometriosis. Ultrasound depends on differences in tissue density of sufficient volume to distinguish one structure from another. Even endometriosis of the cul-de-sac which invades several centimeters beyond the visible peritoneal surface has a tissue density similar to that of the posterior cervix.[10,11] This makes it difficult to distinguish sonographically. Superficial endometriosis lacks sufficient volume to be distinguishable at all.

Although obliteration of the cul-de-sac may be associated with endometriosis of the wall of the rectum, preoperative barium enema or sigmoidoscopy will usually be normal.[8] Bowel endometriosis is primarily a serosal or muscularis lesion that rarely penetrates to the bowel lumen or produces sufficient distortion to be imaged. These studies, however, may be of importance in ruling out intestinal cancer, which begins as a mucosal lesion. Computed tomography or magnetic imaging are too imprecise and too expensive to be warranted in most cases of cul-de-sac endometriosis.

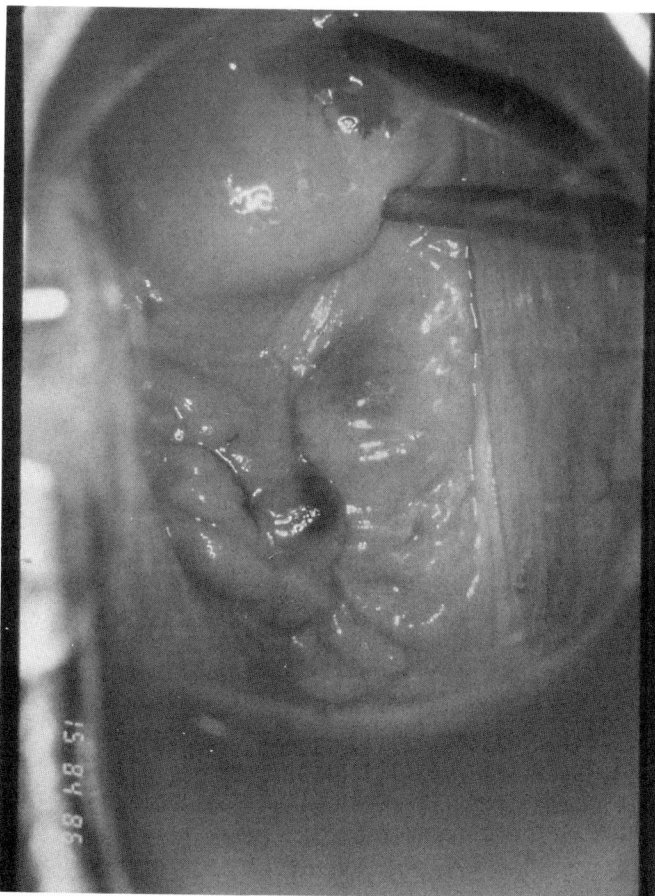

Figure 12.1. Discoloration of the posterior fornix is associated with mucosal invasion by a nodule of endometriosis of the rectovaginal septum. This abnormality was hidden by the posterior blade of a bivalve speculum on a previous pelvic examination. See also color plate.

All imaging studies have only two possible results: normal or abnormal. Even with a normal study result, the patient with marked signs and symptoms is a surgical candidate. An abnormal study result simply reinforces the already apparent need to proceed with surgical diagnosis and treatment.

Preoperative Bowel Preparation

Some symptoms and signs suggest bowel involvement by endometriosis. Patients with these complaints should receive a bowel preparation before surgery. Rectal pain with menses and rectal pain with defecation throughout the month suggest a rectal nodule of endometriosis. Previous surgery revealing bowel disease or obliteration of the cul-de-sac, as well as tender nodularity of the cul-de-sac or uterosacral ligaments, suggests intestinal involvement. Previous operative reports with comments such as "severe cul-de-sac adhesions" or "adherence of the rectosigmoid colon to the uterus" may indicate obliteration of the cul-de-sac. Thus, although a report

may describe the extent of adhesions, the presence of a rectal nodule may be overlooked. If a rectal nodule is described on a previous operative report, this finding increases the likelihood that other intestinal areas may also be involved. Marked uterosacral ligament nodularity on examination may signify partial (Fig. 12.2 and color plate 12.2) or complete obliteration of the cul-de-sac, with the rectosigmoid adhering to one or both uterosacral ligaments.

A bowel prep of 4 L of Oral Colonic Lavage (Abbott, Chicago) (polyethylene glycol 3350, 6g/100 ml) the afternoon before surgery, followed by two enemas the evening before surgery, works well. The lavage can be made more palatable by chilling or by adding flavor crystals. The patient may also use nose plugs. If watery diarrhea results, it is not necessary that she take all 4 L. For patients who have shown a previous intolerance of oral lavage, 150–300 ml of magnesium citrate given the afternoon before surgery is sufficient. A traditional 3-day bowel preparation is rarely necessary. Appropriate antibiotics can be given intraoperatively if you anticipate entry into the bowel lumen. Ampicillin plus sulbactam, 3 gm IV, can be given intraoperatively and postoperatively. For patients allergic to penicillin, administer ceftriaxone, 2 gm, and metronidazole, 1 gm IV.

Vigorous mechanical bowel preparation, followed by prophylactic antibiotics, may result in postoperative antibiotic-mediated pseudomembranous enterocolitis. Anticipate loose stool or diarrhea for several days following bowel preparation and bowel surgery, but if diarrhea persists and is associated with low-grade fever and abdominal discomfort, obtain a stool specimen for

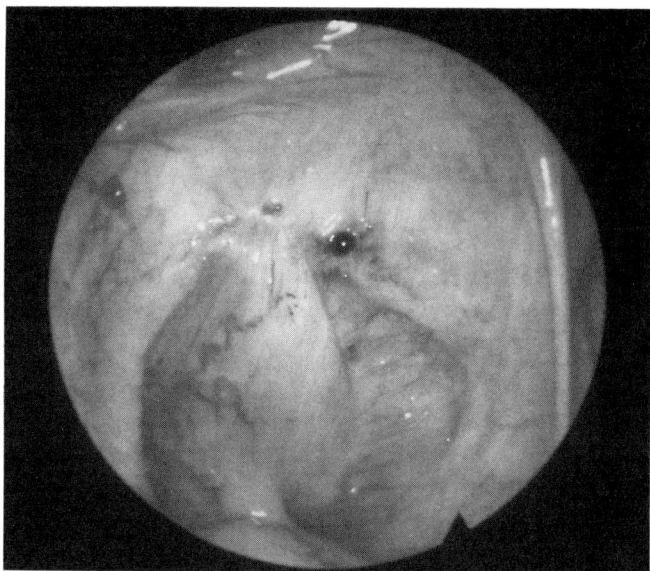

Figure 12.2. The rectosigmoid colon is adherent to the left uterosacral ligament, producing partial obliteration of the cul-de-sac. A significant nodule was palpable in this region on the pelvic examination. See also color plate.

Clostridium difficile toxin titer. If it is positive, the appropriate treatment is either oral vancomycin or oral metronidazole, 500 mg q.i.d. for 7 days.

Adjunctive Medical Therapy

Some clinicians believe that preoperative medical therapy makes endometriosis surgery less bloody and easier to perform. A disadvantage of preoperative ovarian suppression, however, is that it can make endometriosis less apparent to the surgeon.[12] I believe preoperative medical suppression increases the possibility of incomplete identification and incomplete treatment.

It has also been stated that medical therapy may eradicate microscopic deposits of endometriosis. However, recent studies indicate that most patients do not have invisible microscopic endometriosis.[13–18] Further, there is little evidence that medical therapy eradicates endometriosis of any stage. A literature review of medical therapy for endometriosis-associated pain showed that 78% of medically treated patients had persistent endometriosis at the conclusion of therapy while the ovaries were still suppressed.[19] Most patients in the studies reviewed had minimal or mild disease by the revised American Fertility Society (AFS-r) classification system of endometriosis.[20]

In my experience, medical therapy is unnecessary for successful surgical treatment of endometriosis. In a study of 359 patients treated by conservative laparoscopic excision with no adjunctive medical therapy, I found a recurrence rate of minimal endometriosis of 19% at 5 years after surgery.[21] Most patients did not have any visible endometriosis at reoperation. These findings are similar to long-term outcome analysis after laparotomy excision.[22]

While medical therapy may result in temporary relief of any hormonally mediated pain (for example, adenomyosis, leiomyomata, ovulatory cysts, dysmenorrhea, and endometriosis), long-term outcome analysis following medical therapy is lacking.[19] Published results of pain relief following medical therapy can sometimes be misleading.[23] While it is easier to give medical therapy for endometriosis than it is to excise it, this is not a reason to avoid acquiring the skills necessary to treat the disease completely with surgery.

Methods of Surgical Destruction

Some authorities, including The American College of Obstetricians and Gynecologists (ACOG) hold that all methods of destruction of endometriosis are equivalent, particularly for superficial disease.[24,25] I disagree with this view. In the absence of comparative studies showing equivalent rates of persistence or recurrence, such a position has not been documented. Also, nonexcisional techniques (laser vaporization, electrocoagulation, endothermy, or argon beam coagulation) can lead to errors in diagnosis of invasion. A recent study of invasive endometriosis of the cul-de-sac showed that the full extent of invasion could be determined only during the process of surgical excision.[11] Nonexcisional techniques remain unvalidated by any long-term outcome study with respect to how deeply or completely disease can be destroyed. Thus, I consider these methods of treatment unproven at this time. Several authors have mentioned that deeply invasive disease or disease over vital structures preclude electrocoagulation, resulting in a high rate of persistence.[26–28] None of the electrocoagulation reports adequately describe the technique of destruction, equipment, or current density used.[26–29] The results of electrocoagulation, therefore, cannot be easily replicated or validated.

Safe surgery mandates separating diseased tissue and healthy tissue before applying surgically destructive force. Nonexcisional methods of treating endometriosis tempt the surgeon to violate this principle, because the disease may easily be burned in situ (with risk, however, of damage to an underlying vital structure). Or the surgeon may choose not to treat certain pelvic areas at all for fear of damage to underlying structures.

Surgeons normally use sight and touch to ply their trade. Use of laser vaporization or electrocoagulation may compromise both senses. Neither technique has been validated by long-term follow-up to be as effective as excision in eradication of endometriosis.[30] Given the limitations imposed by nonexcisional techniques, I believe that excision of endometriosis is the treatment of choice.

Laparoscopy Versus Laparotomy

Excision of endometriosis can be performed either at laparoscopy or laparotomy. Each approach has certain advantages. The brilliant illumination and magnification of laparoscopy allows all visual manifestations of endometriosis to be identified, increasing the likelihood of complete treatment. Retraction is provided in all directions by the pneumoperitoneum, including a degree of retroperitoneal retraction once the retroperitoneal space is entered. Recovery for the patient usually is faster than with laparotomy. Laparoscopy, however, cannot be used to treat all conditions satisfactorily. Although laparoscopic partial-thickness, full-thickness, or segmental bowel resections for endometriosis can be done with intracorporeal or extracorporeal techniques, laparoscopic segmental bowel resections can last 6 to 8 hours and often require a 4- to 6-day hospital stay and 3 to 8 weeks of convalescence. Segmental resection and anastomosis can be more quickly completed at laparotomy with an identical recovery time.[8,31,32] However, with increasing experience, most cases of endometriosis surgery can be completed laparoscopically (Table 12.3).

Table 12.3. Experience improves successful laparoscopic excision of endometriosis.*

Year	Total cases of endometriosis	Number of cases completed laparoscopically/total cases (%)				
		All stages	Stage 1	Stage 2	Stage 3	Stage 4
<1981	7	2/7 (29%)	2/6 (33%)	0/1 (0%)	0/0	0/0
1981	15	5/15 (33%)	4/13 (31%)	1/2 (50%)	0/0	0/0
1982	18	9/18 (50%)	7/11 (64%)	0/3 (0%)	2/4 (50%)	0/0
1983	19	8/19 (42%)	8/28 (44%)	0/0 (0%)	0/1 (0%)	0/0
1984	20	11/20 (55%)	10/14 (71%)	0/4 (0%)	0/1 (0%)	1/1 (100%)
1985	21	11/21 (52%)	10/15 (67%)	1/5 (20%)	0/0	0/1 (0%)
1986	23	15/23 (65%)	14/17 (82%)	1/3 (33%)	0/1 (0%)	0/2 (0%)
1987	85	63/85 (74%)	38/42 (90%)	18/22 (82%)	4/6 (67%)	3/14 (21%)
1988	182	120/182 (66%)	70/91 (77%)	34/49 (69%)	10/21 (48%)	6/21 (29%)
1989	207	130/207 (63%)	71/92 (77%)	39/55 (71%)	14/24 (58%)	6/36 (17%)
1990	178	134/178 (75%)	74/90 (82%)	31/33 (94%)	14/19 (74%)	15/36 (42%)
1991	184	142/184 (77%)	69/74 (93%)	37/40 (93%)	18/22 (82%)	18/48 (38%)
1992	165	139/165 (84%)	69/75 (92%)	38/44 (86%)	17/20 (85%)	15/26 (58%)

*This table includes patients undergoing hysterectomy.

Nonlaser Versus Laser Techniques

Despite repeated claims of cost savings, laparoscopic surgery can actually increase health care costs both by lengthening the time spent per procedure and by dependence on expensive technology such as disposable items (trocars, suction cannulas, and myriad instruments), videomonitoring equipment, and lasers. A study comparing vaginal hysterectomy with laparoscopic hysterectomy showed that although clinical outcomes were similar, laparoscopic surgery was more expensive.[33] In our cost-conscious world, where laser laparoscopy often seems too slow, many reproductive surgeons are turning toward electrosurgery with reusable instruments.

Modern Monopolar Electrosurgery

The passage of electrons through tissue is what makes monopolar electrosurgery work. The surgical effects of modern monopolar electrosurgery result from tissue resistance to electron flow that produces tissue heat. Vaporization and coagulation are the two most clinically useful tissue effects resulting from electrosurgery.

For practical purposes, the tissue effect occurs only in close proximity to the active electrode, since the density of electrons decreases rapidly farther from the active electrode. For tissue to be a reasonable conductor, it must contain water. Since the human body is 60% to 70% water, distributed relatively evenly except in bones and teeth, electrons do not take any particularly favored path of least resistance from the active to the return electrode.[34] We cannot predict the path of electricity back to the return electrode, since it uses the entirety of tissue in the region. Of course, if tissue is isolated from the rest of the body, and then electricity is passed into it, the isolated tissue becomes a favored path under the active electrode while the tissue is able to conduct electricity.

Once electrons pass into the body, they have an infinite number of paths to take back to the return electrode. The current density in any given tissue volume away from the active electrode is relatively low, so significant heat is not generated. Thus, thermal spread in monopolar electrosurgery is usually limited to "what you see is what you get." If tissue is not being coagulated, it is not getting dangerously hot. Electrical current will, therefore, not selectively follow blood vessels or any other tissue with any important clinical effect. Of course, if a long dwell time is combined with high current density through an electrode in direct contact with a vital structure, that vital structure can be damaged.

Increasing tissue resistance will alter or inhibit the effects of electrosurgery. In the case of total resistance, electron flow (and electrosurgery) almost ceases. Two examples of total resistance in surgery would be tissue that is completely dessicated, as occurs with bipolar tubal coagulation for sterilization, and dessicated tissue that lies between the active electrode and non-dessicated tissue, such as a superficial area of charring occurring during monopolar electrocoagulation of endometriosis.

Dwell Time, Current Density, and Pillowing

In electrosurgery, *dwell time* and *current density* are the two most important electrophysical factors affecting tissue. *Dwell time*, the length of time the active electrode is in contact with a particular tissue site, is a direct consequence of the surgeon's hand-to-eye coordination. Increased dwell time can convert a clean electrosurgical cut into messy coagulation. The better the hand-to-eye coordination, the lower the dwell time; the lower the dwell time, the higher the current density can be; and the higher the current density, the quicker the desired electrophysical effect will occur.

Pillowing of tissue around the active electrode lowers the current density, leading to coagulation effects instead of cutting effects. Pillowing occurs when the surface or edge of the tissue to be cut is not kept under countertension. This allows the active electrode to sink into the tissue. As more of the metal comes into contact with the tissue, dwell time increases and current density drops. Pillowing can also be created by touching the active electrode to the tissue before stepping on the foot pedal. The foot pedal must be activated while the active electrode is still "in the air" above the taut surface to be cut. Thus, when the active electrode comes into contact with tissue, electrons flow instantly and *touch cutting* occurs.

Modern electrosurgery also depends on the surgical principles of tension and countertension provided by traction. The surgeon and/or the assistant must ensure that the tip or cutting edge of the active electrode is always brought against tissue under tension. This will allow the tissue to separate from the active electrode immediately after it is cut. This separation of tissue allows the active electrode to come into contact with fresh tissue (also under tension), which also will separate under the effects of tension after being cut with high-current density. With practice, this action can occur very rapidly by sliding the scissors tip along taut peritoneum (*slide cutting*). Gnawing at tissue with scissors through which current is flowing will produce massive coagulation, which is rarely useful in modern electrosurgery.

Laparoscopic excision of endometriosis provides a pathology specimen and allows removal of deeply invasive disease anywhere in the pelvis. Palpation and handling of the tissue with scissors and graspers results in tactile feedback that enhances the ability to detect deep disease. Since tissues can be cut, bleeders simultaneously coagulated, and tissue handled or repositioned all with one instrument, instrument changes are virtually eliminated. Since the active electrode is typically in contact with tissue, there is no wandering during application of the surgical energy (as can occur with a laser beam, which can be affected by the surgeon's pulse or by the patient's pulse or respirations). These characteristics make electrosurgery precise, and allow it to be used with care around and on vital structures such as the ureter, bowel, bladder, or large vessels. Touch cutting or touch coagulation of tissue under tension allows precise delivery of energy with little dwell time. Electrosurgical excision of endometriosis can be extremely rapid and cost effective. By using a single simple instrument and avoiding the use of disposable instruments such as trocars and staplers, costs can be held down.

Laparoscopic Equipment

Advanced operative laparoscopy of the cul-de-sac requires few instruments (Table 12.4). A triple-puncture technique (10 mm operating laparoscope in the umbilicus, 5.5 mm sheath in the left lower quadrant for a grasper, and a 5.5 mm sheath in the right lower quadrant for a suction-irrigator) is sufficient for virtually all advanced procedures. Although many surgeons operate with video equipment and a monitor, I find that surgery can be done quicker by looking directly down an operating laparoscope with the eyepiece drawn into the nasal bridge with pressure through the scissors handles held in the right hand. This position eliminates the need for triangulation of every movement. A second laparoscope can be inserted for video monitoring if spectators are present.

Patient Positioning for Surgery

The patient is placed in low lithotomy position with a retention catheter in the bladder. Because operative endoscopy can be lengthy, positioning of the legs is particularly important. If knee stirrups are used, extra-thick padding is needed to avoid peroneal nerve paresis. To avoid hypothermia, place a warming blanket under the patient. Also place blankets around the upper torso, head, and arms. The patient's arms are ideally tucked along her side to allow the surgeon (and the assistant if one is used) full mobility. Warmed irrigation fluid is used. An intrauterine manipulator is used and the table is placed in steep Trendelenburg position.

Table 12.4. Laparoscopic equipment used by author.

Manufacturer and device	Model no.
Wolf	
10 mm operating laparoscope	8938.31
3 mm hooked scissors (see ValleyLab below)	8380.02
5 mm needle holder	8383.53
5 mm toothed grasper	8383.447
10 mm trocar sleeve (metal)	934B
10 mm trocar	8934.12
Bipolar coagulation forceps	838.24
Bipolar electric cord	
Monopolar electric cord for 8380.02 (see ValleyLab below)	8106.91
Fiberoptic light cord	8067.55
6 L/minute high-flow insufflator	2054.60
Solos	
5 mm grasper	1011
Cabot	
Corson irrigator	
Wisap	
Needle drivers (2)	7668
ValleyLab	
Force 4 electrosurgical generator	
This device is set at 70 to 90 W pure cutting current and 50 W coagulation current (may be changed depending on the response in the particular patient) and is used with the 3 mm Wolf scissors 8380.02) and the monopolar electrical cord (8106.91).	

Instrument Insertion

After application of an intrauterine manipulator, a vertical incision is made within the umbilicus, where the abdominal wall is thinnest. The abdominal wall is grasped and elevated and a 10 mm sheath with trocar is inserted directly. The tip of the laparoscope is then used to illuminate the avascular space lateral to the right inferior epigastric vessels in a line just above the pubic hair. After a small incision is made, the laparoscope is used to elevate the abdominal wall in this area. The 5.5 mm sheath with trocar is directed *horizontally* beneath the end of the raised laparoscope tenting up the abdominal wall. This horizontal insertion avoids potential damage to the iliac vessels. The same steps are repeated on the opposite side.

All skin incisions are kept small to avoid later leak of pneumoperitoneum and inward travel of the sheaths. If leakage of pneumoperitoneum or sheath travel becomes problematic, an Allis clamp can be applied around the base of the 5.5 mm sheaths or the skin gathered around any of the three sheaths. Disposable sheaths make surgery difficult because they have internal valves that can hinder tissue removal. Also, the 10 mm disposable sheaths do not produce enough friction against the laparoscope to avoid downward travel of the scope during surgery.

Electrosurgical Settings

I use a Valleylab Force 4 (ValleyLab, Boulder, CO) electrosurgical generating unit set at 70 W of pure cutting current and 50 W of coagulation current, which enables me to accomplish most electrosurgical maneuvers. Cutting current can be successfully used on taut peritoneum, while the higher voltage of coagulation current will sometimes be more efficient for cutting through retroperitoneal fat or parenchymal tissue such as the uterosacral ligaments. Depending on the tissue effect, a higher cutting current setting of 90 W or even 110 W may be necessary. Higher current settings, or inadequate surgical response at these settings, may indicate insulation failure of the active electrode. An all-metal umbilical sheath will allow directly or indirectly coupled current to be transmitted into the abdominal wall at a low current density unlikely to result in patient injury.

Electrosurgical Excision of Cul-de-Sac Disease

Separation of diseased tissue from healthy tissue is one of the paramount objectives of surgery. Opening the peritoneum with small electrosurgical scissors is followed by blunt retroperitoneal dissection that helps attain this goal. Once nonvital connections have been encountered between healthy and diseased tissue, they can be severed electrosurgically.

Superficial Peritoneal Resection

Since most patients do not have severely invasive disease, the following technique is commonly used. The tissue to be removed is elevated or dissected away from underlying vital structures and pulled medially toward the center of the pelvis during excision. During palpation with the graspers, small superficial lesions will slide easily over retroperitoneal vessels which can be grasped directly and elevated, whereas invasive endometriosis will seem indurated or nodular and may be difficult to grasp and elevate. The peritoneum is opened with a touch cut, then the lesion is pulled medially, undermined bluntly, and excised with a few peritoneal slide cuts. The rectosigmoid colon passes beneath the cul-de-sac, and its white muscular wall can be inadvertently tented up with the overlying peritoneum. A ring forceps in the colon will keep the surgeon constantly aware of the location of the colon. Since it is more difficult to keep the wall of the bowel taut, pillowing is more likely. Electrosurgical excision involving the bowel wall is frequently problematic and unsafe.

Blunt or sharp dissection should be used to separate involved peritoneum from the bowel. The vascular supply of the lower rectosigmoid colon is supplied in part by vessels coursing through the right and left sides of the cul-de-sac medial to the uterosacral ligaments (Fig. 12.3 and color plate 12.3). These vessels are frequently hidden in the fatty retroperitoneal tissue and can also be inadvertently tented up with the peritoneum.

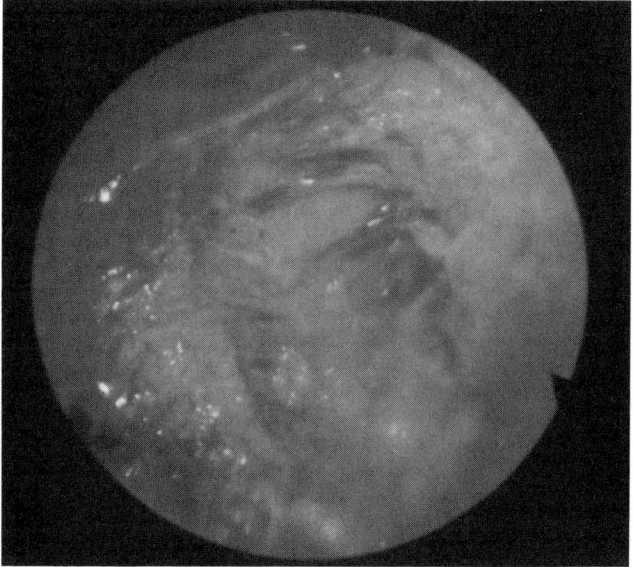

Figure 12.3. The peritoneum of the right side of the cul-de-sac has been excised. The vessels supplying the bowel wall can be seen lying within the retroperitoneal fatty tissue and along the bowel wall. These vessels can be tented up and injured during resection of even superficial cul-de-sac endometriosis. Efforts to control the bleeding with electrocoagulation may lead to damage to the adjacent rectum. See also color plate.

This problem should be anticipated, even during resection of superficial lesions. Unless the peritoneum is meticulously stripped from the underlying fatty tissue, damage to these small vessels is predictable. If the vessels are damaged, blood will quickly pool in the dependent cul-de-sac, obscuring the surgeon's efforts to isolate and coagulate the vessels. Such bleeding increases the likelihood of thermal damage to the bowel wall.

Deep Peritoneal Resection

When a lesion is large, fibrotic, or invading the retroperitoneal area, the peritoneum adjacent to the lesion should be elevated. The resulting taut pleat is opened with a touch cut. The hole is grasped and elevated medially so the scissors can bluntly dissect the lesion away from underlying structures. Then, grasping either the lesion or the adjacent normal peritoneum, slide cuts can extend the line of incision around the lesion, with retroperitoneal dissection working toward the center of the bottom of the lesion. It is only during retroperitoneal dissection that the invasiveness of endometriosis can be appreciated. Coagulation cutting beneath the peritoneum is useful for severing tendrils of tissue left over from blunt dissection. Such invasive lesions will frequently bring the scissors into direct contact with the wall of the rectosigmoid colon and its lateral vascular supply. Blunt and sharp dissection should be used to separate the invasive lesion from these structures before electrosurgery is used.

Resection of the Uterosacral Ligament

Either uterosacral ligament can be involved by invasive endometriosis as large as the volume of a man's thumb, with fibrotic extension down to the sacrum. In such cases, resection of the entire uterosacral ligament will ensure complete removal of all invasive disease. To resect the uterosacral ligament, incise the peritoneum lateral and parallel to it using touch and slide cutting. This incision over the adjacent broad ligament automatically retracts the peritoneum and provides a view of the retroperitoneal structures. The ureter and uterine vessels can then be pushed laterally to ensure that they are not near the uterosacral ligament. The ligament can be partially undermined along much of its length, and this will define much of the ensuing dissection.

With bulky invasive disease, fibrosis may extend laterally to involve the ureter or branches of the uterine vessels descending along the lateral vaginal wall. In this case, the dissection must begin in uninvolved peritoneum more posteriorly along the broad ligament and then proceed around the ureter and uterine vessels toward the uterosacral ligament. Blunt dissection is used adjacent to the ureter, although short bursts of electrosurgery can occasionally be used. Just medial to the point where the uterine vessels cross the ureter are the inferior branches of the uterine vessels. These run adjacent to and parallel with the uterosacral ligaments. Blunt dissection alternating with meticulous use of monopolar current is necessary to separate the uterosacral ligament from these vessels. If bleeding is encountered, it can be safely controlled with unipolar or bipolar coagulation, because the dissection at this point is well medial to the ureter. Once the lateral margin of the uterosacral ligament has been dissected away from these branches of the uterine vessels, a peritoneal incision is made medial and parallel to the ligament.

Next, the insertion of the uterosacral ligament into the posterior cervix is divided with coagulation cutting. The uterosacral ligament is grasped and dissected posteriorly off the pelvic floor using a combination of sharp and blunt dissection and electrodissection. As the dissection retreats from the area of the cervix, and the endometriotic invasion is completely undermined, it will be seen that the uterosacral ligament becomes less dense and spreads out into the surrounding perirectal connective tissue. At this distal point, the ligament is transected with coagulation cutting and removed. The lateral isolation of the uterosacral ligament I have described is key to successful management of the cul-de-sac.

Obliteration of the Cul-de-Sac

Obliteration of the cul-de-sac usually suggests disease invading the wall of the rectum, as well as invasive disease of the uterosacral ligaments and the hidden cul-de-sac. An operative report of a previous surgery may describe "dense cul-de-sac adhesions" or "the rectum adherent to the posterior cervix." In such cases, the floor of the pelvis is probably invaded by endometriosis. Successful surgical treatment of the obliterated cul-de-sac requires more than an attempt at mechanical separation of the rectum from the cervix which only results in persistent disease in most patients.[35] There is a need to remove all invasive endometriosis. Frequently, this will require an en bloc resection of the uterosacral ligaments, posterior cervix, and cul-de-sac, as well as of the rectal nodule.[10]

Laparoscopic surgical treatment of the obliterated cul-de-sac involves specific, consistently reproducible steps. They will allow an experienced laparoscopist to complete this surgery successfully and efficiently.[10] These surgical steps include: lateral isolation of the uterosacral ligaments; transverse incision across the cervix above the adherent bowel; intrafascial dissection down the cervix toward the rectovaginal septum; entry into and blunt development of the rectovaginal septum, with resulting isolation of the uterosacral ligaments; transection of the uterosacral ligaments at their insertion into the posterior cervix; mobilization of the rectum by transection of the lateral rectal attachments; and en bloc resection of the mobilized mass (Figs. 12.4 and 12.5 and color plates 12.4 and 12.5). This may result in partial-thickness, full-thickness, or segmental resection and end-to-end anastomosis of the bowel. Deep partial-thickness resections are repaired with interrupted 3-0 silk sutures in the seromuscularis; whereas full-thickness resections of the bowel wall are repaired with running 3-0 chromic to close the mucosa, and interrupted 3-0 silk sutures to close the seromuscularis.

Segmental bowel resection with end-to-end anastomosis is occasionally required for large nodules or multiple nodules along with a length of bowel.[8,31] Transabdominal stay sutures are used to stabilize and suspend the bowel wall just above and below the point of initial transection. The bowel is transected proximal to the lesion and the proximal segment is retracted against the abdominal wall with a stay suture to avoid spillage. The distal cut edge is elevated with the other stay suture. The open bowel is closed with an endoloop to avoid unnecessary spillage. The bowel is separated from the mesentery by electrosurgical methods. The surgeon works by looking "down the barrel" of the bowel (which is closed by the endoloop) immediately adjacent to the bowel wall. No attempt is made to remove the associated mesentery. A ring forceps in the bowel allows intra-

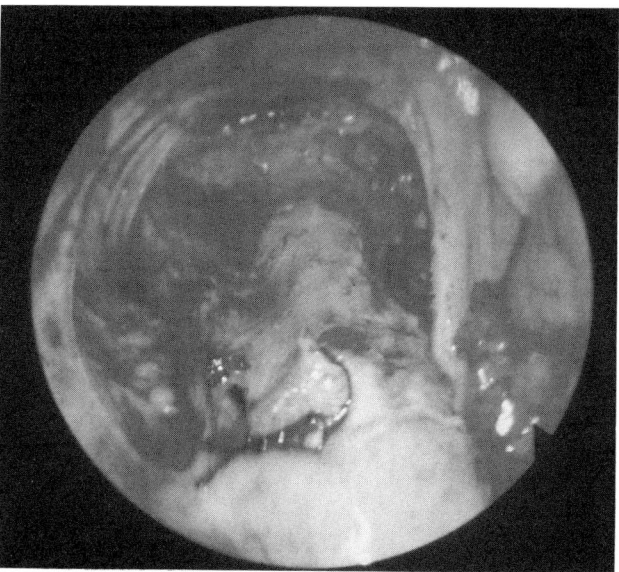

Figure 12.5. The rectal nodule of endometriosis has been removed by partial-thickness bowel resection (mucosal skinning). The seromuscularis has been closed with a single 3-0 silk suture. See also color plate.

operative manipulation. Division with monopolar scissors can be used to isolate the segment to be removed. Once the segment has been sufficiently isolated, the bowel wall distal to the second proposed transection line is held with a grasper or stay suture. The bowel is transected distally and the segment is extracted transanally. A distal purse-string suture of 3-0 Prolene or an Endoloop is applied and an end-to-end anastomosis (EEA) stapler is inserted transanally and into the proximal segment. The proximal purse-string suture or Endoloop is applied, then the stapler is closed and fired to complete the anastomosis. The pelvis is filled with fluid and air is injected through a sigmoidoscope to check for leaks. If bubbles are seen, interrupted 3-0 silk sutures are used to reinforce the bowel wall until the leak is stopped. Segmental bowel resections can also be performed using an extracorporeal technique by video-laser laparoscopy.[32,36]

Complications

If a small hole is created in the unprepared bowel, colostomy need not be performed. Instead, a small defect should be closed with interrupted 3-0 silk. The integrity of the bowel should be checked by underwater air pressure examination. Copious intraoperative irrigation should be performed and postoperative prophylactic antibiotics given. The patient will do well with a simple but properly performed laparoscopic repair.

Recently, a patient of mine who had undergone a partial-thickness, shallow excisional biopsy of the bowel wall without suturing returned to the hospital 6 days

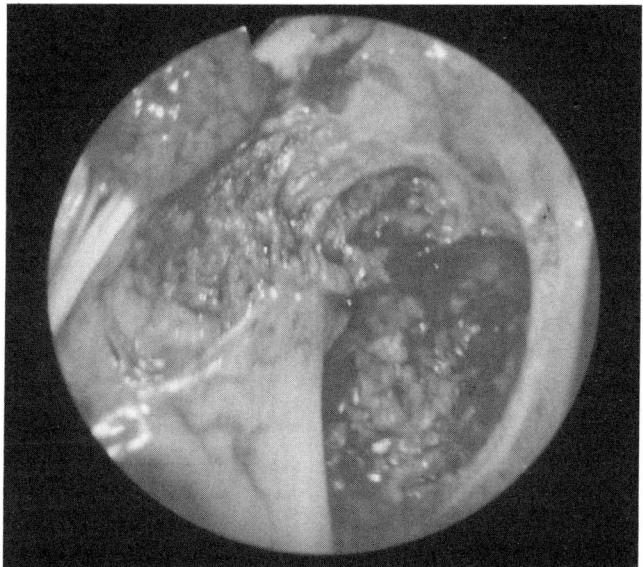

Figure 12.4. The left uterosacral ligament has been isolated by a lateral peritoneal incision and a medial incision in uninvolved peritoneum of the cul-de-sac. An intrafascial dissection down the left side of the posterior cervix has allowed the uterosacral ligament to be transected at its insertion into the posterior cervix. The invasive endometriosis of the left uterosacral and adjacent left posterior cervix and the attached rectosigmoid colon are falling posteriorly away from the cervix. The normal right uterosacral ligament is still intact. See also color plate.

later with acute onset of severe, generalized abdominal pain. She had recovered normally after her initial surgery and had been sightseeing in the mountains at approximately 6,000 feet elevation. X-ray showed free air under the diaphragm, and laparoscopy performed within 2 hours of the onset of her pain showed a pinpoint leak of air from the sigmoid colon. There was no leakage of bowel contents, and the defect was closed with interrupted 3-0 silk sutures tied with intracorporeal knots. The patient recovered without complications. This case shows that if a late bowel perforation does occur and is identified immediately, it can sometimes be handled simply without the need for laparotomy or colostomy. It seems possible that decreased barometric pressure contributed to this patient's late perforation.

Perioperative Patient Management

Modern laparoscopic surgery is major surgery. It bears little resemblance to a simple diagnostic laparoscopy that might have been performed in the 1970s. In my experience, the advisability of performing advanced laparoscopic surgery on an outpatient basis is questionable. Unanticipated admission to the hospital after outpatient surgery has been found strongly associated with the use of general anesthesia and the performance of operative laparoscopy.[37] Minimal recovery critera should be met before patients are discharged from outpatient surgical centers. These criteria include cessation of vomiting, ability to retain both liquids and pain medication by mouth, and the ability to walk to the bathroom with minimal assistance. When patients are discharged too early and have persistent nausea and vomiting, they are unable to retain oral fluids and pain medications. Advanced laparoscopic surgery most commonly results in a hospitalization of 24 hours or less, although laparoscopic segmental bowel resection may require hospitalization of several days.

Full activities may be resumed within 3 weeks by most patients. Sexual intercourse should be delayed for 5 weeks, especially in patients with cul-de-sac or uterosacral ligament resections. The first two menstrual periods may be unusually painful. Some patients may not appreciate the full extent of pain relief for several months.

Patient Outcome

Long-term analysis by life-table techniques of rates of reoperation and recurrent diagnosis of endometriosis after laparoscopic excision indicate a cumulative rate of occurrence of new disease of 19% by the end of the fifth postoperative year.[21] This rate of recurrence is identical with that reported after laparotomy.[22,38]

Complete surgical eradication of endometriosis is possible using excisional techniques. We still await longitudinal follow-up of large numbers of patients treated with laser vaporization or electrocoagulation. These methods have been studied primarily with respect to their effects on symptoms rather than on the disease. Until such follow-up is reported, the long-term benefit of nonexcisional surgery remains unproven.

Complete removal of endometriosis will result in pain relief in patients whose pain is due to endometriosis. If pain persists after identification and aggressive removal of all endometriosis, this does not necessarily indicate a failure of surgical therapy in treating the disease. Persistent pain may be due to other causes, indicating the need for more precision in determining preoperatively which types of pain are due to endometriosis.

References

1. Sampson JA. Perforating hemorrhagic (chocolate) cysts of the ovary. Arch Surg 1921;3:245–323.
2. Sampson JA. Ovarian hematomas of endometrial type (perforating hemorrhagic cysts of the ovary) and implantation adenomas of the endometrial type. Bost Med Surg J 1922;186:445–456.
3. Sampson JA. The development of the implantation theory for the origin of peritoneal endometriosis. Am J Obstet Gynecol 1940;40:549–557.
4. Jenkins S, Olive DL, Haney AF. Endometriosis: pathogenic implications of the anatomic distribution. Obstet Gynecol 1991;67:335–338.
5. Redwine DB. Mulleriosis: the single best fit model of origin of endometriosis. J Reprod Med 1988;33:915–20.
6. Fujii S. Secondary mullerian system and endometriosis. Am J Obstet Gynecol 1991;165:219–25.
7. Redwine DB. The distribution of endometriosis in the pelvis by age groups and fertility. Fertil Steril 1987;47:173–175.
8. Sharpe DR, Redwine DB. Laparoscopic segmental resection of the sigmoid and rectosigmoid colon for endometriosis. Surgical Laparoscopy Endoscopy 1992;2:120–14.
9. Ripps BA, Martin DC. Focal pelvic tenderness, pelvic pain and dysmenorrhea in endometriosis. J Reprod Med 1991;36:470–472.
10. Redwine DB. Laparoscopic en bloc resection for treatment of the obliterated cul-de-sac in endometriosis. J Reprod Med 1992;37:695–698.
11. Koninckx PR, Martin DC. Deep endometriosis: a consequence of infiltration or retraction or possibly adenomyosis externa? Fertil Steril 1992;58:924–928.
12. Evers JLH. The second-look laparoscopy for evaluation of the result of medical treatment of endometriosis should not be performed during ovarian suppression. Fertil Steril 1987;47:502–504.
13. Murphy AA, Green WR, Bobbie D, et al. Unsuspected endometriosis documented by scanning electron microscopy in visually normal peritoneum. Fertil Steril 1986;46:522–54.
14. Jansen RPS, Russell P. Nonpigmented endometriosis. Clinical, laparoscopic, and pathologic definition. Am J Obstet Gynecol 1986;155:1154–1159.
15. Redwine DB. Is "microscopic" peritoneal endometriosis invisible? Fertil Steril 1988;50:665–666.
16. Nisolle M, Paindaveine B, Bourdon A, et al. Histologic study of peritoneal endometriosis in infertile women. Fertil Steril 1990;53:984–988.

17. Redwine DB, Yocom L. A serial section study of visually normal peritoneum in patients with endometriosis. Fertil Steril 1990;54:648–651.
18. Nezhat F, Allan CJ, Nezhat C, et al. Nonvisualized endometriosis at laparoscopy. Int J Fertil 1991;36:340–33.
19. Redwine DB. Treatment of endometriosis-associated pain. In Olive DL, ed. Endometriosis: Infertility and Reproductive Medicine Clinics of North America. Philadelphia, WB Saunders, 1992, pp 697–720.
20. The American Fertility Society. Revised American Fertility Classification system of endometriosis: 1985. Fertil Steril 1985;44:351–352.
21. Redwine DB. Conservative laparoscopic excision of endometriosis by sharp dissection: life table analysis of reoperation and persistent or recurrent disease. Fertil Steril 1991;56:628–634.
22. Wheeler JM, Malinak LR. Recurrent endometriosis. Contr Gynecol Obstet 1987;16:13–21.
23. Redwine DB. Nafarelin vs Danazol vs Surgery. Fertil Steril 1992;58:455–456.
24. Griffin L, Noller K, Kaminetzky H, et al. Personal communications, 1991.
25. Cook AS, Rock JA. The role of laparoscopy in the treatment of endometriosis. Fertil Steril 1991;55:663–680.
26. Sulewski JM, Curcio FD, Bronitsky C, et al. The treatment of endometriosis at laparoscopy for infertility. Am J Obstet Gynecol 1980;138:128–132.
27. Seiler JC, Gidwani G, Ballard L. Laparoscopic cauterization of endometriosis for fertility: a controlled study. Fertil Steril 1986;46:1098–1100.
28. Hasson HM. Electrocoagulation of pelvic endometriotic lesions with laparoscopic control. Am J Obstet Gynecol 1979;135:115–119.
29. Murphy AA, Schlaff WD, Hassiakos D, et al. Laparoscopic cautery in the treatment of endometriosis-related infertility. Fertil Steril 1991;55:245–251.
30. Pitkin R. Operative lapaoscopy: Surgical advance or technical gimmick. Obstet Gynecol 1992;79:441–442.
31. Redwine DB, Sharpe DR. Laparoscopic segmental resection of the sigmoid colon. Journal of Laparoendoscopic Surgery 1991;1:217–220.
32. Nezhat F, Nezhat C, Pennington E. Laparoscopic proctectomy for infiltrating endometriosis of the rectum. Fertil Steril 1992;57:1129–1132.
33. Summitt RL Jr, Stovall TG, Lipscomb GH, Ling FW. Randomized comparison of laparoscopy-assisted vaginal hysterectomy with standard vaginal hysterectomy in an outpatient setting. Obstet Gynecol 1992;80:895–901.
34. Widdowson EM, Dicerkson JWT. Composition of the body. In Diem K, Lentner C, eds. Geigy Scientific Tables, 7th ed. Basle, 1970, pp 517–522.
35. Reich H, McGlynn G, Salvat J. Laparoscopic treatment of cul-de-sac obliteration secondary to retrocervical deep fibrotic endometriosis. J Reprod Med 1991;36:516–522.
36. Nezhat C, Nezhat F, Pennington E. Laparoscopic treatment of infiltrative rectosigmoid colon and rectovaginal septum endometriosis by the technique of videolaser laparoscopy and the CO_2 laser. Brit J Obstet Gynecol 1992;99:664–667.
37. Gold BS, Kitz DS, Lecky JH, et al. Unanticipated admission to the hospital following ambulatory surgery. JAMA 1989;262:3008–3010.
38. Koninckx PR, Meuleman C, Demeyere S, Lesaffre E, Cornillie FJ. Suggestive evidence that pelvic endometriosis is a progressive disease, whereas deeply infiltrating endometriosis is associated with pain. Fertil Steril 1991;55:759–765.

13

Adjunctive Procedures in Treatment of Endometriosis: LUNA, Presacral Neurectomy, and Uterine Suspension

Sanford M. Markham and John A. Rock

Unlike many other diseases of the upper female reproductive tract where total cure involves the removal of part or all of the reproductive organs, endometriosis is generally managed by a variety of more conservative treatments in hopes of preserving reproductive capacity. By accepting this conservative approach, however, endometriosis patients incur higher rates of disease recurrence and persistence of symptoms than with definitive surgery (total abdominal hysterectomy and bilateral salpingo-oophorectomy).[1]

Adjunctive procedures have been proposed to improve the outcome of conservative therapy without requiring total abdominal hysterectomy and bilateral salpingo-oophorectomy. Of the variety of adjunctive procedures available, three have attracted considerable interest in the medical literature: laparoscopic uterine nerve ablation (LUNA), presacral neurectomy (PSN), and uterine suspension. Each has been used with success. Therefore, they should be considered in the management options when reproductive preservation is desired.

Indications for Adjunctive Procedures

Of the symptoms associated with endometriosis, pain is the most frequent and difficult to treat. Central deep pelvic pain, which is often disabling, results from endometriotic infiltration of the posterior cul-de-sac, uterosacral ligaments, posterior uterine wall, and medial aspects of the broad ligaments and/or the adjacent pelvic sidewalls.[1] It occurs when peritoneal endometriosis infiltrates into the subperitoneal fibromuscular tissue where nerve fibers are concentrated.[2] Approximately one-third of patients with endometriosis have lesions penetrating deeper than 4 mm.[3] Deep disease generally involves the area of the pouch of Douglas

(55%), uterosacral ligaments (34%), and the uterovesical fold (11%).[2] Very deep implants (>10 mm) have been found exclusively in patients with disabling pain, whereas more superficial implants are more common in patients with infertility as a primary complaint.[2] Persistent or recurrent pelvic pain may result from deep infiltration of fibromuscular tissue and nerves, not corrected by previous conservative surgical or medical techniques, or by scarring occurring in fibromuscular tissue as a consequence of previous conservative surgical management.

Because of painful recurrent disease, a second operation is often required. In one study, the cumulative 3-year and 5-year recurrence rates of endometriosis were 14% and 40%, respectively.[4] In another, the repetitive surgery rate for recurrent endometriosis exceeded 50%.[5]

Several anatomic factors support the reported benefit of adjunctive surgical procedures including presacral neurectomy, uterine nerve ablation, and uterine suspension in initial management of severe endometriosis and, more frequently, for recurrent symptomatic disease. First, the location of the sensory nerve fibers from the uterus in the superior hypogastric plexus affords the opportunity to transect the presacral nerves. Alternatively, we would expect ligation or ablation of sensory nerve fibers at any point along their tract from the uterus to the hypogastric plexus (specifically fibers of the inferior hypogastric nerves passing through the uterosacral ligaments) to reduce pain from endometriotic implants. Second, because lesions of endometriosis are more common on the posterior surface of the uterus and in the posterior cul-de-sac area, uterine suspension that repositions the uterus anteriorly should reduce the potential for fallopian tube and ovarian entrapment or for marked posterior cul-de-sac adhesions and obliteration, and the pain that results.

Laparoscopic Uterine Nerve Ablation (LUNA)

Pain impulses from the uterus, the cervix, and the proximal fallopian tubes pass through nerve fibers that merge into the uterine plexus, then pass into the paracervical plexus of Frankenhausen at the base of the uterosacral ligaments, and exit through the uterosacral ligaments to the inferior and superior hypogastric plexuses.[6] Because of this sensory pathway, the possibility has been suggested of managing some types of pelvic pain by transecting the uterosacral ligaments, and therefore the uterine nerves. One of the earliest reports appeared in 1915.[7] A more recent report, in 1955, assessed the results of vaginally transecting the uterosacral nerves for dysmenorrhea, with a 70% reduction in pain reported.[8]

The technique for laparoscopic uterine nerve ablation (LUNA) involves surgical principles similar to those for other types of operative laparoscopy. A 10 mm trocar is placed in the subumbilical region, through which an operating laparoscope is passed. Two 5 mm trocars, inserted laterally in the lower abdomen, serve as ports for additional operating instruments. Of major importance is the preoperative placement of a uterine probe through the cervix into the top of the uterine cavity, for use in anteflexing the uterus during the procedure. Grasping instruments are placed through the lateral ports to retract the tubes and ovaries and to allow full visualization of the ureters. The uterosacral ligaments are then put on stretch by markedly anteflexing the uterus with the uterine probe. Ablation of the uterosacral ligaments may be accomplished by one of several techniques. Electrocoagulation of the ligaments at their point of insertion into the cervix, followed by transection of the ligaments by operating scissors, has had good success.[7] Using this technique, the uterosacral ligaments are coagulated until complete blanching is observed before bisecting them with scissors.

More recently, ablation of the uterosacral ligaments using laser vaporization has been reported.[9] This technique, like electrocoagulation, involves complete transection of the uterosacral ligaments at their attachment to the posterior aspect of the cervix, after having identified the ureters before vaporization.

The majority of reports describe uterine nerve ablation in cases of dysmenorrhea without endometriosis. In one study of 39 patients with dysmenorrhea considered for a LUNA procedure, 18 were excluded because of pelvic endometriosis or pelvic inflammatory disease.[7] The remaining 21 were divided into a control group of 10 and test group of 11 receiving a LUNA procedure. Of the 11 patients receiving a LUNA procedure, 9 (82%) reported marked relief of pain, whereas none of the control group reported improvement. In another study of 23 patients with dysmenorrhea treated by CO_2 laser uterine nerve ablation, 3 had minimal endometriosis.[9] The outcome for these 3 patients was not reported; however, 14 of the 20 primary dysmenorrhea patients were available for a 1-year follow-up. Only 5 were free of symptoms. The remaining 9 (64%) had recurrent symptoms.

In another study of 50 patients with chronic pelvic pain who underwent a presacral neurectomy, 44% were found to have endometriosis.[13] Of the total group, approximately half had a presacral neurectomy alone, whereas the others had a presacral neurectomy and uterosacral ligament resection. Results indicated that the addition of uterosacral ligament resection was no more effective than presacral neurectomy alone.

Data are insufficient to determine the effectiveness of LUNA procedure for patients with pelvic endometriosis. Neither tenderness of the uterosacral ligament on pelvic examination, nor pain relief after the application of a local anesthetic agent into the uterosacral ligament, has proven to be a valid indicator of LUNA outcome. Available data on the effectiveness of LUNA in patients with primary dysmenorrhea suggest variable results. These results may or may not be applicable to patients with pelvic endometriosis.

Presacral Neurectomy (PSN)

Presacral neurectomy is a technique that dates back to the 1800s.[10] Early reports addressed the resection of the presacral nerves as a treatment of severe dysmenorrhea.[11] While resection or destruction of endometriotic implants or endometriomas has been found to provide relief of pain in a large percentage of cases, persistent central pain frequently responds well to presacral neurectomy when other conservative measures have failed.[12,13] However, not all studies of endometriosis patients have reported significant relief of pain after presacral neurectomy.[14] Some have reported only short-term improvement in midline menstrual pain, with little difference in the long-term follow-up between patients receiving a presacral neurectomy and those managed by other conservative techniques.[15] Many investigators, however, favor the use of presacral neurectomy in the management of chronic midline pelvic pain associated with pelvic endometriosis. It has been suggested that conflicting results occur because of different criteria for selecting patients or completeness in resecting the presacral nerve plexus.[10]

Complete transection of the presacral nerves is of primary importance for successful outcomes. Failure to identify and transect one or more of the superior hypogastric plexus nerve bundles will result in failure. Figure 13.1 demonstrates the location of the presacral nerves (superior hypogastric plexus) as they pass over the aorta and the common iliac arteries at their bifurcation and enter the pelvis lying above the sacrum in the midline.

The technique of presacral neurectomy may be accomplished by laparotomy or laparoscopy. The route selected should depend on the surgeon's experience and skill. It is important, in either approach, to visualize the posterior pelvis adequately from a level of the fifth lumbar vertebra down to a level of the third or fourth sacral vertebra. At laparotomy, packing the bowel into the upper abdomen and retracting the rectosigmoid colon toward the left pelvic sidewall allows adequate exposure in most cases. At laparoscopy, deep Trendelenburg positioning of the patient and use of a fan retractor (Endo Retract, Auto Suture Co.) placed through a separate port generally allows sufficient exposure. Once adequate visualization of the pelvis has been achieved, key structures of the pelvic anatomy must be identified. These include the right and left common iliac arteries and veins and the middle sacral artery and vein. Bleeding due to injury of the middle sacral vessels is one of the more common complications of presacral neurectomy.[10]

After identifying these pelvic structures, a midline incision in the posterior parietal peritoneum should be made starting at the level of the first or second sacral vertebra and extending the incision cephalad to a level just above the bifurcation of the aorta. The incision should then be extended caudally to a level of the third or fourth sacral vertebra. The peritoneum is carefully dissected from the subperitoneal tissue to develop a peritoneal flap. The edges of the peritoneum should be retracted laterally. This can be accomplished by use of small stay sutures placed at the edge of the peritoneum. At laparoscopy, the peritoneum may be retracted laterally by two grasping instruments placed through the accessory ports.

When the peritoneum has been adequately incised and retracted laterally, the presacral nerves should be identified as they pass over the bifurcation of the aorta. These nerves may enter the pelvis as a single trunk, but they more frequently occur as several trunks (Fig. 13.1). After passing over the bifurcation, the presacral nerves divide into several bundles, which should be isolated and gently dissected away from the retroperitoneal connective tissue. Special care should be taken to avoid trauma to the middle sacral vessels. These commonly lie immediately beneath the right bundle or the middle bundle of the presacral nerves. Elevating the nerve bundles with an umbilical tape or large suture allows easier traction and dissection. The presacral nerve trunks should then be secured with suture ligatures: the first passed superiorly (cephalic) around the nerves close to the bifurcation of the aorta, and the second passed inferiorly (caudal) at the level of the second or third sacral vertebra. This positioning allows excision of 2 to 3 cm of presacral nerve bundles from between the two ligatures. After removal of the presacral nerve tissue, the peritoneum may be closed with a fine absorbable suture (4-0 or 5-0).

The most common immediate complication of this procedure is bleeding from the middle sacral artery or vein or from the inferior mesenteric artery or its superior hemorrhoidal branch. Bleeding can usually be prevented by meticulous surgical technique. If bleeding occurs, control may be accomplished by fine ties, electrocautery, small vascular clips, or by use of bone wax or an orthopaedic thumbtack.

Laparoscopic presacral neurectomy, accomplished in much the same manner, uses a high-resolution laparoscope and video camera and a four- or five-puncture approach. It is useful to place a 10 mm or 12 mm laparoscope with video camera through a suprapubic midline trocar sleeve with two 5.5 mm trocar sleeves 4 to 5 cm lateral to the laparoscope (Fig. 13.1). These two lateral ports serve as the main entry points for the operating instruments, and an additional 10 mm trocar sleeve in a subumbilical position allows passage of a fan retractor to move the rectosigmoid colon to the left

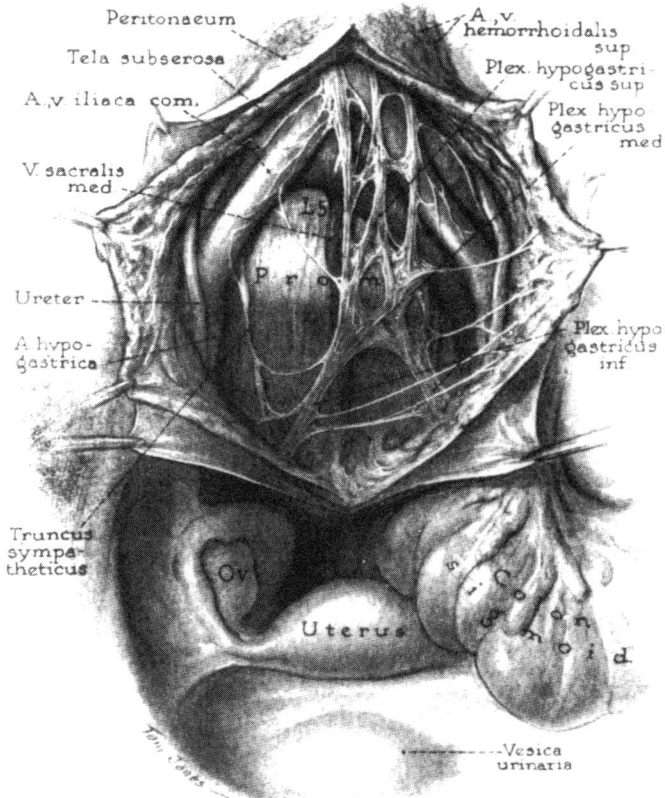

Figure 13.1. *Presacral nerve plexus*: This shows passage of sympathetic trunk over bifurcation of aorta. Note division of trunk into left and right presacral nerves. (Source: DeLancey JOL. Anatomy of the female pelvis. In Thompson JD, Rock JA, eds. TeLinde's operative gynecology, 7th ed., chap. 4. Philadelphia. JB Lippincott Company, 1992, p 53.) With permission from *Surg. Gynecol. Obstet.* 1942; 75:743.

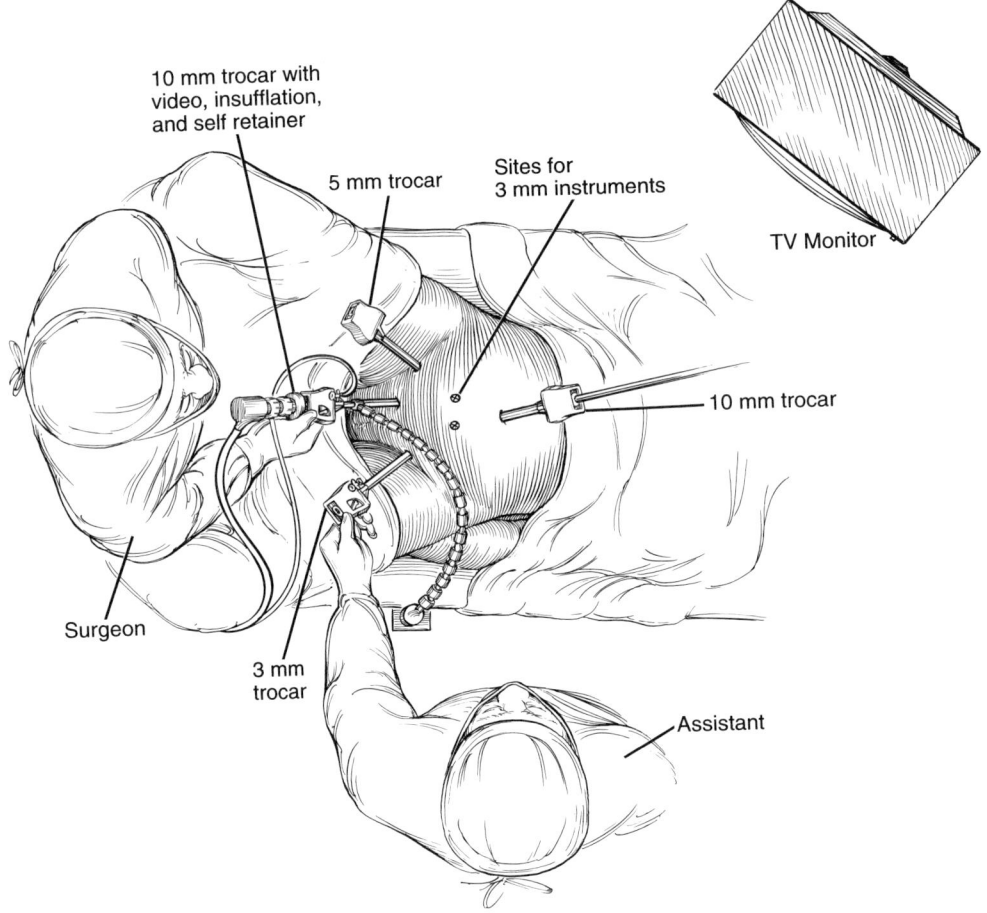

Figure 13.2. Placement of instruments during laparoscopic presacral neurectomy.

(Fig. 13.2). This approach, with the surgeon at the foot of the table, rather than at the patient's side, allows maximal exposure and dexterity by allowing the surgeon to face the operative field directly.

Using laparoscopic technique, identification of essential pelvic anatomy is accomplished in much the same fashion as at laparotomy. The pelvic peritoneum is elevated with a grasping instrument and a midline incision is made from the level of the second or third sacral vertebra superiorly (cephalic) to the bifurcation of the aorta. The underlying retroperitoneal connective tissue is gently dissected away from the peritoneum, and the peritoneum is retracted laterally through two additional mid- and low abdominal entry points using 3 mm trocar sleeve and 3 mm endograsping instruments or endobabcock. The presacral nerve bundles are identified, dissected free, and elevated (Fig. 13.3). At this point, the presacral nerves can be excised by a variety of techniques. These include endoloop suture ligation with excision of intervening nerve bundle, bipolar cauterization of the nerve bundles with resection of intervening segment, or a combination of bipolar cautery and Nd:YAG laser with contact tip to excise

the intervening nerve bundle (Fig. 13.4).[16] After excision of the presacral nerves, the peritoneal edges should be reapproximated utilizing endoloop sutures.

Besides bleeding and injury to the ureter, a variety of postoperative complications have also been reported. These have included adhesions, urinary bladder dysfunction, chronic constipation, vaginal dryness, and painless labor.[10]

Success in the elimination or reduction of pelvic pain in patients with endometriosis generally exceeds 50%, provided the procedure is limited to patients with central deep pelvic pain. In one study of 50 patients undergoing laparotomy presacral neurectomy, 56% reported total pain relief, 14% reported greater than 50% relief of pain, and 10% reported no relief.[13] Of the 50 women, 22 had documented pelvic endometriosis. In another study of patients with endometriosis, 97% reported an improvement in dysmenorrhea after presacral neurectomy.[12] A prospective study of laparotomy presacral neurectomy in patients with AFS stage III and stage IV endometriosis revealed that 15 (88%) of 17 with midline deep pelvic pain reported significant pain relief.[10] In a randomized controlled study of 71

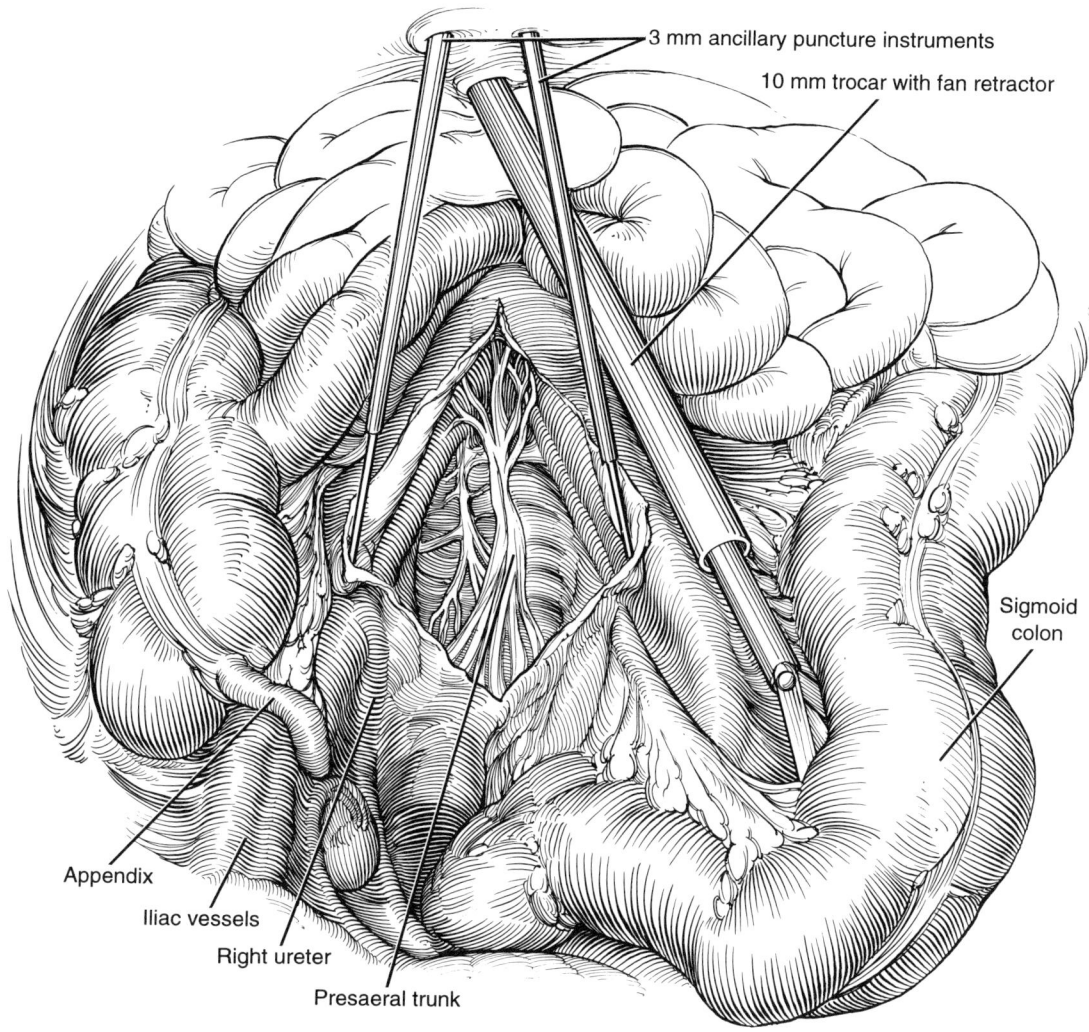

Figure 13.3. Exposure of the presacral nerve trunk in the retroperitoneal space.

patients with moderate to severe endometriosis-associated pelvic pain, 36 underwent conservative surgery and 35 underwent conservative surgery and presacral neurectomy.[15] Postoperative assessment revealed that 8 (23%) of 35 patients receiving a presacral neurectomy experienced recurrent menstrual pain, whereas 15 (42%) of 36 patients receiving only conservative surgery experienced recurrent pain. The authors concluded that presacral neurectomy should be combined with conservative surgery for endometriosis in patients with midline pelvic pain.

Data from laparoscopic presacral neurectomy are limited. In one study of 25 patients undergoing laparoscopic presacral neurectomy, all were reported to have experienced a reduction in symptoms with 2 (8%) becoming pain free and 21 (84%) reporting pain reduction of 50% or more.[16]

These data support the apparent benefit of presacral neurectomy for adjunctive management of patients with pelvic endometriosis who have marked or recurrent

midline deep pelvic pain. Patients with lateral pelvic pain and back pain have shown less improvement with presacral neurectomy. Presacral neurectomy is, therefore, considered a useful adjunct to conservative surgery and medical management of selected patients with endometriosis, namely those suffering from severe midline pelvic pain.

When performing laparoscopic presacral neurectomy, it is essential that the rectosigmoid be mobilized and reflected laterally so that the sacral promontory is completely exposed. If the surgeon is at the level of L_2–L_3, a single nerve bundle may be visualized before it branches into a left and right bundle. Then, an adequate presacral neurectomy may be accomplished. Some surgeons have recommended a neurotomy, or ablation alone, rather than neurectomy. However, regeneration of nerve fibers can occur in some patients if insufficient nerve is removed. It is important, therefore, that a major segment of presacral nerve be removed to minimize the rate of recurrent pain.

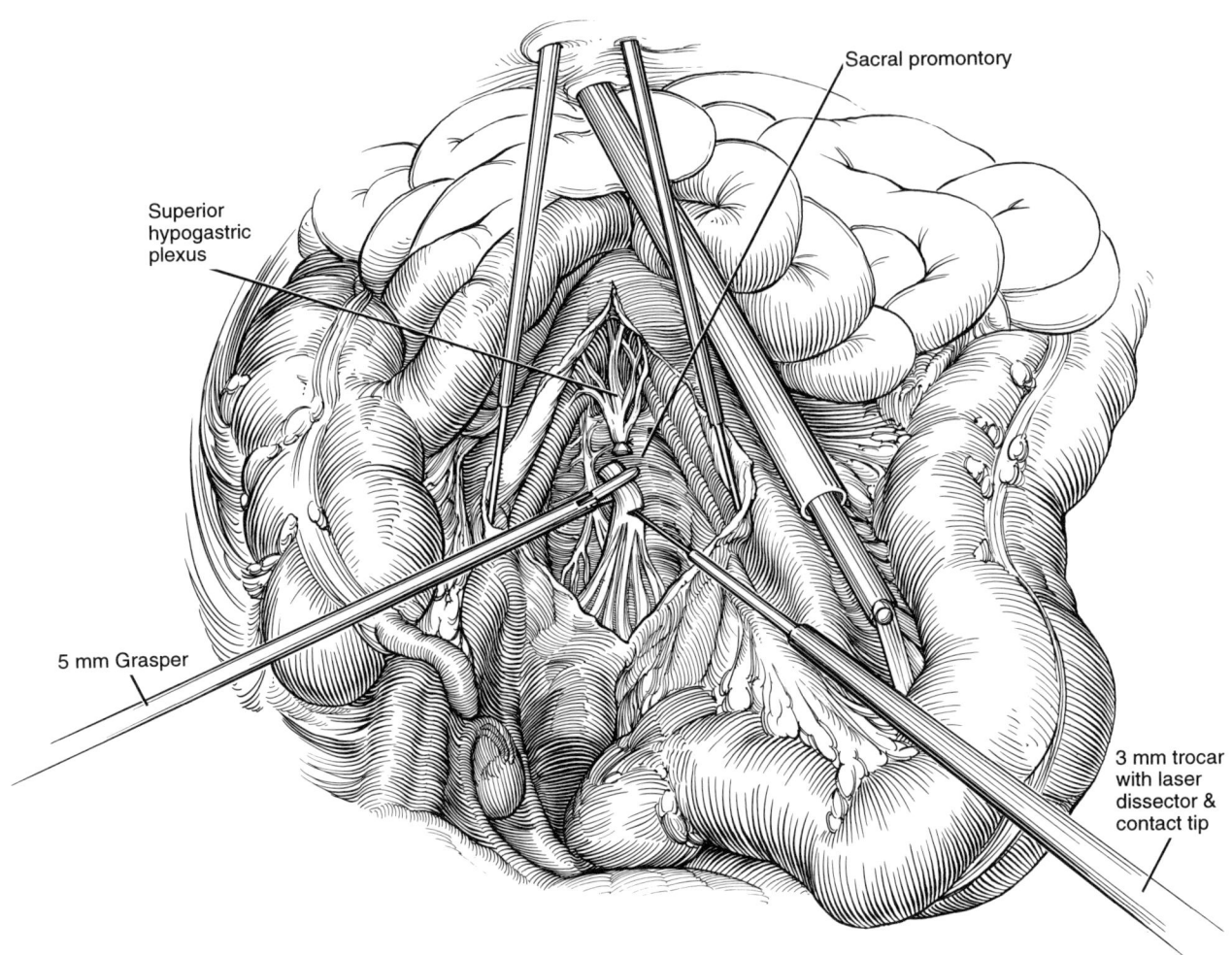

Figure 13.4. Resection of the presacral nerve trunk.

Uterine Suspension

Conservative surgery for endometriosis may include presacral neurectomy, sharp resection of endometrial implants, lysis of adhesions, uterine suspension, and uterosacral ligament plication.[17] This approach remains true today with the addition of laser vaporization and electrocoagulation of endometriotic lesions. Uterine suspension has been considered an adjunctive procedure to prevent entrapment of the ovaries and the fallopian tubes in the posterior cul-de-sac and to prevent adhesions.[18] This procedure becomes particularly important when excision, vaporization, or coagulation is performed in a patient who has a retroflexed uterus and in whom a denuded peritoneum remains at the completion of the conservative procedure. Indications for uterine suspension in the surgical management of endometriosis include: retroflexed uterus, posterior cul-de-sac disease or disease of the posterior uterine wall, and/or a denuded peritoneal surface in the posterior pelvis as a result of conservative surgical procedures.

Uterine suspension may be accomplished at laparotomy or at laparoscopy. A variety of laparotomy choices are possible, the goal of which is to secure the uterus in an anterior position so as to bring the ovaries and fallopian tubes forward and out of the posterior pelvis. The suspension can either shorten or reposition the round ligaments, pulling the uterus anteriorly, or attaching the uterine fundus itself to the anterior abdominal wall. The latter technique is contraindicated in patients wishing to maintain reproductive capacity. Of the round ligament procedures, the modified Gilliam suspension is most often used because of its simplicity. It involves bringing the round ligaments through a small incision in the anterior abdominal wall peritoneum and attaching them to the rectus sheath.

The technique of the modified Gilliam suspension of the uterus is accomplished through a Pfannenstiel incision. A midline incision, however, may be used if such an entry is needed to accomplish the planned conservative surgery. When the abdominal cavity is entered, the uterus is retracted forward and the round ligaments are grasped in the mid-position with a Babcock clamp. A traction suture is then placed around the ligament to replace the Babcock clamp (Fig. 13.5A). The traction suture is best placed at a distance of 3 to 4 cm from the

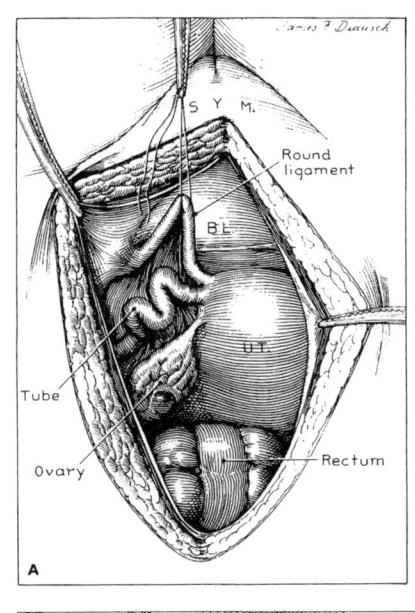

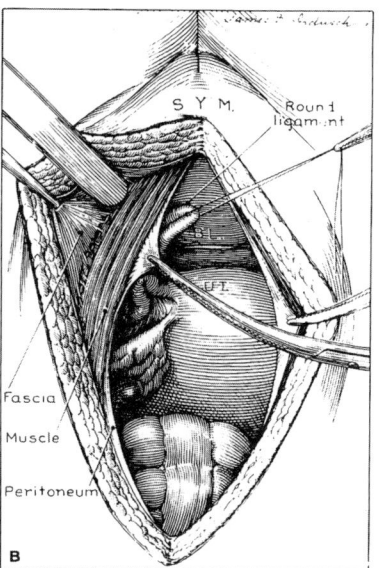

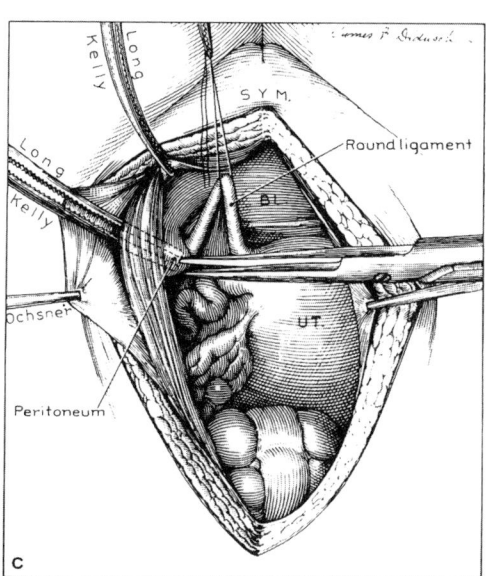

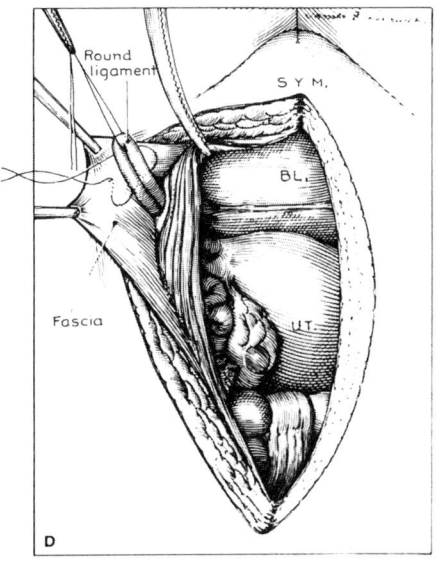

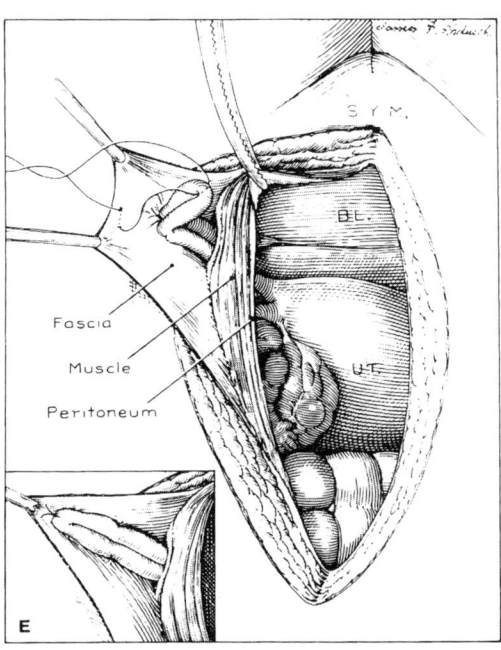

Figure 13.5. Modified Gilliam suspension of uterus through laparotomy incision. (Source: Thompson JD. Malpositions of the uterus. In Thompson JD, Rock JA, eds. TeLinde's operative gynecology, 7th ed., chap. 31. Philadelphia, JB Lippincott Company, 1992, p 825. Reproduced with permission.)

insertion of the round ligament into the wall of the uterus, but the distance may be varied to allow maximal anterior suspension of the uterus. The anterior rectus fascia is grasped with a Kocher or Ochsner clamp and retracted laterally while the peritoneal border is retracted medially. The rectus muscle is dissected from its fascial sheath (Fig. 13.5B). A long Kelly clamp is inserted beneath the lateral border of the rectus muscle remaining above the peritoneum and directing toward the internal inguinal ring (Fig. 13.5C). The tip of the Kelly clamp is then advanced slightly into the peritoneal cavity, tenting the peritoneum. A small incision is made in the peritoneum. Then the clamp is advanced further into the peritoneal cavity. As the traction suture is grasped and pulled back through the peritoneal opening, it brings a loop of the round ligament adjacent to the lateral border of the rectus muscle (Fig. 13.5D). The loop of the round ligament is then sutured to the undersurface of the rectus fascia, using one or two interrupted 2-0 nonabsorbable monofilament sutures (Fig. 13.5E). It is important that the fixation suture include a good bit of the round ligament. Care should be taken not to encircle the ligament and cause strangulation. A similar procedure is carried out on the opposite side. Before closure carefully inspect the fallopian tubes and bowel to exclude any entrapment or malpositioning.

An alternative technique of shortening the round ligaments may be achieved by doubling the ligament on itself and suturing the doubled ligament together with 2-0 nonabsorbable suture. Since insufficient data are available to support the effectiveness of this technique, we prefer the modified Gilliam suspension.

As early as 1942 a report suggested the possibility of performing a uterine suspension without an open abdominal incision.[19] With the development of the modern laparoscope in the late 1960s and early 1970s, a number of reports described laparoscopic uterine suspension.[20-22] In one, a laparoscope and grasping forceps were used to deliver the round ligament to a small skin incision through which the ligament was pulled and sutured to the rectus fascia.[20] Others followed a somewhat similar approach except that the round ligaments were grasped with a tonged forceps and pulled through the operating port and sutured to the rectus fascia (Fig. 13.6).[21,22] A somewhat more novel approach, using Falope rings to shorten the round ligaments and suspend the uterus, has also been reported (Fig. 13.7).[23]

The technique found most effective follows standard laparoscopic procedures for abdominal entry and uses three skin incisions. A 7 mm or 10 mm operating laparoscope with video camera is inserted through a subumbilical skin incision and the patient positioned in a moderate Trendelenburg position. A second skin incision, extended down to the fascia, is made in an avascular region of the lower abdomen approximately three-fourths of the distance from the midline to the inguinal ligament and at the level of the pubic hairline. A third incision is made on the contralateral side, and 5.5 mm trocars are placed through the two incisions. Grasping forceps are passed through the trocar sleeve and the round ligaments are grasped at a point 3 to 4 cm from the uterine attachment point. A portion of the pneumoperitoneum is allowed to escape and a loop of the round ligaments is pulled through the port, removing the grasping instrument and the trocar sleeve at the same time. Appropriate uterine suspension is confirmed by laparoscopic visualization, and the bowel and fallopian tubes are inspected to identify entrapment or abnormal positioning. The round ligaments are then sutured to the rectus fascia using a 2-0 nonabsorbable suture. The skin is closed after evacuation of the remainder of the pneumoperitoneum and removal of the laparoscope. Complications are few. They generally relate to anterior abdominal wall bleeding at the entry sites or to round ligament avulsion.

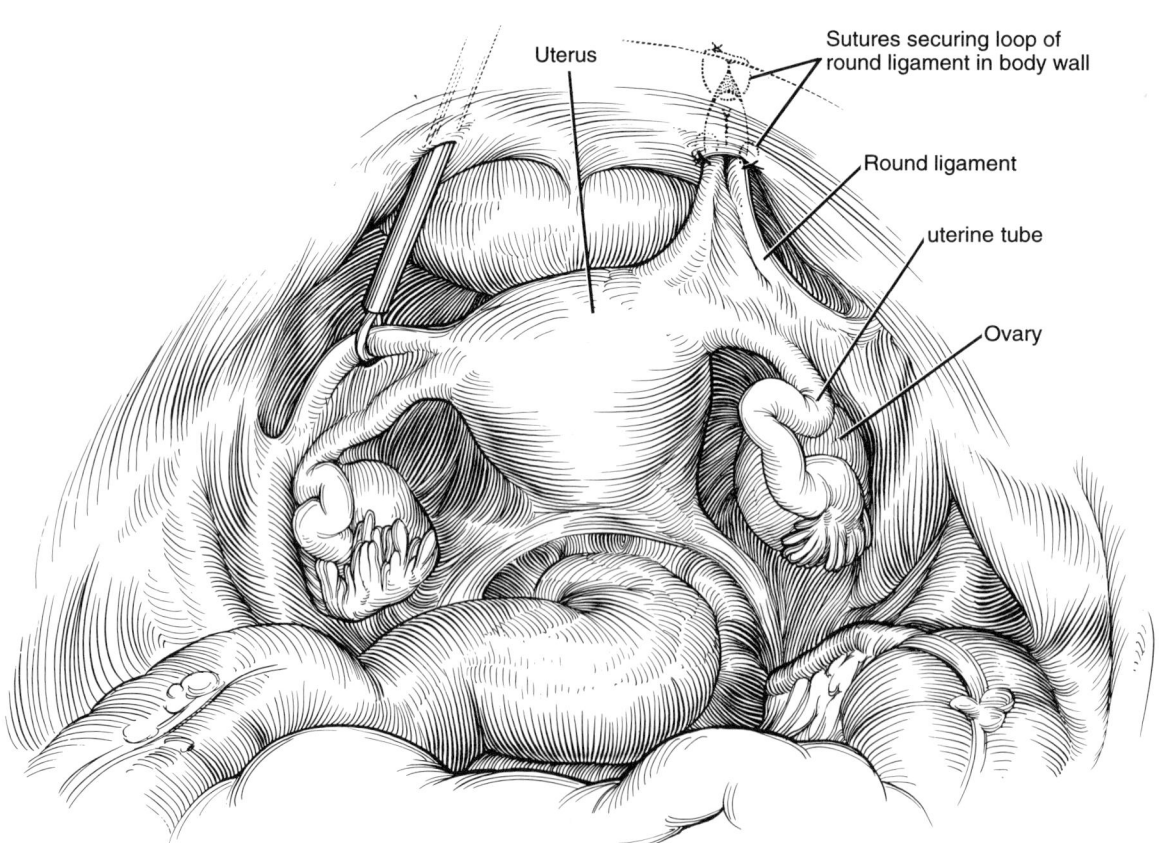

Figure 13.6. Laparoscopist's view of uterine suspension.

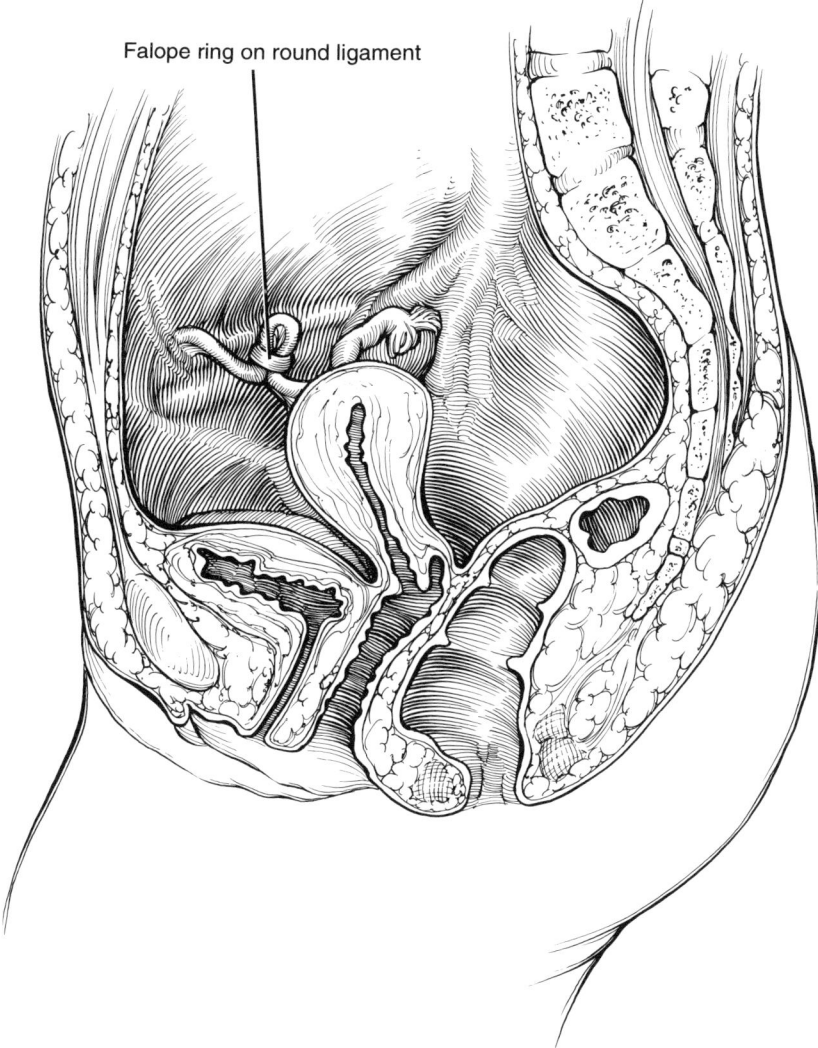

Falope ring on round ligament

Figure 13.7. Pelvic anatomy after application of ring to round ligament.

Conclusion

Management plans for patients with pelvic endometriosis are based on the extent and effect of symptoms and on the desire to maintain reproductive capacity. Conservative management, which includes excision or destruction of surface endometriosis or endometriomas and lysis of adhesions created by the endometriotic process, leaves the uterus, fallopian tubes, and ovaries intact. Conservative management results in an unpredictable but generally high recurrence rate of endometriosis which may cause recurrent pain and frequently requires reoperation. A number of adjunctive surgical procedures to augment conservative management have been proposed. Several appear to have merit in selected cases. Presacral neurectomy (PSN) has been successful in patients with deep pelvic midline pain. This procedure, which works especially well when combined with standard conservative surgical and medical techniques, should be offered to patients suffering progressive and unmanageable midline deep pelvic pain. Complications include hemorrhage and ureteral injury. Complications can be minimized by skill and careful technique. Laparoscopic uterine nerve ablation (LUNA) has also been reported to be effective surgery, but results are not uniform. Its true merit has yet to be proven. Uterine suspension is indicated in selected cases of uterine retroflexion when the posterior pelvic peritoneum is denuded by conservative surgical procedures. This procedure prevents entrapment of the fallopian tubes and ovaries in the posterior cul-de-sac and the resulting symptoms of pain and reduced reproductive capacity.

References

1. Williams TJ, Endometriosis. In Thompson JD, Rock JA, eds. TeLinde's operative gynecology, 7th ed. Chap. 20. Philadelphia: JB Lippincott Co. 1992, pp 463–497.
2. Cornille FJ, Oosterlynch D, Lauweryns JM, et al. Deeply infiltrating pelvic endometriosis: histology and clinical significance. Fertil Steril 1990;53:978–983.
3. Martin DC, Hubert GD, Levy BS. Depth of infiltration of endometriosis. J Gynecol Surg 1989;5:55–60.
4. Wheeler JM, Malinak LR. Recurrent endometriosis: incidence management and prognosis. Am J Obstet Gynecol 1983;146:247–253.
5. Candiani GB, Fedele L, Vercellini P, et al. Repetitive conservative surgery for recurrence of endometriosis. Obstet Gynecol 1991;77:421–424.
6. Malinak LR, Wheeler JM. Conservative surgery for endometriosis. In Wilson EA, ed. Endometriosis. Chap. 8. New York: Alan R. Liss, Inc. 1987, pp 141–160.
7. Lichten EM, Bombard J. Surgical treatment of primary dysmenorrhea with laparoscopic uterine nerve ablation. J Reprod Med 1987;32:37–41.
8. Doyle JB. Paracervical uterine denervation by transection of the cervical plexus for the relief of dysmenorrhea. Am J Obstet Gynecol 1955;70:1–16.
9. Gurgan T, Develioglu O, Urman B, et al. Laparoscopic CO_2 laser uterine nerve ablation for treatment of drug resistant primary dysmenorrhea. Fertil Steril 1992;58:422–424.
10. Tjaden B, Schlaff WD, Kinball A, et al. The efficacy of presacral neurectomy for the relief of midline dysmenorrhea. Obstet Gynecol 1990;76:89–91.
11. Cotte G. Resection of the presacral nerves in the treatment of obstinate dysmenorrhea. Am J Obstet Gynecol 1937;33:1034–1040.
12. Garcia CR, David SS. Pelvic endometriosis: infertility and pelvic pain. Am J Obstet Gynecol 1977;129:740–747.
13. Lee RB, Stone K, Magelssen D, et al. Presacral neurectomy for chronic pelvic pain. Obstet Gynecol 1986;68:517–521.
14. Vercellini P, Fedele L, Bianchi S, et al. Pelvic denervation for chronic pain associated with endometriosis: fact or fancy? Am J Obstet Gynecol 1991;165:745–749.
15. Candiani GB, Fedele L, Vercellini P, et al. Presacral neurectomy for the treatment of pelvic pain associated with endometriosis: a controlled study. Am J Obstet Gynecol 1992;167:100–103.
16. Perez JJ. Laparoscopic presacral neurectomy. J Reprod Med 1990;35:625–630.
17. Schenken RS, Malinak LR. Reoperation after initial treatment of endometriosis with conservative surgery. Am J Obstet Gynecol 1978;131:416–424.
18. Jones HW, Rock JA. Endometriosis externa. In Jones HW, Rock JA, eds. Reparative and constructive surgery of the female generative tract, Chap. 9. Baltimore: Williams & Wilkins 1983;121–144.
19. Donaldson JK, Sanderlin JH, Harrell WB. A method of suspending the uterus without open abdominal incision. Am J Obstet Gynecol 1942;55:537–543
20. Candy JW. Modified Gilliam uterine suspension through the laparoscope. Obstet Gynecol 1976;47:242–243.
21. Smith DB, Kelsey JF, Sherman RL, et al. Laparoscopic uterine suspension. J Reprod Med 1977;18:98–102.
22. Mann WJ, Stenger VG. Uterine suspension through the laparoscope. Obstet Gynecol 1978;51:563–566.
23. Massouda D, Ling FW, Muram D, et al. Laparoscopic uterine suspension with falope rings. J Reprod Med 1987;32:859–861.

14
Extragenital Endometriosis

Robert R. Franklin and George M. Grunert

Nongenital endometriosis has been estimated to occur in 1% to 12% of patients with pelvic endometriosis.[1] The most common sites are the intestine, urinary tract, distal areas in the abdominal cavity, extrapelvic genital structures, lung, skin, and nervous system. In fact, endometriosis has been reported in almost all body structures. That it can occur at these other sites must be considered by gynecologic surgeons treating patients with endometriosis. Extragenital disease can occur in the absence of visible pelvic disease.

Symptoms, though often diverse and puzzling, generally result from functioning endometrial tissue or scarring in the affected site. In general, symptoms of pain, bleeding, or organ dysfunction related to the menstrual cycle offer clues to the presence of endometriosis. Noncyclic symptoms, however, can confuse the diagnostician. Treatment options involve excision of the lesion or ablation or suppression of ovarian function to remove the hormonal support of the ectopic endometrial tissue.

Pathophysiology

The prevailing theories account for its presence on the basis of coelomic metaplasia, activation of embryonic cell rests, or direct transportation and implantation of endometrial tissue. The theory of coelomic metaplasia proposes that multipotential cells, under the proper stimuli, may change from peritoneal epithelium to endometrium.[2] Suggested as stimuli have been cyclic hormonal changes and irritation from menstrual debris. To date, however, there is no experimental work that supports this theory.

Another possibility is that endometriosis may arise from activation of rudimentary cells of Müllerian origin.[3] According to this theory, prolonged hormonal stimulation allows multipotential Müllerian cells to mature into functioning endometrium. This hypothesis was framed to explain the frequent occurrence of endometriosis in peritoneal pockets, defects, and at the base of the broad ligament. This theory, however, would not account for endometriosis in locations other than along the path of the Müllerian ducts.

In the 1920s, Sampson hypothesized that endometriosis results from retrograde menstruation through the fallopian tubes into the pelvis of viable endometrial cells, which then implant in ectopic sites.[4,5] Implantation of endometriosis, in this view, results from the recurrent deposition of viable endometrial tissue, combined with an individual susceptibility to tissue transportation. This hypothesis has the greatest scientific validity because viable endometrial cells have been demonstrated in menstrual flow, endometrium can be experimentally transplanted to the peritoneal cavity, and endometrial cells from menstrual flow can be successfully transplanted.[6–8] Hormonal support is not necessary for implantation of ectopic endometrium.[9] This mode of transmission is further supported by clinical observations that endometriosis is more commonly seen in patients who have increased flow of retrograde menstrual tissue. Specifically, endometriosis has been described in women with incompetence of the uterotubal junction and in women with congenital anomalies that obstruct outflow.[10–13]

Lymphatic dissemination of endometriosis was first described in 1925.[14] Endometriosis has been confirmed in lymphatics and lymph nodes.[15] The demonstration of lymphatic spread to the umbilicus in primates provides further support for this mode of spread.[16] Sampson, who described hematogenous spread of endometriosis, found endometriosis in venous channels.[4] A later researcher confirmed such spread.[15] Hematogenous spread offers the best explanation for the finding of endometriosis in distant, well-vascularized organs. Direct intraperitoneal dissemination follows the flow of peritoneal fluid and represents local transportation and implantation of endometrial tissue. It appears that the incidence of endometriosis decreases with increasing distance from the uterus.[17]

It is apparent, therefore, that there is no one, unifying theory to explain the expansion of endometrial tissue from the uterus to ectopic sites in and beyond the pelvis. The weight of scientific evidence supports the theories of transplantation through retrograde menstruation, direct spread, and lymphatic or hematogenous spread.

The classical histologic appearance of extragenital endometriosis is characterized by endometrial glands and stroma, responding in synchrony with the uterine endometrium. Repeated hemorrhage produces surrounding fibrosis and edema in the involved ectopic site. This action may modify the appearance of the lesions, leaving only glands without active stroma, dilated glands with flattened epithelium, or cysts without epithelium. In some cases, the only clue to endometriosis may be the presence of hemosiderin-laden macrophages, without glands or stroma.[18] As the lesions become more distant from the uterus, there is an increasing tendency for them to lose their hormonal receptors and response, to appear asynchronous with the endometrium, or to exhibit no hormonal response at all.[19] This variation explains why symptoms produced by ectopic endometrium are cyclic and hormonally related in only approximately 50% of patients. It also explains why many distant endometriotic lesions do not respond to hormonal manipulation.

Hormone dependent lesions, similar to those seen in uterine endometrium, can also be seen in ectopic endometrium. Hyperplasia, especially in ovarian endometriosis, has been described as coexisting with endometrial hyperplasia. Rare cases of cytologic atypia, without structural changes characteristic of carcinoma, have been described as atypical endometriosis.[20] It may, on occasion, be difficult to differentiate atypical endometriosis from carcinoma.[21]

Pathologic confirmation of malignant transformation of benign endometriosis requires the contiguous presence of benign and malignant disease. There have been 38 reported cases of malignant change in endometrial implants outside the uterus and ovary, unassociated with other foci of endometrial cancer (28 adenocarcinomas, seven adenoacanthomas, two clear cell carcinomas, and one squamous carcinoma).[22] All cases were in the pelvis, with the majority arising in the rectovaginal septum and vagina. Survival has been poor, with a reported 5-year survival rate of approximately 20%.

Intestinal Endometriosis

It has been estimated that 7% to 37% of patients with endometriosis have involvement of the bowel.[23,24] Up to 50% of patients with severe endometriosis have GI endometriosis.[25,26] The most common sites of bowel endometriosis are: the rectosigmoid (51%), the appendix (15%), the small bowel (14%), the rectum (14%), and the caecum and colon (5%).[27,28]

Symptoms of diarrhea, constipation, perimenstrual changes in bowel habits, rectal bleeding, pain with defecation, tenesmus, abdominal distension, small caliber stools, or colicky abdominal pain should make one suspect large bowel or rectosigmoid endometriosis.[29–31] In more advanced cases, the presenting symptom may be obstruction.[32] Many patients give a history of chronic laxative use or futile attempts at management of symptoms with dietary changes. One must suspect intestinal endometriosis in any patient with a history of cyclic bowel symptoms. Because these patients may have other complaints related to endometriosis, ask specifically about bowel symptoms. In our experience, the truly asymptomatic patient with marked intestinal involvement is rare.

Endometriosis of the appendix has been described in 17% of patients with bowel involvement.[33–35] Appendiceal involvement may present as an incidental finding with or without pelvic disease. Acute symptoms are similar to those of appendicitis, but may not include leukocytosis. The appendix should be inspected in all patients undergoing surgery for endometriosis. Endometriosis has also been found in a Meckel's diverticulum.[36]

Small bowel endometriosis most commonly involves the terminal ileum. Lesions of the small bowel may produce pain, cyclic, partial, or total obstruction, or appear as an upper abdominal mass.[37–40] Appropriate evaluation may include ultrasound, upper GI x-rays, CT scan or MRI, and endoscopy. The absence of pelvic disease does not exclude the possibility of small bowel disease. In approximately 50% of cases of small bowel endometriosis reported, pelvic endometriosis was not seen.

Intestinal endometriosis causes symptoms by producing irritation and inflammation of the bowel wall, or by impairing bowel motility or mobility. Bleeding may occur as a result of the penetration of disease through the bowel wall to the mucosal surface, but can also be seen from mucosal ulceration overlying an area of intramural inflammation. Growth of the endometriosis, which results in progressive fibrosis, leads to narrowing of the bowel lumen and, in its end-stage, bowel obstruction. Obstructive symptoms can result from direct occlusion by transmural endometriosis, or from circumferential constriction from intramural edema, fibrosis, or hemorrhage. Intussusception can result from localized edema or hemorrhage. Perforation can also occur.[41] In post-oophorectomized or postmenopausal patients, symptoms can occur because of active residual disease, or from postendometriotic scarring in the absence of active endometriosis.

A careful bimanual and rectal exam may detect uterosacral nodularity, cul-de-sac fixation or nodularity, immobility of the rectum, or a pelvic mass that cannot be separated from the bowel. Stool should be tested for occult blood. Patients with symptoms or physical findings suggestive of rectosigmoid endometriosis, severe stage endometriosis, or obliteration of the posterior cul-de-sac should have a preoperative colonoscopy and/or barium enema. Suspicious mucosal lesions should be biopsied to exclude malignancy.

Differential diagnoses include appendicitis, regional enteritis, ulcerative colitis, obstruction due to adhesions, and tumors of the GI tract. Laparoscopy is used for diagnosis, staging, prognosis, establishing a treatment plan, and, in selected patients, for corrective surgery. Even with "classical" visual findings consistent with endometriosis, all patients should undergo biopsy to document endometriosis histologically and exclude a malignancy. Palpation with laparoscopic instruments or a rectal finger or probe should be done to outline the extent of endometriotic involvement. In patients not suffering from acute obstruction, we have found it helpful to suppress ovarian function with a gonadotropin-releasing hormone (GnRH) agonist.

Any patient suspected of having intestinal involvement should have a preoperative bowel preparation. Proper preoperative planning, bowel preparation, and consultation with a general or colon-rectal surgeon are essential for appropriate management. The goal of treatment of patients with intestinal endometriosis is to remove the disease and restore normal bowel anatomy and function.

Superficial serosal involvement can be managed by sharp local excision, bipolar electrocautery, or laser excision or vaporization. We prefer excision to ensure complete removal and to obtain a pathologic specimen. This approach eliminates the possibility of vaporizing or cauterizing only the superficial portion of a truly invasive lesion. Intra- or transmural endometriotic lesions should be removed en bloc, either by local excision, or segmental resection and primary anastomosis. Appendiceal endometriosis requires appendectomy. Invasion into the caecum may necessitate removal of the caecum or hemicolectomy. Hysterectomy and bilateral salpingo-oophorectomy is not necessary if the patient wishes to preserve her fertility. In the rare case where the diagnosis has not been suspected preoperatively and the patient is not properly prepared, the best decision is to stop and delay her bowel surgery. Fortunately, even in the emergency situation, such as in the patient with bowel obstruction with an unprepared bowel, colostomy is rarely necessary.[42] With complete removal of all visible disease, and restoration of normal bowel anatomy, the rate of recurrence is low, even in patients preserving ovarian function.[43,44]

Urinary Tract Endometriosis

Endometriotic involvement of the urinary tract has been reported in 16% of women undergoing laparotomy for endometriosis.[45] The bladder is the most common site of implantation. Patients with bladder endometriosis may complain of urgency, frequency, suprapubic pressure, or pain. Hematuria is reported in 33% of cases, but is cyclic in only half of these cases.[46] Occasional patients will also have a pelvic mass that should be evaluated preoperatively.[47] Patients suspected of having bladder endometriosis should be evaluated by cystoscopy and intravenous pyelogram (IVP). Cystoscopy may reveal mucosal involvement, show an extrinsic mass effect, or be normal.[48,49] Any cystoscopically visible lesion should be biopsied. The majority of bladder lesions are superficial peritoneal implants and do not represent involvement of the muscularis or mucosa. They can be approached in the same fashion as other peritoneal lesions.

As with other extragenital endometriotic lesions, if the patient has no acute symptoms and the diagnosis can be established, we prefer to treat these patients with a GnRH agonist prior to surgery. This regimen reduces the volume, edema, and vascularity of the disease. Even with a response to medical therapy, recurrence is common if the area of involvement is not removed.[50,51] Superficial disease can be vaporized or fulgurated, but invasive endometriosis should be excised. This can be performed at laparotomy or laparoscopy depending on the lesion and the skill and experience of the surgeon.[52] Surrounding fibrotic areas should be included in the excision because they may contain disease that could be a source of recurrence.

The most serious area for urinary tract endometriosis is the ureter. Loss of renal function has been described in almost 50% of patients with ureteral endometriosis.[53–55] Lesions have been divided into external (causing compression, deviation, or obstruction of the ureter due to extrinsic endometriosis or fibrosis) and internal endometriosis (where there is invasion of the ureter by the endometriosis). The vast majority of ureteral lesions are in the distal third of the ureter and result from direct extension of pelvic disease.[56] Presenting symptoms include hematuria, flank pain, backache, abdominal pain, or dysuria. Symptoms are not consistently related to menstrual cycles. Occasionally, asymptomatic ureteral involvement may be found only at surgery or on IVP.[57] An IVP should be done in all patients suspected of having ureteral endometriosis or who have peritoneal disease overlying the ureter.[58,59] If the ureter is completely obstructed, retrograde pyelography establishes the location of obstruction, and may allow placement of a ureteral catheter for temporary renal drainage. In cases of hydronephrosis or hydroureter, ultrasound or CT scan may be helpful in excluding the presence of another mass lesion. Patients with renal compromise may benefit from percutaneous nephrostomy for urinary diversion prior to definitive surgery.

GnRH agonist suppression, which may lead to temporary remission of symptoms, can be useful in allowing return of normal renal function before surgery. Therapy discontinuation is associated with a high risk of recurrence.[60–63] Reports of ureteral obstruction in menopausal women support the view that ablation of ovarian function is an insufficient mode of treatment.[64–67]

The aim of surgery for external ureteral endometriosis is to relieve the compression or entrapment of the ureter. To prevent recurrent symptoms, care must be taken to remove the area of scarring along with any active endometriosis. It may also be necessary to relocate the ureter to decrease the possibility of entrapment.

Internal ureteral endometriosis mandates segmental resection of the ureter. Depending on the site of involvement, the procedure of choice is either ureteroureterostomy or ureteroneocystostomy. Although these are usually performed at laparotomy, laparoscopic approaches have been reported.[68] There does not appear to be a specific advantage to hysterectomy and bilateral salpingo-oophorectomy in preventing recurrence.

Direct involvement of the kidney has been reported infrequently.[69–71] Presenting symptoms include flank or back pain, hematuria, hydronephrosis, or a renal mass. Diagnosis has been made at IVP, CT scan, or MRI. Unfortunately, in the absence of a biopsy, there is no definitive diagnosis. Because of the difficulty of accurate preoperative diagnosis and the appropriate concern about malignancy, the majority of patients have been treated by nephrectomy. There is one report of regression of renal endometriosis with GnRH agonist therapy, but follow-up was limited.[72] None of the reports have noted concurrent pelvic endometriosis.

Diaphragmatic Endometriosis

Transportation of viable endometrial cells in peritoneal fluid follows the characteristic clockwise circulation pattern of peritoneal fluid. They move from the pelvis up the right gutter to the diaphragm, across the upper abdomen, and back down the left gutter. Direct spread to the diaphragm, almost exclusively the right hemidiaphragm, has been increasingly reported.[73] Diaphragmatic endometriosis may be asymptomatic or may produce pain in the right upper quadrant of the abdomen or may refer pain to the right shoulder. If there has been penetration of the diaphragm with extension into the pleural space, pneumothorax, hemothorax, or hemop-

tysis may result. In one case, a pregnant patient developed hemoperitoneum because of bleeding from an ectopic pregnancy that had implanted on diaphragmatic endometriosis.[74]

Initially, we use GnRH agonist therapy for these patients and reserve surgery for women who have acute symptoms or who do not respond to hormonal suppression. Resection of the involved area with repair of any associated diaphragmatic defects is the surgical treatment of choice. Prior to surgery, the possibility of pleural or pulmonary involvement should be investigated. Primary laparoscopic treatment of diaphragmatic endometriosis has also been described.[75]

Other Intraabdominal Extragenital Lesions

Direct intraperitoneal spread of endometriosis to almost all organs and structures in the peritoneal cavity has been reported. Direct extension of endometriosis to adjacent omentum is common. Isolated areas of omental involvement can occur by transmission via peritoneal fluid or lymphatics. One patient with isolated omental endometriosis had abdominal pain, abdominal distension, and ascites.[76] Treatment was by excision of the endometriosis and ovarian suppression with medroxyprogesterone acetate (Depo-Provera).

Pancreatic endometriosis has been reported in two patients. One had upper abdominal pain and an abdominal mass; the other had left flank pain and a mass suggestive of renal origin.[77,78] In each case, a partial pancreatectomy and splenectomy were performed. The second patient also underwent left nephrectomy.

One patient with endometriosis of the liver parenchyma has been reported.[79] She had had a history of upper abdominal pain. An endometrioma of the liver was confirmed upon excision of the hepatic mass.

Extraabdominal Genital Tract Endometriosis

Direct extension of endometriosis from the cul-de-sac or down the rectovaginal septum into the vagina is probably more common than has been reported.[80] This condition illustrates the ability of pelvic endometriosis to invade contiguous structures. Symptoms include pain, dyspareunia, pressure, postcoital bleeding, and the presence of a palpable mass.

Cervical endometriosis has been seen as an isolated entity and in association with pelvic or rectovaginal disease.[81,82] These lesions are generally superficial and appear bluish or hemorrhagic. Usually asymptomatic, they are found incidentally at examination, but they may cause pain, dyspareunia, intermenstrual bleeding, or postcoital bleeding.

Vulvar, perineal, and perianal endometriosis is generally reported to occur in episiotomy scars.[83–86] It has also been observed in other vulvar surgical scars.[87]

Characteristically, these genital lesions produce pain and dyspareunia. Examination reveals a painful mass. Depending on the depth of the lesion, bluish or hemorrhagic discoloration can be seen. The majority of patients who have undergone peritoneal exploration have not had peritoneal disease. The most likely explanation for endometriosis in episiotomy scars without concurrent peritoneal disease is direct implantation of endometrial tissue at the time of vaginal delivery.

These lesions should be biopsied to exclude other pathologic processes and malignancy. Treatment is by local excision. Vaginal or cervical disease that results from cul-de-sac or rectovaginal disease should be removed en bloc with the peritoneal endometriosis.

Pulmonary Endometriosis

Presenting signs and symptoms of pulmonary endometriosis include catamenial pneumothorax in 75% of patients, catamenial hemothorax in 11%, or hemoptysis in 8%, although, as with other extragenital lesions, symptoms may be unrelated to menses.[88-93] Occasionally, patients complain of chest or abdominal pain or radiographic findings of a mass lesion without other symptoms.[94] Patients with pneumothorax, thought to result from rupture of a pulmonary bleb or alveolus in the area of endometrial implantation, experience pain and dyspnea.[95] Only 25% of women with pneumothorax have associated pelvic endometriosis in contrast with the finding of pelvic endometriosis in all patients with hemothorax, and one with hemoptysis.[96]

Pulmonary endometriosis can have pleural or parenchymal involvement. Hemothorax or pneumothorax is the most common presenting complaint in pleural disease, whereas hemoptysis was seen predominately in patients with parenchymal disease. The right pleura was involved in 93% of cases. Women with pleural disease tended to be younger than those with parenchymal disease, whereas the latter had a higher incidence of pelvic surgery. There was no difference in previous obstetric history.

At surgery, 35% of patients with pleural disease were found to have endometriosis of the right hemidiaphragm; an additional 33% had fenestrations of the right hemidiaphragm.[96] This finding, combined with the overwhelming predominance of right-sided involvement, suggests that pulmonary endometriosis results from direct spread of endometrial tissue from the peritoneal cavity, through the diaphragm, to the right chest facilitated by diaphragmatic defects, fenestrations, and hernias.[97] Lymphatic transmission, via the predominant right-sided peritoneal drainage pattern, is also a possibility.[98]

Parenchymal disease, without concurrent pleural involvement appears to be equally distributed within the lungs and follows a pattern similar to that seen with pulmonary emboli. A hematogenous pattern of spread seems most likely for parenchymal endometriosis.[96]

Differential diagnosis of pulmonary endometriosis includes carcinoma, infection, rupture of an emphysematous bleb, pulmonary embolism, pulmonary infarction, and vascular malformation. Initial evaluation is by chest x-ray to examine the possibility of a pneumothorax, pleural effusion, or mass. Depending on initial findings and symptoms, a ventilation-perfusion scan, CT scan, or MRI may be indicated. Because of the possibility of malignancy, definitive diagnosis should be made by cytologic examination of fluid recovered at thoracentesis or bronchoscopy with washings or biopsy.[99] In patients with parenchymal disease where bronchoscopy is not diagnostic, thoracotomy is suggested. In young patients with characteristic cyclic symptoms and without risk factors for carcinoma, a presumptive diagnosis can be made on the basis of variation in lesions with the menstrual cycle.[100] Patients with noncyclic symptoms, unchanging lesions, or lack of response to hormonal therapy, must have a histologic diagnosis.

Once the diagnosis is assured, thoracotomy with direct excision of all lesions and pleurodesis has been the traditional therapy. In an attempt to avoid thoracotomy, some patients have been treated with medical suppression of ovarian function.[101-104] One patient benefited during pregnancy.[105] Progestin therapy has been reported to be effective in four patients with parenchymal disease who avoided thoracotomy.[106]

Our approach to treatment is first, to establish the correct diagnosis. With nonacute disease an initial trial of GnRH suppression is warranted. There is little evidence to determine the length of therapy, but remission has been reported following treatment for six months.[107] Careful follow-up is necessary to detect recurrence that may be treated by a second course of GnRH agonist. In the acute situation of pneumothorax or hemothorax, reexpansion of the lung with closed chest drainage is necessary. An attempt at pleurodesis at the time of thoracentesis is reasonable.[108] This is followed by GnRH agonist therapy. Thoracotomy is reserved for patients who fail to respond to medical therapy or who have a lesion that cannot be appropriately diagnosed by other means. Pleural lesions are removed by excisional biopsy followed by chemical or abrasive pleurodesis to reduce the risk of recurrent pneumothorax.[109] Parenchymal lesions are removed by segmental resection of the lung.[110]

A search should be made for diaphragmatic endometriosis, which should be removed, and for fenestrations and hernias, which should be closed meticulously.[111] Because of the frequency of peritoneal endometriosis, it should be sought and treated appropriately to reduce the risk of recurrence. We reserve hysterectomy and salpingo-oophorectomy for patients who do not wish to preserve fertility.[112]

An interesting variation has been described in a patient with postcoital pneumothorax without evidence of diaphragmatic endometriosis. This patient's symptoms resolved following tubal ligation. Presumably, the pneumothorax resulted from transtubal passage of air during intercourse, with transmission of air to the pleural space through a congenital defect or fenestration in the diaphragm.[113]

Cutaneous Endometriosis

Endometriosis involving the skin is limited to the anterior abdominal wall at or below the level of the umbilicus.[114] An Armed Forces Institute of Pathology review of these lesions in 1966 reported 82 cases; 30% involved the umbilicus, 68% were in surgical scars, and 6% were inguinal.[115–117] The majority of abdominal scar lesions were in cesarean section incisions.[118] All patients had a cutaneous mass that, if near the surface, was characteristically blue or black. Other symptoms were variable and included swelling, scar tenderness, pain, and bleeding. Symptoms were cyclic in only half the patients, probably because the ectopic endometrium responds poorly to hormonal changes.[119]

Umbilical endometriosis classically presents as a bluish, tender mass, frequently associated with bleeding.[120–123] Peritoneal disease was present in less than half of patients. These lesions have been evaluated radiographically and by ultrasound.[124] The diagnosis, however, is best evaluated at excision biopsy.

Treatment of cutaneous endometriosis is by wide local excision. Care must be taken to excise endometriosis and the associated scar to reduce the risk of recurrence. Even with apparent complete excision, rapid recurrence has been reported in over 10% of cases.

Inguinal endometriosis presents as a painful mass. Overlying skin changes and cyclic symptoms vary. Endometriosis has been found in hernia sacs, in old inguinal scars, and in the inguinal lymphatics. Direct or lymphatic extension along the course of the round ligament from intraperitoneal endometriosis has been suggested as the mechanism of implantation, but the majority of cases reported have not documented such extension with exploration. The common preoperative diagnosis is inguinal hernia.[125] Treatment is by inguinal exploration and excision.

Other Sites of Extrapelvic Endometriosis

Endometriosis has also been described in virtually every site that can be reached by hematogenous, lymphatic, or direct dissemination. Musculoskeletal endometriosis has been seen in the shoulder, thigh, knee, pubis, thumb, forearm, and bone.[126–132] All patients had pain in the location of the endometriosis and were treated by local excision.

The most common site of endometriosis of the nervous system has been the nerves in or near the pelvis. Sciatic nerve endometriosis presents as sciatic pain, occasionally associated with muscle weakness, sensory deficits, and pelvic pain.[133,134] Cyclic sciatica, which refers to sciatic pain related to menses, should be considered suggestive of endometriosis. Similarly, endometriosis involving the obturator nerve producing pain and proximal muscle weakness has also been described.[135] This case, like those of sciatic nerve endometriosis, was treated by exploration and excision of endometriosis and fibrosis surrounding the nerve. Although the direct spread of pelvic endometriosis to and along nerves coursing through the pelvis seems logical, not all patients were found to have pelvic disease.

A single case of cerebral endometriosis has been reported. A 20-year-old woman had had a history of focal headache and progressive seizures. When a cystic mass, typical for endometrioma, was excised, her symptoms ceased. Pelvic endometriosis was not documented. The authors hypothesized a hematogenous route of spread from the pelvis or endometrium, through the foramen ovale or arteriovenous shunt to the brain.[136]

Experimental transplantation of endometriosis to the eye has been used to establish an easily observed laboratory model to assess response of lesions to therapy.[137] Two patients with endometriosis of the eye have been reported.[138] One patient presented with retinal hemorrhage, which responded only temporarily to medical suppression. The lesion finally resolved after hysterectomy and bilateral salpingo-oophorectomy. The second patient responded only after pituitary stalk section for diabetes. Both of these cases predate the availability of GnRH agonists.

Endometriosis in Men

Lesions characteristic of endometriosis have been reported in men undergoing treatment for prostate cancer by excision, orchiectomy, and high-dose estrogen therapy.[139–141] In 3 cases, lesions in the bladder caused hematuria. A fourth patient had endometriosis in the abdominal wall.[142] He had a painful mass in his surgical scar. All four cases were treated by local excision and repair. The patient with abdominal wall endometriosis required a second excision, and eventually had to discontinue estrogen therapy for relief of pain.

Coelomic metaplasia, induced by the reduction of testosterone production following orchiectomy, and augmented by estrogen therapy, could account for these cases. Similarly, stimulation of endometrial cell rests within the prostatic utricle by the same hormonal milieu could cause true growth of endometrial tissue, which could then spread as it does in females. Support for this latter theory is given by the report of ten cases of prostate cancer with a histologic pattern identical with endometrial cancer, presumed to originate from endometrial cell rests in the prostatic utricle.[143]

Summary

Endometriosis can spread widely throughout the body either by activation or differentiation of local cells, by direct extension from foci of endometrial tissue, by transportation in menstrual flow or peritoneal fluid, by lymphatic dissemination, or by hematogenous spread of endometrial cells. Given that retrograde menstruation occurs monthly in almost all women with patent fallopian tubes, the wonder is that endometriosis in and outside the pelvis is not more common. The presenting signs and symptoms of extragenital endometriosis depend on the pain, bleeding, and fibrosis induced by the implants themselves and the dysfunction in the target organ induced by the endometriosis and scarring. Although cyclic symptoms and organ dysfunction are characteristic (and strongly suggestive) of endometriosis, over half of patients with extrapelvic endometriosis lack catamenial symptoms. This lack is due to the fact that, as endometriosis spreads, it commonly loses its ability to respond to the cyclic production of ovarian hormones.

Suspect endometriosis in any reproductive age woman with cyclic symptoms of pain, bleeding, or dysfunction in sites outside the pelvis. In all cases, histologic confirmation should be sought, because other benign and malignant tumors are always part of the differential diagnosis. The mainstay of therapy is excision of the lesion. If endometriosis can be confirmed, a trial of ovarian suppression with GnRH agonist therapy is warranted in patients with nonlife-threatening lesions that would require major surgical intervention. A short trial of medical suppression may be warranted in patients with classic catamenial symptoms where a tissue diagnosis cannot be made. There is, to date, insufficient follow-up to know if this can suffice as a sole treatment, or should be considered only a temporizing measure. Failure to respond mandates surgical exploration, excision of endometriosis, and removal of associated fibrosis. Entrapment of structures such as ureter or nerves may be more common than actual invasion, but the surgeon must be assured of complete excision of the endometriotic lesions to minimize the chance of recurrence.

Although concurrent pelvic endometriosis is inconsistently found, it should be evaluated in all patients to reduce the risk of recurrence. Because of the reported beneficial effect of pregnancy on extragenital endometriosis, pregnancy should be encouraged in patients desirous of fertility. Patients who have completed their childbearing and who have potentially life-threatening lesions should be considered candidates for bilateral oophorectomy. Because of the many reports of endometriosis occurring in postmenopausal and post-ooph-orectomized patients, the surgeon should not rely on oophorectomy as the sole mode of treatment. We have seen numerous patients with nongenital endometriosis left at the time of hysterectomy and bilateral salpingo-oophorectomy in the mistaken belief that this will cure the patient. The proper course is to remove the disease, if possible, at the same time. With proper diagnostic acumen and forethought, extragenital endometriosis can be diagnosed and treated appropriately, relieving the patient's symptoms, preserving function of the affected site, and minimizing the risk of recurrence.

References

1. Mitchell GW. Extrapelvic endometriosis. In Schenken RS, ed. Endometriosis: contemporary concepts in clinical management. Philadelphia, J.B. Lippincott Co., 1989, pp 307–328.
2. Ridley JH. A review of facts and fancies. Obstet Gynecol Surv 1968;23:1–18.
3. Batt RE, Smith RA. Embryologic theory of histogenesis of endometriosis in peritoneal pockets. Obstet Gynecol Clin North Am 1989;16:15–28.
4. Sampson JA. Metastasis of embolic endometriosis due to menstrual dissemination of endometrial tissue into the venous circulation. Am J Pathol 1927;3:93–96.
5. Sampson JA. Peritoneal endometriosis due to the menstrual dissemination of endometrial tissue to the peritoneal cavity. Am J Obstet Gynecol 1927;14:422–426.
6. Keetel WC, Stein RJ. The viability of the cast-off menstrual endometrium. Am J Obstet Gynecol 1951;61: 440–443.
7. Allan E, Peterson LF, Campbell ZB. Clinical and experimental endometriosis. Am J Obstet Gynecol 1954;68:356–359.
8. Ridley JH, Edwards KL. Experimental endometriosis in the human. Am J Obstet Gynecol 1958;76:783–786.
9. Dizerega GS, Barber DL, Hodgen GD. Endometriosis: role of ovarian steroids in initiation, maintenance, and suppression. Fertil Steril 1980;33:649–653.
10. Ayers JWT, Friedenstap AP. Uterotubal hypotonia associated with pelvic endometriosis. Presented at the 41st Annual Meeting of the American Fertility Society, Chicago, 1985 (abstract 519).
11. Hanton EM, Malkasian GD Jr, Dockerty MB. Endometriosis in young women. Am J Obstet Gynecol 1967; 98:116–118.
12. Schifrin BS, Erez S, Moore JG. Teen-age endometriosis. Am J Obstet Gynecol 1973;116:973–980.
13. Baker ER, Horger EO, Williamson HO. Congenital atresia of the uterine cervix. Two cases. J Reprod Med 1982;27:39–43.
14. Halban J. Metastatic hysteradenosis: lymphatic origin of so-called heterotropic adenofibromatosis. Arch Gynak 1925;125:475–479.
15. Javert CT. Pathogenesis of endometriosis based on endometrial homeoplasia, direct extension, exfoliation and implantation, lymphomatic and hematogenous metastasis. Cancer 1949;2:399–405.
16. Scott RB, Nowak RM, Tindale RM. Umbilical endometriosis and Cullen's sign. Study of lymphatic transport from pelvis to umbilicus in monkeys. Obstet Gynecol 1958;11:556–559.

17. Williams TJ. Endometriosis. In Mattingly RF, Thompson JD, eds. TeLinde's operative gynecology, 6th ed. Philadelphia, J.B. Lippincott, 1985, pp 257–286.

18. Barbieri R, Kistner RW. Endometriosis. In Kistner RW, ed. Gynecology: principles and practice, 4th ed. Chicago, Year Book Medical Publishers, 1986, pp 393–414.

19. Gompel C, Silverberg SG. The female peritoneum. In Gompel C, Silverberg SG, eds. Pathology in gynecology and obstetrics. Philadelphia, J.B. Lippincott Co., 1985, pp 412–417.

20. Czernobilsky B, Morris WJ. A histologic study of ovarian endometriosis with emphasis on hyperplastic and atypical changes. Obstet Gynecol 1979;53:318–323.

21. Lamm D, Gittes R, Benirschke K. Ectopic endometrial glands in lymph nodes masquerading as metastatic adenocarcinoma. J Urol 1974;111:770–774.

22. Mostoufizadeh M, Scully RE. Malignant tumors arising in endometriosis. Clin Obstet Gynecol 1980;29:951–956.

23. Prystowsky JB, Stryker SJ, Ujiki GT, Poticha SM. Gastrointestinal endometriosis: Incidence and indications for resection. Arch Surg 1988;123:855–858.

24. Macafee CH, Greer HL. Intestinal endometriosis: A report of 29 cases and a survey of the literature. J Obstet Gynaecol Br Emp 1960;67:539.

25. Buttram VC Jr, Reiter RC. Endometriosis. In Buttram VC Jr, Reiter RC, eds. Surgical treatment of the infertile female. Baltimore, Williams & Wilkins, 1985, p 89.

26. Kistner RW. Endometriosis. In McElin TW, Sciarra JJ, eds. Gynecology and Obstetrics. Hagerstown, MD, Harper & Row 1981, pp 1–44.

27. FitzGibbons JP. The diagnosis and treatment of endometriosis. III Med J 1951;100:115–118.

28. Jenkins S, Olive DL, Haney AF. Endometriosis: pathogenetic implications of the anatomic distribution. Obstet Gynecol 1986;67:335–338.

29. Farinon AM, Vadora E. Endometriosis of the colon and rectum: an indication for preoperative colonoscopy. Endoscopy 1980;12:136–138.

30. Collin GR, Russel JC. Endometriosis of the colon. Its diagnosis and management. Am Surg 1990;56:275–279.

31. Caccese WJ, McKinley MJ, Bronzo RL, et al. Endoscopic confirmation of colonic endometriosis. Gastrointest Endosc 1984;30:191–193.

32. Forsgren H, Lindhagen J, Melander S, Wagermark J. Colorectal endometriosis. Acta Chir Scand 1983;149:431–435.

33. Langsam LB, Raj PK, Galang CF. Intussusception of the appendix. Dis Colon Rectum 1983;27:387–392.

34. Mann WJ, Fromowitz F, Saycheck T, et al. Endometriosis associated with appendiceal intussusception. A report of two cases. J Reprod Med 1984;29:625–629.

35. Thiel CW. Endometriosis of the cecum associated with acute appendicitis. Minn Med 1986;69:20–21.

36. Won KH. Endometriosis, mucocele and regional enteritis of Meckel's diverticulum. Arch Surg 1969;98:209–212.

37. Teunen A, Ooms EC, Tytgat GN. Endometriosis of the small and large bowel. Study of 18 patients and survey of the literature. Neth J Med 1982;25:142–150.

38. Harty RF, Kaude JV. Invasive endometriosis of the terminal ileum: a cause of small bowel obstruction of obscure origin. South Med J 1983;76:253–257.

39. Herzig B, Smejda J, Steiner I. Endometriosis as a cause of obstruction of the small intestine. Rozhledy V Chirurcii 1990;69:611–614.

40. Bergemann W, Heuer C. Extragenital endometriosis with multiple stenoses of the small intestine. Fortschritte der Medizin 1992;110:281–283.

41. Floberg J, Backdahl M, Silfersward C, et al. Postpartum perforation of the colon due to endometriosis. Acta Obstet Gynecol Scand 1984;63:183–184.

42. Burch JM, Brock JC, Gevirtzman L, et al. The injured colon. Ann Surg 1986;203:701–711.

43. Gray L. Endometriosis of the bowel. Role of bowel resection, superficial excision, and oophorectomy in treatment. Ann Surg 1973;177:580–583.

44. Coronado C, Franklin RR, Lotze EC, et al. Surgical treatment of symptomatic colorectal endometriosis. Fertil Steril 1990;53:411–414.

45. Williams TJ, Pratt JH. Endometriosis in 1,000 consecutive celiotomies: incidence and management. Am J Obstet Gynecol 1977;129:245–252.

46. Vermesh M, Kawasaki N, Oka M, et al. Vesical endometriosis following bladder injury. Am J Obstet Gynecol 1985;153:894–895.

47. Goodman JD, MacChia RJ, MacAsaet MA, et al. Endometriosis of the urinary bladder. Sonographic findings. Am J Roentgenol 1980;35:625–629.

48. Fein RL, Horton BF. Vesical endometriosis: A case report and review of the literature. J Urol 1985;134:539–541.

49. Aldridge KW, Burns JR, Singh B. Vesical endometriosis: A review and 2 case reports. J Urol 1985;134:539–541.

50. Weinberg RW. Vesical endometriosis. Urology 1978;11:72–73.

51. Vaquez MA, Mallett J, Bahsas F. Danazol in the treatment of vesical endometriosis. J Fam Pract 1984;19:117–118.

52. Nezhat CR, Nezhat FR. Laparoscopic segmental bladder resection for endometriosis: a report of two cases. Obstet Gynecol 1993;81:882–884.

53. Kane C, Droulin P. Obstructive uropathy associated with endometriosis. Am J Obstet Gynecol 1985;151:207–211.

54. Miller MA, Morgan RJ. Bilateral ureteric obstruction due to endometriosis resulting in unilateral loss of renal function. Br J Urol 1990;65:421.

55. Ryan JF, Booth CM. Endometriosis of the ureter. Br J Urol 1992;69:430–431.

56. Porena M, Vespasiani G, Virgili G, et al. Ureteral endometriosis: an endoscopic diagnosis. Urology 1985;26:566–567.

57. Moore JG, Hibbard LT, Growdon WA, Schifrin BS. Urinary tract endometriosis: enigmas in diagnosis and management. Am J Obstet Gynecol 1979;134:162–172.

58. Maxson WS, Hill GA, Herbert CM, et al. Ureteral abnormalities in women with endometriosis. Fertil Steril 1986;46:1159–1161.

59. Thomsen H, Schroder HM. Simultaneous external and internal endometriosis of the ureter. Case report. Scand J Urol Nephrol 1987;21:241–242.

60. Klein RS, Cattolica EV. Ureteral endometriosis. Urology 1979;13:477–482.

61. Gantt PA, Hunt JB, McDonough PG. Progestin reversal of ureteral endometriosis. Obstet Gynecol 1981;57:665–667.

62. Gardner B, Whitaker RH. The use of danazol for ureteral obstruction caused by endometriosis. J Urol 1981;125:117–118.

63. Matsuura K, Kawasaki N, Oka M, et al. Treatment with danazol of ureteral obstruction caused by endometriosis. Acta Obstet Gynecol Scand 1985;64:339–343.

64. Dick AL, Lang DW, Bergman RT, et al. Postmenopausal endometriosis with ureteral obstruction. Br J Urol 1975;45:153–155.

65. Plous RH, Sunshine R, Goldman H, et al. Ureteral endometriosis in post-menopausal women. Urology 1985;26:408–411.
66. Ray J, Conger M, Ireland K. Ureteral obstruction in post-menopausal women with endometriosis. Urology 1985; 26:577–578.
67. Kiely EA, Grainger R, Kay EW, et al. Post-menopausal ureteric endometriosis. Br J Urol 1988;62:91–92.
68. Nezhat C, Nezhat F, Green B. Laparoscopic treatment of obstructed ureter due to endometriosis by resection and ureteroureterostomy: a case report. J Urol 1992;148: 865–868.
69. Marshall VF. Occurrence of endometrial tissue in kidney: case report and discussion. J Urol 1943;50:662–664.
70. Hagdu SI, Coss LG. Endometriosis of the kidney. Am J Obstet Gynecol 1970;106:314–316.
71. Bazaz-Malik G, Saraf V, Rana BS. Endometrioma of the kidney: case report. J Urol 1980;123:422–423.
72. Hellberg D, Fors B, Bergqvist C. Renal endometriosis treated with a gonadotropin releasing hormone agonist. Case report. Br J Obstet Gynaecol 1991;98:406–407.
73. Rebound E, Monges H, Salavert JP, et al. Surgical considerations. Apropos of a case of pleurodiaphragmatic endometriosis. Ann Chir Thorac Cardiovasc 1972; 11:423–426.
74. Norenberg DD, Gunderson JH, Janis JF, et al. Early pregnancy on the diaphragm with endometriosis. Obstet Gynecol 1977;49:620–622.
75. Nezhat F, Nezhat C, Levy S. Laparoscopic treatment of symptomatic diaphragmatic endometriosis: a case report. Fertil Steril 1991;58:614–616.
76. Naraynsingh V, Raju GC, Ratan P, et al. Massive ascites due to omental endometriosis. Postgrad Med J 1985; 61:539–540.
77. Marchevsky AM, Zimmerman MJ, Aufses AH Jr, et al. Endometrial cyst of the pancreas. Gastroenterology 1984;86:1589–1591.
78. Goswami AK, Sharma SK, Tandon SP, et al. Pancreatic endometriosis presenting as a hypovascular renal mass. J Urol 1986;135:112–113.
79. Finkel L, Marchevsky A, Cohen B. Endometrial cyst of the liver. Am J Gastroenterol 1986;81:576–578.
80. March CM, Israel R. Rectovaginal endometriosis: An isolated enigma. Am J Obstet Gynecol 1976;125: 274–275.
81. Goodall JR. A study of endometriosis, endosalpingiosis, endocervicitis, and perineo-ovarian sclerosis: a clinical and pathological study. In Goodall JR, ed. Endometriosis. Philadelphia, JB Lippincott Co., 1943, p 14.
82. Novak E, Woodruff JB. Gynecologic and obstetric pathology, Philadelphia: WB Saunders 1979:61.
83. Beischer NO. Endometriosis of an episiotomy scar cured by pregnancy. Obstet Gynecol 1966;28:15–21.
84. Paull T, Tedeschi LG. Perineal endometriosis at the site of episiotomy scar. Obstet Gynecol 1972;40:28–34.
85. Schottler J, Balcos E, Goldberg S. Perianal endometrioma. Dis Colon Rectum 1976;19:260–263.
86. Hambrick E, Abcarian H, Smith B. Perineal endometrioma in episiotomy incision: clinical features and management. Dis Colon Rectum 1979;22:550–552.
87. Sondag PR, Thompson JD, Birch W. Endometriosis occurring at a postoperative radical vulvectomy scar. Med Assoc Georgia 1962;51:430–432.
88. Matsuda Y, Imaizumi K, Makano A, et al. A case of catamenial pneumothorax with endometriosis of the right hemidiaphragm. Nippon Kyobu Shikkan Gakkai Zasshi 1979;17:179–183.
89. Yamazaki S, Ogawa J, Koide S, et al. Catamenial pneumothorax associated with endometriosis of the diaphragm. Chest 1980;77:107–109.
90. Stern H, Toole AL, Merino M. Catamenial pneumothorax. Chest 1980;78:480–482.
91. Wilhelm JL, Scommegna A. Catamenial pneumothorax. Obstet Gynecol 1977;50:277–280.
92. Karpel JP, Appel D, Merav A. Pulmonary endometriosis. Lung 1985;163:151–159.
93. Wilkins SB, Bell-Thompson J, Tyras DH. Hemothorax associated with endometriosis. J Thorac Cardiovasc Surg 1950;131:697–699.
94. Grunewald RA, Wiggins J. Pulmonary endometriosis mimicking an acute abdomen. Postgrad Med J 1988; 64:865–866.
95. Berwanger I, Bonnet R, Jacobsen JP, et al. Die thorakale endometriose—2 fallberichte und literaturubersicht. Pneumologie 1992;45:236–238.
96. Foster DC, Stern JL, Buscema J, et al. Pleural and parenchymal pulmonary endometriosis. Obstet Gynecol 1981;58:552–555.
97. Slasky BS, Siewers RD, Lecky JW, et al. Catamenial pneumothorax: the roles of diaphragmatic defects and endometriosis. Am J Roentgenol 1982;138:639–643.
98. Allen L. On the permeability of the lymphatics of the diaphragm. Anat Rec 1956;124:639–640.
99. Guidry GG, George RB, Payne DK. Catamenial hemoptysis: a case report and review of the literature. J LA State Med Soc 1990;142:27–30.
100. Guidry GG, George RB, Payne DK. Catamenial hemoptysis: a case report and review of the literature. J LA State Med Soc 1990;142:27–30.
101. Rosenberg SM, Riddick DH. Successful treatment of catamenial hemoptysis with danazol. Obstet Gynecol 1981;57:130–132.
102. Ronnberg L, Ylostalo P. Treatment of pulmonary endometriosis with danazol. Acta Obstet Gynecol Scand 1981;60:77–78.
103. Suginami H, Hamada K, Yano K. A case of endometriosis of the lung treated with danazol. Obstet Gynecol 1985;66:68S–71S.
104. Grimm MH, Grady KJ, Golish JA. Bronchopulmonary endometriosis: a rare case of hemoptysis. South Med J 1988;81:1189–9.
105. Lawrence HC III. Pulmonary endometriosis in pregnancy. Am J Obstet Gynecol 1988;159:733–734.
106. Svendstrup F, Husby H. Parenchymal pulmonary endometriosis. J Laryngol Otol 1991;105:235–236.
107. Espaulella J, Armengol J, Bella F, et al. Pulmonary endometriosis: conservative treatment with GnRH agonists. Obstet Gynecol 1991;78:535–537.
108. Bendoff SL, Garfinkle BM Jr. Endometriosis of the pleura. Obstet Gynecol 1965;26:549–551.
109. Ripstein CB, Rohman M, Wallach JB. Endometriosis involving the pleura. J Thorac Surg 1959;37:464–466.
110. Jelihovsky T, Grant AF. Endometriosis of the lung. Thorax 1968;23:434–436.
111. Okaga Y, Handa M, Inaba H, et al. An experience of surgical treatment for catamenial pneumothorax with diaphragmatic and pulmonary endometriosis. Kyobu Geka 1992;45:801–804.
112. Hibbard LT, Schumann WR, Goldstein GE. Thoracic endometriosis: a review and report of two cases. Am J Obstet Gynecol 1981;140:227–232.
113. Muller NL, Nelems B. Postcoital catamenial pneumothorax. Report of a case not associated with endome-

triosis and successfully treated with tubal ligation. Am Rev Respir Dis 1986;134:803–804.

114. Frydman CP, Schwartz JW, Schwartz IS. Endometrioma of the anterior abdominal wall. Mt Sinai J Med 1986; 53:160–162.

115. Steck WD, Helwig EB. Cutaneous endometriosis. Clin Obstet Gynecol 1966;9:373–392.

116. Brenner C, Wohlgemuth S. Scar endometriosis. Surg Gynecol Obstet 1990;177:538–540.

117. Bottino G, Marinello M, Menna C, et al. Endometriosi della parte abdominale inferiore. Descrizione di due dasi secondari a taglio cesareo. Minerva Ginecol 1990;42:283–285.

118. Wolf GC, Singh KB. Cesarean scar endometriosis: a review. Obstet Gynecol Surv 44:89–95, 1989.

119. Tidman MJ, MacDonald DM. Cutaneous endometriosis: a histopathologic study. J Am Acad Dermatol 1988; 18:373–377.

120. Radman H. Endometriosis of the umbilicus. South Med J 1977;70:888–890.

121. Blumenthal NJ. Umbilical endometriosis. S Afr Med J 1981;59:198–200.

122. Michowitz M, Baratz M, Stavorovsky M. Endometriosis of the umbilicus. Dermatologica 1983;167:326–328.

123. Shwayder TA. Umbilical nodule and abdominal pain. Endometriosis. Arch Dermatol 1987;123:106–107.

124. Vincent LM, Mittelstaedt CA. Sonographic demonstration of endometrioma arising in cesarean scar. J Ultrasound Med 1985;4:437–438.

125. Brzezinski A, Durst AL. Endometriosis presenting as an inguinal hernia. Am J Obstet Gynecol 1983;146:982–983.

126. Gennari L, Luciano L. A case of endometriosis of the trapezius muscle. Tumori 1965;51:361–362.

127. Gitelis S, Petasnick JP, Turner DA, et al. Endometriosis simulating a soft tissue tumor of the thigh: CT and MR evaluation. J Comput Assist Tomogr 1985;9:573–575.

128. Patel IV, Samuels H, Abeles E, et al. Endometriosis of the knee. Clin Orthop 1982;171:140–142.

129. Pellegrini VD Jr, Pasternak HS, Macaulary WP. Endometriosis of the pubis: A differential in the diagnosis of hip pain. Am J Bone Joint Surg 1981;63A:1334–1336.

130. Das Gupta S, Pals K, Saha PK, et al. Endometriosis in the thumb. J Indian Med Assoc 1985;83:122–123.

131. Duncan C, Pitney WR. Endometrial tumors in the extremities. Med J Aust 1949;2:715–718.

132. Oei SG, Peters AA, Welvaart K, et al. Aggressive endometriosis in the bone. Lancet 1992;339:1477–1478.

133. Denton RO, Sherril JD. Sciatic syndrome due to endometriosis of the sciatic nerve. South Med J 1955;48:1027–1030.

134. Hibbard J, Schreiber J. Footdrop due to sciatic nerve endometriosis. Am J Obstet Gynecol 1984;149:800–802.

135. Redwine DB, Sharpe DR. Endometriosis of the obturator nerve. A case report. J Reprod Med 1990;35:434–435.

136. Thibodeau LL, Prioleau GR, Manuelidis EE, et al. Cerebral endometriosis. Case report. J Neurosurg 1987; 66:609–610.

137. Rock JA, Prendergast RA, Bobbie D, et al. Intraocular endometrium in the rabbit as a model for endometriosis. Fertil Steril 1993;59:232–235.

138. Franklin RR, Navarro C. Extragenital endometriosis. Prog Clin Biol Res 1990;333:289–295.

139. Pinkert T, Catlow C, Straus R. Endometriosis of the urinary bladder in a man with prostate carcinoma. Cancer 1979;43:1562–1564.

140. Schrodt GR, Alcorn M, Ibanez J. Endometriosis of the male urinary system. J Urol 1980;124:722–724.

141. Martin JD Jr, Hauck AE. Endometriosis in the male. Am J Surg 1985;50:426–430.

142. Miller WB Jr, Melson GI. Abdominal wall endometrioma. Am J Roentgenol 1979;132–134:467.

143. Sufrin G, Gaeta J, Staubitz, et al. Endometrial carcinoma of the prostate. Urology 1980;27:18–21.

15

Endometriosis of the Intestine and Genitourinary Tract

Camran Nezhat, Farr Nezhat, Ceana Nezhat, and Dahlia Admon

The Gastrointestinal Tract

Introduction

As with other organs, the etiology of bowel endometriosis is unknown. Its occurrence was reported as early as 1922 by Sampson.[1] Following his investigation of nineteen cases, he proposed that "implantation adenoma of endometrial type of some portion of the intestinal tract may be present in at least one half of the cases of perforated ovarian hematoma of endometrial type with peritoneal implantations."[1]

Intestinal endometriosis has been reported to affect between 3% and 37% of women with endometriosis (Fig. 15.1).[2-6] In a series of 1,573 women treated consecutively for endometriosis, 5.4% had gastrointestinal involvement; of these, 65% had endometriosis of the rectum and rectosigmoid colon.[2] In another series of 1,000 celiotomies, Williams and Pratt found that in 485 women with endometriosis, 181 (37%) had gastrointestinal involvement. Of these, 172 (95%) had rectosigmoid involvement, 9 (5%) had ileal involvement, and 19 (10%) had appendiceal involvement.[7] Bowel resection with or without castration has been suggested to treat symptomatic patients.[2,6] Coronado et al[8] have reported satisfactory pain relief and pregnancy rates following anterior wall resection of the colon by laparotomy for deeply infiltrating lower colorectal endometriosis.

Bowel involvement is suggested by palpable tumor in the rectovaginal septum, gastrointestinal symptoms such as rectal bleeding, constipation, or diarrhea associated with menses, or pain that persists after surgical removal of all recognizable lesions.

Endometriotic nodularity of the bowel and rectovaginal septum is one of the most difficult aspects of this disease to approach surgically. Because gynecologists maybe uncomfortable operating on the bowel and general surgeons may not be familiar with endometriosis, these cases have frequently required bowel resection or temporary or permanent colostomy. Some have shown that when full-thickness bowel resection and immediate reanastomosis are performed by a surgical team familiar with the disease, low morbidity and good long-term relief of symptoms can be expected.[8]

We have been able to treat most cases involving the rectum and rectovaginal septum laparoscopically.

Women with endometriosis of the lower colon, rectum, uterosacral ligaments or rectovaginal septum often present with chronic pelvic pain, and dysmenorrhea, dyspareunia, back pain, dyschezia, constipation or diarrhea, or infertility with pelvic pain. Most women with small bowel or appendiceal endometriosis are asymptomatic, and rarely experience bowel obstruction.

Surgical Procedures

Operative laparoscopy of the GI tract is performed for the treatment of endometrial implants on the intestinal wall, appendix, or rectovaginal space. Surgical repair of the bowel may be necessary, even in patients whose endometriosis does not invade the lumen of the GI tract, for the repair of incidental injuries occurring during laparoscopic treatment of endometriosis in other areas of the pelvic/abdominal cavity.

Figures reproduced from *Operative Gynecologic Laporoscopy: Principles and Techniques*, C. Nezhat, Editor, 1995. With permission of McGraw-Hill Publishers.

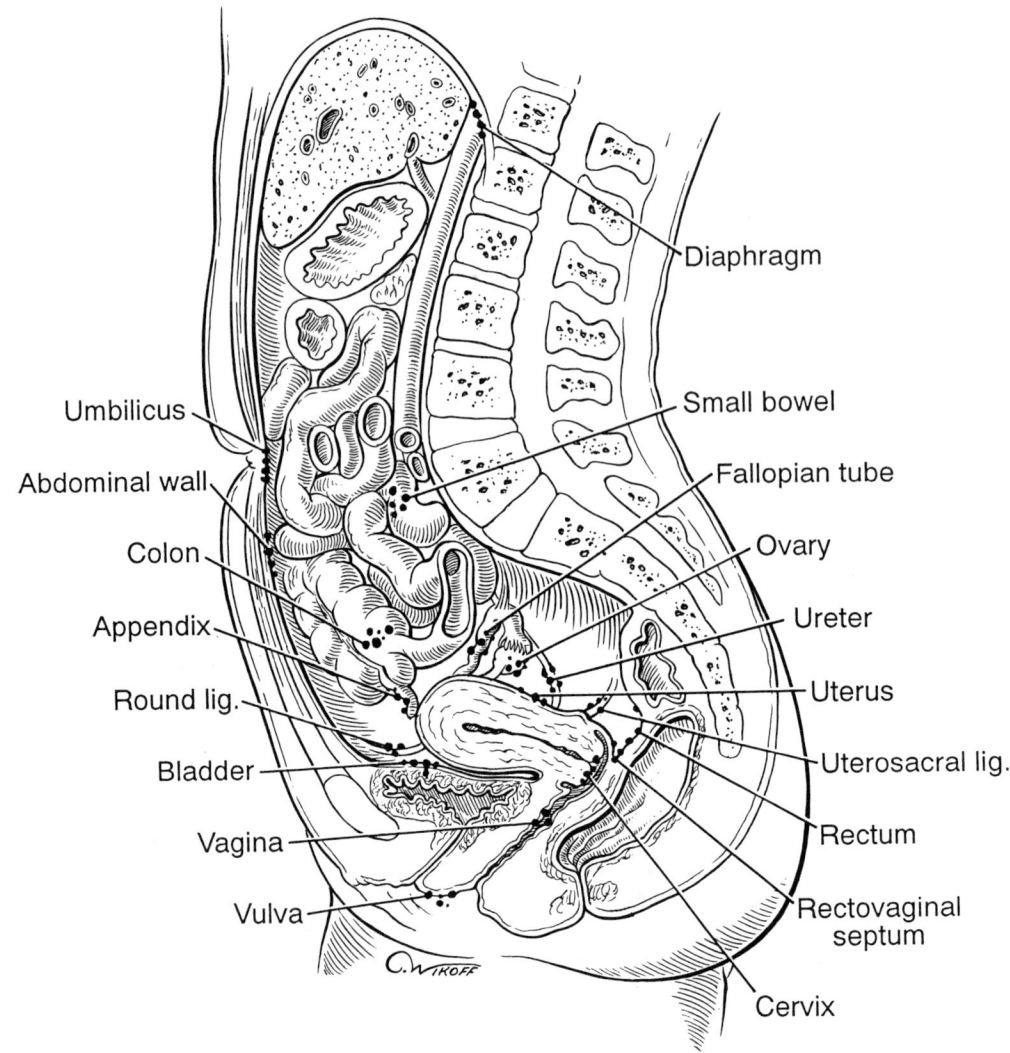

Figure 15.1. Possible sites of endometriosis.

Operative videolaparoscopy of the GI tract includes lysis of bowel adhesions, as well as the treatment of superficial, infiltrative and full-thickness involvement with or without stricture of the appendix, rectosigmoid colon, rectovaginal septum or small bowel.

Preparation for Laparoscopy

To prepare a patient for operative laparoscopy, the surgeon should follow a protocol similar to that for laparotomy, including thorough clinical and laboratory evaluation. Pelvic ultrasound and, in selected cases, hysterosalpingography are recommended to permit the surgeon to evaluate uterine and adnexal abnormalities. Patients with a history of rectal bleeding should be evaluated by sigmoidoscopy before laparoscopy, and a barium enema may be necessary. The procedure should be explained to the patient and proper consent must be obtained. The evening before surgery, patients with

more advanced disease or previous laparotomy receive a bowel preparation consisting of 4 L polyethylene glycol-3350 (Go-LYTELY, Braintree Laboratories, Braintree, MA) and are given 1 g metronidazole at bedtime. As prophylaxis, 1 g cefoxitin is administered preoperatively and postoperatively. Our preferred technique is room setup and system of videolaseroscopy (Figs. 15.2 and 15.3).[9] In describing our surgical techniques we make frequent reference to the CO_2 laser as a cutting modality. Scissors, electrosurgical devices, and fiber lasers are effective and appropriate alternatives.

Lysis of Bowel Adhesions

Bowel adhesions may be thin or thick, vascular or avascular, cohesive or not. Noncohesive adhesions are stretched as much as possible without tearing the tissue, excised with laser or electricity at the points of attachment to the pelvic organs, and removed. Cohesive

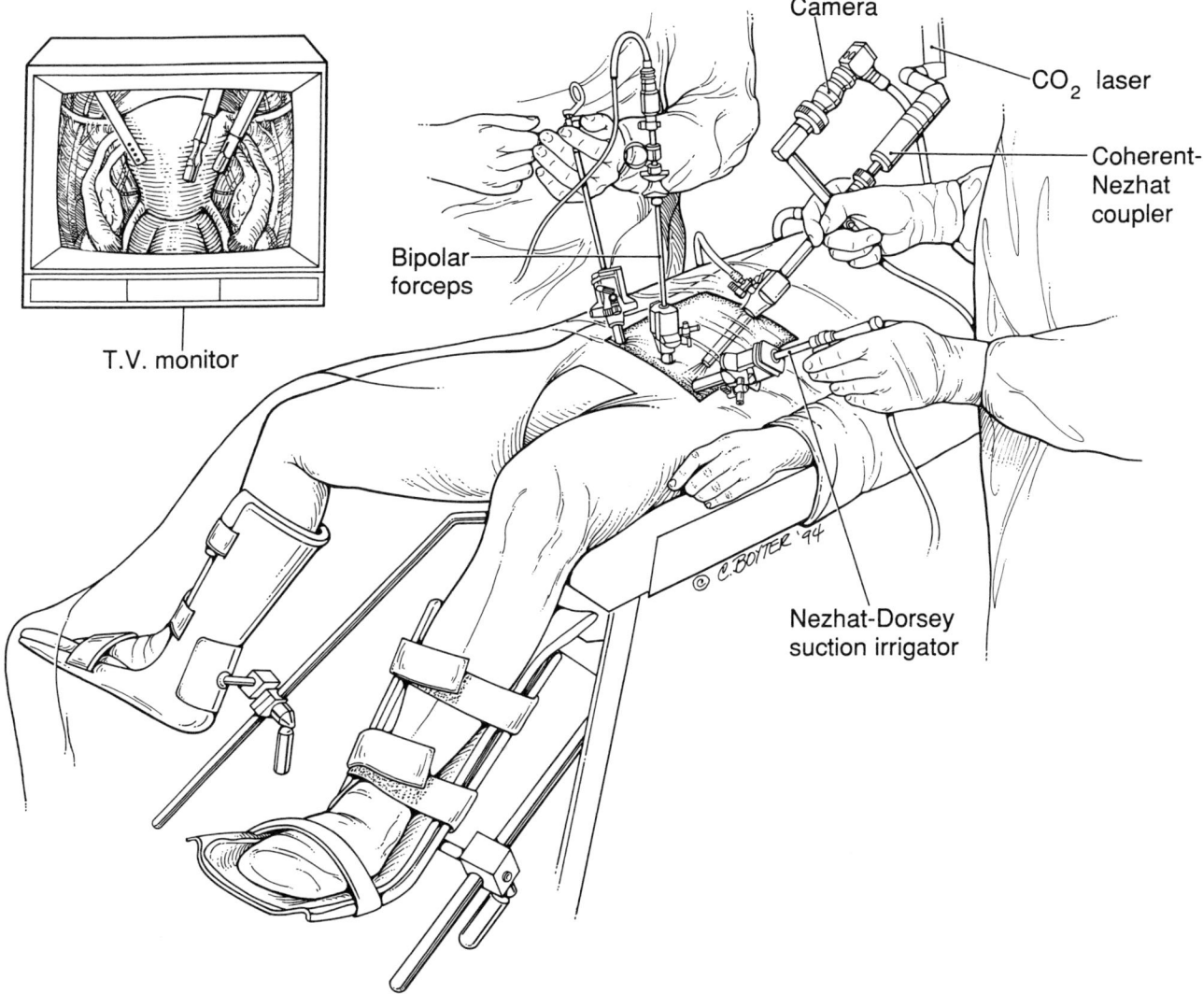

Figure 15.2. Room setup for operative laparoscopy and videolaseroscopy.

adhesions densely adherent to other structures are excised by scissors or CO_2 laser.[10] The latter device has a more controlled and predictable depth of penetration than either electrosurgery or fiber lasers. The ultrapulse laser may be used in conjunction with hydrodissection for lysis of fibrosis and cohesive adhesions. Structures requiring separation are pulled apart with forceps and a cleavage plane is formed. Hydrodissection, which provides atraumatic pressure, may be especially useful in identifying and developing the dissection plane that is laser ablated or excised. The plane may also be dissected sharply or bluntly by opening the scissors while applying pressure.[11]

Treatment of Appendiceal Endometriosis

Because approximately 50% of appendiceal lesions are detected only by palpation and may be missed by visual inspection alone, incidental appendectomy is recommended in patients with severe endometriosis.

Preparation for appendectomy includes mobilization and examination after any necessary lysis of periappendiceal or pericecal adhesions. The surgeon must proceed carefully in case these are attached to the lateral pelvic wall or retrocecal appendix. The bipolar electrocoagulator and the CO_2 laser are used sequentially to dessicate and cut the mesoappendix 0.2 to 0.5 cm from the ileocecal area (Figs. 15.4–15.7).[12] When using the bipolar electrocoagulator in this area, caution should be exercised to prevent thermal damage to the cecum. A backstop is also required when using the CO_2 laser to avoid injuring the external iliac artery and vein.

At this point, the bipolar electrocoagulator is withdrawn, and the Endoloop applicator (Ethicon, Somerville, NJ) is inserted through the suprapubic midline puncture. Two chromic Endoloop sutures (Ethicon)

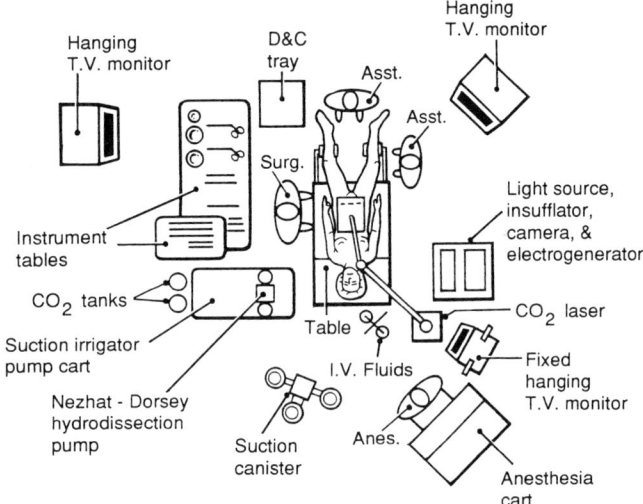

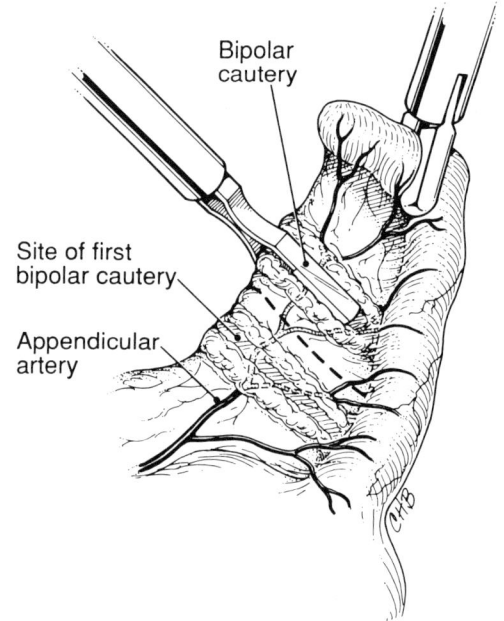

Figure 15.3. System of videolaseroscopy CO_2 laser through operative channel of laparoscopy is used for the purpose of cutting and hemostasis of small blood vessels, bipolar electrocoagulator for hemostasis of large blood vessels and Nezhat-Dorsey suction irrigator probe for hydrodissection and hydrosurgery.

Figure 15.4. Electrodesiccation of mesoappendix.

or polydioxanone sutures (Ethicon) are passed over the base of the appendix 2 to 5 mm from the cecum and then tied, one on top of the other. Both suture ends are cut with the CO_2 laser or scissors. A third endoloop suture is applied less than 2 cm distal to the other sutures

and a 15 cm tail is left to facilitate retrieval should the appendix inadvertently fall into the pelvic well (Fig. 15.6). Using the CO_2 laser, the appendix is cut between the second and third sutures placed. Luminal portions of the appendiceal stump and the removed appendix

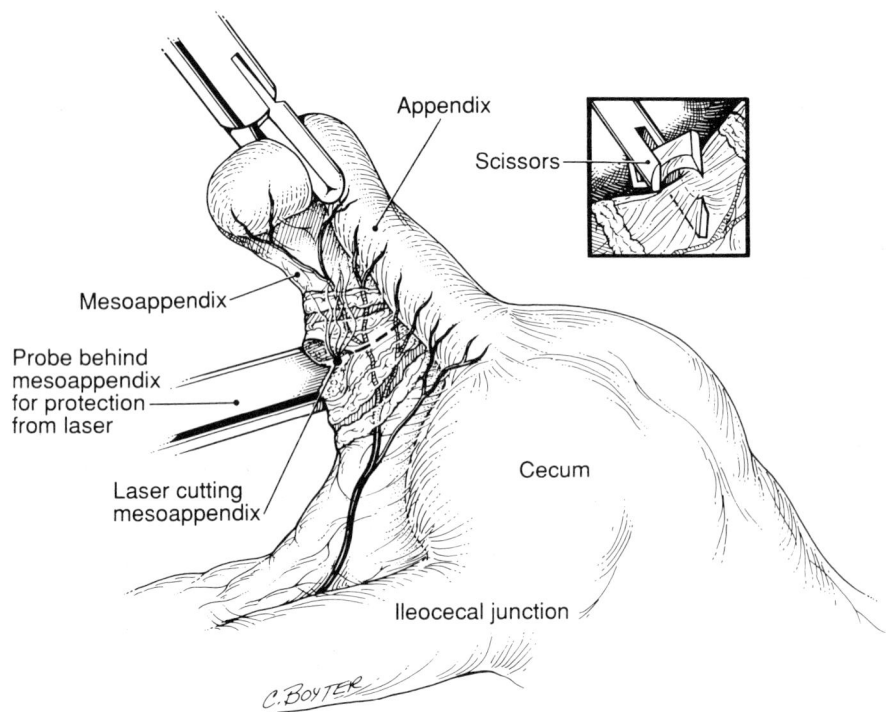

Figure 15.5. Laser or scissors is used to cut the appendix after electrodesiccation of the mesoappendix.

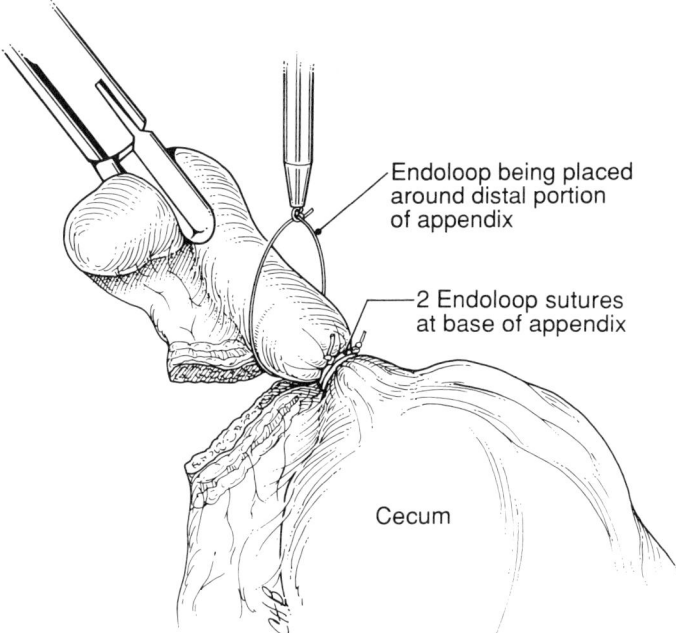

Figure 15.6. Placement of endoloop sutures.

are seared with the CO_2 laser (Fig. 15.7), and the tissues are copiously irrigated with lactated Ringer's solution (Baxter Healthcare, Deerfield, IL). The appendix is removed from the abdomen with a long grasping forceps passed through the operating channel of the laparoscope suprapubically with a short grasping forceps or with an Endopouch tissue removal bag (Ethicon). If appropriate, an appendix extractor may be placed via the sleeve of the 10 mm trocar, replacing the central 5 mm trocar. Instruments that may be contaminated are removed from the surgical area. No adjunctive therapy is

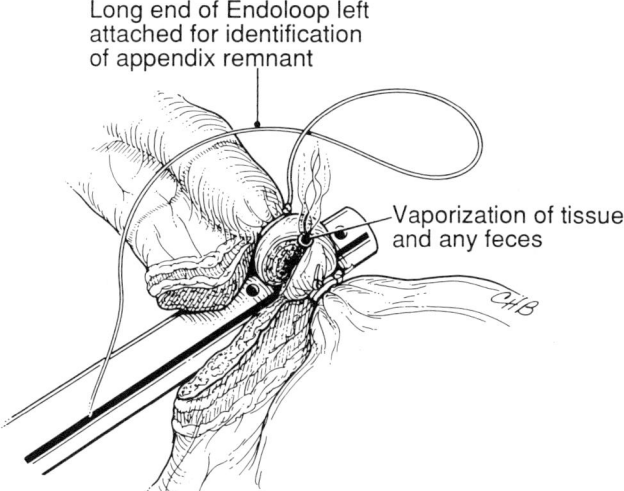

Figure 15.7. Appendix is being cut and seared with CO_2 laser.

necessary. Finally, the appendiceal and other operative sites are inspected for hemostasis and then irrigated with lactated Ringer's solution.[11]

Appendectomies may last from 4 to 21 minutes. Postoperative instructions should include avoiding solid food for 24 hours. Otherwise, instructions are the same as for gynecologic procedures, including an outpatient evaluation the day after surgery. In a series of 100 consecutive appendectomies using the technique of videolaseroscopy, we did not have any major intraoperative complications.[12] One patient had a transient elevated temperature, and one had mild periumbilical ecchymosis. All were discharged within 24 hours.[12] In another series of 254 laparoscopic appendectomies, no major intraoperative complications were noted and again, all were discharged within 24 hours. Postoperatively, one patient developed a small pelvic abscess that required surgical intervention.

We have recently modified our technique for the performance of appendectomy using a single Endoloop suture. The suture is placed over the base of the appendix 2 to 5 mm from the cecum and tied. Using the CO_2 laser, the appendix is cut about 5 mm distal to the suture. Searing of the luminal portion of the appendiceal stump on the removed appendix, irrigation, and removal of the appendix are as described above. Results are comparable to those achieved with our previous technique.

Several other laparoscopic appendectomy techniques have been described. In 1983, Semm reported a procedure incorporating the use of sutures and crocodile forceps.[13] The difference between Semm's technique and ours is that he uses suture ligation for the appendiceal artery rather than bipolar electrocoagulation and scissors or laser. Laparoscopic appendectomy may also be accomplished using a stapling device. The Endocutter (Ethicon) (Fig. 15.8) passes through a 12 mm trocar and allows placement of two triple-staggered lines of staples with a simultaneous cut. The close approximation of the two staple lines to the cutting blade in the cartridge head reduces the risk of spillage from the appendiceal lumen into the peritoneal cavity. The stapling device requires a 12 mm trocar.[14]

Endometriosis of the Rectosigmoid, Rectovaginal Septum, and Cul-de-Sac

Most cases of rectal and rectovaginal septum endometriosis can be managed with outpatient videolaparoscopy and do not require bowel resection.[15] The procedure is performed as follows. An assistant standing between the patient's legs uses one hand to perform rectovaginal examination and the other hand to hold the uterus up with a curette, a dilator, or the Humi rigid uterine elevator. An uninvolved are of peritoneum is identified and injected with 5 to 8 mL of diluted

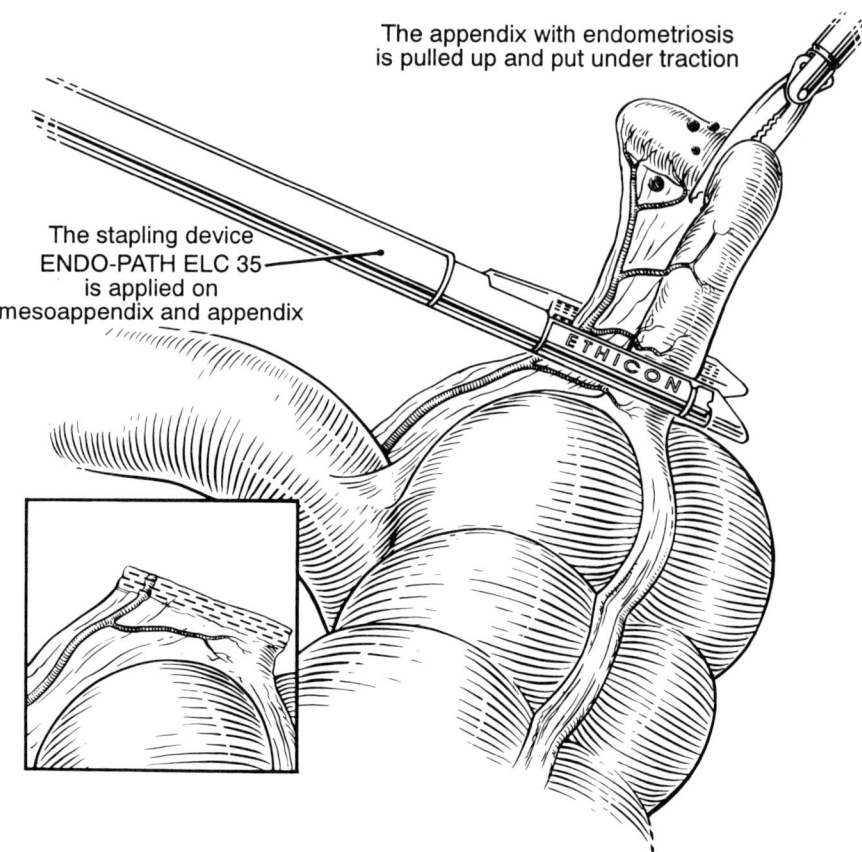

The appendix with endometriosis
is pulled up and put under traction

The stapling device
ENDO-PATH ELC 35
is applied on
mesoappendix and appendix

Figure 15.8. Endo-cutter stapler is used for appendectomy.

vasopressin (10 units in 100 to 200 mL of lactated Ringer's solution) with a 16-gauge laparoscopic needle. Using the CO_2 laser or other cutting modality, an opening is made in the peritoneum. Hydrodissection is performed by means of pressurized lactated Ringer's solution with a Nezhat-Dorsey probe (American Surgical Instruments, Inc., Delray Beach, FL) forming a plane in the rectovaginal septum.[16]

While the assistant examines the rectum, areas of involvement are identified by palpation. CO_2 laser vaporization or excision of rectovaginal implants is continued until no palpable nodules exist. Between 40 and 80 W of CO_2 laser are used to vaporize or excise the endometriosis. An assistant examines the rectum as the involved area is completely excised or vaporized until the loose areolar tissue of the rectovaginal space or normal muscularis layers of the rectum are reached. In patients whose rectum is pulled up and attached behind the cervix between the uterosacral ligaments, the uterus is first anteflexed sharply. Then an incision is made at the right or left pararectal area and extended to the junction of the cervix and rectum (Figs. 15.9 and 15.10). This plane of dissection is continued until the rectovaginal septum is reached (Fig. 15.11). If the rectal involvement is more extensive, a sigmoidoscope may be

used to guide the surgeon, as well as to rule out bowel perforation. The cul-de-sac is filled with irrigation fluid and is observed through the laparoscope while air is introduced into the rectum through the sigmoidoscope. Air bubbles observed in the cul-de-sac fluid indicate perforation. With the assistant guiding the surgeon by rectovaginal examination, the rectum is freed completely from the back of the cervix. At times, generalized ooze or bleeding may occur and can be controlled with an injection of 3 to 5 mL diluted vasopressin solution (1 ampule in 100 mL), laser, or bipolar electrocoagulator. Occasional bleeding from the stalk vessels caused by dissection or vaporization of the fibrotic uterosacral ligaments and pararectal areas is controlled with bipolar electrocoagulator.

Location and assessment of the ureters before proceeding with this procedure is of paramount importance, especially when they are infiltrated by endometriosis. Any alteration in the direction of the ureters should be identified prior to surgery. Because ureters are lateral to the uterosacral ligament, we try to stay between the ligaments as much as possible. Using hydrodissection and making a relaxing incision lateral to the uterosacral ligament allows the ureter to retract laterally. This increases protection of the ureters.

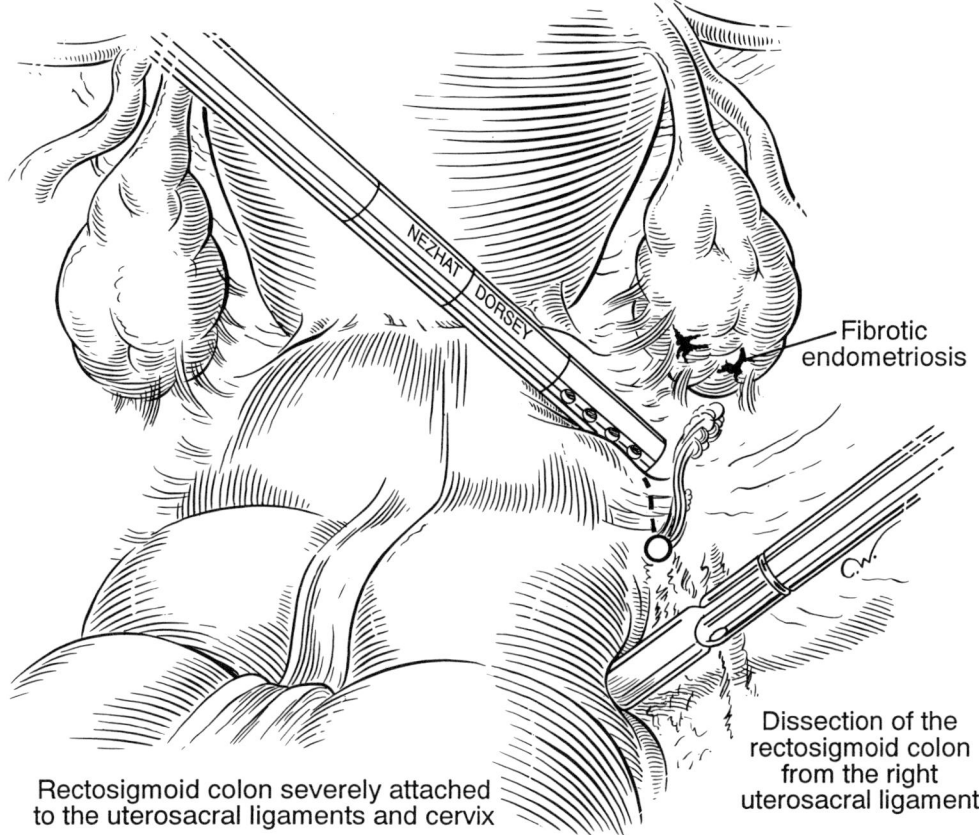

Fibrotic endometriosis

Dissection of the rectosigmoid colon from the right uterosacral ligament

Rectosigmoid colon severely attached to the uterosacral ligaments and cervix

Figure 15.9. Posterior cul-de-sac obliteration. An incision is made at the right pararectal area towards the uterosacral ligament.

For cases in which there is nodularity in the posterior cul-de-sac and infiltration of the endometriosis toward the vagina, vaporization and dissection of the nodularity are continued as an assistant evaluates the nodule by palpation until it is gone.[15,17] Endometriosis rarely penetrates the mucosa of the colon but it commonly involves the serosa, subserosa, and muscularis. The disease can be excised or vaporized thoroughly by an experienced videolaparoscopist. When major portions of both muscularis layers have been excised or vaporized, and the mucosa is reached, the bowel wall may be reinforced by one to three 4-0 polydioxanone sutures. The procedure is very demanding and requires maximal cooperation between the assistant and the surgeon.

This approach was applied to 185 women, aged 25 to 41 years, who had deep, infiltrative endometriosis of the rectovaginal septum, uterosacral ligaments, posterior cul-de-sac, and anterior wall of rectosigmoid colon.[15] Of the 185 patients, 33 had rectovaginal septum involvement, 22 had fibrotic and nodular uterosacral ligaments, and 130 had partial or complete obliteration of the cul-de-sac. Small vaginal perforations, which did not require suturing, occurred in 11 patients who had severe nodularity of the rectovaginal septum. The lumen of the rectosigmoid colon was entered in nine patients.

In eight, the repair was performed laparoscopically; in one, repair was performed after prolapsing the bowel through the anus (this technique is further described below in the section on bowel resection). Of 185 patients, 174 were available for follow-up after 1 to 5 years. Of 31 patients who have undergone second-look laparoscopies for persistent infertility or recurrent pain, 12 (38%) had complete healing of the rectovaginal septum with few filmy adhesions. Nineteen (61%) had dense, vascular adhesions, and 7 (23%) in this group had persistent endometriosis. Moderate to complete pain relief was reported by 162 (93%) of the 174 patients.

Bowel Resection

In cases of severe disease of the bowel wall, bowel resection may be necessary. We first described laparoscopic-assisted anterior rectal wall resection and anastomosis in 1991 to treat symptomatic infiltrative rectosigmoid endometriosis.[17] In 1992, we published the first report of total rectal wall resection by advanced operative laparoscopy.[18] The patient is given a preoperative mechanical bowel preparation as described previously. Three 5 mm suprapubic trocars, one each in the midline, right, and left lower

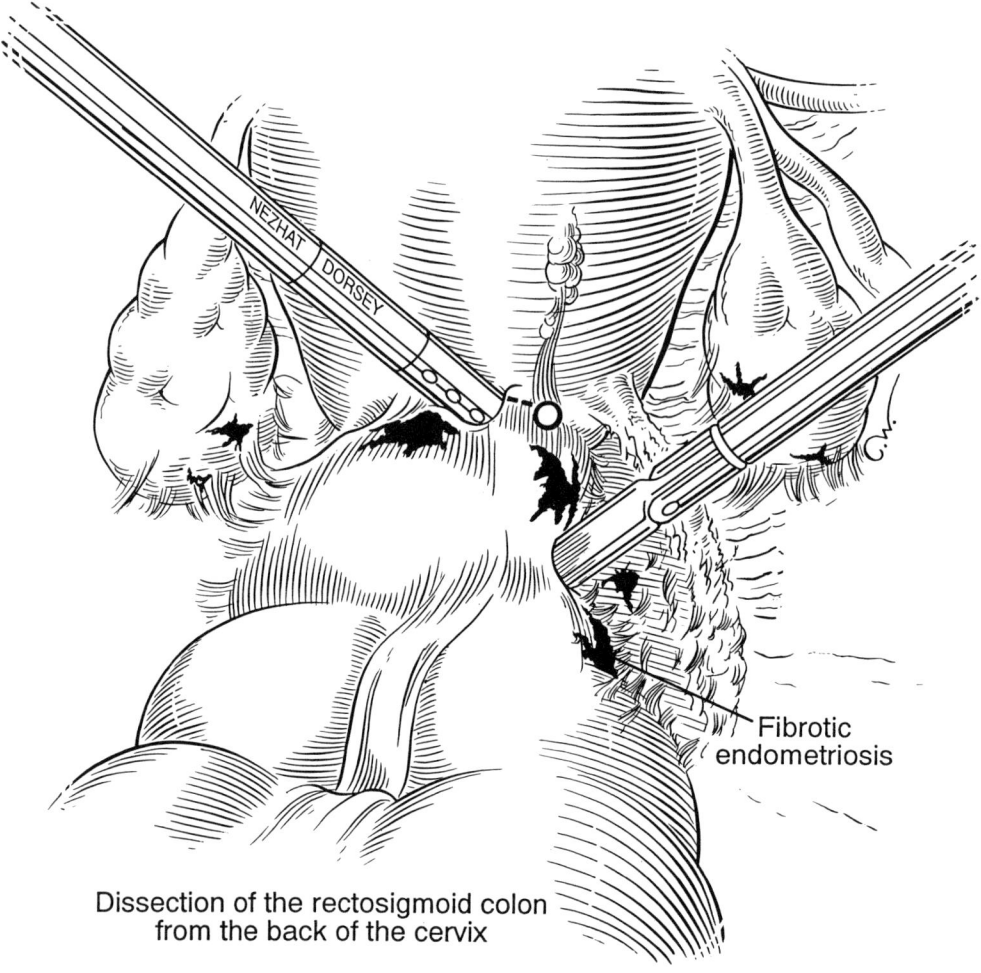

Dissection of the rectosigmoid colon
from the back of the cervix

Figure 15.10. The pararectal incision is extended to the junction of the cervix and rectum. The rectum is separated from the right uterosacral ligament.

quadrants, are used to place grasping forceps, Endo-loop suture applicators, a suction-irrigator probe, and a bipolar electrocoagulator.

The technique includes laparoscopic mobilization of the lower colon, transanal prolapse, resection, and reanastomosis.[17,18] When the lesion involves only the anterior rectal wall near the anal verge, the rectovaginal septum is delineated by simultaneous vaginal and rectal examinations performed by an assistant. The rectum is mobilized along the rectovaginal septum anteriorly to within 2 cm of the anus, using the CO_2 laser or other cutting modality, and hydrodissection. Mobilization continues along the left and right pararectal spaces by electrodesiccating and dividing branches of the hemor-rhoidal artery, and partially posteriorly, as well. When the rectum is sufficiently mobilized, the tumor is pro-lapsed to the level of the anus, the perineal body is retracted, and an RL 30 (Ethicon) multifire stapler is applied across the segment of the anterior rectal wall containing the nodule. Two staple applications may be required to traverse the width of the involved mucosa.

The tumor nodule is excised using electrosurgery, and two additional interrupted 2-0 polyglactin sutures are inserted along the staple line. The rectum is returned to the pelvis under direct visualization, and closure is confirmed by insufflating the rectum while the cul-de-sac is filled with lactated Ringer's.

In patients with more extensive and circumferential lesions, the entire rectum is mobilized, the lateral rectal pedicles are electrodesiccated, and the presacral space is entered to the level of the levator ani muscles to be able to mobilize the bowel. The branches of the inferior mesenteric vessels of the bowel segment to be resected are electrodesiccated and cut. The rectum is transected proximal to the lesion, and the proximal limb is pro-lapsed into the distal limb, using Babcock clamps (Fig. 15.12A). A 2-0 purse-string suture is inserted to the end of the proximal bowel to secure the opposing anvil of an ILS 29 or 33 stapler (Ethicon) (Fig. 15.12B–C). The anvil is then replaced transanally into the pelvis along with the proximal bowel. The rectal stump containing the endometrial lesion and fibrosis is then prolapsed out

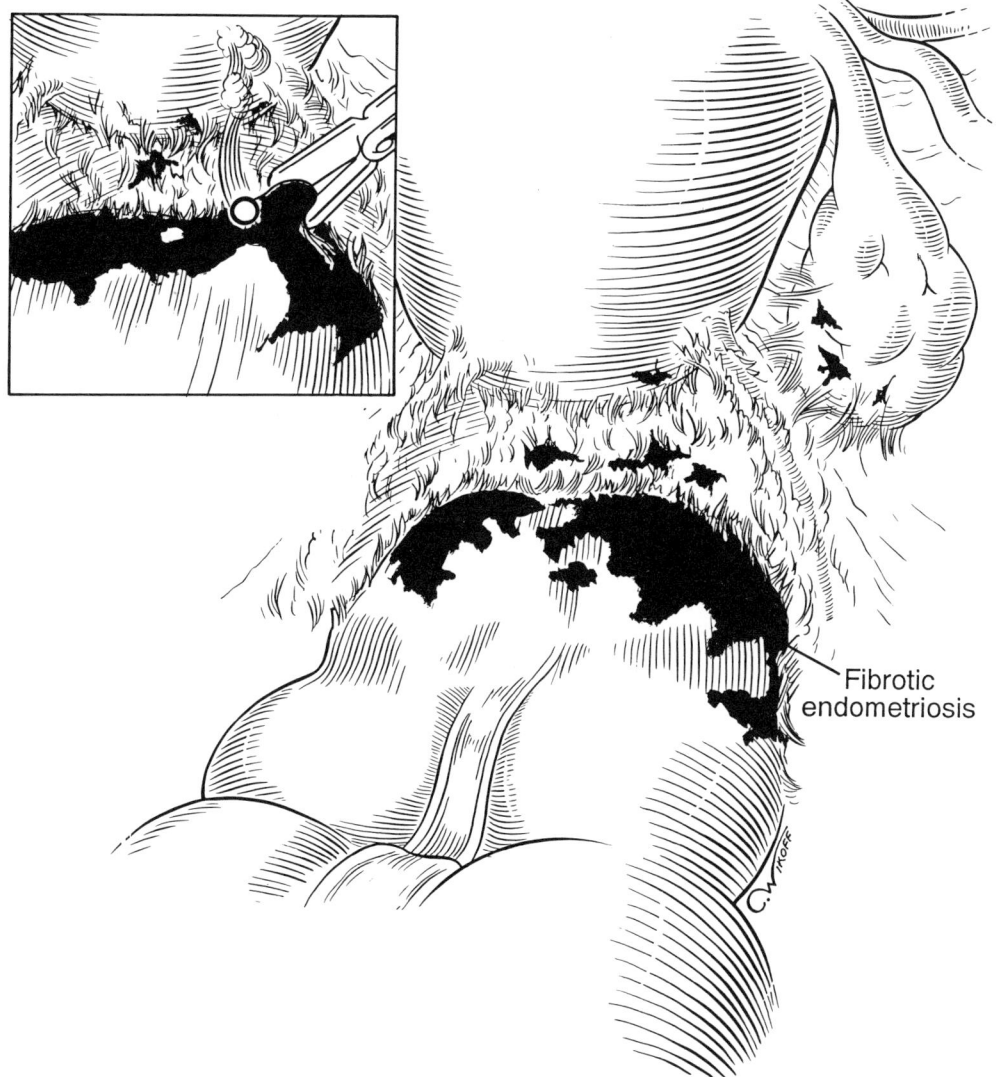

Figure 15.11. The rectosigmoid colon is completely separated from the back of the uterus, cervix and uterosacral ligaments. Then the anterior rectosigmoid colon fibrosis and endometriosis is vaporized or excised (inset).

of the anus by grasping the transected end of the rectal stump with Babcock clamps (Baxter Mueller, Chicago, IL) and pulling it through the anal canal. The rectum is stapled shut with an RL60 linear stapler (Ethicon) and the rectal specimen is resected and sent to surgical pathology (Fig. 15.13). The rectal stump is reduced inside the pelvis and an end-to-end double stapled anastomosis is performed with the ILS 33 stapler (Ethicon). A trocar in the gun is passed through the stapled end of the rectum (Fig. 15.14A). The laparoscope is then used to attach the opposing anvil in the proximal bowel (Fig. 15.14B). The bowel ends are approximated, and the stapler is fired to complete the anastomosis. Intact "doughnut" margins should be present (Fig. 15.14C). A proctoscope is used to examine the anastomosis for structural integrity and bleeding. Lactated Ringer's solution is inserted into the pelvis and visualized with

the laparoscope as air is insufflated into the rectum to check for leakage. Air leaks may be corrected using transanally placed 2-0 Vicryl sutures. Laparoscopic bowel resection by this technique is identical with resection at laparotomy with the bipolar electrocoagulator and laser replacing the suture and scissors.[19]

A simplified method for resection of severe endometriosis of the anterior wall of the colon[20] is as follows. The extent of the lesion is evaluated visually and by palpation using the tip of the suction-irrigator probe. If the lesion is low enough, an assistant can identify it by performing a rectal examination. A sigmoidoscope is used to further delineate the lesion and guide the surgeon.

After identification of the ureters in order to avoid inadvertent injury, the lower colon is mobilized in all

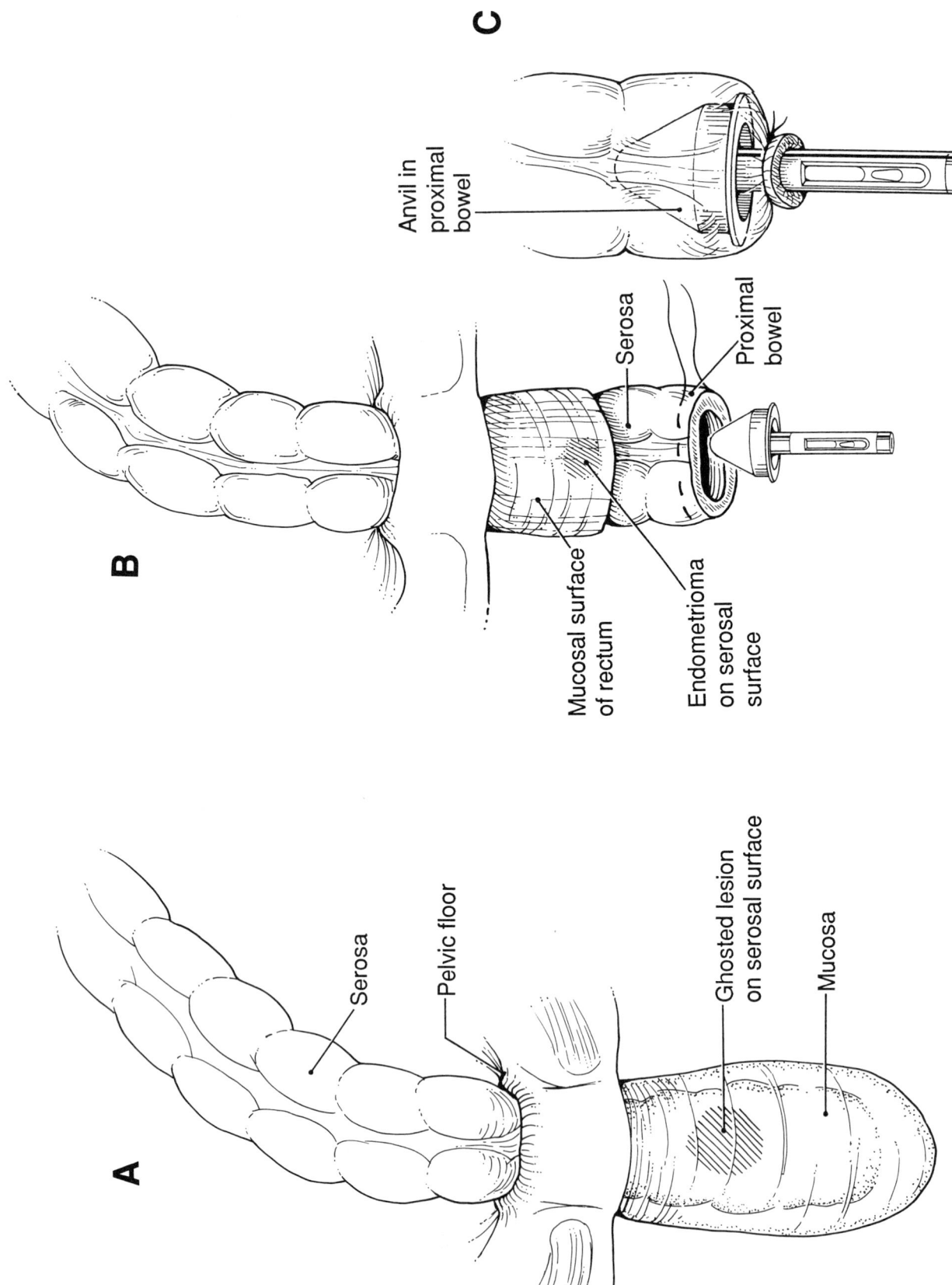

Figure 15.12. A. Fibrosis and endometriosis. Narrowing of lower rectosigmoid colon. **B.** After rectosigmoid colon is transected distal to the lesion, the proximal colon has been prolapsed anally via the distal colon. Purse-string suture has been placed. **C.** Anvil of stapler is placed through the pursestring into the proximal bowel.

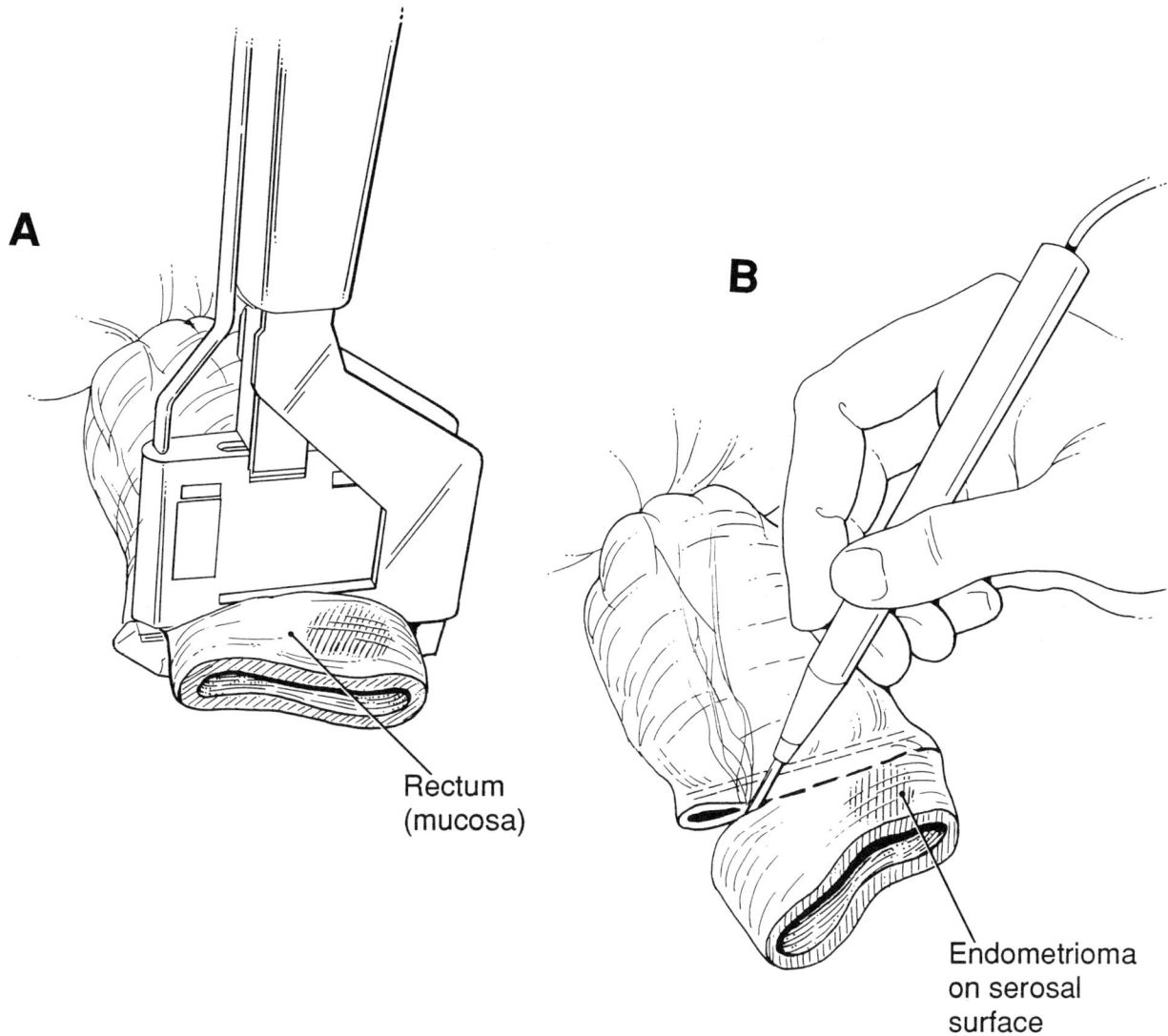

A

Rectum
(mucosa)

B

Endometrioma
on serosal
surface

Figure 15.13. A. The rectum is stapled shut with an RL 60 linear stapler above the lesion. **B.** A portion of colon with endometriosis involvement removed.

aspects except posteriorly. Depending on the location of the lesion, the right pararectal area, left pararectal area, or both are entered using the CO_2 laser and hydrodissection. The colon is separated from the adjacent organs. Full-thickness excision is carried out, beginning above the area of visible disease. After identifying the normal tissue, the lesion is held at its proximal end with grasping forceps. An incision is made using the CO_2 laser through the bowel serosa and muscularis, and the lumen is entered (Fig. 15.15A). The lesion is excised from the anterior rectal wall (Fig. 15.15B). The suction-irrigator probe is used as a backstop for the laser and to evacuate the laser plume. After complete excision of the lesion, the pelvic cavity is irrigated and suctioned. Resected pieces of bowel are extracted through the operative channel of the laparoscope using a long grasping forceps, or from the anus using polyp forceps, and submitted for pathology. The bowel is repaired transversely in one layer. Two traction sutures are applied to each side of the defect, transforming it to a transverse opening (Fig. 15.16A). The stay sutures are brought out through the right and left lower quadrant incisions. The sleeves are removed, then replaced in the peritoneal cavity next to the stay sutures, and the sutures are secured outside the abdomen. The bowel is then repaired by placing several interrupted through-and-through sutures in 0.4 to 0.6 cm increments until it is completely reanastomosed (Fig. 15.16B). We use 0-Vicryl or PDS laparoscopic sutures with a straight or curved needle (Ethicon) with extracorporeal knot tying (Fig. 15.17). When the lesion is not very extensive and the bowel defect after resection is less than 4 cm, the bowel can be repaired vertically without causing stricture. At the end of the procedure, sigmoidoscopy is performed to ensure that the closure is airtight and that there in no bowel stricture.[20]

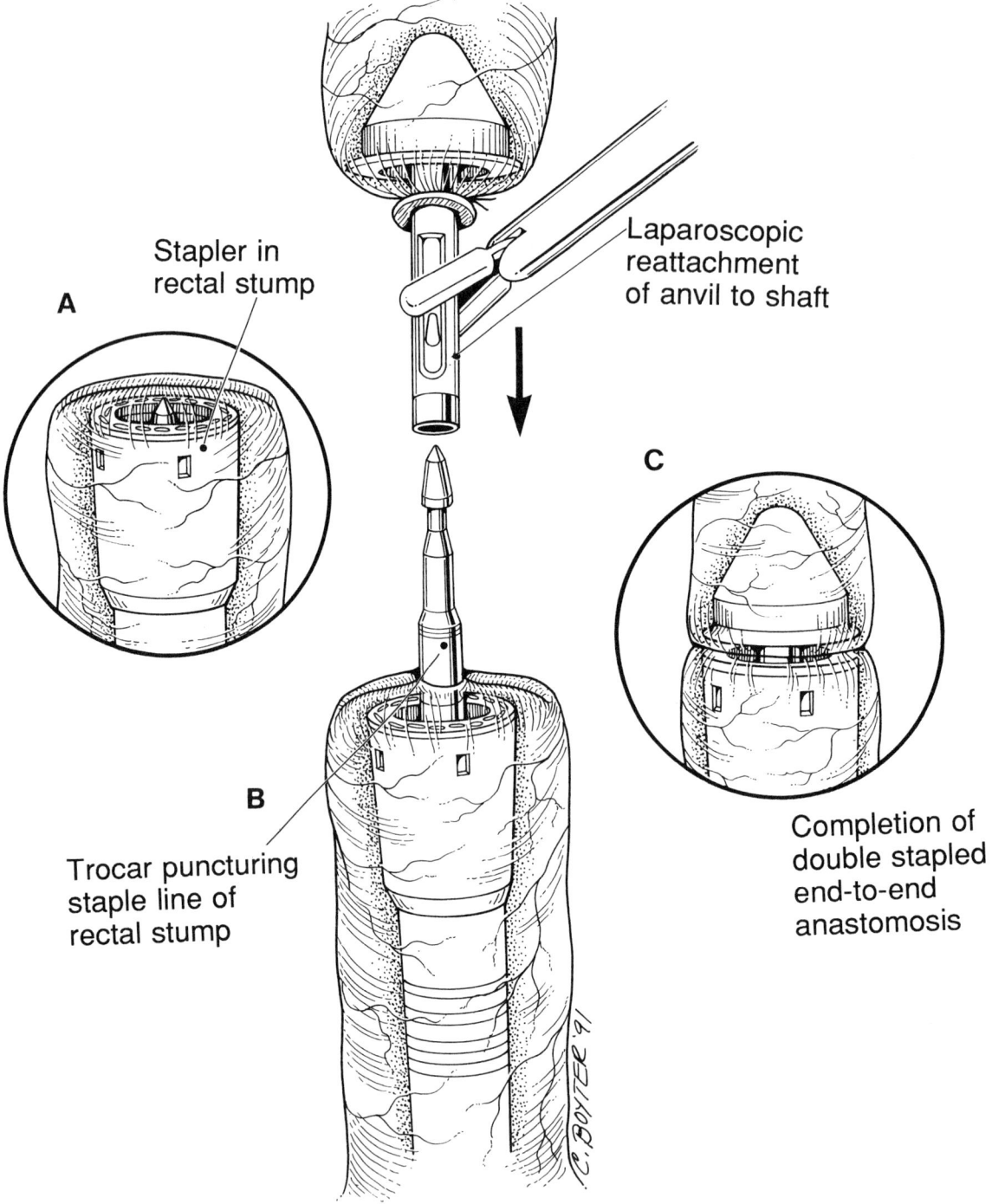

A. Stapler in rectal stump

Laparoscopic reattachment of anvil to shaft

C

B. Trocar puncturing staple line of rectal stump

Completion of double stapled end-to-end anastomosis

Figure 15.14. A. Distal portion of colon with anvil inside of it is placed into the pelvic cavity. **B.** Distal and proximal portion of bowel were attached together laparoscopically. **C.** Reanastomosis is completed.

In a series of 356 women who underwent laparoscopic treatment of bowel endometriosis using different techniques, two patients required intraoperative laparotomy early in our experience. The first patient underwent laparotomy for repair of enterotomy after treatment of infiltrative rectal endometriosis. The other patient required laparotomy for anastomosis due to an unsuccessful attempt to place a purse-string suture around the patulous rectal ampulla. Significant postoperative complications occurred in 1.7% of patients. Two women developed leaks and pelvic infections. One required a laparoscopic temporary colostomy with subsequent takedown and repair, and one was managed by prolonged drainage under CT scan guidance. One woman had bowel stricture requiring resection and reanastomosis. One developed

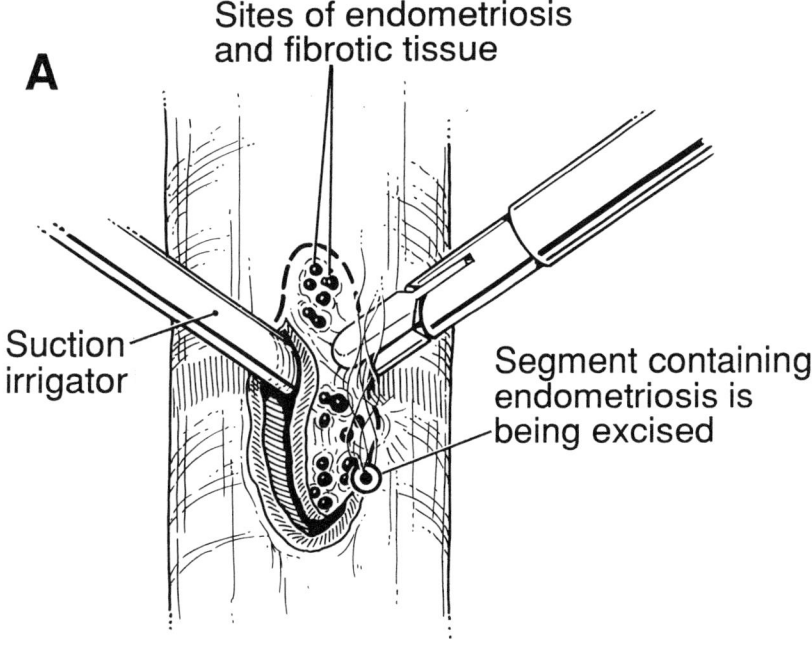

A

Sites of endometriosis
and fibrotic tissue

Suction
irrigator

Segment containing
endometriosis is
being excised

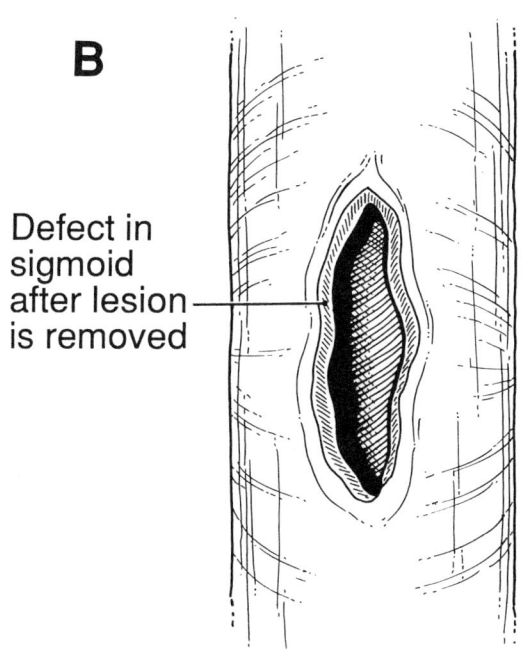

B

Defect in
sigmoid
after lesion
is removed

Figure 15.15. A. Segment of anterior colon involved with severe endometriosis is being excised using CO_2 laser. **B.** Sigmoid colon defect after the lesion is removed.

a pelvic abscess which after failed drainage required subsequent laparoscopic right salpingo-opphorectomy. One patient who had anterior wedge resection of the recturn experienced an immediate rectal prolapse which was reduced without surgical management. Her original bowel symptoms persisted, and she finally had a colectomy.

Minor complications included skin ecchymosis, temporary urinary retention, temporary diarrhea or constipation, and dyschezia.

Small Bowel

The small bowel has the least involvement with endometriosis. The most common location is the ileocecal

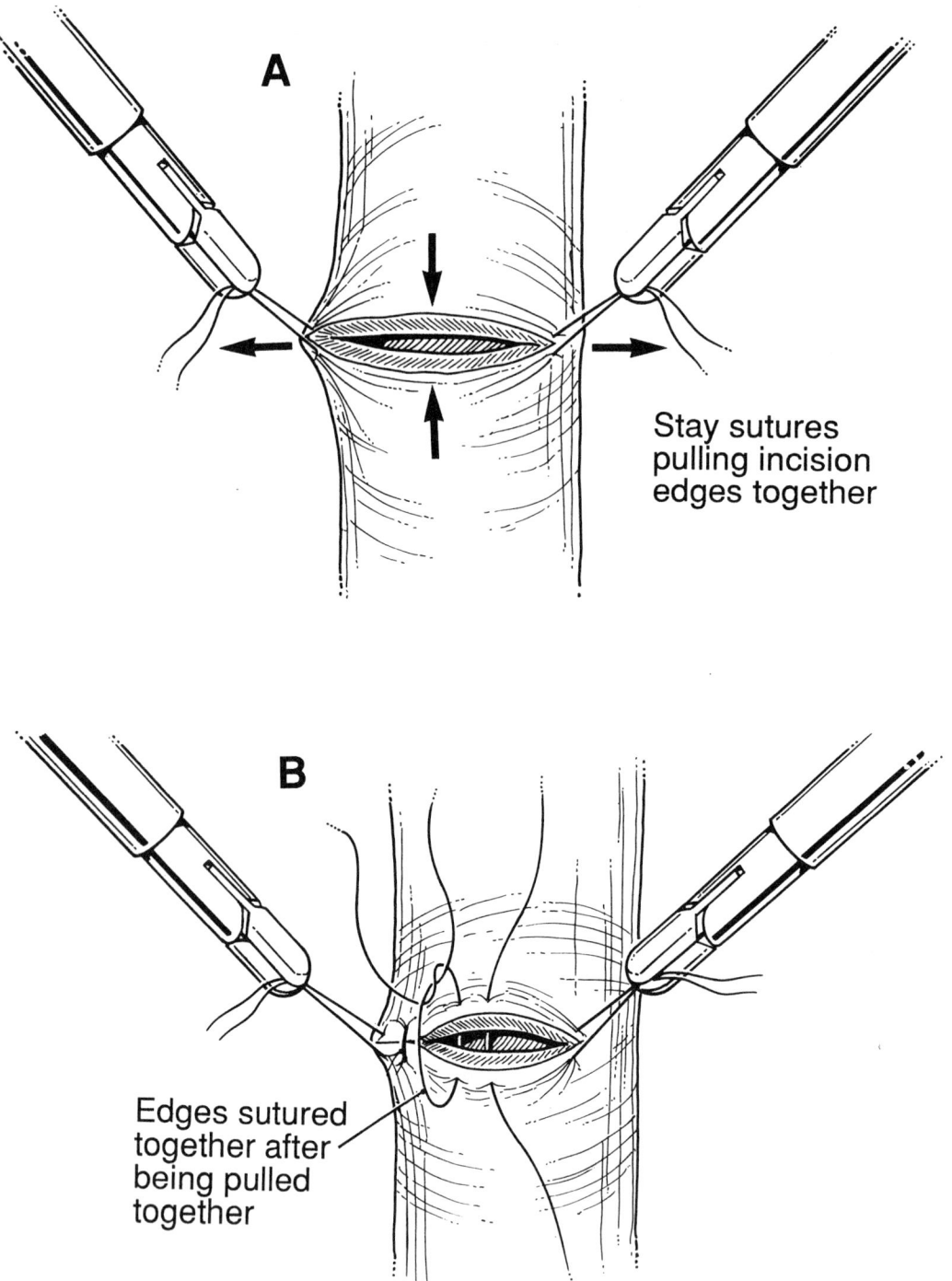

Figure 15.16. A. Two stay traction sutures are applied to each side of the defect, transforming it to a transverse opening. **B.** The bowel is then repaired by placing several interrupted sutures.

area. Superficial spots of endometriosis can be vaporized with low power CO_2 laser (15–25 watts). Occasionally, the lesion is deep and entry into the lumen of bowel is necessary. If the entry is less than 1 cm, it can be repaired using one Endoloop suture.[21] After thorough irrigation of the perforation is performed, the Endoloop is tied over the defect and the perforation is brought

inside the loop using anastomotic grasping forceps and tied below the perforation leaving adequate stump. The repair is immersed in the lactated Ringer's and observed for air bubbles to be sure it is airtight.

A defect of more than 1 cm is repaired in one layer using through-and-through 0 Vicryl or PDS suture as was described before (Figs. 15.16 and 15.17).[21] When

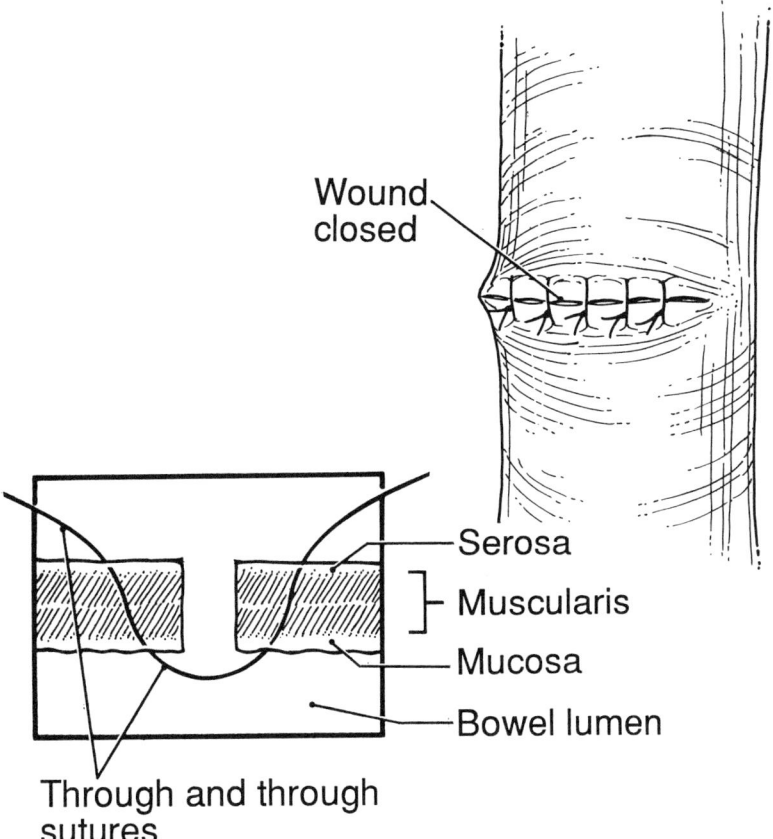

Figure 15.17. One layer through-and-through sutures placed until the bowel is completely repaired.

the involvement is more extensive and complete resection and reanastomosis is required, the bowel is completely mobilized laparoscopically and brought out through McBurney incision or vaginal posterior colpotomy, resected and reanastomosed.

We have treated three such cases laparoscopically. In the first, the patient had cecal and appendiceal endometriosis. Following laparoscopic mobilization of the bowel, the cecum was resected and reanastomosed through a McBurney incision. An appendectomy was then performed. The other two women had small bowel endometriosis which was causing partial stricture. The mesentery was coagulated and cut, and the bowel exteriorized through a Pfannenstiel incision in one case and through a posterior colpotomy in the other. Resection and reanastomosis were then completed with no intraoperative or postoperative complications, and the women are doing well.

The Genitourinary Tract

Variable ureteral and bladder involvement have been reported in 1% to 11% of women diagnosed with endometriosis.[22] As the disease becomes more advanced, the ureter is vulnerable to endometriotic implant involvement. Endometriosis of the urinary tract can be superficial or invasive, and in sporadic cases, may even completely obstruct the ureter. The bladder wall is one of the sites least frequently involved with endometriosis. In fact, fewer than 180 cases have been reported.[23] Management options include hormone suppressive therapy, oophorectomy, hysterectomy, and/or segmental cystectomy.[24,25]

Decreased bladder capacity and bladder instability unresponsive to conventional therapy may be due to endometriosis. Goldstein and Brodmann reported one case of bladder endometriosis that they monitored cystometrically over a 4-year period.[26] They found that decreased bladder capacity and bladder instability, both unresponsive to conventional parasympatholytic agents, were corrected after surgical destruction of superficial endometriosis. When bladder symptoms recurred 2 years later, a course of danazol again reversed bladder instability. It is important that clinicians consider endometriosis in cases of refractory and unexplained urinary complaints.

If endometriosis of the urinary tract is suspected, a complete preoperative evaluation should be performed including an intravenous pyelogram, ultrasound scan of the kidneys, and routine blood and urine workup.

In selected cases where patients present recurrent hematuria, cystoscopy may be indicated.

Treatment of Genitourinary Tract Implants

Most superficial implants of endometriosis over the ureter and the bladder can be safely treated by operative laparoscopy, utilizing hydrodissection and the CO_2 laser. Before the introduction of hydrodissection to the operative laparoscopic treatment of endometriosis, sensitive areas at risk of injury, such as bowel, ureter, bladder, and major blood vessels, were often excluded from surgical intervention.[27,28] This omission was serious because the patient often continued to have symptoms after surgical therapy. Hydrodissection makes treatment with the CO_2 laser in these high-risk areas safer. Because the CO_2 laser beam does not penetrate fluid, treatment can be confined to the endometrial lesion yet leave adjacent normal tissue unharmed. By creating a bed of water beneath the peritoneum, the risk of laser beam penetration to underlying tissue is reduced.

Superficial implants over the ureter can generally be treated by a variation of hydrodissection. Approximately 20 to 30 mL of lactated Ringer's solution is injected subperitoneally on the lateral pelvic wall, elevating the peritoneum and backing it with a bed of fluid. The CO_2 laser is then used to create a 0.5 cm opening on this elevation. The peritoneum is opened anteriorly and laterally, close to the corresponding round ligament. The hydrodissection probe is then inserted into the opening and approximately 100 mL of lactated Ringer's is injected under 300 mm/Hg pressure into the retroperitoneal space along the course of the ureter (Fig. 15.18). The fluid surrounds the ureter, moves it posteriorly, and allows superficial CO_2 laser dissection or vaporization of the area.

After creating the water bed, a superpulse or ultrapulse mode of the CO_2 laser of between 20 and 80 W is used for vaporization or excision of the lesion, which should be performed with a circumference of 1 to 2 cm. When the lesions are large and excision is preferred, a circular line with a 1 to 2 cm margin is made around the lesion. The peritoneum is then grasped with an atraumatic grasping forceps and peeled away with the

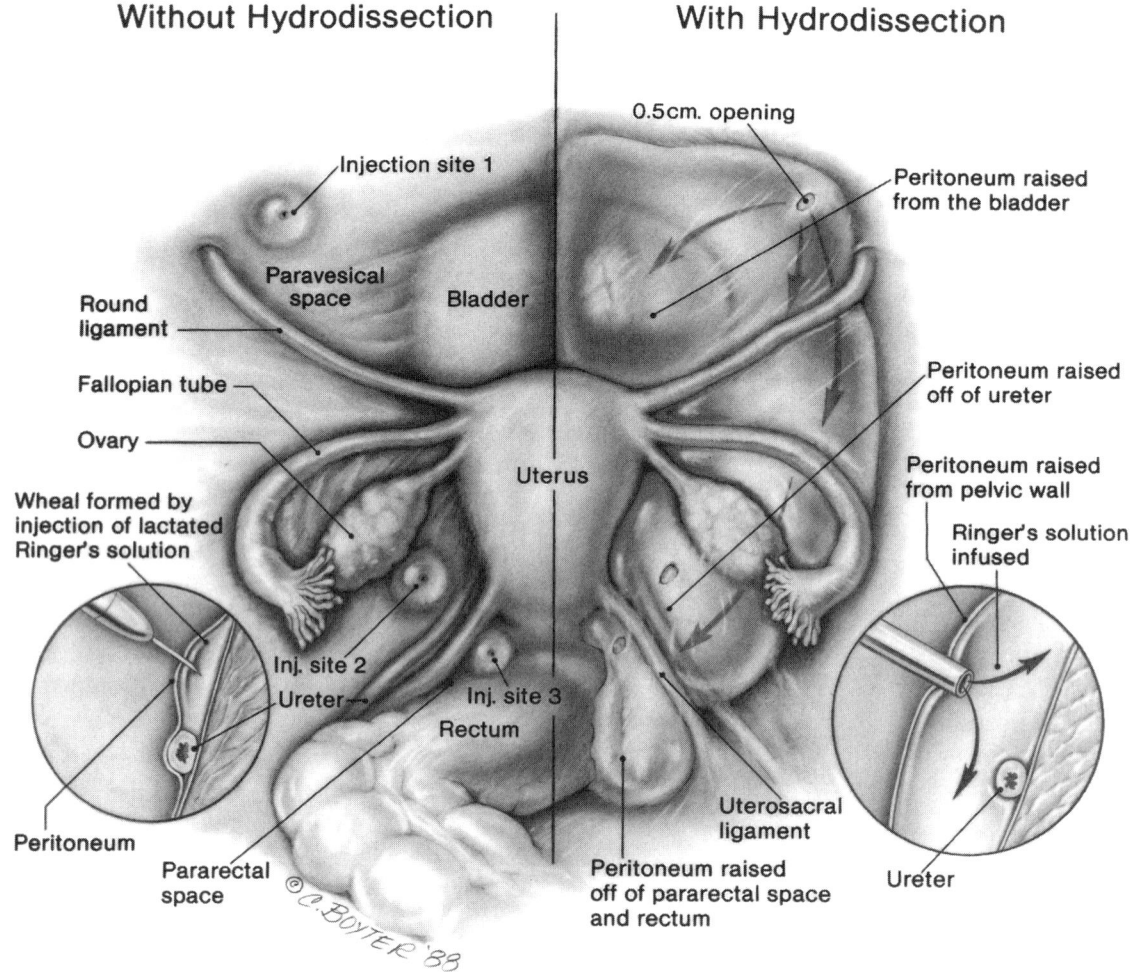

Figure 15.18. Hydrodissection.

help of the CO_2 laser and the tip of the suction-irrigation probe. If the endometrial implant is firmly embedded and has formed scarring down to the subperitoneal connective tissue, hydrodissection should be extended. By injecting fluid around the lesion, water "tunnels" beneath the lesion, and often separates the scar tissue. The lesion can then be safely treated. After vaporization or excision of these lesions, the area must be carefully irrigated to remove all remaining charcoal and verify that all remaining endometriosis has been properly treated.

Nezhat and Nezhat reported over 500 sites of genitourinary implants treated by this method. There have been no major complications involving injury to the bladder or ureters. Two patients were unable to void immediately following surgery; this problem was resolved with an indwelling catheter which was removed the day after surgery. Four patients with endometriosis of the bladder had postoperative hematuria which cleared within several hours. Following hydrodissection of the broad ligaments and the pelvic side wall, about 5% of the patients had swelling of the external genitalia. This is most likely because of the penetration of water through the inguinal canal to the labia. This swelling resolved in most cases within one to two hours, and did not leave any permanent sequelae.

Obstructed Ureter

In severe cases of endometriosis, the implants may invade the periureteral tissue or ureter and cause obstruction. The incidence of ureteral obstruction due to endometriosis is low. Most gynecologists will never encounter this entity. However, as this complication has severe effects on the patient's quality of life, any surgeon treating endometriosis must be thoroughly acquainted with the modes of treatment available. Conventional therapy consists of laparotomy and resection of the obstructed segment of the ureter.

We first performed a ureteroureterostomy by laparoscopy in 1989 in a 36-year-old woman with long-term ureteral obstruction caused by endometriosis.[29] The condition had been previously diagnosed at laparoscopy, but the patient refused to undergo treatment by laparotomy. When the patient came to us, she had had a nephrostomy tube in place for 4 years. Laparoscopic findings included a 3 to 4 cm fibrotic nodule over the left ureter, approximately 4 cm above the bladder, distorting the course of the ureter (Fig. 15.19). This corresponded to the level of the obstruction previously diagnosed by radioimaging techniques. Under direct visualization by laparoscopy, we attempted to place a retrograde catheter, but were unsuccessful. We decided to excise the nodule using videolaseroscopy and hydrodissection.

The left retroperitoneal space was entered at the

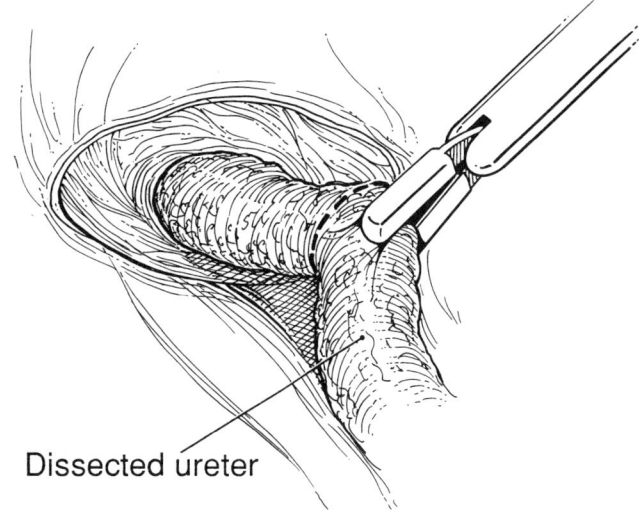

Figure 15.19. Fibrotic nodule of left ureter 4 cm above ureter.

pelvic brim and after treating all associated lesions, such as endometriosis, fibrosis, or adhesions, the ureter was dissected with the CO_2 laser. During dissection, when we discovered that the nodule involved the entire thickness of the ureter, we elected to do a partial resection (Fig. 15.20).[29]

Under cystoscopic guidance, a 7F ureteral catheter was passed through the ureterovesical junction, and the CO_2 laser was used to enter the ureter at this level.

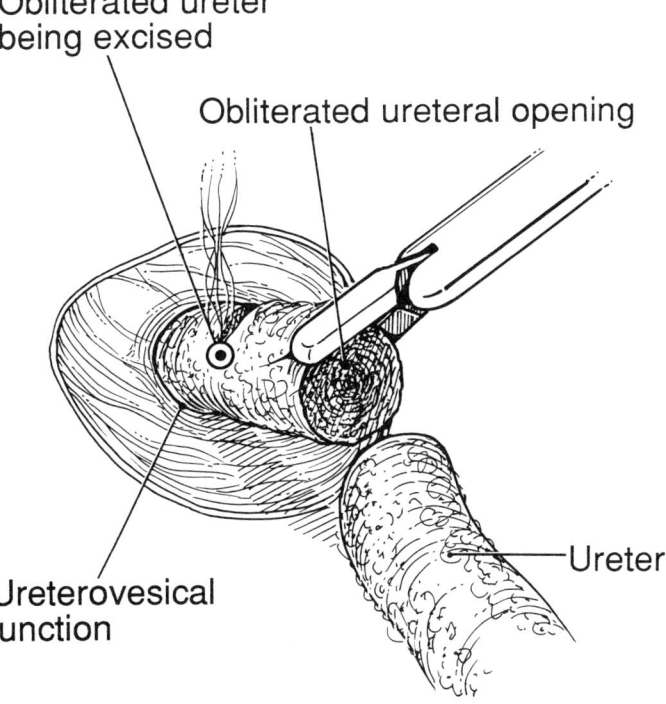

Figure 15.20. Partial resection of a completely obstructed ureter.

Indigo carmine was injected into the patient's IV to test the ureter's patency. The distal ureter was transected over the stent, and the obstructed portion of the ureter was removed. When this was completed, the ureteral stent was introduced into the proximal ureter and advanced into the renal pelvis (Fig. 15.21). Finally, the edges of the ureter were reapproximated using four 4-0 PDS sutures placed in an interrupted fashion at the 6, 12, 9, and 3 o'clock positions to approximate the proximal and distal ureteral edges (Fig. 15.22). In this case, an external ureteral stent was left in the ureter for a minimum of 4 weeks, at which time it was exchanged cystoscopically for an internal stent. This stent remained in place for approximately 2 months postoperatively. The patient's follow-up included IVP, ultrasound, and nephrostogram. All showed function of the kidney and patent ureter.

This patient went home the day after surgery. Her postoperative course was uncomplicated. An intravenous pyelogram confirmed ureteral patency and renal function. Estimated blood loss was less than 100 mL and the duration of the procedure was just under 2 hours. The length of the removed/vaporized segment was 3 to 4 cm. The pathology report confirmed severe endometriosis and fibrosis of the resected ureter.

Since then we have treated 12 more cases of severe endometriosis of the ureter in which the endometriosis and fibrosis caused partial or complete ureteral obstruction. All patients had a known history of endometriosis and underwent different surgical and medical treat-

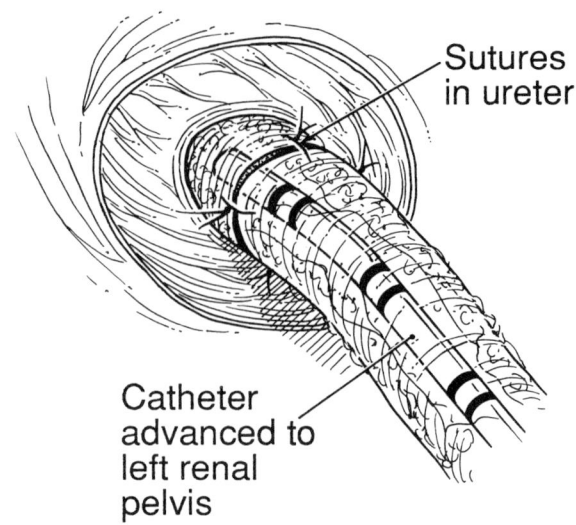

Sutures in ureter

Catheter advanced to left renal pelvis

Figure 15.22. Reanastomosis has been accomplished by applying suture at 6, 12, 9, and 3 O'clock.

ments. In four women, the ureteral endometriosis was removed completely without entering the ureteral lumen. In three women, the obstructed ureter required a complete segmental resection. One right and one left ureteroureterostomy and one reanastomosis of the left ureter to the bladder (ureteroneocystostomy) were performed using four through and through interrupted 4-0 polydioxanone (PDS) sutures to reapproximate the edges over the ureteral catheter. In five women, the ureter was partially involved. The severe peritoneal and ureteral endometriosis was cautiously vaporized using the CO_2 laser until ureterotomy occurred.

In three women, the ureterotomy was very small and was detected by intravenous injection of indigo carmine. A ureteral stent was left in place and no suture was required. In two patients, the ureterotomy was repaired using 4-0 PDS to overlap the laceration after stent placement. Histological examination of the resected specimen revealed fibrosis, endometriosis or both in all women. A rare case of endometriosis with focal severely atypical hyperplasia was found in the specimen of a 46-year-old woman. She had undergone total abdominal hysterectomy and bilateral salpingo-opphorectomy followed by hormonal replacement therapy at another institution. All patients had an uneventful intra- and postoperative course and reported symptomatic relief of their symptoms. Imaging techniques demonstrated patent ureters with a functioning kidney in all patients except for one. She was a 24-year-old woman who underwent treatment at another institution of chronic pelvic pain. She had been diagnosed several months earlier with pelvic endometriosis which was partially treated at laparoscopy followed by GnRH analog therapy postoperatively. During our laparoscopy, she was found to have severe left uterosacral and left pelvic

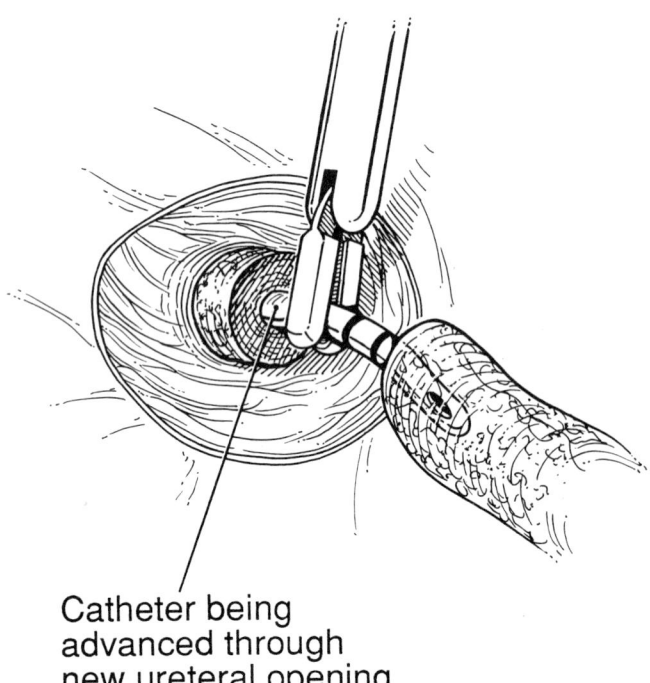

Catheter being advanced through new ureteral opening

Figure 15.21. Ureteral stent is introduced to the proximal ureter and advanced to the renal pelvis.

sidewall endometriosis which had caused complete obstruction of the ureter. Segmental resection and ureteroureterostomy was performed. Intraoperative intravenous injection of indigo carmine did not reveal any leakage from the ureter and raised the question of a nonfunctioning kidney. Postoperative follow up and imaging revealed a 5–10% functioning kidney. However, the ureter was patent.

Bladder Endometriosis

If the lesions of the bladder serosa are superficial, hydrodissection and vaporization will adequately remove them. However, different management is necessary when the involvement is deep within the muscularis or mucosa. The efficacy of conservative therapy varies. Some regard it as palliative and temporary. When conservative medical and surgical therapy fails, segmental cystectomy is necessary to remove the lesions.

We have successfully performed laparoscopic segmental cystectomy on six patients. Operative laparoscopy was performed using a laparoscope, video camera, and three suprapubic portals.[30] We thoroughly evaluate the abdominal and pelvic cavities to assess the extent of the endometriosis. Simultaneous cystoscopy is performed. Bilateral ureter catheters are inserted to better identify the ureters.

The bladder dome is held near the midline with the grasping forceps and the endometriotic nodule is excised 5 mm beyond the lesion (Fig. 15.23). The incision is made with the CO_2 laser using the suction irrigation probe as a backstop (Fig. 15.24). The specimen is removed from the abdominal cavity with the assistance of a long grasping forceps through the operative channel of the laparoscope. The excised tissue is held by a previously placed grasping forceps. The lesion is then regrasped and removed with the laparoscope as one unit. The CO_2 gas distends the bladder cavity and pro-

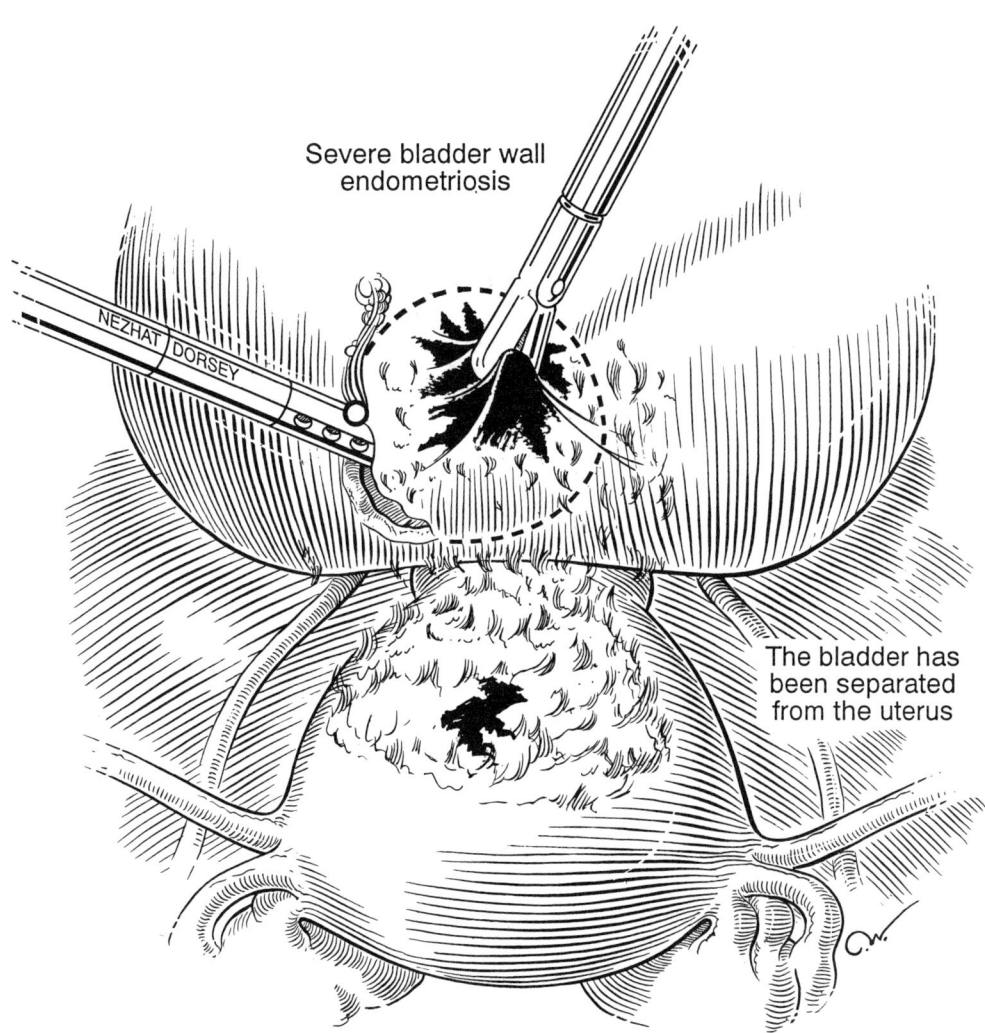

Severe bladder wall endometriosis

The bladder has been separated from the uterus

Figure 15.23. The bladder dome is held near the midline with the grasping forceps and the endometriotic nodule is excised beyond the lesion.

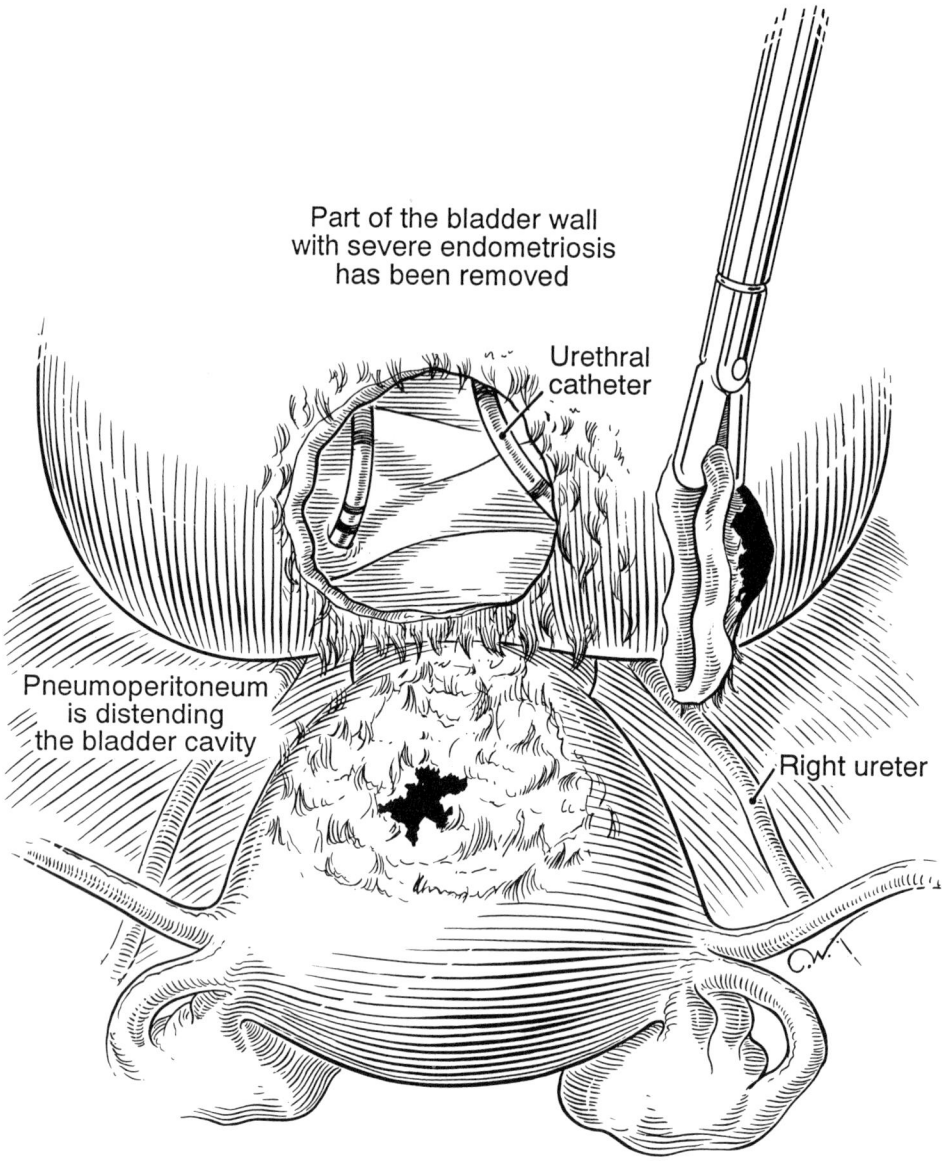

Part of the bladder wall
with severe endometriosis
has been removed

Urethral
catheter

Pneumoperitoneum
is distending
the bladder cavity

Right ureter

Figure 15.24. The lesion and partial cystectomy is performed using the CO_2 laser.

vides excellent visualization of the bladder interior. After again identifying the ureters, and careful examination of the bladder mucosa, the bladder is closed. This is performed with several interrupted polydioxanone or Vieryl through-and-through sutures using extracorporeal or intracorporeal knotting (Fig. 15.25). Cytoscopy is then performed to check for possible leaks. Laparoscopic segmental cystectomy takes approximately 35–45 minutes. Each woman was discharged from the hospital the following day and instructed to take trimethoprim and sulfamethoxazole for 2 weeks. The Foley catheter was removed 7–14 days later, at which time the cystograms were normal. The average estimated blood loss was less than 150 mL. The pathology report confirmed severe endometriosis and fibrosis of the resected bladder wall in all six cases. No intraoperative or postopera-

tive complications were noted. Ten to 23 months postoperatively, the patients are doing well, with no hematuria at menstruation.

Summary

In experienced hands, the laparoscopic approach provides an excellent route for diagnosis and treatment of endometriosis of the intestine and genitourinary tract. Endoscopic magnification of the bowel and bladder wall planes, coupled with hemostasis facilitated by pneumoperitoneum and the CO_2 laser, allows excellent identification of anatomic structures with this laparoscopic technique. Bipolar electrocoagulation and laser replace conventional dissection techniques and sharp instruments. Our short-term and long-term follow-up have

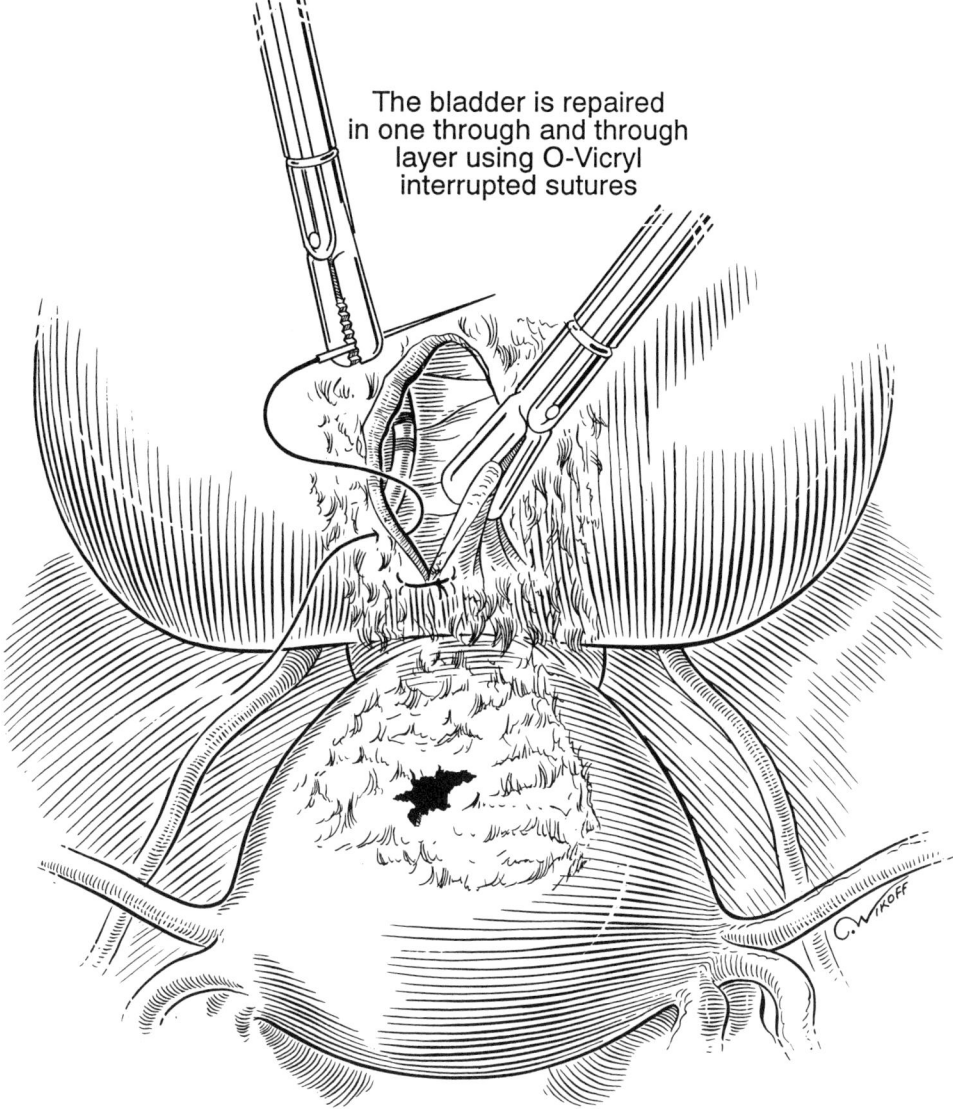

The bladder is repaired
in one through and through
layer using O-Vicryl
interrupted sutures

Figure 15.25. The bladder wall is repaired in one layer with several interrupted 4.0 polydioxanone through-and-through sutures.

been promising. The key point in adequate laparoscopic treatment of endometriosis in addition to the surgical skill is the operator's knowledge of this disease and its natural history and availability of proper instruments.

References

1. Sampson JA. Intestinal adenomas of endometrial type. Arch Surg 1922;5:217–280.
2. Prystowsky JB, Stryker SJ, Ujiki GT, et al. Gastrointestinal endometriosis. Arch Surg 1988;123:855–858.
3. Samper ER, Slagle GW, Hand AM. Colonic endometriosis: its clinical spectrum. South Med J 1984;77:912–914.
4. Cattell RB. Endometriosis of the colon and rectum with intestinal obstruction. N Engl J Med 1987;217:9–16.
5. Forsgren H, Lindhagen J, Melander S, et al. Colorectal endometriosis. Acta Chir Scand 1983;149:431–435.
6. Meyers WC, Kelvin FM, Jones RS. Diagnosis and surgical treatment of colonic endometriosis. Arch Surg 1979;114:169–175.
7. Williams TJ, Pratt JH. Endometriosis in 1,000 consecutive celiotomies: Incidence and management. Am J Obstet Gynecol 1977;129:245–250.
8. Coronado C, Franklin RR, Lotze EC, et al. Surgical treatment of symptomatic colorectal endometriosis. Fertil Steril 1990;53:411–416.
9. Nezhat C, Nezhat F, Nezhat CH. Operative laparoscopy (minimally invasive surgery): state of the art. J Gynecol Surg 1992;8:111–141.
10. Nezhat C. Videolaseroscopy for the treatment of endometriosis. In John Studd, ed. Progress in Obstetrics and Gynecology. Churchill Livingstone, London, 1989, pp 293–303.
11. Nezhat C, Nezhat F, Winer W. Salpingectomy via laparoscopy: a new surgical approach. J Laparosc Surg 1991;1:91–95.

12. Nezhat C, Nezhat F. Incidental appendectomy during videolaseroscopy. Am J Obstet Gynecol 1991;165:559–566.
13. Semm K, Friedrick E. Operative manual for endoscopic abdominal surgery. Chicago: Yearbook Medical, 1987.
14. Nezhat C, Nezhat F, Silfen SL. Laparoscopic hysterectomy and bilateral salpingo-oophorectomy using multifire GIA surgical stapler. J Gynecol Surg 1990;6:287–288.
15. Nezhat C, Nezhat F, Pennington E. Laparoscopic treatment of infiltrative rectosigmoid colon and rectovaginal septum endometriosis by the technique of videolaparoscopy and the CO_2 laser. Br J Obstet Gynecol 1992;99:664–667.
16. Nezhat C, Nezhat F. Safe laser endoscopic excision or vaporization of peritoneal endometriosis. Fertil Steril 1989;52:149–151.
17. Nezhat C, Pennington E, Nezhat F. Laparoscopically assisted anterior rectal wall resection and reanastomosis for deeply infiltrating endometriosis. Surg Laparosc Endosc 1991;1:106–108.
18. Nezhat C, Nezhat F, Pennington E. Laparoscopic proctectomy for infiltrating endometriosis of the rectum. Fertil Steril 1992;57:1129–1132.
19. Nezhat F, Nezhat C, Pennington E, et al. Laparoscopic segmental resection for infiltrating endometriosis of the rectosigmoid colon: a preliminary report. Surg Laparosc Endosc 1992;2:212–216.
20. Nezhat C, Nezhat F, Pennington E, et al. Laparoscopic disk excision and primary repair of the anterior rectal wall for the treatment of full-thickness bowel endometriosis. Surg Endosc 1994;8:682–685.
21. Nezhat C, Nezhat F, Ambroze W, et al. Laparoscopic repair of small bowel, colon, and rectal endometriosis: a report of twenty-six cases. Surg Endosc 1993;7:88–89.
22. Stanley KE, Utz DC, Dockerty MB. Clinically significant endometriosis of the urinary tract. Surg Gynecol Obstet 1965;120:491.
23. Fianu S, et al. Surgical treatment of post abortum endometriosis of the bladder and postoperative bladder function. Scand J Urol Nephrol 1980;14:151–155.
24. Anderson WC, Larsen GD. Endometriosis: treatment with hormonal pseudopregnancy and/or operation. Am J Obstet Gynecol 1975;118:643–651.
25. Neto WA, Lopes RN, Cury M, et al. Vesical endometriosis. Urology 1984;24:271–274.
26. Goldstein MS, Brodmann ML. Cystometric evaluation of vesical, endometriosis before and after hormonal or surgical treatment. Mt Sinai J Med 1990;57:109–111.
27. Davis GD, Brooks RA. Excision of pelvic endometriosis with the carbon dioxide laser laparoscope. Obstet Gynecol 1988;72:816.
28. Martin DC, Vander Zwaag R. Excisional techniques for endometriosis with the CO_2 laser laparoscope. J Reprod Med 1987;32:754.
29. Nezhat C, Nezhat F, Green B. Laparoscopic treatment of obstructed ureter due to endometriosis by resection and ureteroureterostomy. A case report. J Urol 1992;148:865–868.
30. Nezhat F, Nezhat C. Laparoscopic segmental bladder resection for endometriosis: A report of two cases. Obstet Gynecol 1993, pp 81.

16
Recurrent Endometriosis

Giovanni B. Candiani, Luigi Fedele, and Stefano Bianchi

Endometriosis is generally defined as a progressive disease that may be locally invasive and tends to recur after treatment. Based on this concept, definitive surgery was considered for years as the only logical treatment option. However, various studies, particularly that of Meigs published in 1953, demonstrated a low recurrence rate after conservative surgery.[1] This finding suggested that recurrence might not be inevitable and raised the question of which conservative procedures were most appropriate.

The natural history of endometriosis, however, is still unclear and poorly documented. That it is progressive is widely accepted, but data supporting this view are not unequivocal. The currently most accredited pathogenetic theory, that of retrograde menstruation, would explain progression of the disease and the occurrence of ex novo lesions after conservative treatment. The implantation of refluxed endometrial cells and the subsequent growth and spread of lesions would depend on the efficacy of the woman's immune response. Therefore, even after all foci apparent at treatment are eliminated, the patient would remain at risk of developing new implants because of the persistence of retrograde menstruation. The appearance of ex novo endometriotic lesions after adequate treatment, however, is also compatible with the theory of coelomic metaplasia. The mechanisms, including metaplasia of cells originating from the coelomic epithelium, may be repetitive.

The only prospective study on the evolution of lesions was performed by Thomas and Cooke on 17 untreated women with minimal or mild endometriosis.[2] Follow-up laparoscopy after six months of placebo treatment demonstrated disease progression in eight patients, improvement in five, and total disappearance of the lesions in four. It is unclear, however, whether the authors were aware of the possible change in color of some endometriotic lesions, which may give a false impression of disease progression and spread.[3] These findings support the hypothesis that endometriosis is progressive in about 50% of the cases. In contrast, two cross-sectional studies suggest that the disease is static. Redwine observed that the number of pelvic areas involved in the disease does not rise with age; Konickx and co-workers reported that the total pelvic area affected by endometriosis does not increase with age, although the depth of infiltration of implants and the incidence of endometriomas do.[4,5] One particular feature of the natural history of the disease is color modifications of age-related lesions. Jansen and Russel found that nonpigmented lesions had progressed to typical pigmented foci in six untreated patients at repeat laparoscopy.[6]

Thus, available data seem to suggest that the formation of ex novo implants is a relatively limited phenomenon whereas single foci appear able to evolve, at least in some women. An important aspect of endometriosis that has recently been confirmed by various authors is the existence of macroscopically invisible, but histologically demonstrable, lesions in apparently intact peritoneal areas.[7,8] Such microscopic foci have been detected also in women apparently free of endometriosis. They could progress and give rise to clinically appreciable lesions, interpreted as new areas of ectopic endometrium.

Based on these considerations, it is clear that many endometriosis recurrences could represent evolution of lesions invisible at time of treatment. Disease persistence may also be due to lack of recognition of visible but subtle lesions (frequently documented in recent years), lack of identification of subperitoneal lesions, or incomplete surgical treatment.

Diagnosis of Recurrence

Clinical suspicions of endometriosis recurrence arise when, despite treatment, the symptoms and/or signs that led to the initial diagnosis persist or return. Symptom reappearance, physical examination, ultrasound findings, and magnetic resonance imaging (MRI) have a greater sensitivity and specificity in correctly identifying disease recurrence in the case of a woman already treated for endometriosis than in one without previously recognized disease. Transvaginal ultrasonography is particularly useful for identifying deep multilocular ovarian endometriomas (Fig. 16.1). A possible noninvasive diagnostic aid is serum CA-125 measurements. In our experience, CA-125 levels of $\geq 35\,U/mL$ have a specificity of 100% in the diagnosis of recurrence but, unfortunately, the sensitivity is very low (15%).[9]

The clinical findings and results of noninvasive examinations should be considered together when deciding the most appropriate time to perform a repeat laparoscopy or a laparotomy that is required for a definitive diagnosis of recurrent endometriosis.

Recurrence Rates After Surgical Therapy

The exact recurrence rate of endometriosis after conservative surgery is not known. Rates from 2% to over 50% have been reported in the literature. The uncertainty surrounding the true recurrence rate after conservative surgery is due primarily to the lack of specific prospective long-term studies. Only a few trials have included a systematic repeat laparoscopy to document any recurrences; unfortunately, in most cases the second laparoscopy was generally performed too soon to obtain long term data.

Other studies have provided results based on the reappearance of symptoms as a measure of disease recurrence. In most cases, follow-up was variable and

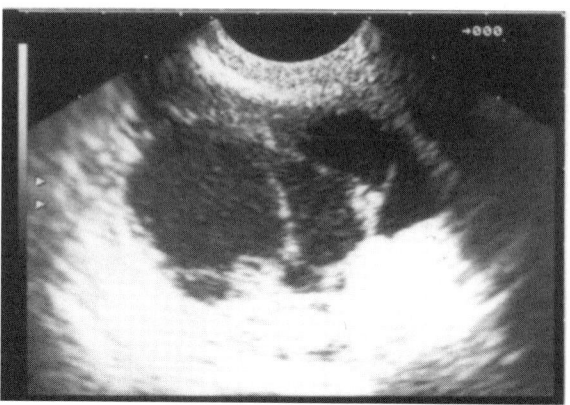

Figure 16.1. In this transvaginal ultrasound scan of a patient with recurrent ovarian endometriosis, the endometrioma appears multilocular with three contiguous compartments.

incomplete, and visual documentation of endometriosis recurrence by laparoscopy or laparotomy was obtained only in selected patients in whom pain returned, infertility persisted, or reoperation was required for other disease.

The wide variability in reported recurrence rates may also be due to other factors. The stage of disease at initial surgery may be important. Extensive endometriosis can cause greater surgical problems and thus be associated with a greater probability of persistence. It could also reflect less efficacious immune defenses of the patient against ectopic endometrium. Last, it must be emphasized that only recently have the subtle aspects of endometriosis been generally appreciated. Very likely, in the earlier studies, the rate of persistence was higher than was recognized, due to underdiagnosis of subtle lesions.

Recurrence Rates

The recurrence rates after surgery for endometriosis at laparotomy reported in the literature are shown in Table 16.1. The reoperation rate after conservative surgery at laparotomy (CSL) was 0 in a few small series published in the 1940s.[10–12] In 1949, Bacon described a large series of women with endometriosis who, between 1905 and 1941, underwent surgical treatment with preservation of childbearing function.[13] Of these, 41 (30%) required further treatment; hysterectomy in 26, other procedures at laparotomy in 5, and radiotherapy in 10. A histologic diagnosis was available in 20 cases, which showed recurrent endometriosis in 9 (45%) and other diseases in the other 11. According to Bacon, these findings indicated that the disease is not always progressive and that conservative intervention is appropriate.

In 1953, Meigs observed the return of symptoms and/or objective findings in 15 (7%) of 215 women, but he did not consider reoperation necessary in any.[1] Similar results were reported by McCoy and Bradford, who found only one case of recurrent endometriosis in 13 patients reoperated after CSL, and by Ranney in whose series reoperation for endometriosis was required by 3 (4%) of 77 women and 1 (0.8%) of 129 who had undergone CSL and hysterectomy with excision of the implants, respectively.[14,16] The recurrence rate was 13% in Spangler and co-workers' study of 105 infertile women who underwent CSL.[17] Five of the 13 reoperated patients had conceived after their first operation. The reoperation rates for endometriosis reported by Andrews and Larsen in women followed for over two years were 39% after combined CSL and pseudopregnancy regimen and 35% after surgery alone.[18] Hammond's group obtained even more unfavorable results with combined medical and surgical treatment compared with surgery alone (recurrences in 51% and 25% of the cases, respectively).[19] These authors had to

Table 16.1. Recurrence rates of endometriosis after surgery at laparotomy.

Author	Year	No.of patients	Treatment	Recurrence of symptoms No. (Rate)	2nd operation Patients No. (Rate)	Follow-up (years)	Recurrence No. (Rate)	Subsequent treatment
Dannreuther[10]	1941	18	CSL H	2 (11%)	0	?	0	—
Holmes[11]	1942	24	CSL	4 (17%)	0	?	0	Irradiation
		35	H + UO	1 (3%)	0	0	0	—
Beecham[12]	1946	32	CSL	2 (6%)	0	?	0	—
		14	H	0	0	?	0	—
Bacon[13]	1949	138	CSL	41 (30%)	31 (22%)	4.8	9 (7%)	H
Meigs[1]	1953	215	CSL	15 (7%)	0	?	—	—
McCoy & Bradford[14]	1963	60	CSL	?	13 (22%)	1–15	1 (2%)	H
Sheets et al.[15]	1964	39	CSL	13 (33%)	11 (28%)	5	11 (28%)	11H; 2Med
		40	H	1 (3%)	1 (3%)	5	0	Med
Ranney[16]	1970	77	CSL	?	16 (21%)	9.7	3 (4%)	?
		129	H	?	1 (1%)	1	1 (1%)	
Spangler et al.[17]	1971	101	CSL	?	13 (13%)	>1	13 (13%)	11H; 2CSL
Andrews & Larsen[18]	1974	80	CSL	?	29 (36%)	>2	29 (36%)	?
		36	CSL + EP	?	14 (39%)	>2	14 (39%)	?
		86	H + UO	?	3 (4%)	>2	3 (4%)	?
Hammond et al.[19]	1976	12	CSL	3 (25%)	3 (25%)	2.9	3 (25%)	?
		35	CSL + EP	19 (54%)	18 (51%)	?	18 (51%)	
		13	H + UO	11 (85%)	11 (85%)	1–5	11 (85%)	BO
Williams & Pratt[20]	1977	64	CSL	26 (41%)	21 (33%)	?	10 (16%)	?
		153	H	11 (7%)	12 (8%)	?	9 (6%)	BO
Shenken & Malinak[21]	1978	117	CSL	?	28 (24%)	>3	28 (24%)	26CSL; 2H
Buttram[22]	1979	138	CSL	?	?	3.8	6 (4%)	H + BO
Punnonen et al.[23]	1980	903	CSL	?	132 (15%)	6–10	132 (15%)	58H; 10BO; 64CSL
Rock et al.[24]	1981	214	CSL	65 (30%)	29 (14%)	2.5	29 (14%)	?
Wheeler & Malinak[25]	1983	423	CSL	?	62 (15%)	1–9	42 (10%)	15H; 20CSL; 7LPS
Gordts et al.[26]	1984	176	CSL	?	39 (22%)	>1.5	11 (6%)	?
Chong & Baggish[27]	1984	54	Laser CO_2	?	8 (15%)	0.3	0	—

H: hysterectomy; UO: unilateral ovariectomy; BO: bilateral ovariectomy; CSL: conservative surgery at laparotomy; MED: medical therapy.

reoperate on 11 of the 13 women in whom one or both ovaries were left when the uterus was removed. These findings raise questions regarding the mechanisms underlying recurrence after hysterectomy. Ex novo lesions due to transtubal reflux cannot be hypothesized in such women, and reappearance of endometriosis must be attributed to evolution of persistent foci or the disease has another pathogenesis.

Williams and Pratt observed recurrent endometriosis in 10 of 21 patients who were reoperated after conservative surgery; reoperation for endometriosis was required also in 9 (6%) of the 153 women who had undergone hysterectomy with conservation of ovarian tissue.[20] In a follow-up of 117 infertile women after conservative surgery, Shenken and Malinak found that 28 (24%) required reoperation, repeat conservative surgery in 26, and total abdominal hysterectomy and bilateral salpingo-oophorectomy in 2.[21] There were no absolute criteria for reoperation; all the patients except one wanted children, only two conceived after their first

operation, and all complained of pain. Three became pregnant after the second operation, and three others required a third operation for recurrent symptomatic endometriosis. These authors indicated that the severity of disease at the first operation, and failure to conceive after it, were important risk factors for recurrence. In 1979, Buttram observed recurrence requiring definitive surgery in 6 (4%) of 138 infertile women without infertility factors other than endometriosis.[22] The pregnancy rate was particularly high in these women (72%).

In the largest study published so far, Punnonen observed a reoperation rate of 15% in a six- to ten-year follow-up of 903 surgically treated patients.[23] Most reoperations were performed within one to five years. Gestagen therapy after initial surgery had no effect on the recurrence rate. At reoperation 14 patients had bilateral ovarian endometriosis, which was treated with bilateral ovarian resection; two were operated for a third time for recurrence of ovarian endometriosis, and three received clomiphene citrate and had a normal pregnancy. In Rock and co-workers' series of 214 infertile women given surgical treatment for endometriosis 65 (30%) had recurrent symptoms suggestive of persistent or recurrent disease and 29 (14%) required a second operation for recurrent endometriosis.[24] Pregnancy was less likely to occur in patients with recurrence. Reoperation for endometriosis was more frequent in patients with extensive disease at first surgery.

In 1983, Wheeler and Malinak published their classic paper on the incidence and management of recurrent endometriosis.[25] Of the 423 patients studied, 62 required reoperation for persistent infertility or recurrent pelvic pain and 41 (10%) had documented recurrent endometriosis. The annual recurrence rate (number of patients with recurrent endometriosis within a given 12-month period divided by the total number of patients followed over the same period) varied from 1% in the first year of follow-up to 14% in the eighth year, and the cumulative recurrence rate was 14% at 3 years and 40% at 5 years. However, these authors subsequently revised their original life-table analysis and calculated that the cumulative recurrence rate at 5 years was 20%.[28] In their initial calculation of the 5-year recurrence rate, the numerator was the number of patients reoperated in the first 5 years of follow-up and the denominator the number of patients at risk in the fifth year only. A weakness of the study was the large number of patients lost to follow-up. Therefore, extrapolation from the rates calculated in the last years of follow-up should be performed with caution. These authors also attempted to identify risk factors for recurrence, but obtained results contrary to those reported in Shenken and Malinak's previous study.[21] They did not find significant differences between disease stage and conception after the first operation among the patients with recurrence, those who were reoperated but did not have endometriosis, and those not requiring reoperation. Of the 41 patients with recurrence, 20 underwent a second conservative operation, 15 a hysterectomy, and 6 a diagnostic laparoscopy only.

In 1984, Gords and others used an atraumatic, microsurgical technique on 176 infertile women with endometriosis, mostly stages II (99 women) and III (53 women) of the original American Fertility Society (AFS) classification.[26,29] Repeat laparoscopy was performed 18 months or more after initial surgery in 39 women, which revealed recurrence of peritoneal endometriotic implants in 11 (28%), adhesions in 13, and a normal pelvis in 17. In Chong's study, 8 of 54 women who underwent CO_2 laser treatment at laparotomy for stage III/IV endometriosis subsequently underwent a laparoscopy three months later at which no lesions were detected.[27]

Recurrence Rate After Laparoscopic Surgery

The recurrence rates after laparoscopic surgery for endometriosis published in the literature are given in

Table 16.2. In 1979 Hasson reported the results of laparoscopic electrocoagulation of pelvic endometriosis in 19 patients, eight infertile, and 11 with pelvic pain.[30] Five were subsequently reoperated, and recurrence was documented in only one, 18 months after the first operation. The following year, Sulewsky's team described 100 infertile women with mild or moderate endometriosis treated with laparoscopic cautery.[31] Of 34 who did not become pregnant and were followed for at least 12 months, recurrence was observed in two at repeat laparoscopy. Daniell and Christianson treated 60 infertile women with AFS stage II/III endometriosis by laparoscopic cautery followed by danazol 600 mg/day for 6 months.[32] Follow-up laparoscopy was performed five months after the end of treatment in 19 who did not conceive, and endometriosis was observed in six (32%). Of 71 women with ovarian endometriomas of 1 to 10 cm in diameter treated at laparoscopy by Reich and McGlynn, 15 were reoperated at laparoscopy or laparotomy, and 14 (20%) had endometriosis.[35] The procedure consisted of simple draining of the endometrioma followed in some cases by fulguration of the cyst wall and in others by stripping of the whole cyst.

Seiler's group described 45 infertile women with moderate endometriosis who underwent unipolar cautery of implants.[34] Six were reevaluated surgically 9 to 28 months after the initial operation, and two were disease-free, three had recurrent ovarian endometriomas, and one an endometrioma in an ovary previously considered unaffected by the disease. Davis did not detect recurrent endometriosis in 29 women at repeat laparoscopy performed within ten weeks of laparoscopic CO_2 laser treatment.[33] Donnez used the same operative procedure in 70 women with stage II/III endometriosis (AFS-r), and observed no residual lesions or adhesions in eight who underwent follow-up laparoscopy within three months of laser surgery.[36] Of 66 women treated by CO_2 laser laparoscopy by Davis and Brooks, laparoscopy was repeated 4 to 15 months later in 14, and recurrent endometriosis was observed in four.[37]

In 1988, Fayez and co-workers published their study of 162 infertile women with revised AFS (AFS-r) stage I/II endometriosis treated by laparoscopic excision alone (82 subjects) or followed by danazol 600 mg/day for 6 months (80 subjects).[38,47] This was not a randomized study as the two treatment modalities were used in different, successive periods. Follow-up laparoscopy performed 12 months later in 19 women of the former group and 28 of the latter revealed recurrent endometriosis in 3 (4%) and 7 (9%) of the women, respectively. These findings confirm the impression that postoperative danazol does not reduce the risk of recurrence.

Corson's team performed a repeat laparoscopy on four of 43 women treated for stage I/II endometriosis (AFS-r) with Nd-YAG laser laparoscopy two to four

Table 16.2. Recurrence rates of endometriosis after operative laparoscopy.

Author	Year	No.of patients	Treatment	Recurrence of symptoms No. (Rate)	2nd operation Patients No. (Rate)	2nd operation Follow-up (months)	2nd operation Recurrence No. (Rate)	Subsequent treatment
Hasson[30]	1979	19	Cautery	5 (26%)	5 (26%)	1–48	1 (5%)	3H; 1CSL; 1LPS
Sulewski et al.[31]	1980	100	Cautery	18 (18%)	2 (2%)	17.7	2 (2%)	?
Daniell & Christianson[32]	1981	60	Cautery + Dan	" "	19 (32%)	6	6 (10%)	2 CSL; 1 LPS
Davis[33]	1986	158	Laser CO_2	11 (7%)	29 (18%)	15	0	—
Seiler et al.[34]	1986	45	Cautery	?	6 (13%)	7–28	4 (9%)	?
Reich & McGlynn[35]	1986	71	Cautery Lining stripping	11 (15%)	15 (21%)	>6	14 (20%)	6H; 6CSL; 2LPS
Donnez[36]	1987	70	Laser CO_2	?	8 (11%)	3	0	—
Davis & Brooks[37]	1988	66	Laser CO_2	4 (6%)	14 (21%)	4–15	4 (6%)	?
Fayez et al.[38]	1988	82	Excision	?	19 (23%)	12	3 (4%)	LPS
		80	Excision + Dan	?	28 (35%)	12	7 (9%)	LPS
Corson et al.[39]	1989	43	YAG laser	1 (2%)	4 (9%)	4	2 (5%)	?
Sutton[40]	1989	181	Laser CO_2	" "	33 (18%)	" "	18 (10%)	" "
Kojima et al.[41]	1990	30	YAG Laser	1 (3%)	10 (33%)	?	10 (33%)	?
Daniell et al.[42]	1991	47	KTP, CO_2, Argon laser	7 (15%)	11 (23%)	?	9 (19%)	3H; 1CSL; 5LPS
Fayez & Vogel[43]	1991	26	Excision + Dan	?	26 (100%)	2	6 (23%)	?
		24	Lining stripping + Dan	?	24 (100%)	2	6 (25%)	?
		30	Lining vaporization + Dan	?	30 (100%)	2	10 (33%)	?
		44	Aspiration + Dan	?	44 (100%)	2	13 (30%)	?
Marrs[44]	1991	31	KTP laser	?	4 (13%)	6–21	1 (3%)	CSL
Redwine[45]	1991	359	Excision	?	81 (23%)	24	35 (10%)	?
Canis et al.[46]	1992	42	Stripping & cautery	?	42 (100%)	3–6	4 (10%)	?

H: hysterectomy; CSL: conservative surgery at laparotomy; LPS: laparoscopy; DAN: danazol.

months previously and minimal persistent disease was found in two.[39] In 1989, Sutton reviewed 181 women who underwent laparoscopic CO_2 laser treatment for pelvic pain associated with endometriosis.[40] He performed a repeat laparoscopy to evaluate the results of treatment in 33 women, and recurrence was detected in 18 (55%) at sites different from those of the original lesions. The other 15 women were free of disease. The same laparoscopic procedure was used by Kojima's team in 1990 on 30 women with AFS-r stage III/IV endometriosis.[41] Recurrence was documented in ten cases; a recurrent ovarian endometrioma was treated by alcoholization. The following year, Daniell and co-workers reported the results of laparoscopic laser (CO_2, KTP, or argon) treatment given to 47 women with ovarian endometriomas of over 3 cm in diameter.[42] Subsequently, three patients underwent hysterectomy for persistent pain symptoms; repeat laparoscopy was performed on eight others, revealing recurrent ovarian endometriosis in five and only peritoneal lesions in one. Recurrence of ovarian endometrioma at four months was reported by Marrs in one out of 31 women with ovarian endometriomas treated by KTP laser laparoscopy; no endometriosis was detected at laparoscopy performed later in three women in a gamete intrafallopian transfer (GIFT) program.[44]

Redwine recently calculated the interval and cumulative recurrence rates in 359 women with stages I–IV endometriosis treated by excision through the laparoscope and followed for a mean of 2 years.[45] He demonstrated recurrence or persistence of the disease in 35 (43%) of 81 reoperated women, for a five-year cumulative recurrence rate of 10% among the original group of 359 women. Unlike Wheeler and Malinak, Redwine did not find that the interval recurrence rate increased with length of follow-up, which he interpreted as demonstrating the static nature of the disease.[25] Redwine attributed the lesions detected at reoperation, which were mainly in areas other than those treated previously, to foci not identified and removed at initial surgery. In another recent study, Canis and co-workers systematically performed repeat laparoscopy on 42 women three to six months after laparoscopic cystectomy for ovarian endometriomas of over 3 cm in diameter.[46]

Four patients (10%) had deep ovarian endometriomas that they considered were persistent lesions after dissection of very large cysts and/or friable cyst walls. Fayez and Vogel carried out a randomized prospective study comparing different laparoscopic procedures in the treatment of ovarian endometriomas.[43] At repeat procedures performed two months after initial surgery, they observed residual endometriosis in 23% of the patients in whom the lesion was excised, in 25% treated by opening and stripping the lining, in 33% in whom the endometriomas were opened and the lining evaporated by CO_2 laser, and in 30% who underwent only cyst drainage. However, recurrent/persistent ovarian endometriomas were detected only in the last three groups, in 22%, 22%, and 21% of cases, respectively. All patients received danazol for 2 months after the initial surgery.

Endometriosis Recurrence After Medical Treatment

It is unclear whether the reappearance of endometriosis after surgical treatment at laparotomy or laparoscopy is attributable to ex novo implant formation or to persistent lesions. There is, however, little doubt that endometriosis present after medical treatment alone constitutes disease persistence. Although there was initial enthusiasm for the use of hormonal therapies (progestins, danazol, gestrinone, GnRH agonists), it has been shown that these drugs induce a temporary regression but are unable to eradicate the disease. In most studies on the various medical treatments, repeat laparoscopy was performed at the end of the treatment when gonadal activity was still suppressed, with the result that lesions disappeared in a large proportion of cases. However, as clearly demonstrated by Evers, follow-up laparoscopy performed after resumption of ovarian activity does not demonstrate important regression of the disease.[48] In accordance with Evers' observation, Fayez's group found persistent endometriotic foci 12 months after the end of treatment in all 36 infertile women with stage I/II endometriosis (AFS-r) treated with danazol 800 mg/day for six months.[38] In a study of 116 women after hormonal treatment with lynestrenol, gestrinone, or buserelin, Nisolle-Pochet and co-workers reported a high prevalence of active ovarian endometriotic lesions without signs of degeneration at histologic examination; the mitotic index of the ectopic endometrial cells was similar to that of a group of untreated women.[49]

In summary, currently available medical treatments do not cure endometriosis. The results of clinical studies, however, indicate that at least partial resolution of symptoms is often obtained and that second treatment is not always required.[50]

Management of Endometriosis Recurrence

A visual and preferably also histologic diagnosis of recurrence is mandatory before treatment decisions are made. This is important since return of pain symptoms and persistent infertility may be due to other causes other than endometriosis, the most frequent being postsurgical adhesions, pelvic inflammation, and adenomyosis.

The available therapeutic options for recurrent endometriosis are substantially the same as those used to treat the disease initially. No pathogenetic or histologic difference has been demonstrated between initial and recurrent disease lesions. However, in the case of recurrent endometriosis, the gynecologist will obviously choose therapeutic measures that carry the least risk of further recurrence. Thus, definitive surgery may be considered even for women under 40 and those with such extensive disease that complete resection is not feasible. Also, unilateral adnexectomy may be deemed appropriate if the condition of the ovary appears inconsistent with normal function or if anatomically abnormal tubo-ovarian relations would not allow ovum pickup. This operation may be performed with greater confidence if the contralateral adnexa appear normal, taking into account the patient's age and desire for offspring. In women with severe pain symptoms, pelvic denervation should be combined with conservative surgery.

With the aim of providing a definitive solution, laparotomy appears preferable to laparoscopy in repeat conservative surgery for extensive endometriosis and suspected deep subperitoneal lesions. The treatment of recurrent endometriosis may present specific problems. Residual ovarian parenchyma may have to be completely isolated, and it often involves the corresponding pelvic part of the ureter. In these circumstances, it may be necessary to dissect out a portion of the ureter to avoid causing it mechanical or vascular damage. Therefore, the ureter should be identified from where it enters the pelvis; that is, where it crosses the iliac vessels.

Another common finding at the second operation is involvement of the pouch of Douglas, due to adhesions formed with the adnexa and/or posterior wall of the uterus. In these cases, meticulous adhesiolysis is necessary. Attention must be given to the fibromuscular component of the rectum, which may be extensively involved in the disease. It is prudent to follow the course of the ureter to avoid damaging its lower pelvic part.

A third possible finding at reoperation is involvement of the rectovaginal septum, which may not have been evident at the first operation but may have developed progressively since. This is typically a subperitoneal manifestation accompanied, in some cases, by disease of the pouch of Douglas and the last part of the rectum with spread into the posterior vaginal fornix. This type of recurrence requires an operation that starts at laparotomy, dissects the pouch of Douglas peritoneum from the rectum, and the latter from the vagina. Once the posterior vagina fornix is open via the vaginal route, complete ablation of the affected part of the fornix can be performed by stretching the uterine cervix upward (Fig. 16.2 and color plates 16.2A,B,C).

The possibility must also be considered of endometriotic lesions of the uterine ligaments. Localization of endometriosis on the uterosacral ligaments is frequent, and the remedies proposed, to be carried out during laparoscopy, range from simple unipolar cauterization to vaporization or resection of superficial foci. Laparoscopic uterine nerve ablation (LUNA) should be performed in women with midline pain. Total removal of the uterosacral ligaments, performed at laparotomy, is a more difficult technique but useful in cases of extensive disease.[51]

Last, although rare, nodules may occur in parametrium in the presence of subperitoneal disease. This is difficult to diagnose, although it can be done if rectovaginal pelvic exploration is performed at the start of the laparotomy. MRI may make a useful diagnostic contribution. Surgery appears the only option for treatment of parametrial endometriosis. A technique is required similar to the classical preparation of parametrium according to Meigs.[52] The paracervical and pararectal fossae are identified and the corresponding portion of the ureter is isolated. It may be dilated proximally because of pressure from the endometriotic process and terminate in a "rattail" at its junction with the bladder. Thus, it is evident that only destruction of the entire parametrium will be efficacious. Damage suffered by the ureter may necessitate its implantation in the bladder (Fig. 16.3 and color plates 16.3B,C,D).

Based on the above considerations, the choice of therapy for recurrent endometriosis should take the following factors into account: the patient's symptoms, the extent of disease, and the desire to maintain menstrual and/or reproductive function. Furthermore, the presence of important associated pelvic diseases may influence treatment decisions.

Infertile Patients

In women in whom recurrence is classified as AFS-r stages I or II, the main therapeutic option is endoscopic surgery (laser, cautery, excision) at the time of diagnosis. No specific results have been reported on the use of such procedures in the treatment of recurrent endometriosis associated with infertility, but it seems logical that operative endoscopy in these patients should have the same advantages as demonstrated in new cases. Of the therapeutic alternatives, medical treatment may be

given with interruption to attempt conception for six months or longer; assisted reproduction techniques presumably have a better yield if preceded by the elimination of implants. In these patients, assisted reproduction techniques seem to have a similar success rate to that in women with tubal or unexplained infertility.[53,54] In women of 35 or over, in our opinion, inclusion in an in vitro fertilization and embryo transfer (IVF-ET) or GIFT program is indicated immediately after laparoscopy; whereas, in younger women, this should be considered only after six to 12 months of follow-up after laparoscopic treatment.

Moderate or severe recurrent endometriosis in a woman wanting offspring constitutes an indication for operative laparoscopy provided that the operator is expert and the disease is completely identifiable and resectable. In women not fulfilling these conditions, particularly in the presence of suspected subperitoneal disease and deep, multilocular ovarian endometriomas (generally an expression of partial persistence and fibrosis secondary to the first operation), surgery at laparotomy seems to be the most appropriate approach. Various data appear to support the use of repeat CSL in patients with extensive endometriosis. Wheeler and Malinak observed a crude pregnancy rate of 47% at 18 months of follow-up after reoperation for recurrent endometriosis in 15 women wanting offspring.[25] Two of Ranney's ten patients who underwent a second conservative operation achieved a pregnancy.[55] Three of Evers' eight patients who had repeat conservative surgery for endometriosis became pregnant.[56]

Recently, we reported the results of a prospective study involving 42 patients with endometriosis, 39 (93%) with AFS-r stage III/IV disease, who had a conservative reoperation.[57] Of the 28 women wanting children, eight (29%) succeeded in becoming pregnant, for a cumulative pregnancy rate at 27 months of 31% and a corrected rate of 35%. These findings seem to indicate that the reproductive prognosis of patients reoperated for endometriosis is less than that reported in the literature for infertile women with moderate or severe endometriosis after a first operation (pregnancy rates of 50% and 39%, respectively). Unfortunately, six of our patients (14%) and 30% of Wheeler and Malinak's series had to undergo a third operation because of further recurrence.[25]

Many authors suggest the use of hormonal therapy to complement surgery, but data are still lacking on whether such treatment, given pre- or postoperatively, is efficacious. Another possible treatment for the infertile woman with recurrent moderate or severe endometriosis consists of assisted reproductive techniques. This approach avoids surgery in patients without bulky ovarian endometriomas and/or severe pain symptoms. However, the results of IVF-ET have been disappointing in women with advanced endometriosis, yielding cycle

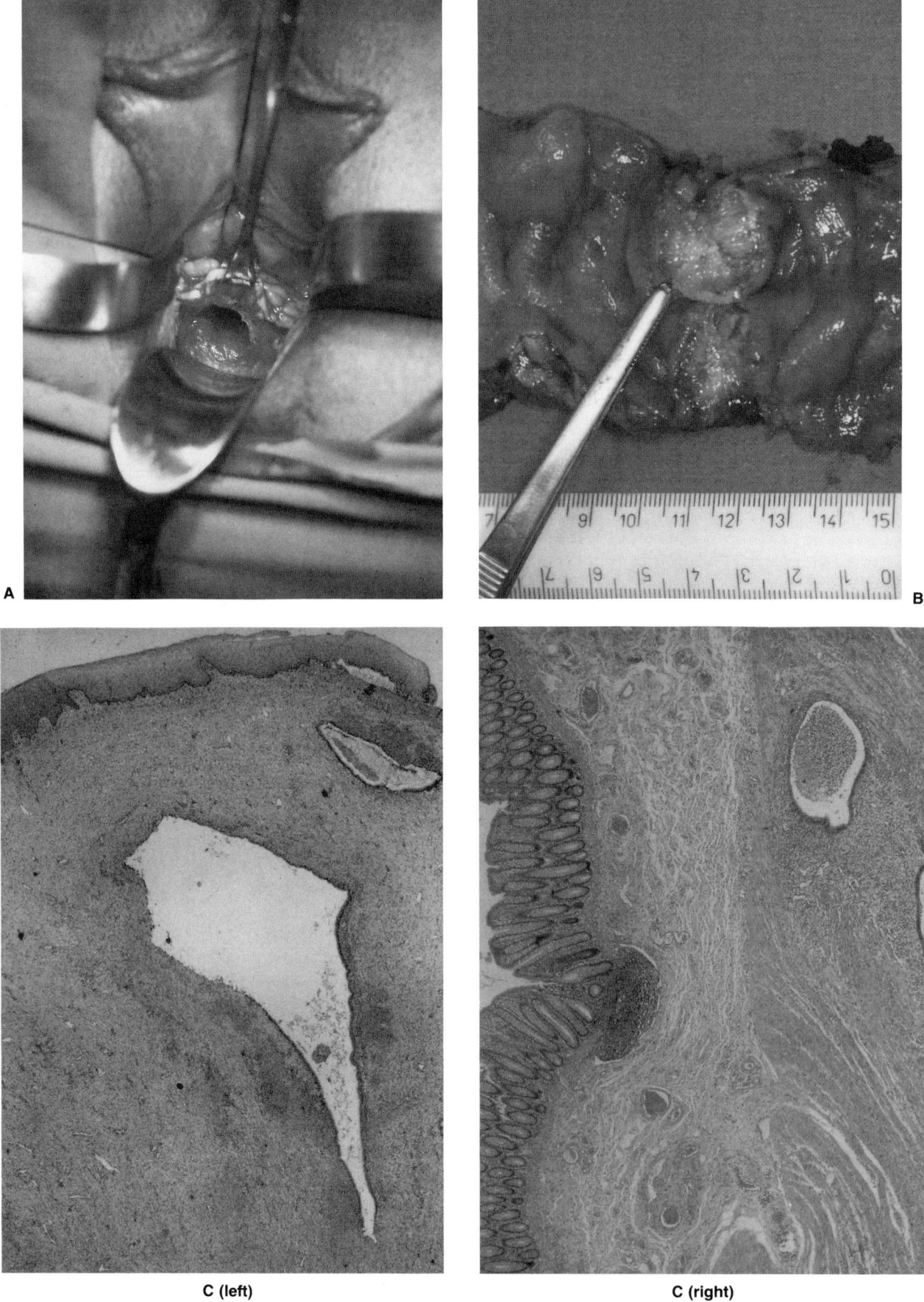

C (left)   C (right)

pregnancy rates of only 2% to 7%.[58,59] This low rate is possibly due to embryo implantation defects and/or to difficulties in oocyte retrieval because of adnexal adhesions and ovarian endometriomas. The former hypothesis is confirmed by the results of a recent randomized study performed by Dicker's team.[60] Of 67 women with severe endometriosis, the cycle pregnancy rate was 25% among women treated with the GnRH analogue decapeptyl for six months before IVF, compared with a cycle pregnancy rate of only 4% in women who under-

went IVF immediately. Eight preclinical pregnancies were observed in the latter subgroup and only one in the former. In view of these observations, for infertile women with stage III/IV (AFS-r) recurrent endometriosis, we prefer to perform conservative surgery (at laparoscopy or laparotomy according to the operator's preference) when complete removal of the disease and restoration of pelvic anatomy compatible with recovery of fertility is possible. In other cases, it is useful when performing diagnostic laparoscopy to carry out surgical

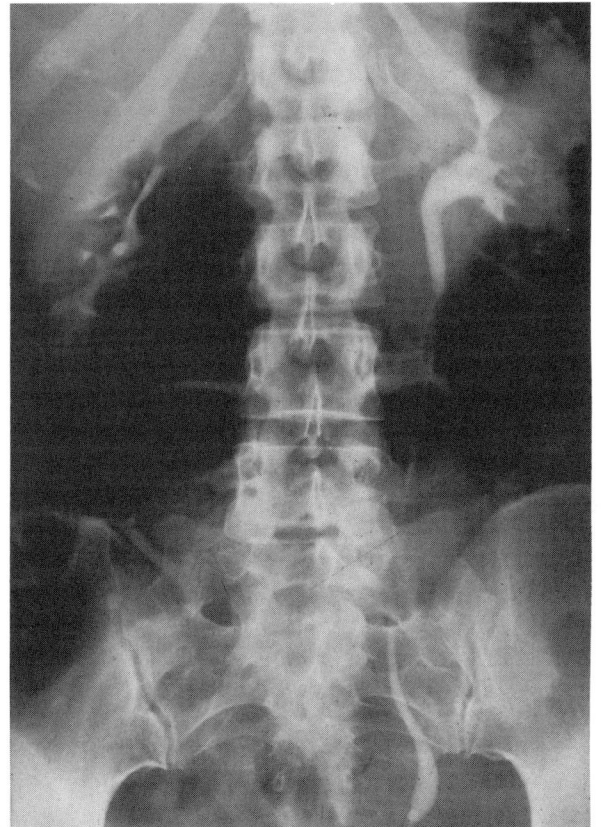

A

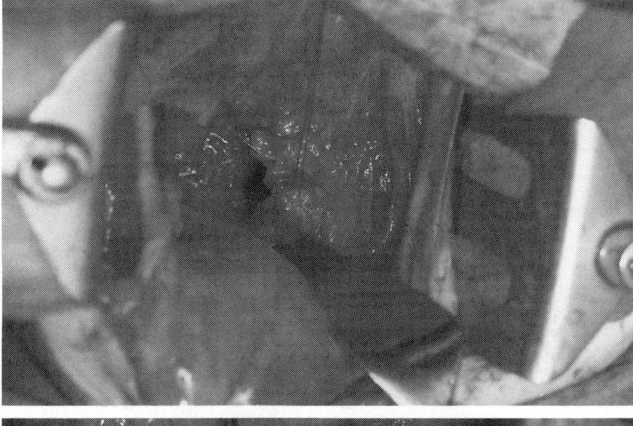

B

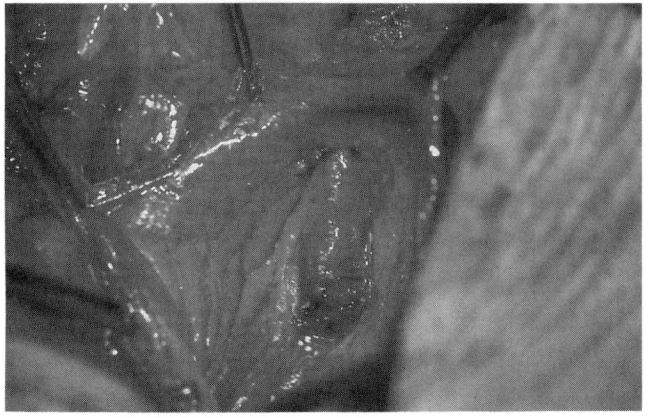

C

Figure 16.3. A multipara, aged 41, previously underwent right adnexectomy for rupture of an endometrioma with peritoneal irritation at age 28. Six years later, she developed severe left pelvic pain and hematuria. Vaginal and rectal examination revealed extensive thickening of the left parametrium, and complete resection of the left parametrium, partial resection of the left angle of the vesical dome and ureteral

implantation according to Landbetter-Politano was performed. **A.** Preoperative pyelogram shows left ureteral obstruction with moderate hydronephrosis. **B.** Endometriotic nodule of parametrium appears after surgical exposure. **C.** View of ureteral implantation is after partial resection of the vesical dome.

Figure 16.3. *Continued*

←

Figure 16.2. A 30-year-old nullipara underwent enucleation of left ovarian endometrioma at laparotomy, and after 18 months had a term delivery. Five years later, rectal pain, rectal bleeding, and deep dyspareunia developed, all closely related to the menstrual cycle. Posterior vaginal fornix and colorectal endometriosis was diagnosed. Vaginoabdominal

surgery was performed with segmental removal of the posterior fornix and low anterior rectosigmoid resection with end-to-end anastomosis. **A.** The vaginal implants are removed. **B.** Rectosigmoid endometriosis. **C.** Histologic results reveal: (left) rectosigmoid endometriosis and (right) vaginal endometriosis. See also color plates.

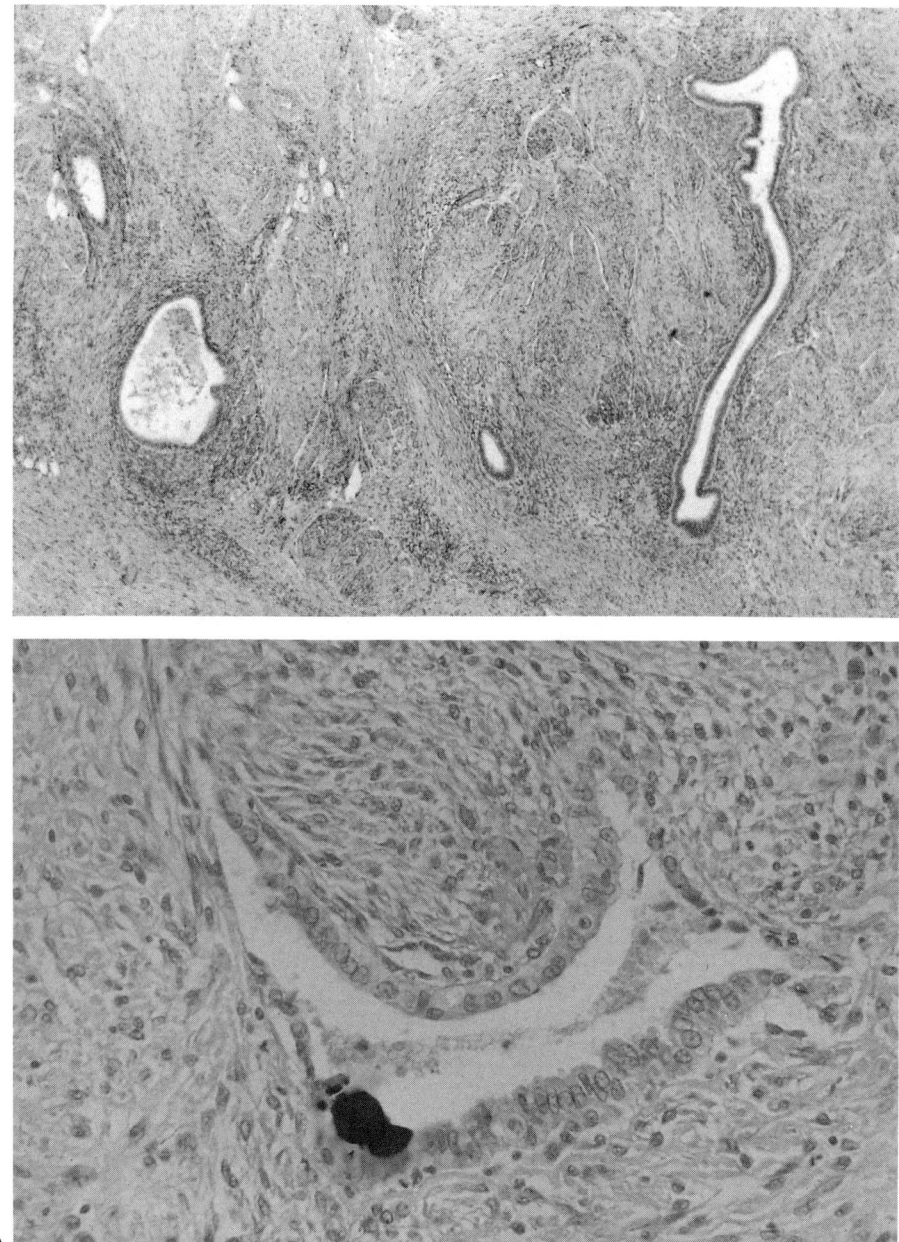

Figure 16.3. *Continued* **D.** Histologic findings shown are of: (top) detrusor muscle, and (bottom) parametrial specimens. Note the presence of endometrial glands. See also color plates.

maneuvers (mobilization of the ovaries, lysis of adhesions, emptying the endometriomas) that may favor the success of a subsequent IVF-ET.

Patients With Pelvic Pain and Infertility

The therapeutic choice for patients who present with pelvic pain and infertility is not substantially different from that for patients with infertility alone. There is a high rate of recurrence of pain after surgical removal of adhesions and implants whether by laparoscopy or laparotomy.[22,24,40] There is also a positive correlation between amount of disease and severity of pain symptoms.[61] When treating endometriosis recurrence in patients with pelvic pain and infertility, consider pelvic denervation procedures such as uterosacral ligament resection or ablation and presacral neurectomy at the time of conservative surgery. These adjunctive procedures may be performed at either laparotomy or laparoscopy, but what must be clearly established is the existence of the indication. Patients who benefit from pelvic denervation are those in whom the main pain component is midline.[62] In other patients, the advantages offered by these interventions are probably out-

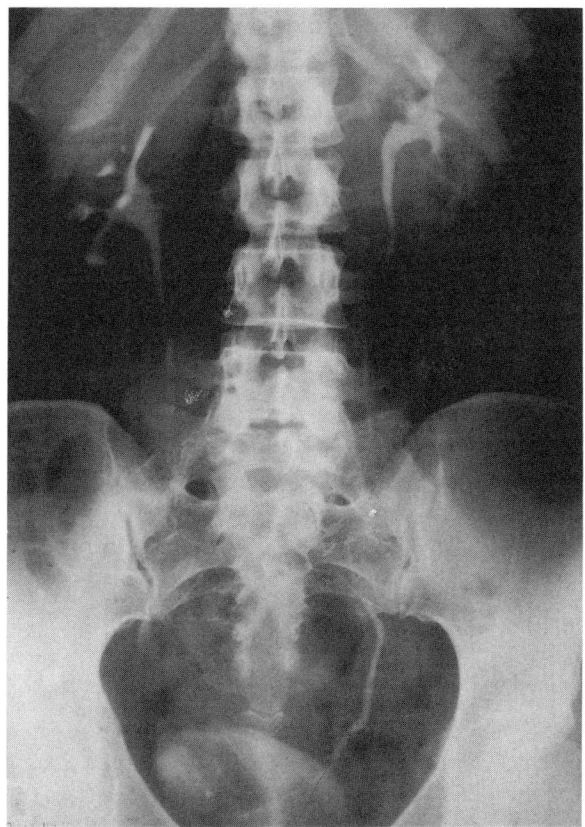

E

Figure 16.3. *Continued* **E.** Postoperative pyelogram shows restored left ureteral patency and resolution of left hydronephrosis.

weighed by the associated intra- and postoperative morbidity. The indications for assisted reproductive techniques in these women are the same as for those patients with infertility alone.

Patients With Pelvic Pain

In patients who have completed their family, and in whom endometriosis recurrence is associated with pelvic pain, treatment decisions depend mainly on age. For women of 35 or under, the choice will be conservative surgery at laparoscopy or laparotomy combined with pelvic denervation if the pain is midline. When it is uncertain that the disease has been completely eliminated, a postoperative six-month course of medical treatment with a GnRH agonist or danazol is appropriate. A similar treatment may be useful also in the case of incomplete remission of symptoms after only surgical reoperation.

In our view, medical treatment alone for recurrence has a limited role because pain returns at suspension of the therapy in a large proportion of patients.[63,64,65] In patients older than 35, conservative treatment is indicated only in the case of limited recurrence that allows complete removal of the lesions. In all other cases,

definitive surgical treatment is indicated, and should include bilateral adnexectomy. This is justified by the important risk of return of pain symptoms in women in whom the adnexae have been conserved (mean 10% in the literature). We believe that estrogen replacement therapy rarely stimulates the growth of residual ectopic endometrium afer bilateral adnexectomy and does not seem to constitute an important risk factor for recurrence. If childbearing is still desired, the uterus may be spared, if the presence of adenomyosis can be excluded, and oocyte donation can then be performed.

References

1. Meigs JV. Endometriosis—etiologic role of marriage and parity; conservative treatment. Obstet Gynecol 1953; 2:46–53.
2. Thomas EJ, Cooke ID. Impact of gestrinone on the course of asymptomatic endometriosis. Br Med J 1987;294:272–274.
3. Redwine DB. Age-related evolution in color appearance of endometriosis. Fertil Steril 1987;48:1062–1063.
4. Redwine DB. The distribution of endometriosis in the pelvis by age groups and fertility. Fertil Steril 1987;47:173–175.
5. Konninckx PR, Meuleman C, Demeyere S, et al. Suggestive evidence that pelvic endometriosis is a progressive disease, whereas deeply infiltrating endometriosis is associated with pelvic pain. Fertil Steril 1991;55:759–765.
6. Jansen RPS, Russel P. Nonpigmented endometriosis: clinical, laparoscopic and pathologic definition. Am J Obstet Gynecol 1986;155:1154–1159.
7. Murphy AA, Green WR, Bobbie D, et al. Unsuspected endometriosis documented by scanning electron microscopy in visually normal peritoneum. Fertil Steril 1986; 46:522–524.
8. Brosens IA, Cornillie FJ, Vasquez G. Etiology and pathophysiology of endometriosis. In Rolland R, Chadha DR, Willemsen WNP, eds. Gonadotropin down-regulation in gynecological practice. New York, Alan R. Liss, Inc., Publ., 1986, pp 81–102.
9. Fedele L, Arcaini L, Vercellini P, et al. Serum CA-125 measurement in the diagnosis of endometriosis recurrence. Obstet Gynecol 1988;72:19–22.
10. Dannreuther WT. The treatment of pelvic endometriosis. Am J Obstet Gynecol 1941;41:461–472.
11. Holmes WR. Endometriosis. Am J Obstet Gynecol 1942; 43:255–256.
12. Beecham CT. Conservative surgery in endometriosis. Am J Obstet Gynecol 1946;52:707–715.
13. Bacon WB. Results in 138 cases of endometriosis treated by conservative surgery. Am J Obstet Gynecol 1949;57:953–958.
14. McCoy JB, Bradford WZ. Surgical treatment of endometriosis with conservation of reproductive potential. Am J Obstet Gynecol 1963;87:394–398.
15. Sheets JL, Symmonds RE, Banner EA. Conservative surgical management of endometriosis. Obstet Gynecol 1964;23:625–628.
16. Ranney B. Endometriosis. I. Conservative operations. Am J Obstet Gynecol 1970;107:743–753.
17. Spangler DB, Jones GS, Jones HW Jr. Infertility due to endometriosis. Conservative surgical therapy. Am J Obstet Gynecol 1971;109:850–857.

18. Andrews WC, Larsen GD. Endometriosis treatment with hormonal pseudopregnancy and/or operation. Am J Obstet Gynecol 1974;118:643–651.
19. Hammond CB, Rock JA, Parker RT. Conservative treatment of endometriosis: the effects of limited surgery and hormonal pseudopregnancy. Fertil Steril 1976;27:756–766.
20. Williams TJ, Pratt JH. Endometriosis in 1,000 consecutive celiotomies: incidence and management. Am J Obstet Gynecol 1977;129:245–250.
21. Shenken RS, Malinak RL. Reoperation after initial treatment of endometriosis with conservative surgery. Am J Obstet Gynecol 1978;131:416–424.
22. Buttram VC Jr. Surgical treatment of endometriosis in the infertile female: a modified approach. Fertil Steril 1979;32:635–640.
23. Punnonen R, Klemi P, Nikkanen V. Recurrent endometriosis. Gynecol Obstet Invest 1980;11:307–312.
24. Rock JA, Guzick DS, Sengos C, et al. The conservative surgical treatment of endometriosis: evaluation of pregnancy success with respect to the extent of disease as categorized using contemporary classification systems. Fertil Steril 1981;35:131–137.
25. Wheeler JM, Malinak LR. Recurrent endometriosis: incidence, management and prognosis. Am J Obstet Gynecol 1983;146:247–253.
26. Gordts S, Boeckx W, Brosens I. Microsurgery of endometriosis in infertile patients. Fertil Steril 1984;42:520–525.
27. Chong AP, Baggish MS. Management of pelvic endometriosis by means of intraabdominal carbon dioxide laser. Fertil Steril 1984;41:14–19.
28. Wheeler JM, Malinak LR. Recurrent endometriosis. Contemp Gynecol Obstet 1987;16:13–21.
29. American Fertility Society. Classification of endometriosis. Fertil Steril 1979;32:633–634.
30. Hasson HM. Electrocoagulation of pelvic endometriotic lesions with laparoscopic control. Am J Obstet Gynecol 1979;135:115–121.
31. Sulewski JM, Curcio FD, Bronitsky C, et al. The treatment of endometriosis at laparoscopy for infertility. Am J Obstet Gynecol 1980;188:128–132.
32. Daniell JF, Christianson C. Combined laparoscopic surgery and danazol therapy for pelvic endometriosis. Fertil Steril 1981;35:521–525.
33. Davis GD. Management of endometriosis and its associated adhesions with the CO_2 laser laparoscope. Obstet Gynecol 1986;68:422–425.
34. Seiler JC, Gidwani G, Ballard L. Laparoscopic cauterization of endometriosis for fertility: a controlled study. Fertil Steril 1986;46:1098–1100.
35. Reich H, McGlynn F. Treatment of ovarian endometriomas using laparoscopic surgical techniques. J Reprod Med 1986;31:577–584.
36. Donnez J. CO_2 laser laparoscopy in infertile women with endometriosis and women with adnexal adhesions. Fertil Steril 1987;48:390–394.
37. Davis GD, Brooks RA. Excision of pelvic endometriosis with the carbon dioxide laser laparoscope. Obstet Gynecol 1988;72:816–819.
38. Fayez JA, Collazo LM, Vernon C. Comparison of different modalities of treatment for minimal and mild endometriosis. Am J Obstet Gynecol 1988;159:927–932.
39. Corson SL, Unger M, Kwa D, et al. Laparoscopic laser treatment of endometriosis with Nd:YAG sapphire probe. Am J Obstet Gynecol 1989;160:718–723.
40. Sutton C. CO_2 laser laparoscopy in the treatment of endometriosis. Baillière's Clin Obstet Gynecol 1989;3:499–523.
41. Kojima E, Morita M, Otaka K, et al. Nd:YAG laser laparoscopy for ovarian endometriomas. J Reprod Med 1990;35:592–596.
42. Daniell JF, Kurtz BR, Gurley LD. Laser laparoscopic management of large endometriomas. Fertil Steril 1991;55:692–695.
43. Fayez JA, Vogel MF. Comparison of different treatment methods of endometriomas by laparoscopy. Obstet Gynecol 1991;78:660–665.
44. Marrs RP. The use of potassium-titanyl-phosphate laser for laparoscopic removal of ovarian endometrioma. Am J Obstet Gynecol 1991;164:1622–1628.
45. Redwine DB. Conservative laparoscopic excision of endometriosis by sharp dissection: life table analysis of reoperation and persistent or recurrent disease. Fertil Steril 1991;56:628–634.
46. Canis M, Mage G, Vattiez A, et al. Second-look laparoscopy after laparoscopic cystectomy of large ovarian endometriomas. Fertil Steril 1992;58:617–619.
47. American Fertility Society. Revised American Fertility Society classification of endometriosis: 1985. Fertil Steril 1985;43:351–355.
48. Evers JLH. The second-look laparoscopy for evaluation of the result of medical treatment of endometriosis should not be performed during ovarian suppression. Fertil Steril 1987;47:502–504.
49. Nisolle-Pochet M, Casanas-Roux F, Donnez J. Histologic study of ovarian endometriosis after hormonal therapy. Fertil Steril 1988;49:423–426.
50. Fedele L, Bianchi S, Bociolone L, et al. Buserelin acetate in the treatment of pelvic pain associated with minimal and mild endometriosis: a controlled study. Fertil Steril 1993;49:516–521.
51. Buttram VC Jr. Surgical treatment of endometriosis in the infertile female: a modified approach. Fertil Steril 1979;32:635–640.
52. Meigs JV. The Wertheim operation for carcinoma of the cervix. Am J Obstet Gynecol 1945;49:542–553.
53. Lin Tan S, Royston P, Campbell S, et al. Cumulative conception and livebirth rates after in vitro fertilization. Lancet 1992;339:1390–1394.
54. Damewood MD. The role of the new reproductive technologies including IVF and GIFT in endometriosis. Obstet Gynecol Clin North Am 1989;16:179–191.
55. Ranney B. Reoperation after initial treatment of endometriosis with conservative surgery (discussion). Am J Obstet Gynecol 1978;131:416–421.
56. Evers JLH, Dunselman GAJ, Land JA, et al. Endometriosis: the management of recurrent disease. In Shaw RW, ed. Endometriosis. Carnforth, Parthenon Publ., 1990:93–105.
57. Candiani GB, Fedele L, Vercellini P, et al. Repetitive conservative surgery for recurrence of endometriosis. Obstet Gynecol 1991;77:421–424.
58. Chillik CF, Acosta AA, Garcia JE, et al. The role of in vitro fertilization in patients with endometriosis. Fertil Steril 1985;44:56–61.
59. Yovich JL, Matson PL. The treatment of infertility associated with endometriosis by in vitro fertilization. Fertil Steril 1986;46:432–438.
60. Dicker D, Goldman JA, Levy T, et al. The impact of long-term gonadotropin-releasing hormone analogue treatment on preclinical abortions in patients with severe endometriosis undergoing in vitro fertilization-embryo transfer. Fertil Steril 1992;57:597–600.

61. Fedele L, Bianchi S, Bocciolone L, et al. Pain symptoms associated with endometriosis. Obstet Gynecol 1992;79: 767–769.

62. Candiani GB, Fedele L, Vercellini P, et al. Presacral neurectomy for the treatment of pelvic pain associated with endometriosis: a controlled study. Am J Obstet Gynecol 1992;167:100–103.

63. Fedele L, Bianchi S, Viezzoli T, et al. Gestrinone versus danazol in the treatment of endometriosis. Fertil Steril 1989;51:781–785.

64. Fedele L, Bianchi S, Arcaini L, et al. Buserelin versus danazol in the treatment of endometriosis associated infertility. Am J Obstet Gynecol 1989;161:871–876.

65. Buttram VC Jr, Betts JW. Endometriosis. Curr Probl Obstet Gynecol 1979;2:11–18.

17

Laparoscopically Assisted Vaginal Hysterectomy, Laparoscopic Hysterectomy, and Bilateral Salpingo-Oophorectomy

Camran Nezhat, Farr Nezhat, Ceana Nezhat, and Dahlia Admon

The use of hysterectomy, one of the most frequently performed major surgical procedures, for treatment of endometriosis doubled between 1965 and 1984. This rise, which exceeded the increase for any other indication, probably reflected not only an increased recognition of endometriosis, but also an increase in the frequency and/or severity of disease.[1,2] About 75% of all hysterectomies are accomplished abdominally and 25% vaginally.[3,4]

Abdominal hysterectomy is usually reserved for women who have pelvic disease that may complicate a vaginal approach. These diseases include endometriosis and adhesions or other pelvic abnormalities that cannot be treated during vaginal hysterectomy.[5] In comparing vaginal and abdominal approaches, the latter are associated with more febrile morbidity, blood transfusions, and longer postoperative hospitalization and convalescence.[4,6] In theory, if a greater percentage of hysterectomies could be performed vaginally, therapeutic, economic, and social benefits would result.[7–10]

Vaginal hysterectomy is usually contraindicated in cases of severe endometriosis, poor uterine descent, possible adhesions from previous abdominal surgery such as cesarean section, or large leiomyomas. Women with these conditions may benefit from a laparoscopic approach which avoids some of the disadvantages of either abdominal or vaginal operations (Table 17.1).

There are many variations of laparoscopic-assisted hysterectomy. To differentiate the varying degrees of laparoscopic and vaginal dissection, we propose the following terminology: (1) *total laparoscopic hysterectomy (TLH)*: all steps, including vaginal cuff closure, are performed laparoscopically; (2) *subtotal laparoscopic hysterectomy (SLH)*: supracervical hysterectomy in which all steps are performed laparoscopically; (3) *vaginally assisted laparoscopic hysterectomy (VALH)*: most steps are performed laparoscopically, and the procedure is completed by a vaginal approach; and (4) *laparoscopically assisted vaginal hysterectomy (LAVH)*: a hysterectomy begun by laparoscopy but most steps are performed by the vaginal approach. The seven basic steps of hysterectomy are summarized in Table 17.2.

Patients with suspected pelvic endometriosis should undergo a diagnostic laparoscopy to allow inspection of the pelvis. Marked pelvic disease can be treated endoscopically and, if necessary, the ovaries can be removed. The hysterectomy is completed vaginally (combined diagnostic and/or operative laparoscopy and vaginal hysterectomy).[7]

In most cases, a combined laparoscopic and vaginal approach is used to dissect and remove uterine attachments.[8–11] The extent of laparoscopic and vaginal dissection should be based on the surgeon's preference and experience with laparoscopic and vaginal surgery. A more experienced endoscopist can perform the entire hysterectomy laparoscopically.[10–12] TLH, however, requires more surgical expertise. It can also be time-consuming, especially if the uterus is more than 16 to 18 weeks gestational size. Laparoscopic hysterectomy is useful when: (1) the vagina is narrow; (2) there is severe, infiltrative pelvic endometriosis; and (3) when the surgeon is very experienced in operative laparoscopy, including laparoscopic suturing. It is preferable to finish the procedure vaginally whenever the surgeon feels more comfortable in doing so. We can convert almost all abdominal hysterectomies for endometriosis to LAVH, VALH or TLH. We believe that other

Figures reproduced from *Operative Gynecologic Laporoscopy: Principles and Techniques*, C. Nezhat, Editor, 1995. With permission of McGraw-Hill Publishers.

Table 17.1. Advantages and disadvantages of laparoscopic-assisted hysterectomy.

	Advantages	Disadvantages
Abdominal hysterectomy	Good visualization and access Ability to treat abdominal and pelvic pathology More surgical expertise	Abdominal incision Greater morbidity Long recovery
Vaginal hysterectomy	Short recovery Less painful Less expensive	Limited by uterine size, associated pathology Unable to explore abdomen
LAVH, VALH, and LH	Good visualization and access Ability to assess and treat abdominal and pelvic pathology Quick recovery Low level of pain	Longer operating time Endoscopic complications Less surgical expertise among current gynecologists Can be more expensive than both vaginal and abdominal

surgeons will be able to do so with experience.[10] Candidates for traditional vaginal hysterectomy, however, should not undergo LAVH, VALH, or LH. All these approaches are more difficult to perform and are expensive.[13,14]

Preoperative Evaluation

All patients should be evaluated as they would be for hysterectomy by any route, either abdominal or vaginal. Routine preoperative tests include CBC with differential, serum electrolytes, bleeding time, and urinalysis. More comprehensive blood chemistry, thrombin time, partial thrombin time, ECG, chest x-ray, and endometrial biopsy may be ordered as indicated. All women undergoing a laparoscopic approach are given a mechanical and antibiotic bowel preparation (Tables 17.3 and 17.4). Consultations with a urologist, bowel surgeon, and oncologist are sought as necessary. Appropriate informed consent is obtained from the patient after she receives a thorough explanation of the planned operation, its potential risks and benefits, the possibility of conversion to laparotomy, and therapeutic alternatives. Following an overnight fast, patients are admitted to the ambulatory surgical unit the morning of surgery.

Table 17.2. Seven basic steps of hysterectomy.

1. Severing the round ligaments and dissection of the upper portion the broad ligament.
2. Severing the tubouterine junction and the utero-ovarian ligament if the adnexa are to be preserved, or severing the infundibulopelvic ligaments.
3. Severing the uterine vessels.
4. Preparation of the bladder flap and severing the bladder pillars.
5. Severing the cardinal-uterosacral ligament complex.
6. Performing anterior and posterior culdotomy and separation of the cervix from the vaginal membrane.
7. Closure of the vaginal cuff.

Positioning Patient

The patient's initial positioning is the same for standard laparoscopy. The 10 mm trocar is inserted infraumbilically for placement of the operative laparoscope, and two to four accessory trocars are positioned subumbilically. For the vaginal portion, the patient's legs are readjusted to allow vaginal access (we prefer Allen Universal stirrups). With an adjustment under the drapes, the legs can be flexed and abducted without redraping.

Laparoscopic and Operative Technique

Every operative laparoscopy begins with a thorough exploration of the abdominal and pelvic cavity to assess the extent of disease. Important anatomic landmarks, anomalies, distortions, and alterations are identified. The location of the bladder, ureters, colon, rectum, and major blood vessels are noted. The omentum and small bowel are evaluated for disease and checked for Verres needle or trocar injury.

After the diagnostic portion of the examination is completed, the surgeon uses the CO_2 laser and hydrodissection to resect, ablate, or coagulate any endometriosis implants. An electrocoagulator, clips, staplers, or Endoloops (Ethicon) may be used for coagulating or ligating large vessels. Monopolar electrodes or fiber lasers may also be used. We prefer to use the CO_2 laser via the operative channel of the laparoscope as a long knife and the bipolar electrocoagulator. We have used both with few complications.[15] Other instruments we use include bipolar forceps (middle port), suction-irrigator probe (left), and grasping forceps (right). The bowel is freed from the pelvic organs to expose the pelvic cavity. The ovaries and tubes are then dissected from the cul-de-sac or pelvic sidewall, and any endometriosis or other pathology is excised. Once the uterus and adnexa are separated from adhesions, hysterectomy is performed.[10]

Table 17.3. One-day bowel preparation.

Clear liquid day before surgery
1 gallon Nu-LYTELY or Go-LYTELY consumed over 3 hours evening
   before surgery
One Fleet enema at bedtime
1 gm metronidazole (Flagyl) by mouth at 11:00 pm
1 gm cefoxitin IV 1/2 hour before procedure

Ureteral Evaluation and Dissection

The direction and location of both ureters are identified from the pelvic brim to the cardinal ligaments, where they are no longer visible. When the ureters cannot be clearly identified, because of severe scarring or endometriosis, they are dissected retroperitoneally, using sharp dissection, blunt dissection, or hydrodissection.[16] For extensive endometriosis, very wide dissection is performed during radical hysterectomy as necessary.[17] To identify the ureters at the level of the cardinal ligaments, the peritoneum is opened above or below the ureter and hydrodissection is performed. A peritoneal incision is made and the ureter is identified toward its course to the bladder. Small bleeders are controlled by laser or electrosurgery. If the uterosacral ligaments are dissected, the ureter is retracted laterally and the uterosacral ligaments are dissected at their connection to the back of the cervix. The uterine vessels, which run superiorly, are isolated and safely coagulated. When pelvic anatomy is severely distorted, it may be easier to perform a cystoscopy and place catheters in both ureters. This may ensure better identification.

Upper Broad Ligament and Adnexa

If adnexectomy is indicated, the infundibulopelvic ligament is electrodesiccated and cut by taking progressive bites of tissue starting at the pelvic brim and moving toward the round ligament. If the endoscopic linear stapler is used, the adnexa are grasped with forceps. The device is retracted medially and caudally to stretch

Table 17.4. Three-day bowel preparation.

Day 1
   100 mL Fleet phospo-Soda by mouth at bedtime
Day 2
   Clear liquid diet
Day 3
   Clear liquid diet
   10 mg prochlorperazine by mouth at noon
   Begin drinking 1 gallon Go-LYTELY at 2:00 pm
   1 g neomycin by mouth at 6:00 pm and 11:00 pm
   1 g erythromycin base by mouth at 6:00 pm and 11:00 pm
   One Fleet enema at bedtime
Day of surgery
   Two tap water enemas before reporting to hospital

and outline the infundibulopelvic ligament, which is grasped and secured with the stapler. The stapler is not fired until the contained tissue is identified and the ureter's safety is confirmed. Once transected, the staple line should be closely examined for placement and hemostasis. After infundibulopelvic ligament transection, the adnexa and uterine fundus are retracted in the opposite direction and the tissue of the upper broad ligament, including the round ligament, is grasped, secured, and cut once safe margins are established. The infundibulopelvic and the round ligaments may occasionally be cut with a single staple application.

Preserving the Adnexa

If the adnexa are to be preserved, the round ligament is electrodesiccated and cut approximately 3 cm from the uterus. Using hydrodissection, the anterior and posterior leaves of the broad ligament are opened toward the vesicouterine fold and the bladder flap is developed. The utero-ovarian ligament, proximal tube, and mesosalpinx are progressively electrodesiccated and cut. Similarly, the round ligament, fallopian tube, and utero-ovarian ligament may be grasped close to their insertion into the uterus with the endoscopic linear stapler, then secured, stapled, and severed. The distal end of the stapler or bipolar forceps must be kept free from the bladder and ureter.

Developing the Bladder Flap

After the broad ligaments are severed, the anterior leaf of the broad ligament is grasped with forceps and elevated and dissected from the anterior lower uterine segment with hydrodissection and CO_2 laser. The uterovesical junction is identified, grasped, and elevated with forceps while being cut with scissors, laser, or electrode. The bladder pillars are identified, desiccated, and cut. The bladder is completely freed from the uterus by pushing downward with the tip of a blunt probe along the vesicocervical plane until the anterior cul-de-sac is exposed.

In cases of severe anterior cul-de-sac endometriosis, previous cesarean section, or adhesions, sharp dissection of the vesicouterine fold is often necessary. Injecting 5 mL of indigo carmine in the patient's IV may help you detect bladder trauma.

Uterine Vessels

After dissecting the bladder from the anterior cervix, the uterine vessels, which vary in size, number, and location, are identified, desiccated, and cut to free the lateral borders of the uterus. It is important to skeletonize the vessels to prevent slippage of the clips or staples. As the uterine vessels are severed and cut, the safety and position of the ureters should be periodically checked. This can be done more easily if they have been marked, exposed, or catheterized at the beginning of the procedure.

The hysterectomy may now be completed vaginally. However, in patients with extensive adhesions and/or endometriosis involving the cul-de-sac and rectum, it may be best to continue the dissection laparoscopically. This approach involves resecting the cardinal ligaments and performing a culdotomy.

Vaginal Portion of the Hysterectomy

Once the dissection is extended to the lower uterine segment or to the level of the cardinal ligaments, dissecting and resecting the uterus can be completed vaginally using standard techniques. Once the uterus is removed, the vaginal cuff is closed in standard fashion. To ensure support of the vaginal vault, the vaginal angles are attached to the uterosacral and cardinal ligaments with absorbable sutures. The vaginal cuff is closed transversely, and any coexisting cystocele or rectocele is repaired. Once the vaginal surgery is completed and the cuff closed, any additional necessary laparoscopic surgery may resume.

Hysterectomy for Extensive Pelvic Endometriosis With Adhesions

In women who have extensive endometriosis, the rectosigmoid colon is often densely adherent to the posterior aspect of the uterus. The rectosigmoid colon is separated from the posterior uterus incrementally, and the bowel endometriosis is resected or vaporized (Figs. 17.1 and 17.2). Since the high-power Ultrapulse CO_2 laser is very

precise,[18] and with a penetration of $100\,\mu m$, the possibility of delayed bowel necrosis is very low. Any excessive bleeding not controlled by the CO_2 laser can be stopped with cautious application of the bipolar electrocoagulator. Endometriosis of the rectum, rectovaginal septum, and uterosacral ligament is treated by vaporization, excision, or a combination of the two. The posterior cul-de-sac is completely freed (Figs. 17.3 and 17.4). Bipolar forceps are carefully used for achieving hemostasis. If the endometriosis has penetrated deeply to the bowel muscularis or mucosa and caused stricture requiring anterior or complete resection and repair, this step will be performed after the hysterectomy.[19,20]

The hysterectomy starts with electrodesiccation and transection of the round ligament close to the pelvic sidewall (Fig. 17.5). The peritoneum is opened, and the paravesical spaces are dissected by blunt dissection, hydrodissection, and CO_2 laser. This technique allows excellent skeletonization of the obliterated hypogastric artery (Fig. 17.6).[17]

The bladder serosa is injected with lactated Ringer's.[16] The bladder flap is developed using the CO_2 laser and countertraction.[9,10,13] After division of any scar tissue in the vesicouterine fold, the suction-irrigator probe is used for blunt dissection and mobilization of the bladder (Fig. 17.7). The infundibulopelvic ligaments are electrodesiccated with bipolar electrocoagulation and transected with the laser or other cutting modality (Fig. 17.8).

The uterine vessels are retracted medially and removed from the ureter using the CO_2 laser. The anterior parametrium is transected using the laser. The suction-

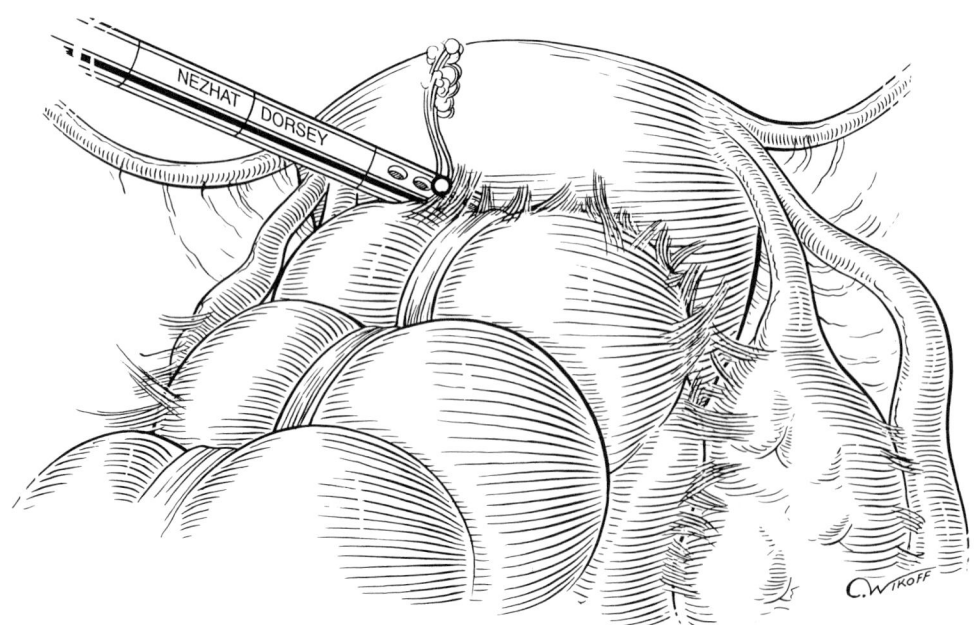

Figure 17.1. The rectosigmoid colon is severely attached to the posterior aspect of the uterus.

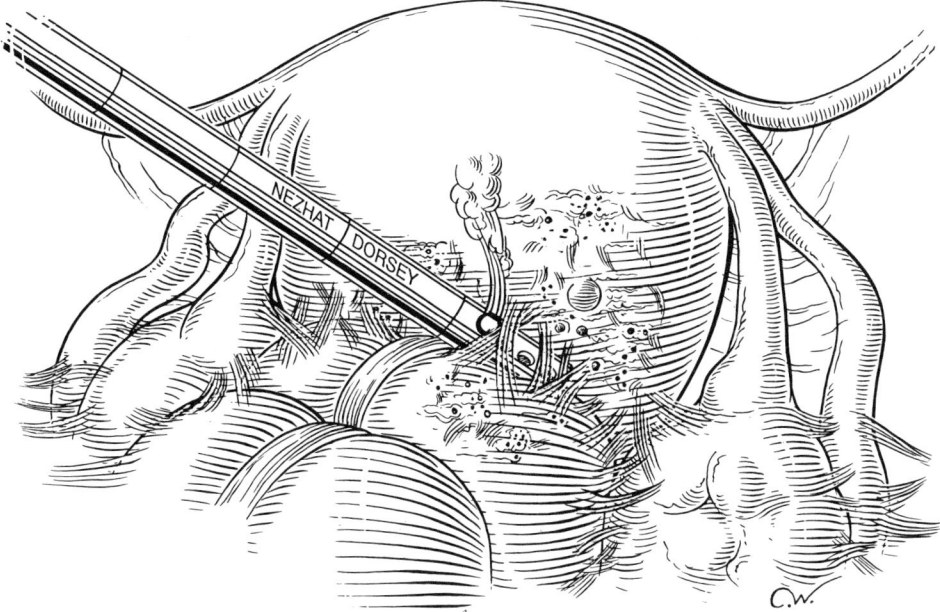

Figure 17.2. The rectosigmoid colon is dissected from the posterior aspect of the uterus using hydrodissection and a CO_2 laser.

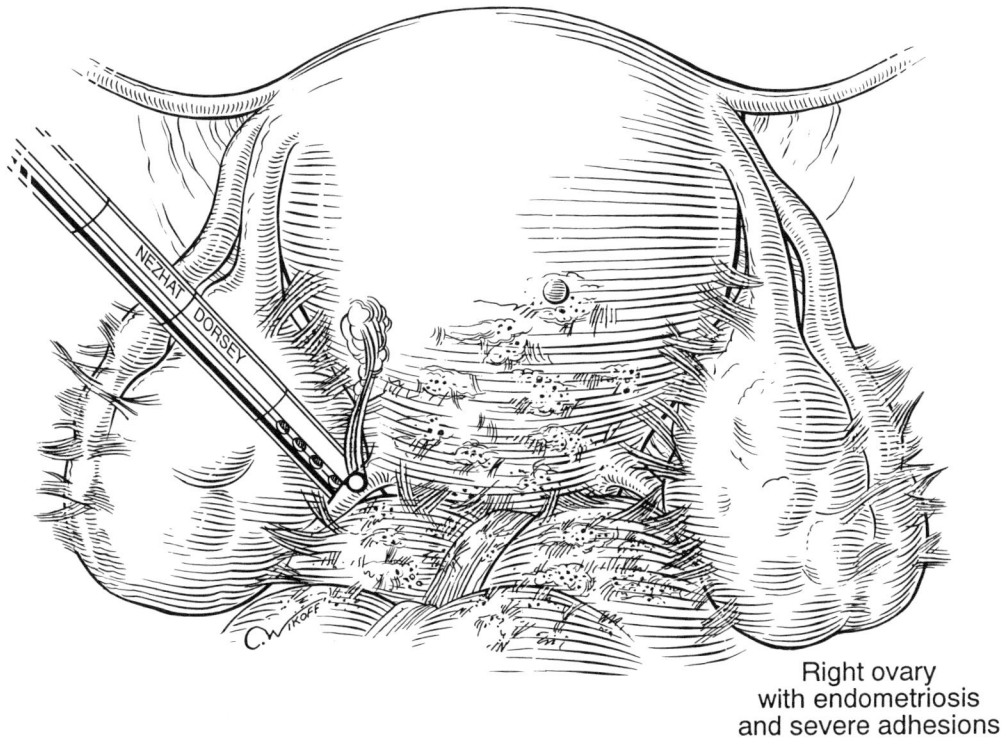

Right ovary
with endometriosis
and severe adhesions

Figure 17.3. The rectum is dessicated from the back of the cervix and uterosacral ligaments.

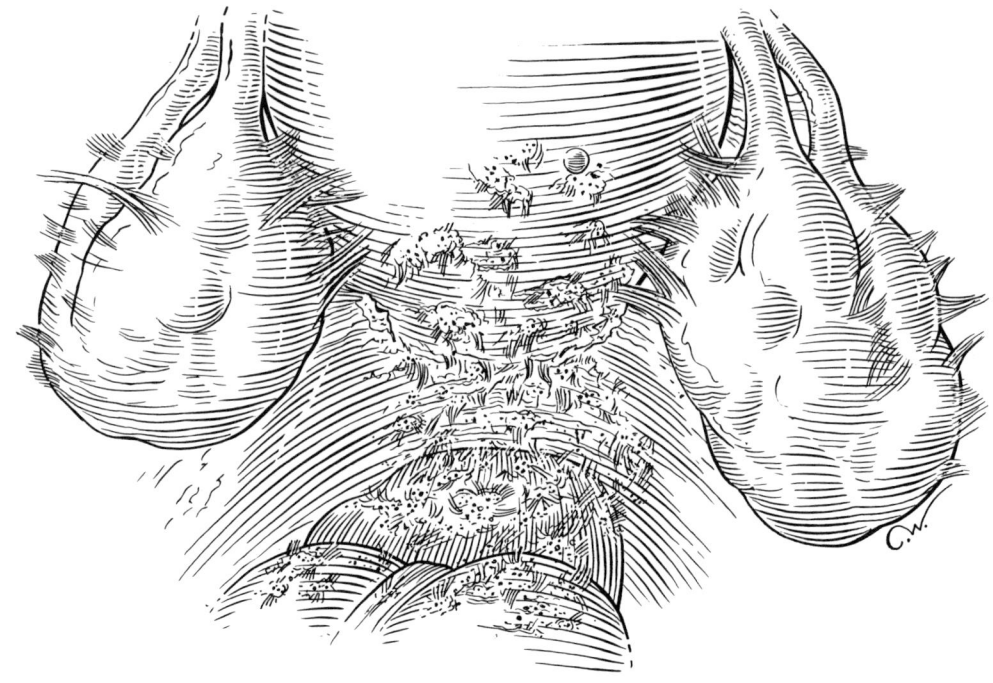

Figure 17.4. The posterior aspect of the uterus is completely freed from the rectosigmoid colon.

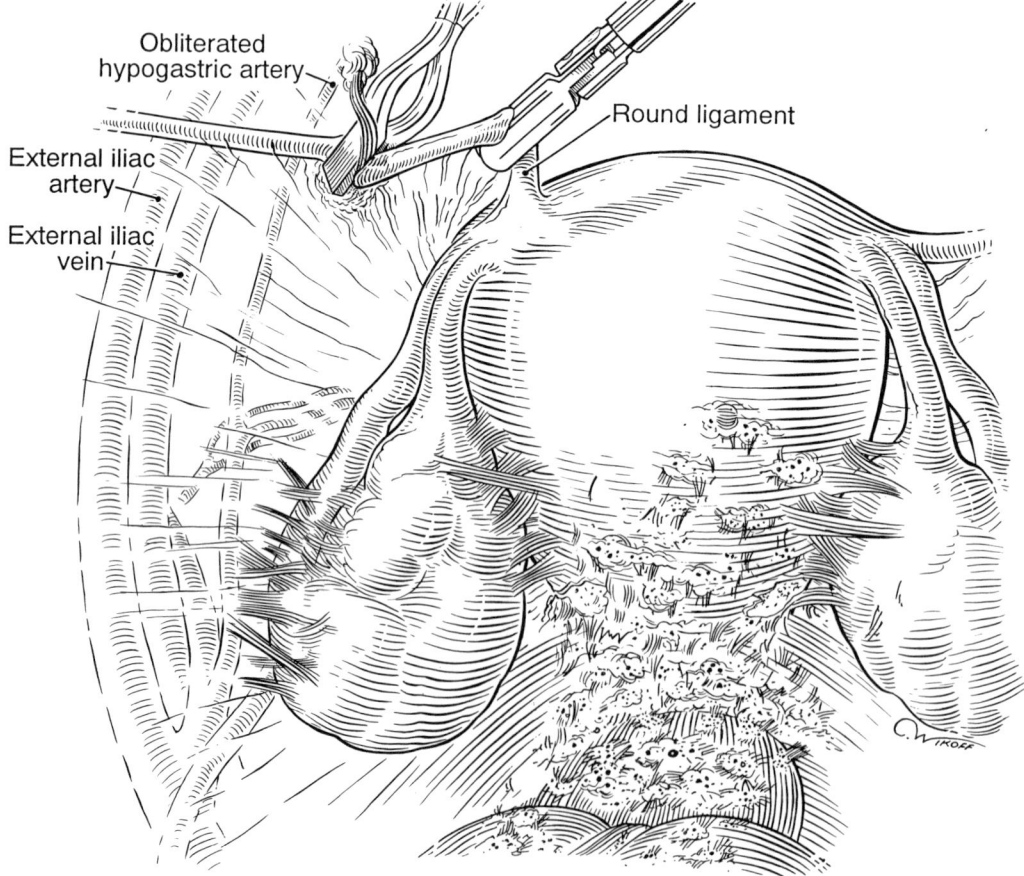

Figure 17.5. The round ligament is electrodessicated and cut.

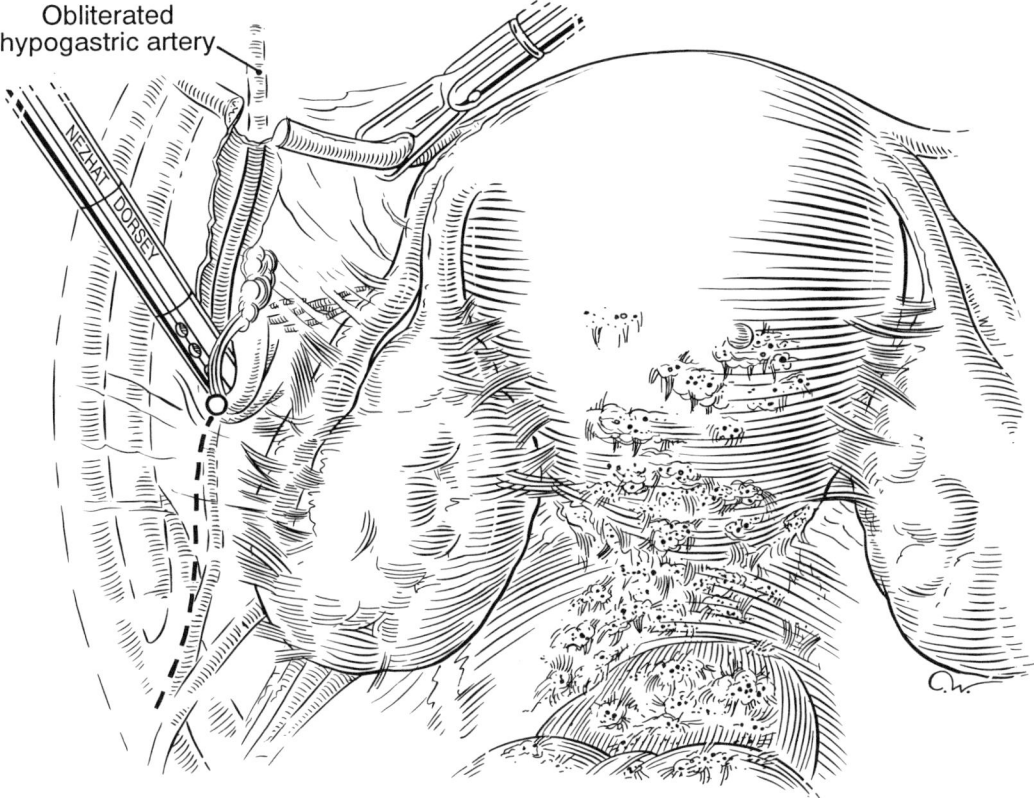

Figure 17.6. Developing the paravesical space allows excellent skeletonization.

irrigator probe acts as a backstop to protect the ureter. The ureters are freed from the peritoneum and skeletonized down to the bladder using the suction-irrigator probe and the laser. The uterine vessels are electrodesiccated close to the hypogastric artery (Fig. 17.9).

Cardinal Ligaments

At the level of the cardinal ligaments, the ureter and the descending branches of the uterine artery are close to one another and the cervix. Therefore, cardinal ligament dissection must be precise to prevent bleeding and ureteral injury. The linear stapler should be used only if the parametrium has been dissected with ample margins, as for cervical malignancy. The linear stapler is 12 mm wide. Considering the short distance between the cervix and ureter, use of the stapler in this area increases the risk of ureter injury.[21] Using contralateral retraction of the uterus, the cardinal ligament is carefully dissected to identify tissue planes, vessels, and the ureter (Fig. 17.10). Once the ureter is displaced laterally, the cardinal ligament tissue closest to the cervix is electrodesiccated and resected (Fig. 17.11). The bladder pillars, which can be very thick and involved with endometriosis, are transected close to the cervix (Fig. 17.12).

Culdotomy With Cuff Closure

After the uterosacral ligaments are completely dissected, a folded wet gauze in a sponge forceps, or the tip of a right-angle Heaney retractor, is used to mark the anterior or posterior vaginal fornix. The vaginal wall is tented and transected horizontally with laser or electrode (Figs. 17.13 and 17.14). Bipolar electrocoagulation can be used to control bleeding. The remainder of the procedure can be performed vaginally, if it is possible or if the operator prefers.

Total Laparoscopic Hysterectomy

If TLH is performed, we place a surgical glove containing two 4 × 4 wet sponges into the vagina (Ceana's glove) to prevent loss of pneumoperitoneum. By applying contralateral retraction to the uterus, the vaginal wall surrounding the cervix is outlined, coagulated with unipolar scissors or bipolar forceps, and cut circumferentially until the cervix is separated (Fig. 17.15). The specimen is pulled to the mid-vagina but not removed, to preserve pneumoperitoneum. The vaginal cuff is copiously irrigated and inspected for bleeding. Once hemostasis is achieved, vaginal angles are sutured to the adjacent cardinal and uterosacral ligaments. Care is taken to avoid the ureters. The rest of the vaginal

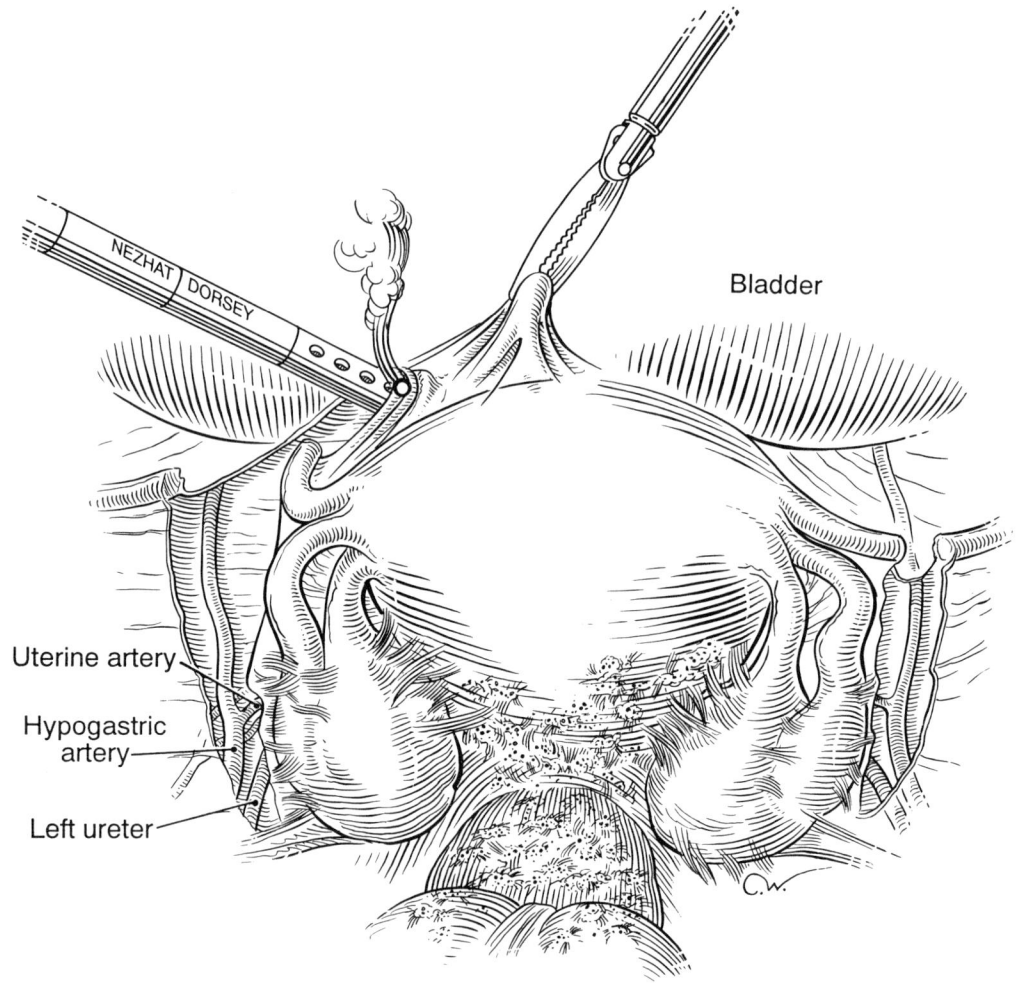

Figure 17.7. The suction-irrigator probe is used for blunt dissection of the bladder.

cuff can be closed with 0 Vicryl (Ethicon) suture on a straight or curved needle using extracorporeal knotting (Figs. 17.16 and 17.17). Endoscopic suturing can be time-consuming and should be done by experienced endoscopists who are comfortable with laparoscopic suturing. Bipolar electrocoagulation should be used cautiously at the vaginal cuff to prevent tissue necrosis and subsequent wound breakdown should sutures be placed in nonviable tissue.

Final Laparoscopic Evaluation

After the vaginal cuff is closed, whether from below or above, and the pneumoperitoneum is restored, the pelvic and abdominal cavities are evaluated, copiously irrigated, and cleared of blood clot and debris, and reevaluated laparoscopically. The pelvis is filled with 300 to 500 mL of lactated Ringer's before inspecting the pedicles and vaginal cuff for bleeding under low pneumoperitoneal pressure.[10,22] The vaginal cuff is examined to ensure that no small bowel or omental

tissue is included in its closure. At this point, the fluid in the pelvis should be clear. A final look at the ureters should confirm normal peristalsis and anatomic integrity. If the stapling device has been used, the stapler line should be very carefully evaluated under low pneumoperitoneal pressure to be sure there is no bleeding. To avoid incisional omental or bowel strangulation after the removal of any trocar(s) more than 5 mm in size, the fascia is repaired with delayed absorbable sutures.[21] Interceed Tc 7/(Johnson and Johnson) is applied to the vaginal apex to prevent or decrease adhesion formation.

Subtotal Hysterectomy (SLH)

Although supracervical hysterectomy is generally in disfavor at present, we perform this operation on occasion at the patient's request, following appropriate consultation and thorough evaluation for history of cervical dysplasia. Some believe that the cervix helps provide better vaginal support and sexual response. The

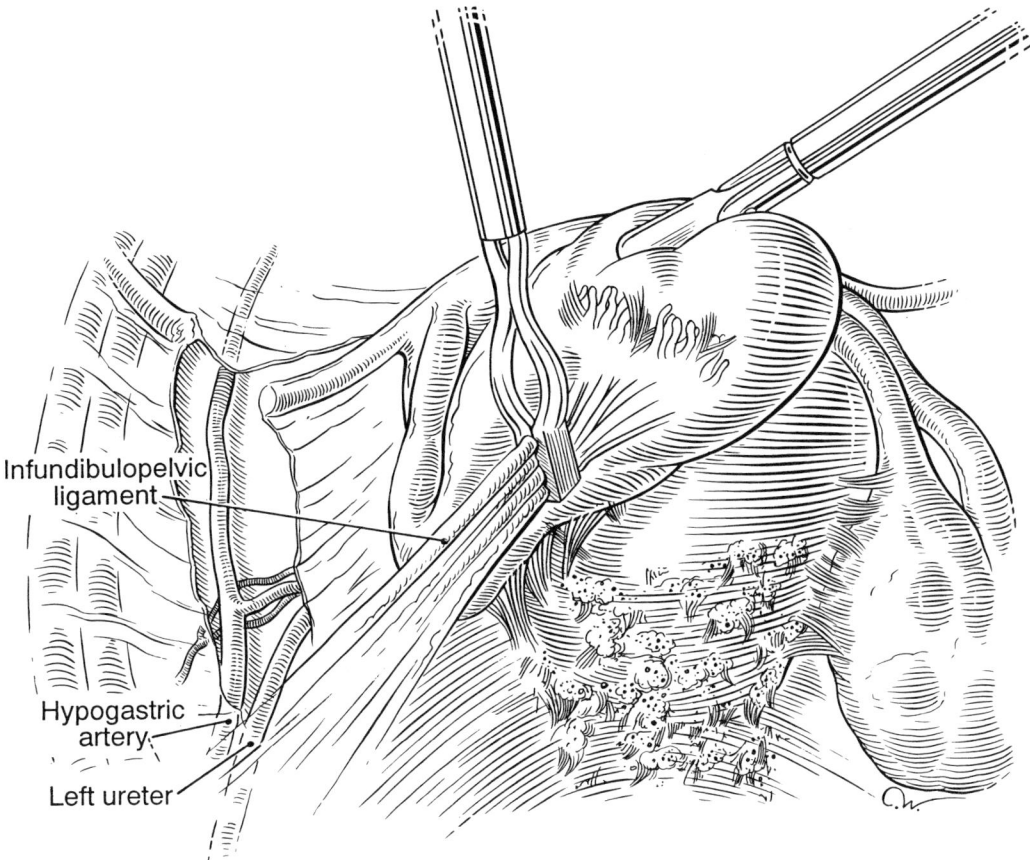

Figure 17.8. The infundibulopelvic ligaments are electrodessicated and cut.

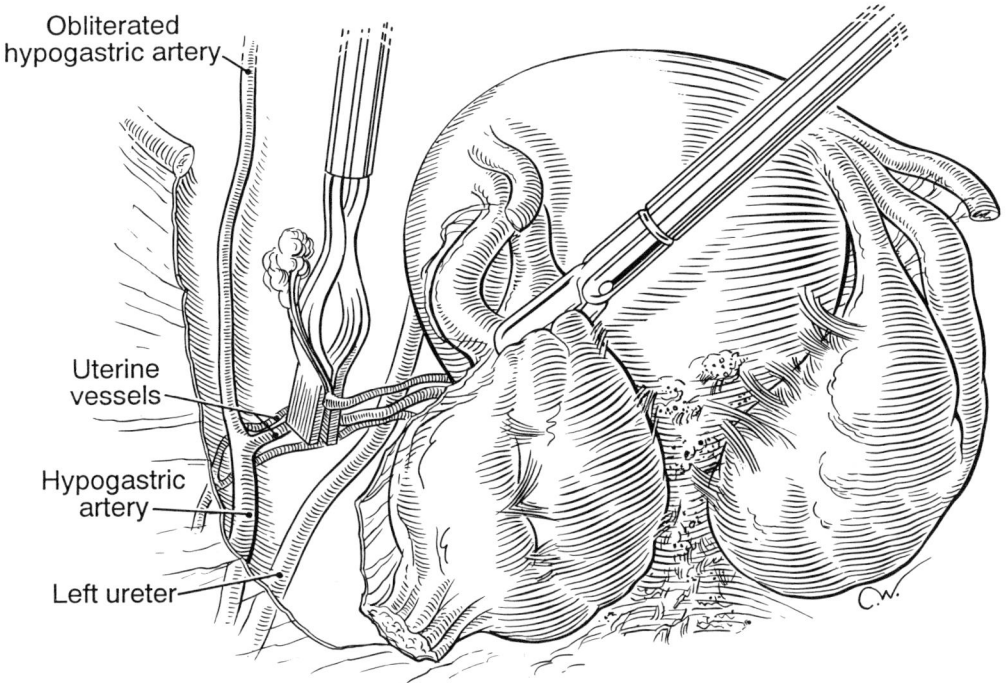

Figure 17.9. The uterine vessels are electrodessicated close to the hypogastric artery.

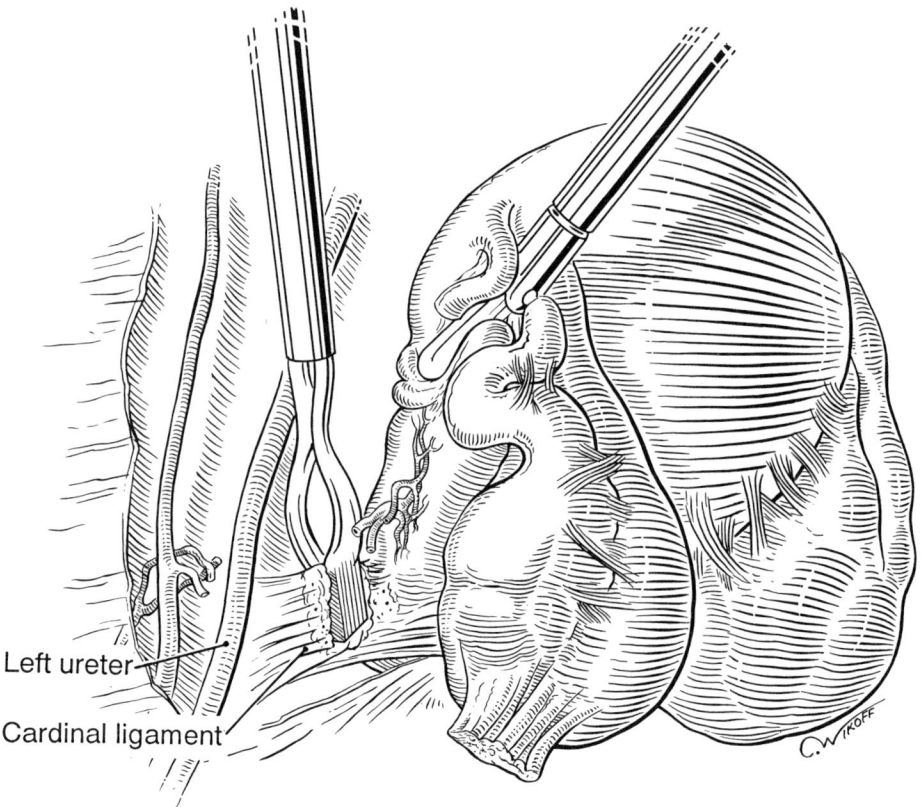

Left ureter

Cardinal ligament

Figure 17.10. The cardinal ligament tissue closest to the cervix is electrodessicated.

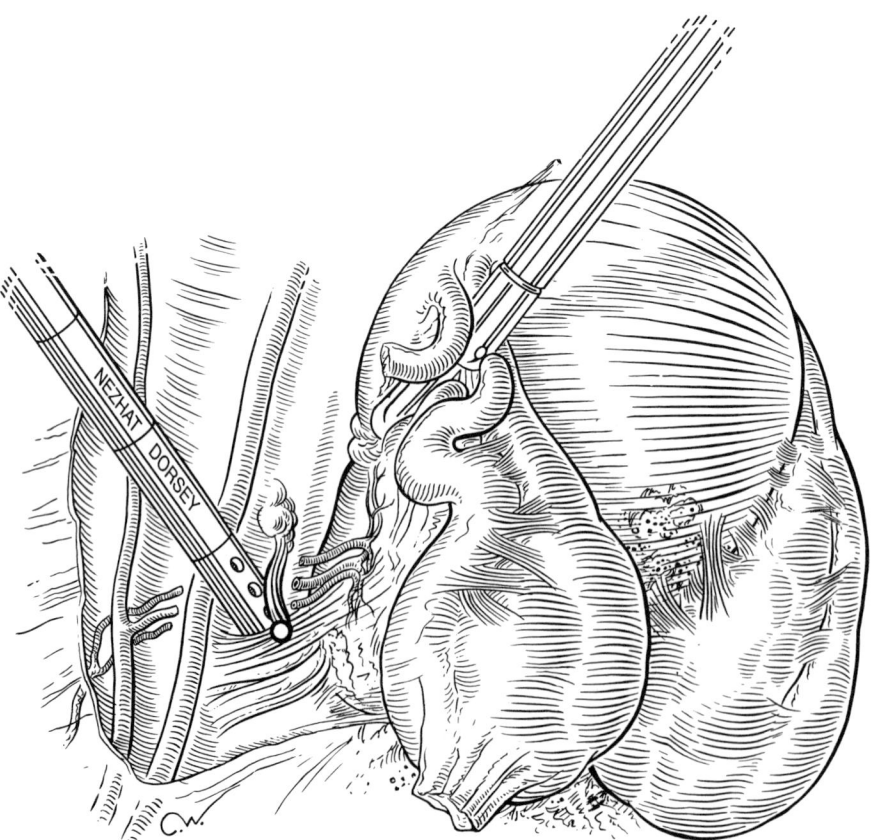

Figure 17.11. The cardinal ligament is dissected.

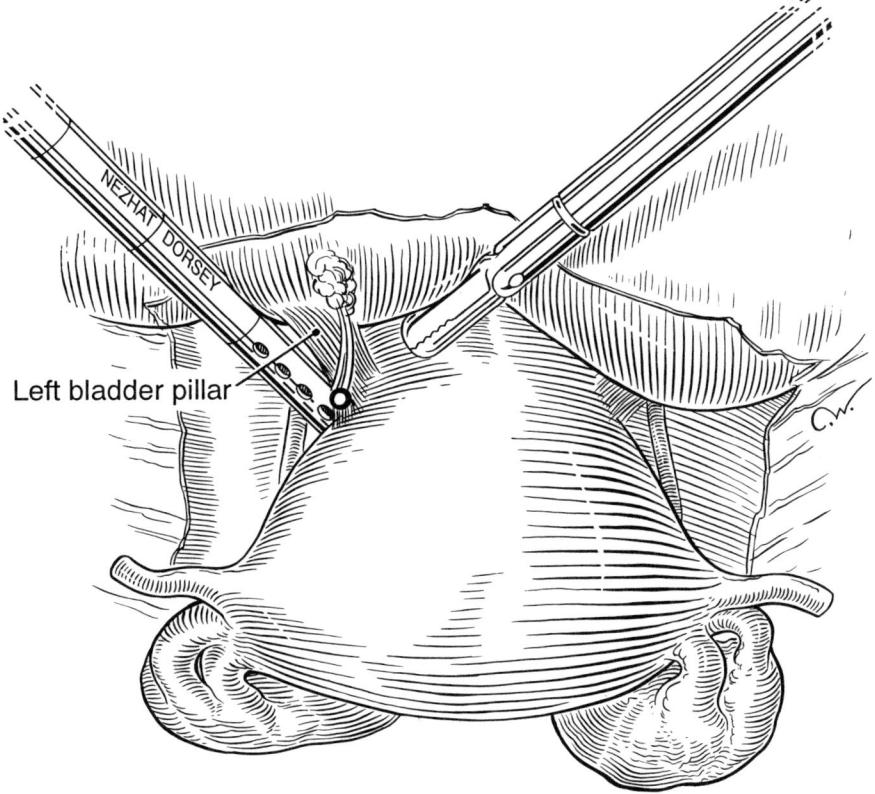

Figure 17.12. The bladder pillars are transected close to the cervix with a CO_2 laser.

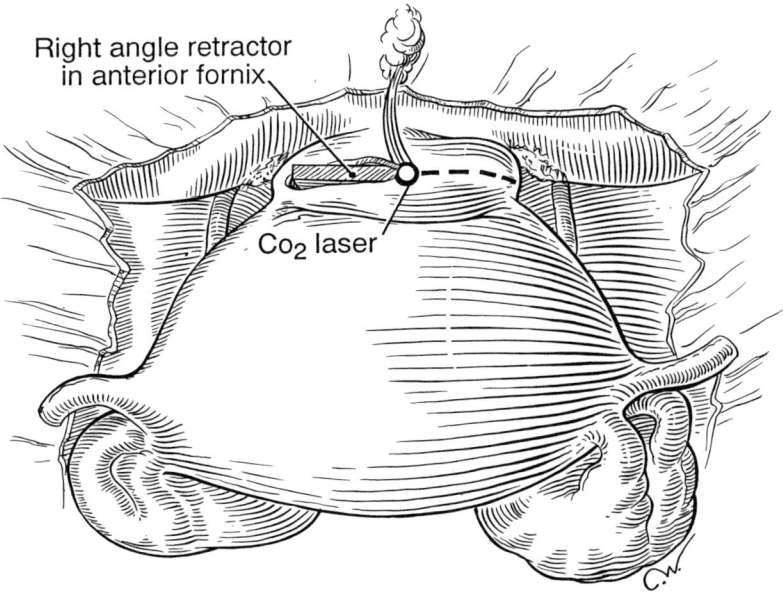

Figure 17.13. An anterior culdotomy is performed.

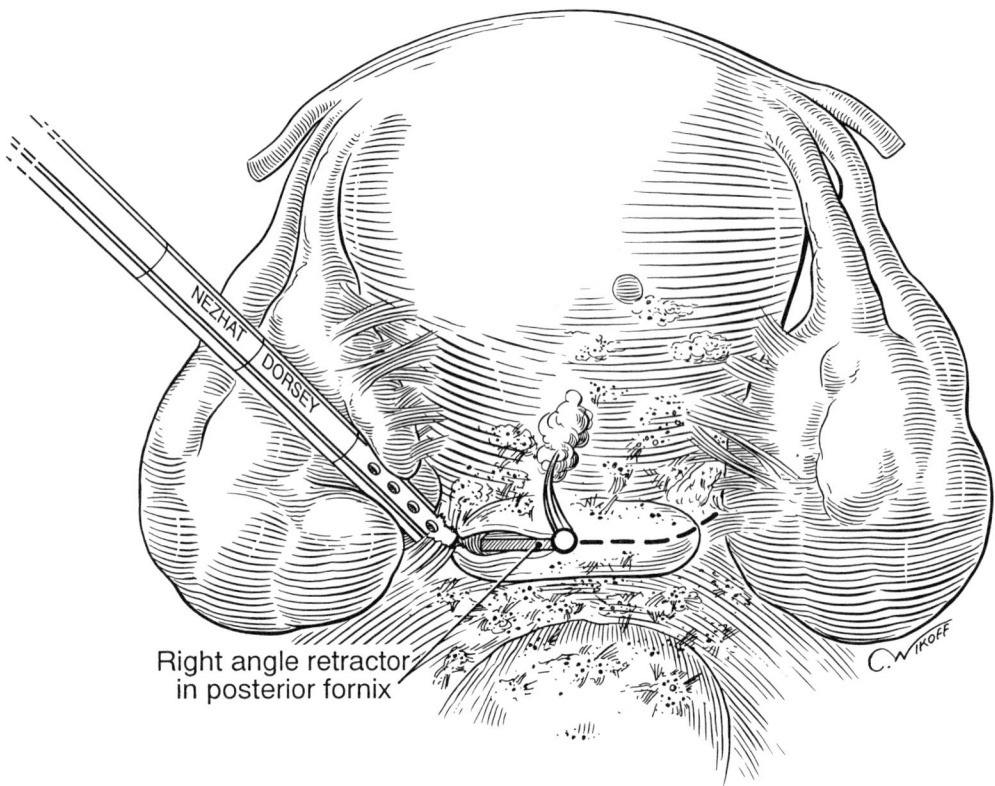

Figure 17.14. A CO_2 laser is used to perform a posterior culdotomy.

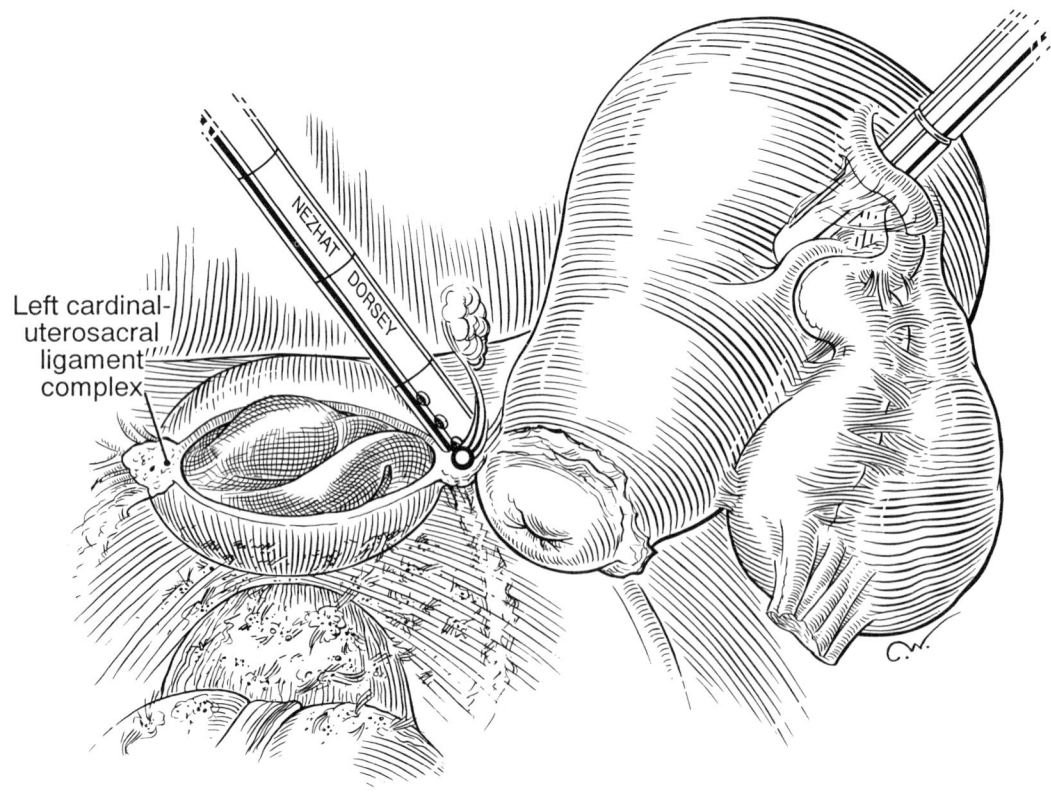

Figure 17.15. The vaginal wall is outlined, then cut circumferentially until the cervix is separated.

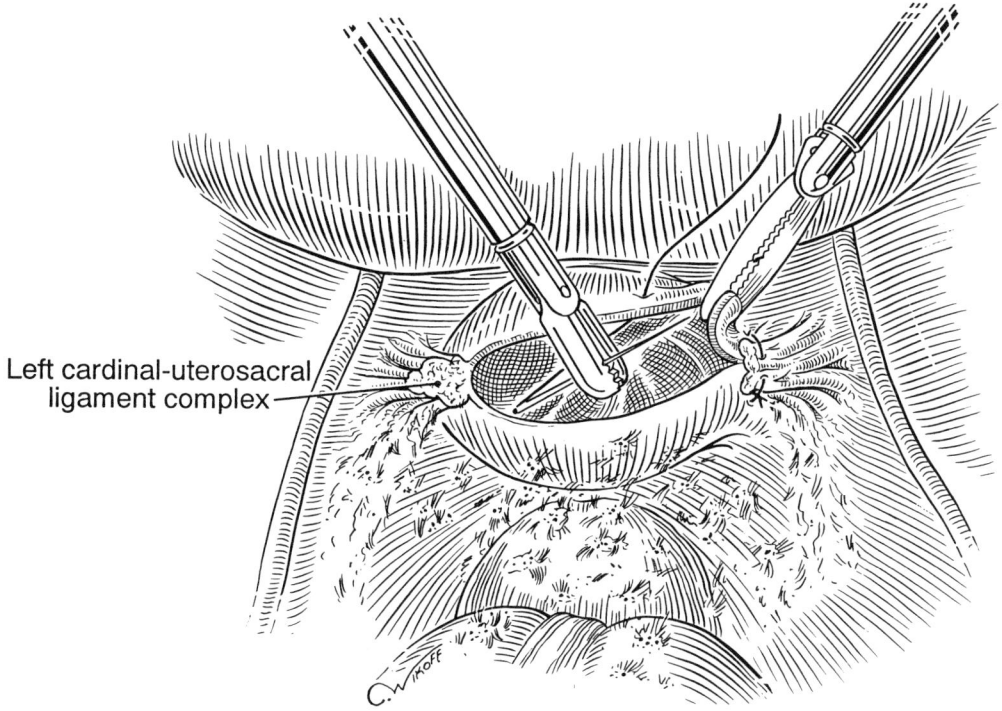

Figure 17.16. The right vaginal angle is sutured to the adjacent cardinal and uterosacral ligaments.

procedure can be performed laparoscopically, albeit with the additional difficulty of removing the specimen through the small incision.

After desiccating and cutting the uterine vessels at the level of the cardinal ligaments about the uterosacral ligaments, the uterus is retracted and its lower segment amputated with scissors, unipolar endoscopic electrode, or laser. After transecting the uterus from the cervix, the uterine manipulator is removed vaginally, the cervical stump copiously irrigated, and any bleeding is controlled. Once hemostasis is achieved, the endocervical epithelium lining the cervical canal is vaporized or

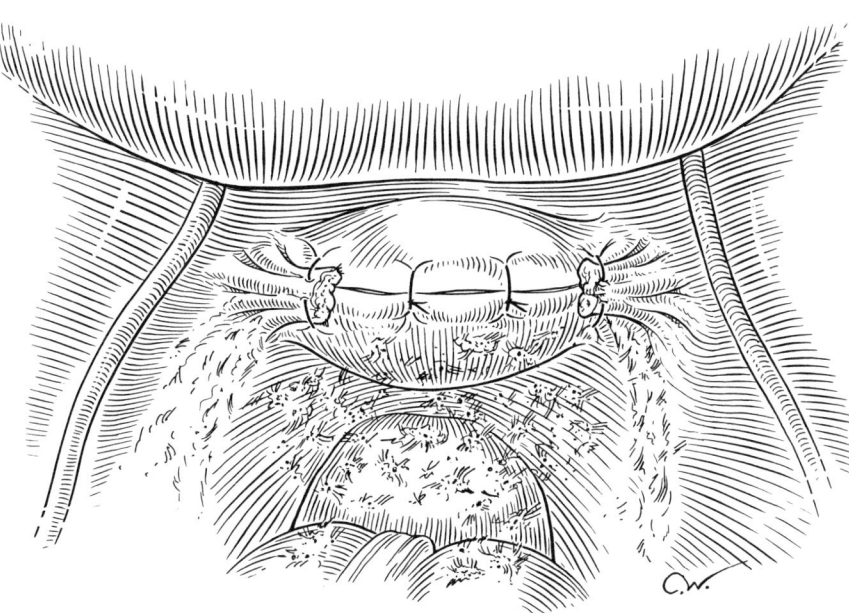

Figure 17.17. The vaginal cuff is closed.

Table 17.5. Distribution of patients by stage of endometriosis (AFS-r).

Stage	Patients
1	31 (15%)
2	42 (20%)
3	49 (23%)
4	90 (42%)
All stages	212 (100%)

Table 17.7. Method of hysterectomy and adnexectomy among 212 patients with endometriosis.

Type	Hysterectomy ($N = 212$)	BSO ($N = 129$)	RSO ($N = 21$)	LSO ($N = 34$)
LAVH	11%	11%	10%	9%
VALH	24%	24%	38%	18%
TLH	62%	62%	52%	70%
SLH	3%	3%	0%	3%
Total	100%	100%	100%	100%

coagulated laparoscopically with laser or electricity as far down as possible. The rest of the endocervical canal can be ablated vaginally to reduce the risk of intraepithelial cervical neoplasia. The cervical stump is closed with interrupted absorbable sutures and may be covered with peritoneum, which is sewn transversely with either continuous or interrupted sutures. The uterus is morcellated and removed through a 10mm trocar, small mini-laparotomy, or posterior colpotomy.[23] Copious peritoneal washing and thorough inspection of the pelvis and abdomen should be performed at the end of the procedure. These patients should be advised of the continued risk of cervical neoplasia and the need for annual examinations and Pap smears. The remaining procedure is similar to regular hysterectomy which is performed either vaginally or completely laparoscopically as described.

Endometriosis Cases

From July 1987 through July 1992, we performed a total of 361 hysterectomies for benign disease using the laparoscopic techniques described; 212 of these women had cases of endometriosis. Tables 17.5 and 17.6 summarize the staging and intraoperative and pathologic findings of these patients. Table 17.7 indicates the type of hysterectomy and number of salpingo-oophorectomies performed in these 212 patients. Table 17.8 lists the concomitant procedures (excluding salpingo-oophorectomy). Many women required ureterolysis when endometriosis involved the pelvic wall (Table

17.8). Bowel resection was performed when there was severe involvement of the bowel.[19,20] Average operating room time in this group was 105 minutes (Table 17.9). The mean age was 41.7 years (between 25 and 67 years old). The average blood loss was 73mL (between 50 and 800mL). Two patients had ovarian remnant. Four patients had previous laparotomy for hysterectomy that failed due to extensive pelvic and bowel endometriosis and adhesions. Average hospital stay was 21 hours (between 20 hours and 5 days). The overall complication rate was 10%. Table 17.9 lists the complications in these patients. During the dissection of the bladder from the cervix, bladder injury occurred in one patient with severe endometriosis and fibrosis between the bladder and the cervix. In another patient, the small bowel was severely attached to the posterior aspect of the uterus, and enterotomy occurred while lysing dense adhesions between the bowel and the uterus. Both complications were repaired laparoscopically. There were no ureter injuries.

There were two incidents of postoperative vaginal cuff bleeding between 2 to 4 weeks; one in the VALH group, and one in the TLH group. Both were controlled with sutures, and neither patient needed transfusion. Two patients with extensive pelvic endometriosis and severe ovarian attachment to the bowel developed ovarian remnant syndrome. One patient complained of pain and, because medical therapy was unsuccessful, she underwent laparoscopic resection of ovarian remnant.[24] The other patient responded to medical therapy and, at present, has a functioning piece of ovary without

Table 17.6. Adjunctive diagnoses among 212 patients with endometriosis at laparoscopic hysterectomy.

Pathology	Patients
Adhesions	152 (72%)
Leiomyomas	98 (46%)
Adenomyosis	61 (29%)
Endometriomas	22 (10%)
Uterine polyps	10 (5%)
Paratubal and ovarian cysts (except endometrioma)	9 (4%)
Hydrosalpinx	7 (3%)
Ovarian remnants	4 (2%)
Endometrial hyperplasia	1 (0.5%)
Cervical dysplasia	1 (0.5%)

Table 17.8. Adjunctive procedures among 212 patients with endometriosis performed at laparoscopic hysterectomy.

Procedure	Patients (No.)
Uterolysis	118
Appendectomy	34
Moschcowitz procedure	33
Marshal-Marchetti-Krantz procedure	13
Bowel resection	11
Rectocele repair	8
Removal of ovarian remnant	4
Cystocele repair	2
Cholecystectomy	1

Table 17.9. Descriptive statistics of 212 laparoscopic hysterectomy patients with endometriosis.

Characteristics	Average	Range
Age (years)	41.7	25–67
Parity	1.1	0–5
OR time (minutes)	105	55–330
Estimated blood loss (ml)	73	50–800
Uterine weight (gm)	165	36–1070
Hospital stay (days)	1	1–5
Use of pain medication postop (days)	3.3	0–21
Postop full recovery (weeks)	3.3	<1–13

pain. One patient with extensive pelvic endometriosis and a medical history of afibrinogenemia experienced bleeding from the umbilical incision 20 hours postoperatively. This was managed by resuturing the incision and applying pressure. She was discharged on postoperative day 2 in stable condition. But 10 days later, this patient complained of a vaginal serosanguinous discharge. Speculum exam revealed an intact vaginal cuff. Because the source of bleeding was unknown, the patient underwent second-look laparoscopy. The laparoscopy showed that she had apparently bled from the umbilical incision postoperatively. The bleeding had ceased but had formed a hematoma extending from the umbilicus to the pelvis. The hematoma was dissolving, and the blood clots were evacuated. There was no active bleeding, and she was discharged the following day.

Conclusion

Currently, about one in four hysterectomies are performed vaginally. Among the remaining patients, LAVH and TLH are excellent alternatives to abdominal hysterectomy as long as the surgeon is experienced and trained. However, the endoscopic approach is not without limitations or complications. It is difficult in women with extensive endometriosis, adhesions, or an enlarged uterus. We have replaced the laparotomy approach in performing hysterectomies. At the Center for Special Pelvic Surgery, our efforts are no longer directed at validating the role of endosurgery, but rather providing other gynecologic surgeons with opportunities for proper training and supervised experience.

Table 17.10. Complications of 212 patients with endometriosis undergoing hysterectomy.

Intraoperative
- Inferior epigastric vessel injury   1
- Transfusion   1
- Small bowel injury   1
- Bladder injury   1

Postoperative
- Vaginal cuff bleeding   2
- Delayed incisional bleeding   1
- Abdominal wall ecchymosis   2
- Cystitis   2
- Urinary retention   2
- Fever   3
- Transient tachycardia   1
- Pneumonia, bronchitis   3
- Ovarian remnant syndrome   2

References

1. Porkas R, Hufnagel VG. Hysterectomy in the United States, 1964–84. Am J Public Health 1988;78:852.
2. Nezhat C, Berger GS, Nezhat F, Buttram VC, Nezhat CH., eds. Modern Surgical Management of Endometriosis. New York, Springer-Verlag, 1993.
3. Bachmann GA. Hysterectomy: A critical review. J Reprod Med 1990;35:839.
4. Dicker RC, Scally MJ, Greenspan JR, et al. Hysterectomy among women of reproductive age. JAMA 1982;248:323.
5. White SC, Wartel OLJ, Wade ME. Comparison of abdominal and vaginal hysterectomy—1a review of 600 operations. Obstet Gynecol 1971;37:350.
6. Wingo PA, Huezo CM, Rubin GL, et al. The mortality risk associated with hysterectomy. Am J Obstet Gynecol 1985;152:803.
7. Kovac RS, Cruikshank SH, Retto HF. Laparoscopy-assisted vaginal hysterectomy. J Gynecol Surg 1990;6:185.
8. Nezhat C, Nezhat F, Silfen SL. Laparoscopic hysterectomy and bilateral salpingo-oophorectomy using multifire GIA surgical stapler. J Gynecol Surg 1990;6:287.
9. Nezhat C, Burrell MO, Nezhat FR, et al. Laparoscopic radical hysterectomy with para-aortic and pelvic node dissection. Am J Obstet Gynecol 1992;166:864–865.
10. Nezhat C, Nezhat F, Gordon S, et al. Laparoscopic versus abdominal hysterectomy. J Reprod Med 1992;37:247–250.
11. Carter J, Ryoo J, Katz A. Laparoscopic-assisted vaginal hysterectomy: A case control comparative study with total abdominal hysterectomy. J Am Assoc Gynecol Lap 1994;2:116–121.
12. Nezhat C, Nezhat F, Nezhat CH. Operative laparoscopy (minimally invasive surgery): State of the art. J Gynecol Surg 1992;8:141.
13. Summitt RL, Stovall TG, Lipscomb GH, et al. Randomized comparison of laparoscopy-assisted vaginal hysterectomy with standard vaginal hysterectomy in an outpatient setting. Obstet Gynecol 1992;80:895.
14. Nezhat C, Bess O, Admon D, et al. Hospital cost comparison between abdominal, vaginal, and laparoscopy-assisted vaginal hysterectomies. Obstet Gynecol 1994;83:713–716.
15. Nezhat F, Nezhat C, Levy JS. A report of laparoscopic injuries and complications over a 10 year period. Presented at 41st annual clinical meeting of American College of Obstetricians and Gynecologists, Washington, D.C., May 3–6, 1993.
16. Nezhat C, Nezhat F. Safe laser endoscopic excision or vaporization of peritoneal endometriosis. Fertil Steril 1989;52:1:149–151.
17. Nezhat C, Nezhat F, Burrell MO, et al. Laparoscopic radical hysterectomy and laparoscopically assisted vaginal radical hysterectomy with pelvic and paraaortic node dissection. J Gynecol Surg 1993;9:105.

18. Nezhat C, Nezhat F. Laparoscopic surgery with a new tuned high-energy pulsed CO_2 laser. J Gynecol Surg 1992; 8:251–255.
19. Nezhat F, Nezhat C, Pennington E, et al. Laparoscopic segmental resection for infiltrating endometriosis of the rectosigmoid colon: a preliminary report. Surg Laparosc Endosc 2:212–216.
20. Nezhat C, Nezhat F, Pennington, et al. Laparoscopic disk excision and primary repair of the anterior rectal wall for the treatment of full-thickness bowel endometriosis. Surg Endosc 1994;8:682–685.
21. Nezhat C, Nezhat F, Bess O, et al. Injuries associated with the use of a linear stapler during operative laparoscopy: review of diagnosis, management, and prevention. J Gynecol Surg 1993;3:145–150.
22. Nezhat C, Nezhat F, Winer W. Salpingectomy via laparoscopy: a new surgical approach. J Laparosc Surg 1991;1:91–95.
23. Schwartz R. Hysterectomy. Relevant Issues and Reproductive Medicine.
24. Nezhat F, Nezhat C. Operative laparoscopy for the treatment of ovarian remnant syndrome. Fertil Steril 57: 1003–1007.

18

Management of Recurrent Endometriosis After Hysterectomy and Bilateral Salpingo-Oophorectomy

Lisa A. Hasty and Ana A. Murphy

Persistent or recurrent endometriosis after a total abdominal hysterectomy and bilateral salpingo-oophorectomy (TAH BSO) has been reported by several investigators.[1-3] Although many aspects of endometriosis are incompletely understood, the stimulation and growth of endometrial implants by cyclic ovarian steroids has been demonstrated. Therefore, removing this cyclic stimulation should permit the disease to regress. We don't know the exact incidence of recurrent endometriosis after "definitive" surgery, but it is thought to be extremely rare following TAH BSO even when the woman takes hormone replacement therapy.[4] Several investigators have published reviews with small patient numbers. In 1970, Ranney reported no recurrences when estrogen replacement was not given but a 3% recurrence rate if replacement was given.[5] In the same decade, Gray reported no recurrence without hormonal replacement therapy compared with a 20% rate if estrogen therapy was initiated.[6] Interestingly, the majority of patients with recurrence in the latter series had bowel involvement with endometriosis. If recurrent disease exists after resection of endometriosis with TAH BSO, then this surgery is not "definitive" for this group of patients.

It is important to try to distinguish new endometriotic lesions from persistent disease in which implants are not adequately treated. Sometimes this condition may be determined only by the presence of new locations of endometriotic lesions. After TAH BSO, however, these two entities (persistent disease vs recurrent disease) are managed in the same manner.

A related phenomenon of postmenopausal endometriosis has been reported.[4,7,8] Sampson observed that incompletely resected endometriotic lesions atrophied after castration.[9] But there is no agreement on the best approach if surgical or natural menopause fails to alleviate symptoms.[2]

Definitive Surgery

It has been said that to prevent persistent or recurrent disease, we must completely remove or ablate the uterus, ovaries, and all endometriosis. The use of an operating microscope, loupes, or near-contact laparoscope may help in the complete excision. Some experts prescribe progestin therapy before TAH BSO in an effort to make dissection easier with decidualization of implants.[10] Others report that progestin therapy results in increased friability of the implants and increased bleeding.[11] By shrinking implants, GnRH analogs may mask disease and keep surgeons from recognizing lesions.

Failure to recognize the extent of endometriosis may prevent complete removal of the disease. The appearance of endometriosis varies greatly. Atypical or nonpigmented lesions may appear as red lesions, yellow-brown patches, or vesicular lesions.[12-14] Retroperitoneal disease may also go unrecognized or increase the complexity of the surgery and hinder the full removal of this disease.[13]

The most common presenting symptoms for recurrent disease after surgery are pelvic pain and dyspareunia. Vaginal or rectal bleeding may also be present. The differential diagnosis includes ovarian remnant syndrome and adhesive disease as well as recurrent endometriosis. In these patients, it is often difficult to determine the exact cause of persistent or recurrent pain.

Serum gonadotropin and estrogen determination will help establish whether an ovarian remnant exists. If the patient is taking hormonal replacement therapy, this should be discontinued until a diagnosis is made. A trial of danazol or GnRH agonist therapy may be attempted before surgery if imaging studies show remaining ovarian tissue. Progestational agents may also be helpful.[10] If the symptoms persist despite medical management, surgical reexploration may be necessary, especially if there are obstructive signs. Because of the possibility of occlusive sigmoid disease in these patients, they must have preoperative bowel preparation. Malignancy arising from endometriosis must also be considered in these patients. It is rare, but several reports have been published on malignant transformation of endometriosis.[15,16]

Ovarian Remnant Syndrome

If all or part of an ovary remains after surgery, then the procedure was not truly definitive. Ovarian remnant syndrome is often associated with surgery for endometriosis. Failure to remove an ovary completely may occur where a portion of the ovary or the entire ovary is located in the retroperitoneum. Complete removal may also be difficult when the ovary is densely adherent to the pelvic sidewall, ureter, hypogastric vessels, or the bladder base. Failure to excise even a small part of ovarian capsule may lead to recurrent pain or persistent endometriosis.

The diagnosis of ovarian remnant syndrome requires documentation of a previous bilateral oophorectomy and histologic evidence of ovarian tissue obtained at reoperation.[17] In a report on 31 such cases, 14 had endometriosis. The most common presentation is pain. In attempting to diagnose ovarian remnant syndrome, a follicle-stimulating hormone (FSH) determination may be helpful. The ovarian remnant may contain functional ovarian tissue and therefore an FSH value would be in the normal range. However, some remnants may not have active tissue and FSH may be elevated.

The treatment options for ovarian remnant syndrome include reoperation and removal of the tissue, medical management, or radiation. If imaging studies clearly demonstrate a mass, then reoperation is recommended. If no mass is evident, then medical management, including progestin therapy, danazol, or GnRH agonist, may be in order. Radiation therapy is rarely used, if ever, but may be considered if FSH levels are normal and no mass is demonstrated.

Steroid Receptors in Endometriosis

The cause of recurrent endometriosis after TAH BSO is unknown. Abnormal hormonal responsiveness of endometrial implants has been postulated. Metzger and co-workers have clearly demonstrated that the hormonal responsiveness of endometrial implants is unpredictable and inconsistent.[18] Specifically, estrogen and pro-

gesterone receptor content in endometriotic tissue was highly variable and did not undergo cyclic change throughout the menstrual cycle (Figs. 18.1 and 18.2).

The unpredictable levels of estrogen and progesterone receptors in implants indicate faulty regulation of steroid hormone receptors. Paracrine and autocrine factors may be important in delineating the differences in regulation. The site of implantation may also be a contributing factor. Poor vascularity, fibrosis, or exposure to various inflammatory cells may be responsible for hormonally nonresponsive endometriotic implants. An alteration in the basic regulatory and cellular processes within the endometrial implant may explain these findings.[19]

Extrapelvic Endometriosis

Extrapelvic endometriosis is frequently seen in patients whose endometriosis persists following radical surgery. In the few cases of postmenopausal endometriosis reported, vesical or retroperitoneal disease has been found.[8] Extrapelvic disease can be defined as endometriotic lesions of the cervix, vagina, vulva, intestinal tract, urinary tract, abdominal wall, thoracic cavity,

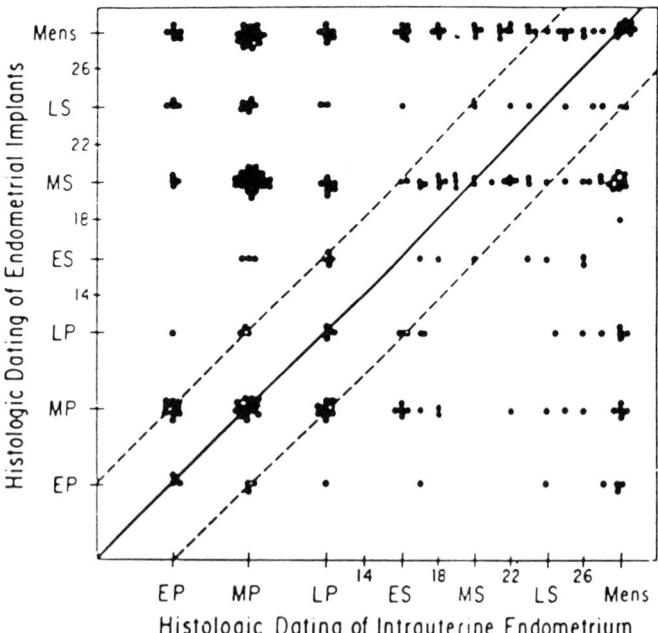

Figure 18.1. In this scatter plot of the histologic dating of ectopic endometrium and the corresponding intrauterine endometrium, the solid line represents those implants in phase. The dotted line encompasses those implants synchronous with the endometrium within one cycle stage or dating subdivision. EP, early proliferative; MP, mid-proliferative; LP, late proliferative; ES, early secretory (days 16 through 19); MS, mid-secretory (days 20 through 23); LS, late secretory (days 24 through 27); Mens, menstrual. (Source: Metzger et al.[18] with permission.)

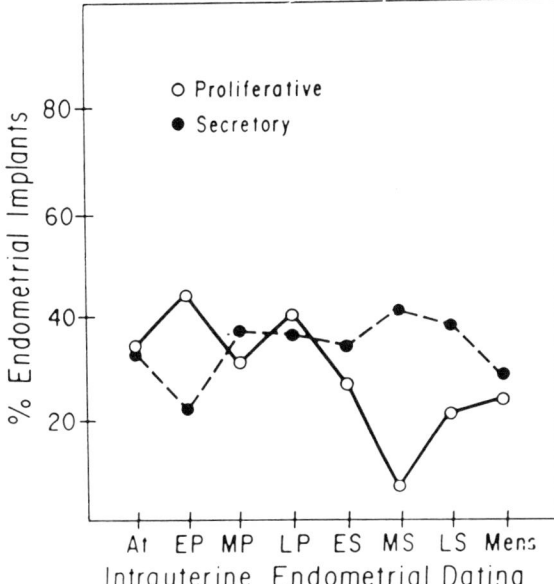

Figure 18.2. The distribution of proliferative and secretory ectopic endometrium is shown relative to the corresponding intrauterine endometrial dating. EP, early proliferative; MP, mid-proliferative; LP, late proliferative; ES, early secretory (days 16 through 19); MS, mid-secretory (days 20 through 23); LS, late secretory (days 24 through 27); Mens, menstrual. (Source: Metzger et al.[18] with permission).

extremities, central nervous system and other sites.[20] The intestinal tract and the urinary system are common sites for extrapelvic endometriosis. Intestinal lesions have been reported in up to 25% of women with pelvic endometriosis.[21] The descending colon, sigmoid, and appendix are the most common locations. Symptoms include pain, abdominal distension, diarrhea, nausea, vomiting, constipation, and rectal bleeding. Intestinal obstruction is also a complication. Treatment depends on the location and extent of the disease. If the lesions are nonobstructive, then conservative medical management is in order (Table 18.1). More advanced lesions or failure to respond may require surgery and complete excision of the disease, including a possible segmental bowel resection.[20] Urinary tract endometriosis includes

Table 18.1. Hormonal therapy of extrapelvic endometriosis.

Continuous progestins
  Medroxyprogesterone acetate, 40 to 60 mg daily po; 200 mg IM
    every other week (Provera, Depo-Provera)
  Norlutate, 30 mg po daily
  Megestrol acetate (Megace) 20 to 40 mg po daily
Combined oral estrogen-progestin
  Ethinyl estradiol, 0.03 to 0.05 mg, with norgestrel, 0.3 to 0.5 mg po
    daily without interruption (Lo Ovral, Ovral)
Continuous testosterone
  Ethinyltestosterone (danazol), 400 to 800 mg po daily
  19-Nortestosterone derivatives (gestrinone), 2.5 to 5.0 mg po 2 or 3
    times per week

surface implants of the bladder. More important, it may involve the ureter and may extend intrinsically to the ureteral orifice and bladder wall. These extensive lesions may or may not respond to medical or surgical oophorectomy. Complete surgical excision of the disease is often required. Cases of obstruction may require segmental resection with ureteral implantation or anastomosis.[20]

Unanswered Questions

Does extrapelvic endometriosis arise from the same source as pelvic endometriosis? Does extrapelvic disease represent tissue arising from coelomic metaplasia? And does disease arising from this source have a limited hormonal responsiveness and a more autonomous nature? Do as yet unidentified risk factors exist for recurrent disease following "definitive" therapy? Should modifications of estrogen replacement therapy be investigated in these patients? Who would benefit from these modifications? These questions remain to be answered in order for us to deal effectively with the problem of recurrent disease after TAH BSO.

References

1. Schram JD. Endometriosis after "Pelvic Cleanout." Southern Med J 1978;71(11):1419–1420.
2. Dmowski WP, Radwanska E, Rana N. Recurrent endometriosis following hysterectomy and oophorectomy: the role of residual ovarian fragments. Int J Gynecol Obstet 1988;26:93–103.
3. Metzger DA, Lessey BA, Soper JT, et al. Hormone-resistant endometriosis following total abdominal hysterectomy and bilateral salpingo-oophorectomy: correlation with histology and steroid receptor content. Obstet Gynecol 1001;78(5):946–950.
4. Punnonen R, Klemi PJ, Nikkanen V. Postmenopausal endometriosis. Europ J Obstet Gynec Reprod Biol 1980; 11:195–200.
5. Ranney B. Endometriosis. Conservative Operations. Am J Obstet Gynecol 1970;107:743–753.
6. Gray LA. Endometriosis of the bowel: role of bowel resection, superficial excision, and oophorectomy in treatment. Ann Surg 1973;177:580–587.
7. Kempers RD, Dockerty MB, Hunt AB, et al. Significant postmenopausal endometriosis. Surg Gyn Obstet 1960; (91):348–356.
8. Vorstman B, Lynne C, Politano VA. Postmenopausal vesical endometriosis. Urology 1983;22(5):540–542.
9. Sampson JA. Intestinal adenomas of the endometrial type. Arch Surg 1922;5:217.
10. Schlaff WD, Dugoff L, Damewood WD, et al. The use of megestrol acetate in the treatment of endometriosis. Obstet Gynecol 1990;75(4):647.
11. Henzl MR, Corson SC, Moghissi K, et al. Administration of nasal nafarelin as compared with oral danazol for endometriosis. N Engl J Med 1988;318:485.
12. Martin DC, Hubert GD, Vander Zwaag R, et al. Laparoscopic appearances of peritoneal endometriosis. Fertil Steril 1989;51:63.

13. Cornillie FJ, Oosterlynck D, Lanneryns JM, et al. Deeply infiltrating pelvic endometriosis: histology and clinical significance. Fertil Steril 1990;53:978.

14. Jansen RP, Russell P. Nonpigmented endometriosis: clinical, laparoscopic, and pathologic definition. Am J Obstet Gynecol 1986;155:1154.

15. Heaps JM, Nieberg RK, Berck JS. Malignant neoplasms arising in endometriosis. Obstet Gynecol 1990;75:1023–1028.

16. Addison WA, Hammond CB, Parker RT. The occurrence of adenocarcinoma in endometriosis of the rectovaginal septum during progestational therapy. Gynecol Oncol 1979;8:193–197.

17. Pettit PD, Raymond AL. Ovarian remnant syndrome: diagnostic dilemma and surgical challenge. Obstet Gynecol 1988;71:580.

18. Metzger DA, Olive DL, Haney AF. Limited hormonal responsiveness of ectopic endometrium: histologic correlation with intrauterine endometrium. Hum Path 1988;19:1417–1424.

19. Lessey BA, Metzger DA, Haney AF, et al. Immuno-histochemical analysis of estrogen and progesterone receptors in endometriosis: comparison with normal endometrium during the menstrual cycle and the effect of medical therapy. Fertil Steril 1989;51(3):409–414.

20. Markham SM, Carpenter SE, Rock JA. Extrapelvic endometriosis. Obstet Gynecol Clin N Amer 1989;16(1):193–219.

21. Jenkinson EL, Brown WH. Endometriosis. A study of 117 cases with special reference to constricting lesions of the rectum and sigmoid colon. JAMA 1943;122:349.

19
Prevention of Postoperative Adhesions

Anthony A. Luciano

Peritoneal adhesions may give rise to bowel obstruction, pelvic pain, and infertility.[1-3] The association between peritoneal adhesions and infertility has long been known. It was firmly established in 1979 by Caspi and associates who reported an inverse relationship between the grade of adhesions and pregnancy rates.[2]

Since a major detriment to the success of infertility surgery is postoperative adhesions at and beyond the surface of the wound, it is important that gynecologic surgeons understand the mechanism of adhesion formation, implement optimal surgical techniques for adhesiolysis, and appropriately apply agents or devices that may reduce adhesions. In this chapter, I will review the pathophysiology of adhesion formation, mention techniques and adjuvants that have been used in managing pelvic adhesions, and describe my approach to laparoscopic adhesiolysis.

Adhesion Formation

Tissue trauma from infection, endometriosis, or surgery results in immunologic defenses that lead to the immediate formation of fibrinous attachments between adjoining structures covering the peritoneal defect. Normal fibrinolytic activity usually lyses these fibrous attachments (fibrinous exudate), within 72 to 96 hours of the injury. Simultaneously, connective tissue cells carry on mesothelial repair so that, within 5 days after an injury, a single cell layer of mesothelium covers the injured raw area and replaces the fibrinous exudate. However, if the fibrinolytic activity of the peritoneum is suppressed, fibroblasts will migrate, proliferate, and form fibrous adhesions with collagen deposition and vascular proliferation.[1]

Table 19.1 lists factors that suppress fibrinolytic activity and promote postoperative adhesions. When performing reconstructive pelvic surgery, these factors must be kept to a minimum by applying optimal microsurgical principles, avoiding the use of reactive sutures and foreign substances, and implementing effective medical adjuvants.

Postoperative Adhesion Formation and Reformation

Microsurgery connotes not only the use of magnification but also the concept of delicate surgery, which embodies gentle handling and constant irrigation of tissues, meticulous hemostasis, use of microsurgical instruments and fine sutures, and precise tissue approximation. Microsurgery was specifically developed to minimize factors that contribute to postoperative adhesions. Although microsurgery has been successful in uterotubal and tubo-tubal anastomosis, failures persist at disappointing rates, especially for distal tubal disease.[4-6]

Even when properly applied, microsurgical techniques frequently produce adhesions. Indeed, in all published reports to date, adhesion reformation is found at 37% to 72% of surgical sites.[5,6] New adhesions develop in 51% of patients after reproductive surgery at laparotomy.[6] Therefore, reproductive pelvic surgery performed by laparotomy is frequently followed not only by adhesion reformation but also by de novo adhesion formation.[5,6]

Although useful and versatile in pelvic reconstructive surgery, lasers do not seem to have marked advantages over the more traditional mechanical or electrosurgical tools.[7,8] However, we do believe that the use of CO_2 laser beam through the operative channel of the laparoscope acts as a "long sharp knife," and it is practical and safe as described by the Nezhats.[9,10]

Table 19.1. Contributors to adhesion formation.

- Blood clots retained in peritoneal cavity
- Drying of serosal surfaces
- Suture material
- Instrumentation of adnexa
- Ischemia
- Prolonged operating time
- Omental patches
- Traction of peritoneum

With the development of improved endoscopic instruments, optics, and video systems, the gynecologic surgeon has been able to perform more complex operative procedures via laparoscopy. Several controlled animal and clinical studies comparing postoperative adhesion formation and reduction after reproductive surgery by laparoscopy versus laparotomy have concluded that the former results in less adhesion reformation and new adhesion formation.[11-14] Even in the hands of the most experienced laparoscopists, however, adhesion recurrence is observed in 30% to 45% of patients.[12]

These results are consistent with the observations made a century ago by Von Dembrowski and by Franz, and later confirmed by Ellis, who reported that uncomplicated peritoneal injury, such as that likely to occur at operative laparoscopy, heals without adhesion formation. However, with tissue drying or bleeding, as is often the case at laparotomy, significant adhesion formation follows peritoneal injury. The finding of the studies listed in Table 19.2 hold true regardless of whether we use laser, electricity or scissors, through laparoscopy, or laparotomy.

Adjuvants to Minimize Adhesion Formation/Reformation

The benefits derived from medical adjuvants remain controversial, despite their widespread use by reproductive surgeons. Table 19.3 lists the most commonly used techniques aimed at preventing postoperative adhesion formation.

The use of steroids and antihistamines has been abandoned by most reproductive surgeons because of their questionable efficacy and potential adverse effects of delayed healing and risk of wound dehiscence.[15] Dextran 70 (Hyskon) is absorbed slowly from the peritoneal cavity, over a period of 7 to 10 days. During that time, its osmotic effect draws sufficient fluid into the peritoneal cavity to float mobile peritoneal organs, thus allowing them to avoid close contact and to reduce adherence between intraperitoneal structures. Several studies in animals and humans have demonstrated therapeutic effects of dextran 70 in postoperative adhesion reduction.[16-19] However, inconsistent results also suggest limited efficacy, with the more favorable effects being reported in the more dependent portions of the pelvis.[17] Reports of allergic reactions, infections, and complications of fluid overload have tempered the use of this agent in reproductive surgery.

Recent studies on barrier methods, some using absorbable surgical membranes, seem more promising. The mechanism by which barriers may reduce adhesions relates to separation of interposing peritoneal surfaces, which prevents fibrous bands from binding different structures.

In a multicenter clinical study, oxidized regenerated cellulose (Interceed) was randomly placed on one of the two sidewalls treated for comparable disease/adhesions.[20] At second-look laparoscopy, significantly fewer adhesions reformed on the treated side. However, postoperative adhesions were not prevented in all cases. A more recent multicenter clinical study from Japan reported similar efficacy of this barrier in reducing, but not eliminating, postoperative adhesion formation.[21] Although animal studies using either rats[22] or mice[23] did not find Interceed to be effective in preventing postoperative adhesion formation, the more relevant clinical studies recently conducted both in the United States and in Europe have consistently reported that Interceed barrier reduces the incidence, extent, and severity of postoperative adhesion reformation.[24,25] In a prospectively randomized multicenter clinical study, Franklin et al.[24] showed that following the surgical treatment of ovarian defects, Interceed reduced adhesions by 75.36% versus 53.3% for the contra lateral control. Similarly, in a multicenter clinical study conducted in Sweden by Larsson et al,[25] Interceed was found to reduce the adhesion scores by 48% when compared to control side.

Gore-Tex is a nonabsorbable, nonreactive surgical membrane that has been extensively used for repair and reconstruction of the pericardium or peritoneum.[26] Animal studies demonstrated that the Gore-Tex surgical membrane was effective in reducing primary adhesions after pelvic injuries.[27] In a recent multicenter pilot

Table 19.2. Historical perspective of peritoneal adhesions.

1. Peritoneal defects in dogs heal mostly without adhesions. (Von Dembrowski T. Arch Klin Chir 1898; 37:745); (Franz K. Geburtshilfe Gynaekol 1902;47:64)
2. Ischemia is a major etiologic factor in adhesion formation. (Benzi and Boeri. Berl Klin Wochenschr 1903;40:773)
3. Oversewing serosal defects increases rather than decreases adhesion formation. (Thomas J. et al. Proc Soc Exp Biol Med 1950;74:497)
4. Excision of parietal peritoneum from rats resulted in healing without adhesion formation in 52/58 experiments. But "meticulous" repair of peritoneal defects resulted in fibrinous adhesions in 16/19 experiments. (Ellis H. Surg Gynecol Obstet 1971,133:497)
5. The combination of tissue drying and bleeding is a major promoter of adhesion formation. (Ryan et al. Amer J Path 1971;65:117-148)
6. Postoperative adhesion formation and reformation occur more frequently when surgery is performed by laparotomy than by laparoscopy. (Luciano et al.[11])

Table 19.3. Adjuvants proposed to minimize postoperative adhesions.

Agent	Action
Corticosteroids/antihistamines	Inhibit fibroblast migration, stabilize lysosomal membranes, decrease vascular permeability, and antagonize effects of histamine
Antibiotics	Reduce risk of infections
Nonsteroidal, anti-inflammatory agents	Decrease foreign body reaction
Dextran-70 (Hyskon)	Induces hydroflotation of peritoneal organs by drawing fluid into peritoneal cavity and reducing adherence between peritoneal structures
Surgical membranes	Separeate interposing peritoneal surfaces

study, Gore-Tex membrane was applied over the raw surface of the peritoneal wall or uterus after adhesiolysis or myomectomy by laparotomy. At second-look laparoscopy, when the surgical membrane was removed, the mean postoperative adhesion score had been reduced from 10.1 to .8 ($P < .001$).[27]

These preliminary studies suggest that membrane barriers are effective in reducing postoperative adhesions. If further studies substantiate these claims, we may finally approach adhesion-free surgery.

Laparoscopic Adhesiolysis

For adequate laparoscopic adhesiolysis, a three- or four-puncture technique is required in most cases; the intraumbilical incision for the operative laparoscope and two suprapubic punctures, one on either quadrant. Four punctures are occasionally required.

Atraumatic grasping forceps are placed through the suprapubic port on the side of the assistant to grasp the adhesion and stretch it in order to identify its boundaries and avascular planes (Fig. 19.1). The opposite suprapubic port, on the side of the surgeon, should be used either for microscissors for cutting or for the irrigator-aspirator to serve as a manipulator or as a backstop when the laser is used.

Adhesions should be cut close to the affected organ at both ends and totally removed whenever possible. Vascular adhesions can be coagulated and ablated simultaneously with either lasers or microelectrodes. When scissors are used, filmy and avascular adhesions can be stretched and cut (Fig. 19.2). When separating thick, vascular adhesions, it is best to coagulate (Fig. 19.3) and then cut (Fig. 19.4).

We recommend a systematic approach: first, sever bowel adhesions; then, perform adhesiolysis of the ovaries; and, finally, free the fallopian tubes. This

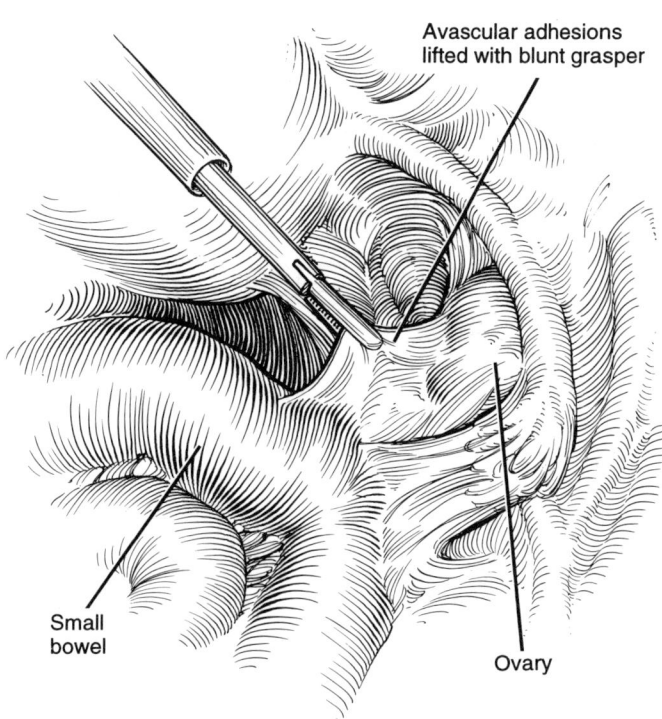

Avascular adhesions
lifted with blunt grasper

Small
bowel

Ovary

Figure 19.1. Avascular adhesions between small bowel and right adnexa are stretched before dissection with scissors.

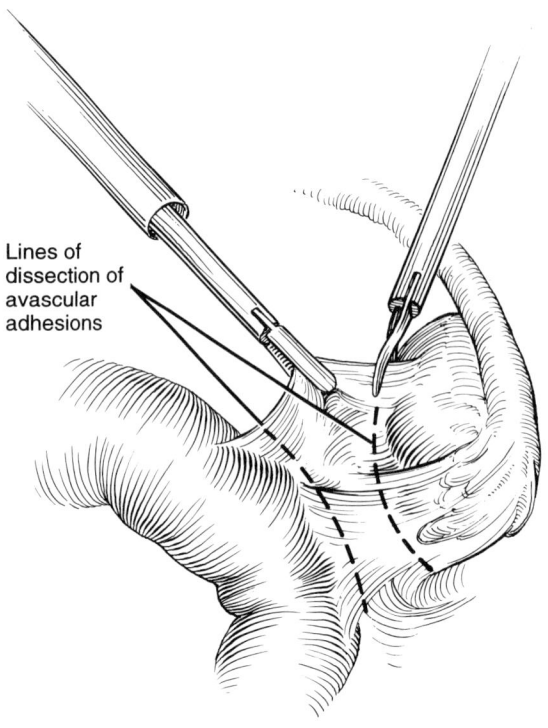

Lines of
dissection of
avascular
adhesions

Figure 19.2. Avascular adhesions are dissected with scissors.

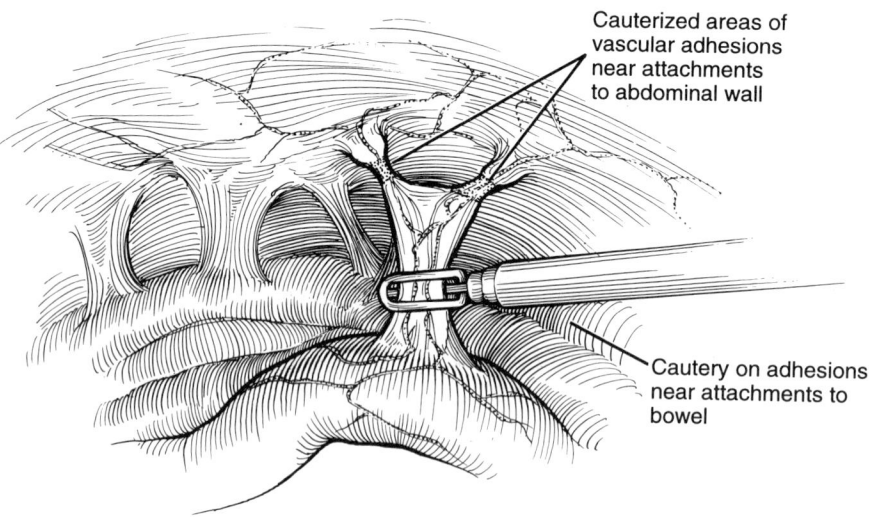

Cauterized areas of
vascular adhesions
near attachments
to abdominal wall

Cautery on adhesions
near attachments to
bowel

Figure 19.3. Thick, vascular adhesions are coagulated before dissection.

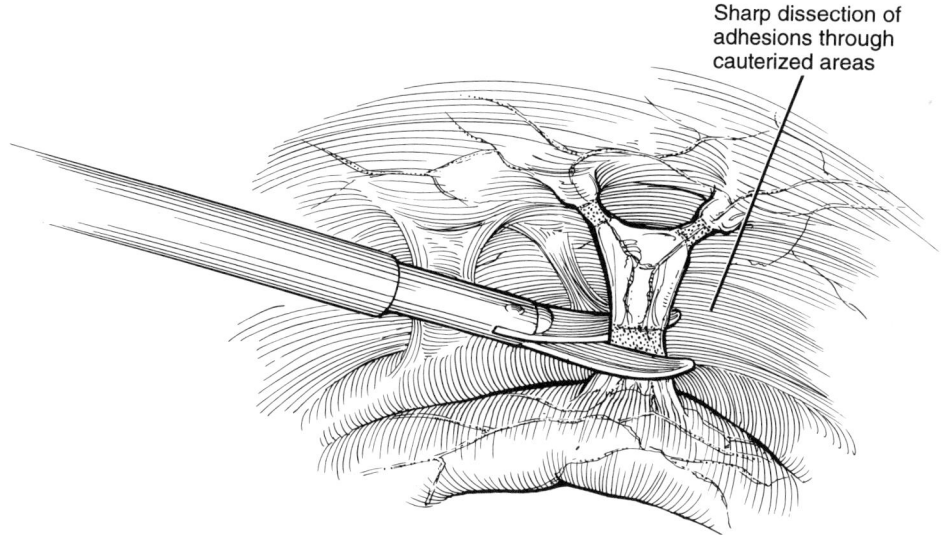

Sharp dissection of adhesions through cauterized areas

Figure 19.4. A coagulated vascular adhesion is lysed with scissors.

approach allows for progressive exposure of the pelvic structures as the surgery unfolds. Once the bowel is freed from adjacent structures, it can be gently pushed cephalad, away from the operative field, allowing for subsequent exposure of the uterus, ovaries, tubes, and cul-de-sac. The ovaries are freed from the pelvic sidewall or from the broad ligament. Grasping forceps are used for applying traction on the ovary, tube, bowel, and abdominal wall so that a plane of dissection can be identified and cut.

Bleeders are immediately coagulated with laser or bipolar energy so that vision is never compromised by a bloody operative field. Whenever possible, to reduce ovarian tissue trauma, grasp either the adhesions or ovarian ligaments instead of the ovarian cortex. Once the ovaries are lifted from the cul-de-sac and completely freed, the ipsilateral fallopian tube is relieved of adhesions throughout its length.

Adhesions can be effectively coagulated and incised with CO_2 laser, superpulse (40 W), ultrapulse (20–80 W and 25–200 mJ), fiber laser (15–25 W) or microelectrode (15–20 W) cutting mode. When there are dense adhesions between different organs (bowel and uterus, ovaries, pelvic sidewall, and anterior abdominal wall), hydrodissection is useful in creating tissue planes before dissection.

Because enterotomies may occur during enterolysis, patients who have a history of laparotomy or severe endometriosis should undergo bowel preparation. Enterorrhaphy may be accomplished by an experienced endoscopist. We use a 1 layer closure of 5-0 polyglactin (Vicryl, Ethicon) or an Endoloop. The integrity of the closure is checked under fluid by looking for air bubbles.[28]

Once the pelvic structures are freed and hemostasis is achieved, the cul-de-sac is filled with lactated Ringer's solution and the adnexae are allowed to float in the clear fluid (Fig. 19.5).[29] Filmy adhesions, which are usually difficult to identify on the surface of the ovary, will be clearly visible, because they float away from the ovarian cortex in the solution. These adhesions can now be grasped with the forceps and sharply cut and removed from their attachments, preferably using laparoscopic microscissors. Since these adhesions are generally filmy and avascular, the coagulating properties of electricity or lasers are not required. Under fluid, microsurgical adhesiolysis with sharp scissors can be precise, effective, and totally atraumatic, since only the floating filmy adhesions will be grasped and resected.

Fimbrioplasty, where the fimbrial folds are agglutinated by fine avascular adhesions without tubal obstruction, is best performed under fluid. As the fimbrial folds float and disperse in the water, the adhesions between them become clearly visible and are grasped, stretched, and sharply cut with fine scissors or ultrapulse laser. The nonultrapulse laser beam delivered through the laparoscope is at least 1 mm in diameter, which is too wide for these narrow bands of adhesions and frequently injures the involved fimbrial folds. Similar thermal damage may be inflicted with electricity and, to a greater extent, with the fiber laser (Nd:YAG, KTP, or argon). Thus, for the most delicate microscopic procedures of fimbriolysis and salpingo-ovariolysis, the microscissors or ultrapulse laser are best. After adhesiolysis, pregnancy rates vary according to the extent of adnexal damage and, to a lesser degree, according to the severity of the adhesions.[2,3,12,30]

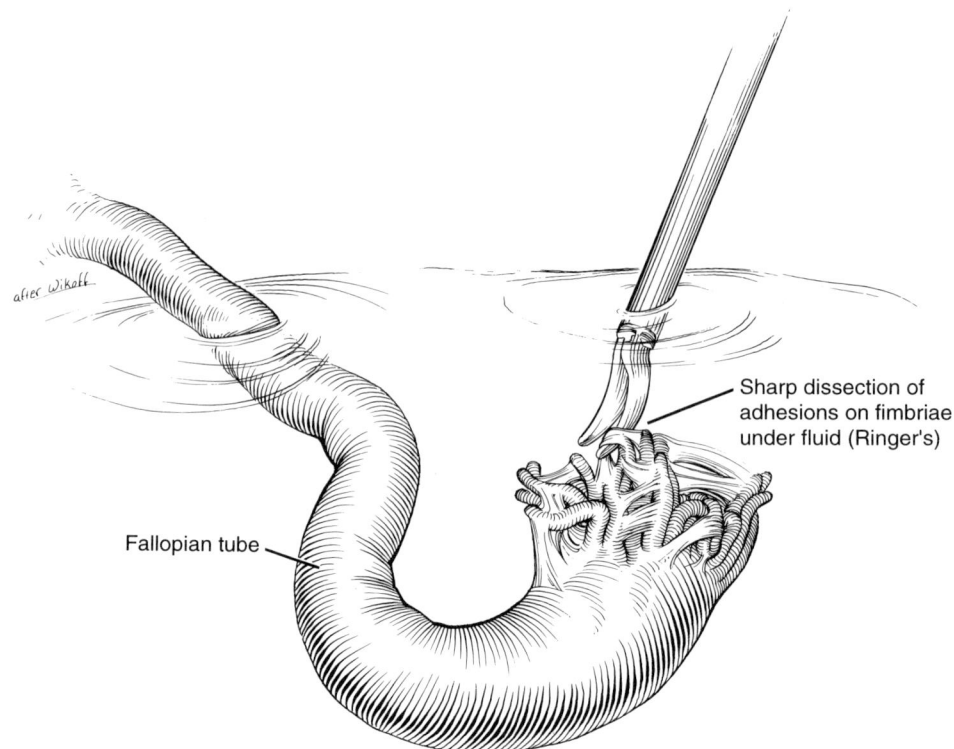

after Wikoff

Sharp dissection of
adhesions on fimbriae
under fluid (Ringer's)

Fallopian tube

Figure 19.5. Hydroflotation of the tube and fimbria permits detection and removal of filmy adhesions.

Conclusion

Postoperative adhesions continue to plague reproductive surgeons. Although progress has been made toward understanding the pathophysiology of postoperative adhesion formation, efforts at prevention have not eliminated the problem. Until we discover the ideal adjuvant, which should prevent adhesions without impeding healing or inducing adverse effects, we rely on "time-honored" microsurgical principles. Recent data from both animal studies and clinical reports indicate operative laparoscopy is more effective than laparotomy in reducing peritoneal adhesion formation and reformation.[11-14] When possible, adhesiolysis is best performed by laparoscopy.

References

1. diZerega GSD, Holtz G. Cause and prevention of post-surgical pelvic adhesions. In Osofsky H, ed. Advances in Clinical Obstetrics and Gynecology. Baltimore, Williams & Wilkins, MD, 1982, pp 277–289.
2. Caspi E, Halperin Y, Bukovski I. The importance of periadnexal adhesions in tubal reconstruction surgery for infertility. Fertil Steril 1979;31:296–300.
3. Hulka JF. Adnexal adhesions: a prognostic staging and classification system based on a five year survey of fertility surgery results at Chapel Hill, North Carolina. Am J Obstet Gynecol 1982;144:141–145.
4. Diamond MP, Daniell SF, Feste J, et al. Adhesion reformation and de novo formation after reproductive pelvic surgery. Fertil Steril 1987;47:864–866.
5. Trimbos-Kemper TCM, Trimbos JB, van Hall EV. Adhesion formation after tubal surgery: results of the 8 day laparoscopy in 188 patients. Fertil Steril 1985;43:395–400.
6. Gomel V, McComb P. Microsurgery in gynecology. In Silver JS, ed. Microsurgery. Baltimore, Williams & Wilkins, MD, 1979, pp 143–183.
7. Luciano AA, Whitman G, Maier DB, et al. A comparison of thermal injury, healing patterns, and postoperative adhesion formation following CO_2 laser and electromicrosurgery. Fertil Steril 1987;48:1025–1029.
8. Tulandi T. Salpingo-ovariolysis: a comparison between laser surgery and electrosurgery. Fertil Steril 1986;45:489.
9. Nezhat C, Nezhat F. Laparoscopic management of appendectomy, myomectomy, endometriosis of the rectovaginal spectrum and presacral neurectomy. In Soderstrom RM, ed. Operative Laparoscopy—The Master's Techniques. New York, Raven Press, 1993, pp 143–150.
10. Nezhat C, Nezhat F, Nezhat CH. Operative laparosacopy (minimaly invasion surgery): state of the art. J Gynecol Surg 1992;8:111.
11. Luciano AA, Maier DB, Koch EL, et al. A comparative study of postoperative adhesions following laser surgery by laparoascopy versus laparotomy in the rabbit model. Obstet Gynecol 1989;74:220–224.
12. Nezhat C, Metzger MD, Nezhat F, et al. Adhesion formation following reproductive surgery by videolaseroscopy. Fertil Steril 1990;53:1008–1011.
13. Operative laparoscopy study group. Postoperative adhesion development after operative laparoscopy: evaluation

at early second-look procedures. Fertil Steril 1991;55: 700–704.

14. Lundorff P, Hahlin M, Kallfelt B, et al. Adhesion formation after laparoscopic surgery in tubal pregnancy: a randomized trial versus laparotomy. Fertil Steril 1991; 55:911–915.

15. Jansen BPS. Failure of intraperitoneal adjuncts to improve the outcome of pelvic operations in young women. Am J Obstet Gynecol 1983;363–371.

16. Luciano AA, Hauser KS, Benda J. Evaluation of commonly used adjuvants in the prevention of postoperative adhesions. Am J Obstet Gynecol 1983;146:88–92.

17. Rosenberg SM, Board JA. High molecular weight dextran in human fertility surgery. Am J Obstet Gynecol 1984; 148:380–384.

18. diZerega GS, et al. Reduction of postoperative pelvic adhesions with intraperitoneal 32% dextran 70: a prospective randomized clinical trial. Fertil Steril 1983;40: 612–619.

19. Borten M, Seibert CP, Taymor ML. Recurrent anaphylactic reaction to intraperitoneal dextran 75 used for prevention of postsurgical adhesions. Obstet Gynecol 1983;61:755–757.

20. Interceed (TC7) Barrier Adhesion Study Group. Prevention of postsurgical adhesions by Interceed (TC7), an absorbable adhesion barrier: a prospective randomized multicenter clinical study. Fertil Steril 1989;51:933–938.

21. Sekiba K & the obstetrics & gynecology adhesion prevention committee. Use of Interceed (TC7) absorbable adhesion barrier to reduce postoperative adhesion reformation in infertility and endometriosis surgery. Obstet Gynecol 1992;79:518–522.

22. Pagidas K, Tulandi T. Effects of Ringer's lactate, Interceed (TC7) and Gore-Tex surgical membrane on PST surgical adhesion formation. Fertil Steril 1992;57:199.

23. Haney AF, Doty E. Murine peritoneal injury and de novo adhesion formation caused by oxidized-regenerated cellulose (Interceed*[TC7]) but not expanded polytetrafluoroethylene (Gore-Tex* surgical membrane). Fertil Steril 1992;57:202.

24. Franklin R, Jansen R, Larsson B, et al. A multicenter clinical evaluation of interceed (TC7) absorbable adhesion barrier in the treatment of ovarian defects. American Fertility Society Annual Meeting, Montreal Canada, 1993, abstract O-063, supplement S31.

25. Larsson B, Thorburn BJ, Hogsetk, et al. Beneficially Effects of Interceed (TC7) as adjuvant therapy and prevention of postoperative adhesions on ovaries and oviducts in microsurgical operations for fertility. American Fertility Society Annual Meeting, Montreal Canada, 1993, Abstract 172, supplement S159.

26. Minale C, Nikol S, Hollweg G, et al. Clinical experience with expanded polytetrafluoroethylene Gore-Tex surgical membrane for pericardial closure: a study of 110 cases. J Cardiac Surg 1988;3:193–201.

27. Boyers SP, Diamond MP, DeCherney AH. Reduction of postoperative pelvic adhesions in the rabbit with Gore-Tex surgical membrane. Fertil Steril 1988;49:1066–1070.

28. Nezhat C, Nezhat F, Ambroze W, et al. Laparoscopic repair of small bowel, colon, and rectal endometriosis: a report of twenty-six cases. Surg Endosc 1993;7:88–89.

29. Nezhat F, Winer WK, Nezhat C. Fimbrioscopy and salpingoscopy in patients with minimal to moderate pelvic endometriosis. Obstetrics & Gynecology 1990; 75.

30. Donnez J, Casanas-Roux F. Prognostic factors of fimbrial surgery. Fertil Steril 1986;45:778–782.

Addendum: The Effect of INTERCEED® (TC7) Absorbable Adhesion Barrier on the Development of Adhesions in Patients With Endometriosis

D.M. Wiseman, H.J. Van Geldorp, M.G. Marks, and M.P. Diamond

Endometriosis and the creation of peritoneal trauma, for example in the removal of endometriotic lesions, are widely regarded as causes of peritoneal adhesions. The general pathologic mechanism underlying the formation of adhesions centers around traumatization of the peritoneum, generation of peritoneal inflammation, and compromise of peritoneal fibrinolytic activity.[1-3]

Some attention has been paid recently to characterization of the inflammatory response in patients with endometriosis.[4] However, other than the obvious connection between peritoneal inflammation and adhesions, surprisingly little attention has been paid to the specific pathophysiology of adhesion formation in patients with, or at sites of, endometriosis. Furthermore there has been no evaluation of the relationship between the severity of endometriosis and adhesion formation. In fact, most patients with Stage III or IV endometriosis must have adhesions in order to obtain a score high enough to meet the criteria set by the AFS.[5]

Implicit in a recently proposed classification of adhesions[6] is that differences in the mechanism of adhesion formation exist between de novo and reformed adhesions, both at sites of surgical injury and sites of injury (such as endometriosis). In this regard, answers to two questions might help us improve the surgical outcome for surgical treatment of endometriosis by reducing adhesion formation: Does the presence or severity of endometriosis influence the incidence or extent of adhesions? and Does the presence or severity of endometriosis influence the efficacy of adhesion prevention agents?

Although no data have been collected prospectively, several studies contain data that may help answer these questions by providing the basis for clinical hypotheses. This addendum will be limited to reviewing these studies for a specific adhesion prevention agent, INTERCEED® (TC7) Absorbable Adhesion Barrier. However, before assessing the influence of endometriosis, it is important to understand the clinical efficacy of INTERCEED Barrier, whether endometriosis is present or not.

Clinical Efficacy of INTERCEED Barrier

INTERCEED, a physical barrier composed of oxidized regenerated cellulose (Johnson & Johnson Medical, Inc., Arlington, Texas) has been shown to reduce the formation or reformation of pelvic adhesions in eight clinical studies.[7-14] Six of these studies were controlled and included patients with endometriosis,[7-12] one study specifically excluded patients with endometriosis,[13] and one study lacked an untreated control and did not describe the patient population.[14] These clinical studies show consistently that INTERCEED Barrier reduces the incidence of postoperative adhesions compared to the contralateral untreated control side (Table A.1). In virtually all cases the number of surgical sites treated with INTERCEED Barrier that are adhesion free at a second look observation (~50%) is approximately double the number (~25%) of adhesion free surgical sites not treated with INTERCEED Barrier. The consistency of these clinical data contrasts with data from animal studies that show INTERCEED Barrier is both effective[14-19] and ineffective[20-24] at preventing adhesions; this contrast further illustrates that conclusions concerning the efficacy of adhesion adjuvants should be based on clinical trials.

Two of these clinical studies[8,11] included enough patients with a primary diagnosis of endometriosis to permit post hoc analysis for the purpose of formulating

Table A.1. Clinical studies with INTERCEED Barrier.

Investigator	N	Surgical region	Adhesion-free untreated control (%)	Adhesion-free INTERCEED (%)
Azziz et al.[7]	134	Sidewall	24	51
Sekiba et al.[8]	63	Sidewall	24	59
Franklin et al.[9]	55	Ovary	25	47
Li & Cooke[10]	27	Pelvic Peritoneum	33*	48*
Van Geldorp[11]	20	Ovary	15	30
Keckstein et al.[12]	17	Ovary (laparoscopy)	35	76
Larsson et al.[13]	66	Ovary, Fimbria, Tubes	29*	52*

*Adhesion-free results based specifically on sites of adhesiolysis. Results for all other studies based on entire surgical region.

Table A.2. The reduction of sidewall adhesions by INTERCEED Barrier in patients with severe endometriosis.

Group	N	Sidewalls adhesion-free at second look (%)		Reduction in extent of adhesions (mean ± SEM) (%)	
		Control	INTERCEED	Control	INTERCEED
Patients with severe endometriosis (AFS Class III/IV)	28	18*	50	34 ± 8	73 ± 8**
Patients with no endometriosis	31	29*	61	49 ± 8	86 ± 8**

*Differences between control and INTERCEED were statistically significant (chi-square, $p < 0.05$).
**Differences between control and INTERCEED were statistically significant (paired t test, $p < 0.05$).
From Sekiba et al.[8]

further hypotheses about adhesions in patients with endometriosis and the action of INTERCEED Barrier therein; these analyses are described below.

Effect of INTERCEED Barrier When Placed on Sidewalls of Patients With Severe Bilateral Endometriosis. Sekiba et al.[8] reported the results of a study in which 63 patients from 12 investigational centers in Japan were randomized to receive INTERCEED Barrier on one sidewall, and no treatment on the contralateral sidewall, after the lysis of sidewall adhesions at laparotomy. The initial area of adhesions was expressed as the area of deperitonealization at laparotomy after completion of adhesiolysis. At second look, laparoscopy 10 days to 14 weeks later, the presence or absence of adhesions was noted, and the area of adhesions was measured using a calibrated probe. For each sidewall, the percent reduction in the extent of adhesions was calculated as

$$100 \times \frac{(\text{deperitonealized area at laparotomy} - \text{area of adhesions at laparoscopy})}{\text{deperitonealized area at laparotomy}}.$$

The reductions in adhesions for treated and untreated sidewalls were compared using a paired t test.

Of the 63 patients in this study, 32 patients had bilateral endometriosis and 31 patients had no endometriosis. The severity of endometriosis, classified according to the revised AFS classification was: Class I, 2 patients; Class II, 2 patients; Class III, 8 patients; Class IV, 20 patients. This permitted a post hoc analysis of the results for two main study populations: those patients ($n = 28$) with severe endometriosis (AFS III or IV) and those patients ($n = 31$) with no endometriosis (Table A.2). The number of patients with endometriosis of Class I or II was too small ($n = 4$) to permit analysis.

Does the presence or severity of endometriosis influence the incidence or extent of adhesions? Although not statistically significant ($p > 0.15$ at $\alpha = 0.05$, power to detect difference $= 0.23$), a greater percentage of patients with no endometriosis tended to have a lower incidence of adhesions at second look laparoscopy compared to those with severe endometriosis, regardless of treatment (INTERCEED Barrier or untreated control). When considering reduction in the extent of adhesions, patients

Table A.3. Extent of ovarian adhesions in patients with bilateral endometriosis.

Treatment	Deperitonealized ovarian area (cm²) (mean ± SEM)		Mean reduction*	Mean reduction (%)**
	Laparotomy	Laparoscopy		
INTERCEED	2.60 ± 0.41	0.86 ± 0.46	1.75 ± 0.46	66.9
Control	2.25 ± 0.38	3.04 ± 0.57	−0.78 ± 0.35	−35.1
Difference	0.35 ± 0.36+	−2.18 ± 0.41	2.54 ± 0.57^	

*Defined as the mean of reductions for each patient.
**Defined as [(area at laparotomy) − (area at laparoscopy)]/(area at laparotomy).
+$p = 0.16$, paired t test.
^$p < 0.001$, paired t test.
From Van Geldorp.[11]

Table A.4. Severity of ovarian adhesions in patients with bilateral endometriomas.

Severity	Laparotomy		Laparoscopy	
	Control	INTERCEED*	Control	INTERCEED**
None	2	2	3	6
Filmy	2	2	2	6
Organized	9	8	9	2
Severe	1	2	0	0

*p = 0.942, chi-square, vs. control.
**p = 0.024, chi-square, vs. control.
From Van Geldorp.[11]

with no endometriosis tended to have a greater percent reduction compared to those with severe endometriosis, regardless of treatment.

Does the presence or severity of endometriosis influence the efficacy of adhesion prevention agents? Regardless of the presence or absence of endometriosis, the number of adhesion-free pelvic sidewalls at second look for INTERCEED Barrier was at least twice the number of the untreated control. When assessing the effects of treatment on the reduction in the extent of adhesions, there was a greater percent reduction when INTERCEED Barrier was used, although the percent reduction was greater in patients with no endometriosis. Baseline data for this parameter were not reported so as to permit a quantitative comparison. No significant difference was identified comparing efficacy of INTERCEED Barrier in patients with severe endometriosis from those with no endometriosis. This result for pelvic sidewalls is consistent with studies in the same or other surgical regions.[7,9-13]

Effect of INTERCEED Barrier When Placed on Ovaries of Patients After Removal of Bilateral Endometriomas. A study was reported recently by Van Geldorp[11] in which 20 patients underwent ovarian surgery. INTERCEED Barrier was randomly assigned to one of the two ovaries. Of the 20 patients, 14 had bilateral endometriomas, permitting a subgroup analysis. At second look laparoscopy, the extent of ovarian adhesions was assessed by measuring the raw serosal area after adhesiolysis (Table A.3). The severity of adhesions was also assessed (Table A.4).

Does the presence or severity of endometriosis influence the incidence or extent of adhesions? The number of patients without endometriosis was insufficiently large to permit comparisons to be made. Does the presence or severity of endometriosis influence the efficacy of adhesion prevention agents? Ovaries treated with INTERCEED Barrier formed adhesions less extensively and of lesser severity than those left untreated. There is a reduction in the incidence of adhesions, although not statistically significant, compared with the untreated control.

These data are qualitatively similar to those found by

Franklin et al.,[9] who used an almost identical protocol, except of the 55 patients, only 28% of them had a secondary diagnosis of endometriosis. The data are also qualitatively similar to those obtained by Larsson et al.,[13] who specifically excluded patients with endometriosis from their study of 66 patients.

Discussion

A retrospective analysis in one study[8] gives evidence of a slight trend towards increased adhesion reformation in patients with severe endometriosis undergoing adhesiolysis. This must be confirmed by a controlled prospective study in which the relationship between the site of adhesiolysis, and the severity and site of endometriosis are well defined.

There is some debate as to whether the pathologic processes present in Stage I or II endometriotic lesions represent a more active inflammatory process than exists in Stages III or IV. Because it has been argued that it is more of a challenge for an adhesion barrier to reduce adhesion formation at ablated sites of Stage I or II endometriosis, further studies are warranted to determine the role of adhesion barriers in these settings.

Conclusion

Further studies are needed to establish whether endometriosis influences the extent or incidence of adhesions, any more than other pathologies. However, regardless of the presence of endometriosis, INTERCEED Barrier is able to reduce the formation of surgical adhesions.

References

1. Jansen RPS. Prevention of peritoneal adhesions. Curr Opin Obstet Gynecol 1991;3:369.
2. Grainger DA. Incidence and causes of pelvic adhesions. Infertil Reprod Med Clin North Am 1994;5:391.
3. Rodgers K. Pathophysiology of adhesion formation. Infertil Reprod Med Clin North Am 1994;5:413.
4. Haney AF. Endometriosis, macrophages and adhesions. Prog Clin Biol Res 1993;381:19.

5. The American Fertility Society. Revised American Fertility Society classification of endometriosis: 1985. Fertil Steril 1985;43;351.

6. Diamond MP, Nezhat F. Adhesions after resection of ovarian endometriomas. Fertil Steril 1993;59:934–935; discussion 935–936.

7. Azziz R, INTERCEED(TC7) Adhesion Barrier Study Group II. Microsurgery alone or with Interceed absorbable adhesion barrier for pelvic sidewall adhesion re-formation. Surg Gyn Obst 1993;177:135.

8. Sekiba K, Obstetrics and Gynecology Adhesion Prevention Committee. Use of Interceed (TC7) absorbable adhesion barrier to reduce postoperative adhesion reformation in infertility and endometriosis surgery. Obstet Gynecol 1992; 79:518.

9. Franklin R, Jansen R, et al. A multicenter clinical evaluation of Interceed® absorbable adhesion barrier in the treatment of ovarian defects. Fertil Steril 1993;Suppl:31S.

10. Li TC, Cooke ID. The value of an absorbable adhesion barrier, Interceed®, in the prevention of adhesion reformation following microsurgical adhesiolysis. Br J Obstet Gynecol 1994;101:335.

11. Van Geldorp H. Interceed® absorbable adhesion barrier reduces the formation of postsurgical adhesions after ovarian surgery. 1994 Annual Meeting of the American Fertility Society, Suppl.: S212.

12. Keckstein J, Karageorgieva E, Roth A, Sasse V, Tuttlies F, Ulrich U. Reduction of postoperative adhesion formation after laparoscopic ovarian cystectomy. Int J Gynecol Obstet 1994;46(Suppl 1):8.

13. Larsson B, Bryman I, et al. Beneficial effect of Interceed (TC7) as adjuvant therapy in prevention of postoperative adhesions on ovaries and oviducts in microsurgical operations. Fertil Steril 1993;Suppl:159S.

14. The Adhesion Barrier Study Group. Prevention of pelvic sidewall adhesion reformation using surgical barriers: expanded-polytetrafluoroethylene (Gore-Tex® surgical membrane) is superior to oxidized regenerated cellulose (Interceed® TC7). 1994 Annual Meeting of the American Fertility Society, Suppl.: S210.

15. Diamond MP, Linsky CB, Cunningham T, et al. Interceed(TC7) as an adjuvant for adhesion reduction: animal studies. Prog Clin Biol Res 1990;358:131–141.

16. Diamond MP, Linsky CB, Cunningham T, et al. Development of a model for sidewall adhesions in the rabbit and their reduction by an absorbable barrier. Microsurgery 1987;8:197–200.

17. Linsky CB, Diamond MP, Cunningham T, et al. Effect of blood on the efficacy of barrier adhesion reduction in the rabbit uterine horn model. Infertility 1988;11:273–280.

18. Linsky CB, Diamond MP, Cunningham T, et al. Adhesion reduction in the rabbit uterine horn model using an absorbable barrier, TC7. J Reprod Med 1987;32:17–20.

19. Montz FJ, Monk BJ, Lacy SM. Effectiveness of two barriers at inhibiting post-radical pelvic surgery adhesions. Gynecol Oncol 1993;48:247–251.

20. Steinleitner A, Lopez G, Suarez M, Lambert H. An evaluation of Flowgel as an intraperitoneal barrier for prevention of postsurgical adhesion reformation. Fertil Steril 1992;57: 305–309.

21. Haney AF, Doty E. Expanded-polytetrafluoroethylene but not oxidized regenerated cellulose prevents adhesion formation and reformation in a mouse uterine horn model of surgical injury. Fertil Steril 1993;60:550–558.

22. Best CL, Rittenhouse D, Sueldo CE. A comparison of TC7 and 32% dextran 70 for prevention of postoperative adhesions in hamsters. Obstet Gynecol 1991;78:858–860.

23. Best CL, Rittenhouse D, Vasquez C, et al. Evaluation of Interceed(TC7) for reduction of postoperative adhesions in rabbits. Fertil Steril 1992;58:817–20.

24. Pagidas K, Tulandi T. Effects of Ringer's lactate, Interceed (TC7) and Gore-Tex Surgical Membrane on postsurgical adhesion formation. Fertil Steril 1992;57:199–201.

25. Maxson WS, Herbert CM, Oldfield EL, and Hill GA. Efficacy of a modified oxidized cellulose fabric in the prevention of adhesion formation. Gynecol Obstet Invest 1988;26: 160–165.

20

Laparoscopy Versus Laparotomy in the Treatment of Endometriosis

Guomundur Arason and Anthony A. Luciano

Although the term endometriosis was first introduced in Sampson's classic publication in 1921, much about this disease remains uncertain.[1] Prevalence, etiology, and pathogenesis are still speculative and symptoms are varied. Although pelvic pain and infertility are the predominant presenting problems, endometriosis frequently produces no symptoms. It is diagnosed in more than 10% of fertile women undergoing sterilization procedures.[2] Since the basic knowledge of its pathophysiology is lacking, therapy remains controversial and, in many cases, palliative. Treatment may be medical, surgical, or both. Surgery may be conservative or radical therapy, and may be performed by open laparotomy or by operative laparoscopy.

Some concerns have been expressed about the adequacy of laparoscopic surgery for endometriosis. Four technical limitations have been mentioned: (1) the lack of depth perception with monocular telescopes and limited resolution of the video camera; (2) operating from a distance may impede the surgeon's ability to carry out fine movements for precise dissection of tissue planes; (3) the inability to palpate tissue in the assessment of the extent and depth of disease; and (4) the limited supply and versatility of endoscopic instruments compared with the microsurgical instruments available for laparotomy. These issues have led some gynecologic surgeons to conclude that "certain difficult microsurgical cases cannot be adequately performed laparoscopically" because of "the inability to safely dissect between tissue planes and the need for improved access to the tissue for atraumatic manipulation and strict adherence to the principles of good surgical technique."[3] However, many of these limitations have been overcome by improved instruments and the high resolution of modern video cameras. Moreover, with extended experience in laparoscopic surgery, "atraumatic ma-

nipulation and strict adherence to the principles of good surgical technique" may be accomplished by laparoscopy as well as by laparotomy.[4]

Since the principal reasons for treating endometriosis are pain and/or infertility, we may define surgical success by the degree of pain resolution or by the attainment of viable pregnancy. Neither of these goals is easy to quantify: pain relief is subjective and may be only temporary; viable pregnancy rates depend on factors difficult to assess and control. Nevertheless, the literature abounds with studies reporting on the therapeutic efficacy of the various surgical approaches to endometriosis for the relief of pain or infertility. Most claim positive results. However, the majority of these studies are retrospective, usually uncontrolled and none randomized.

Endometriosis-Associated Pain

The most common complaint of patients with endometriosis is pain. As a presenting symptom, it is three times more frequent as a complaint than infertility.[5] Furthermore, pain is responsible for a great deal of physical and emotional suffering.[6] Although pain can occur with typical or atypical lesions, superficial or deep implants, and with minimal or extensive disease, the exact mechanism is unknown.[7,8] Intraperitoneal bleeding by endometriotic implants has long been suggested as a cause of pain and adhesions. But, unlike normal endometrium, endometriosis tissue bleeds unpredictably, noncyclically, or not at all, according to its content of estrogen and progesterone receptors, which may differ markedly from those of intrauterine endometrium.[9] Other factors that may be responsible for the pain of endometriosis include paracrine substances secreted by the implants (prostaglandins, interleukins;

peritoneal accumulation of inflammatory cells and debris; location, invasion, and fibrosis of implants; and, finally, the psychosocial makeup of patients.[10] All of these factors may play a role and must be considered in order to develop a better understanding of the patho-physiology of endometriosis-associated pain.

The surgical treatment of endometriosis-associated pain has ranged from complete removal of the reproductive organs to the more conservative approach of resection of implants and associated adhesions to restore the normal anatomic relationship and function of the affected organs. The degree of pain relief seems linked to the extent of extirpative surgery. Hysterectomy and bilateral oophorectomy appears to be the most curative procedure in most cases.[7,8] Less radical surgical procedures are usually palliative and associated with variable recurrence rates of 10% to 40%.[11]

Conservative surgical treatment of endometriosis by laparotomy has been reported to result in complete relief of pain in 49% to 89% of patients. The others experience mild improvement or no change in their symptoms.[8] The addition of presacral neurectomy or uterosacral nerve ablation may yield better results in appropriately selected patients. The efficacy of presacral neurectomy at laparotomy for midline pelvic pain and dysmenorrhea was recently confirmed in a prospectively randomized controlled study.[12] Laparoscopic presacral neurectomy could be extremely useful for patients with central pain.

The conservative management of endometriosis-associated pain by laparoscopy results in complete relief of pain in 25% to 97% of patients which is comparable with the results obtained by laparotomy.[8] In a series of 190 patients with endometriosis treated by video-laseroscopy, Nezhat and co-workers reported total pain relief in 97% of patients at one month and 82% of patients at 12 months after surgery.[13]

To determine the long-term outcome after laparoscopic excision of endometriosis, Redwine used life-table analysis in the follow-up of 359 patients whose endometriosis (including deeply invasive disease) was completely excised laparoscopically, without using adjunctive medical therapy.[14] The cumulative rate of recurrent or persistent disease was 19% in the fifth postoperative year, which is identical with the five-year recurrence rate reported by Wheeler and Malinak after conservative excision of endometriosis by laparotomy.[15]

The results of studies to date, albeit uncontrolled and retrospective, suggest surgery is moderately effective for the treatment of endometriosis-associated pain. The recurrence rate approaches 20% by 5 years after treatment, regardless of surgical approach. Therefore, it appears that the results from laparotomy and laparoscopy are identical in the treatment of endometriosis-associated pain.

Endometriosis-Associated Infertility

The relationship between endometriosis and infertility is complex and poorly understood. The disease is encountered in some form in 25% of infertile women and 60% of women with endometriosis suffer from infertility.[16] In a study from the Mayo Clinic, endometriosis was found at laparoscopy in 21% of infertile women, but in only 2% of fertile controls.[16] The disease was also more severe in the infertile group. These observations led the authors to conclude that the risk of infertility is 20 times greater in women with endometriosis than in those without it.[17] Jansen reported that in women undergoing artificial insemination by donor, the cycle fecundity rate was 2% in women with endometriosis versus 12% in women without endometriosis.[18] Thus, women with endometriosis take considerably longer to conceive. However, many women with endometriosis achieve pregnancy and never perceive that they have any gynecologic disease or fertility problem.[2,16]

In the more severe cases of endometriosis, with extensive pelvic adhesions that distort the normal anatomy and limit ovarian and tubal mobility, the mechanism of infertility can easily be imagined as a compromise in ovum pickup and gamete transfer. Many infertile patients, however, have relatively mild endometriosis with neither alterations of the pelvic anatomy nor compromise of tubo-ovarian mobility. In such patients, their infertility is more difficult to explain, and the indications for therapy are not readily apparent. Although some studies have suggested that therapy for mild endometriosis may not be necessary, others have noted that conception seems to improve after surgical therapy.[16] Some have reported fertility rates of up to 70% after surgery.[19-23] Moreover, progression of disease is greater in untreated (64%) than in treated (25%) patients.[24] Therefore, most clinicians treat infertile patients who have minimal or mild disease.[19-23]

A variety of mechanisms have been suggested to explain endometriosis-associated infertility; prostaglandin-induced tubal and ovulatory dysfunction, spontaneous abortion, luteinized unruptured follicle syndrome, alterations in the immune system, and intraperitoneal inflammation.[16] Although all of these mechanisms emphasize different pathophysiologic events, they all rely on the presence of ectopic endometrial implants as the basis for the infertility. Therefore, eradication of implants should restore fertility to normal.

Because medical treatment does not eradicate endometriosis, the traditional treatment has been surgery by laparotomy.[25-27] The concomitant development of improved endoscopic instruments, optics, and video systems has allowed the gynecologic surgeon to perform progressively more complex operative procedures via laser laparoscopy for the treatment of pelvic disease.[19-23] This ever expanding use of operative laparoscopy in gynecologic surgery is justified by its acknowledged advantages of convenience, quick recovery, and supposed cost savings. But the most important goals of reconstructive pelvic surgery, results and success rates, have not been adequately addressed in the published clinical studies.

The clinical results of surgical treatment of endometriosis have been reported as crude pregnancy rates with variable length of patient follow-up in their study population. Since pregnancy rates increase with length of follow-up, it is easy to improve pregnancy rates by merely extending the study period. The monthly fecundity rate (MFR), however, describes a woman's chances of conceiving in one month. Although the MFR removes some of the bias of the follow-up period, it has drawbacks. Its underlying assumption, that the monthly probability of getting pregnant remains the same throughout the study period, is not true. A woman's chance of conceiving varies markedly with her age, previous fertility history, and with the time spent in attempting conception.[28] Moreover, the chance of pregnancy in previously infertile women is best immediately after completing the therapy and decreases thereafter.[29] This is especially true for infertile women after surgical treatment of their endometriosis.[30] A much better way to assess therapeutic efficacy and compare results from different studies is the use of cumulative pregnancy rates derived from life-table analyses. Unfortunately, few studies have used this statistical tool.

To conclusively assess the therapeutic efficacy of any given regimen, a study must prospectively randomize comparable patients to different treatment arms. The patients in each therapeutic arm should be of about the same age, have the same extent of disease, symptoms, and similar infertility factors. No such "ideal" study has yet been published for endometriosis-associated infertility. Therefore, existing studies must be considered imperfect if not anecdotal, and the value of their data should be viewed as suggestive and not definitive.

Following conservative surgery for endometriosis by laparotomy, the pregnancy rate is generally related inversely to the severity of disease. When Olive and Haney summarized the results of ten studies, published from 1973 to 1986, on conservative surgery by laparotomy in the treatment of endometriosis-associated infertility, the reported crude pregnancy rates were 60% for mild endometriosis, 50% for moderate, and 39% for severe disease.[16] Similarly, in a recent review of 500 cases of endometriosis-associated infertility, Wheeler and Malinak reported pregnancy rates of 65% in mild, 55% in moderate, and 40% in severe disease.[31]

Unlike the results obtained from laparotomy, where pregnancy rates decrease with severity of disease, pregnancy rates reported after operative laparoscopy are similar for mild, moderate, and severe stages of endometriosis.[19-23,30,33] Olive and Martin reported that laser laparoscopic vaporization of endometriosis is associated with a cumulative pregnancy rate similar to those achieved with laparotomy.[30] In this series of 129 patients, the pregnancy rates were 39% for stage I, 46% for stage II, and 50% for stage III disease. Even more impressive are the results published by Nezhat's group.[20] They reported that of 243 infertile patients with mild to severe disease, 69% became pregnant following treatment via laparoscopy. The pregnancy rates were 72% for stage I, 70% for stage II, 67% for stage III, and 69% for stage IV. These results confirmed those of Olive and Martin: with laser laparoscopy, the pregnancy rates are not inversely related to the severity of disease. Similarly, in a study of 60 patients with stage III (36 patients) and stage IV disease (24 patients), the cumulative pregnancy rates were 71% for each group.[23]

It is possible that, in experienced hands, laparoscopic surgery may be so precise that the disease and associated adhesions can be completely eradicated without inflicting serious trauma to the adjacent structures. The excellent visualization and the easy access to tissue achieved with the laparoscope, even deep in the pelvis, allows the reproductive surgeon to see tissue planes and vascular areas so that endometrial implants can be clearly identified and thoroughly removed, without disturbing adjacent organs. The experienced endoscopic surgeon practices state-of-the-art microsurgery by atraumatically removing diseased tissue while restoring the reproductive organs to their normal anatomic relationship and function. When all identifiable endometriosis and adhesions are removed, near-normal reproductive functions may be expected, regardless of the stage of disease.[20]

At laparotomy, a large abdominal incision is required to gain access to the deep pelvis, which is usually involved with severe cases of endometriosis. Unless magnification is used with loupes or microscope, which is extremely difficult deep in the pelvis and sidewalls, precise dissection of tissue planes and strict adherence to microsurgical principles are nearly impossible. Therefore, conservative surgery for endometriosis by laparotomy is invariably a macro- instead of a microsurgical procedure. Furthermore, it may be bloody and incomplete because of poor visualization and limited access to the pelvic structures. It is not surprising, then, that the results from laparotomy for severe endometriosis are worse than those obtained for less severe disease or from the results obtained when comparably severe disease is treated by laparoscopy.

Table 20.1 lists several studies published in the more recent literature which report crude pregnancy rates

Table 20.1. Pregnancy rates following surgical treatment of endometriosis.

Study	Mild		Moderate*		Severe	
	Cases	Rate	Cases	Rate	Cases	Rate
Laparotomy						
Buttram[26]	88	69%	50	45%	68	47%
Rock et al.[37]	45	62%	88	54%	81	48%
Rantala et al.[38]	44	59%	39	56%	46	30%
Gordts et al.[39]	20	40%	99	42%	47	35%
Olive & Lee[40]	11	45%	43	51%	34	29%
Chong et al.[32]	—	—	—	—	13	54%
Fayez & Collazo[31]	—	—	—	—	42	36%
Adamson et al.[19]	—	—	—	—	52	34%
Total	208	61%	319	50%	383	39%
Laparoscopy						
Feste[41]	47	51%	6	66%	5	40%
Martin et al.[21]	27	26%	19	16%	4	25%
Nezhat et al.[4]	24	75%	51	63%	27	44%
Olive & Martin[30]	59	37%	48	35%	21	52%
Nezhat et al.[20]	39	72%	153	69%	51	69%
Chong et al.[32]	—	—	—	—	11	55%
Fayez & Collazo[31]	—	—	—	—	106	58%
Adamson et al.[19]	—	—	—	—	48	38%
Luciano et al.[23]	—	—	36	61%	24	58%
Total	196	50%	313	59%	297	57%

*Stages II and III of AFS-r classification.

after treatment of endometriosis by either laparotomy or operative laparoscopy. They were performed with different patient populations and surgeons, at different locations and times. Therefore, they cannot be adequately compared and only suggestive conclusion can be drawn from them. Nevertheless, the overall results indicate the transition from laparotomy to operative laparoscopy has not resulted in significant improvements of pregnancy rates, except for the more severe stages of disease.

The study by Fayez and Collazo included two groups of patients treated by operative laparoscopy followed immediately with danazol treatment for four to six months or six to ten weeks.[31] A third group was treated by laparotomy followed immediately with danazol therapy for six to nine months. The laparotomy group underwent uterine suspension, nerve ablative procedures (uterosacral or presacral neurectomy), and suturing of peritoneal defects. These procedures were not performed in the laparoscopy groups. Consequently, although the authors did not specifically state it, laparotomy was more likely to have been chosen for the patients with more severe disease. The same surgeons performed both procedures and they obtained significantly better pregnancy rates in the laparoscopy groups (58%) than the laparotomy group (36%).[31]

Chong and Luciano assessed the relative efficacy of CO_2 laser surgery by laparoscopy versus laparotomy in the treatment of infertile patients with severe endometriosis.[32] They reported mean AFS-r classification scores of 59 and 58 for the laparoscopy and laparotomy

groups, respectively. All laparotomies were performed by Chong, whose expertise is in microlaser surgery by laparotomy. All operative laparoscopies were performed by Luciano, who has extensive experience in endoscopic techniques. Thus, although this study was neither randomized nor controlled and involved two different surgeons, it has value because each surgeon used the technique that he does best. The pregnancy rates were the same for both groups.

In the study by Adamson and co-workers, the results from CO_2 laser laparoscopy were compared with those obtained from laparotomy in the treatment of infertility associated with severe endometriosis.[19] In this study, the authors stated that the indications for laparotomy rather than laparoscopy were: (1) larger endometriomata (>4 cm); (2) significant tubal or fimbrial damage requiring microsurgery; or (3) myomata requiring laparotomy for removal. Thus, the patients in the laparotomy group had more severe disease than the patients in the laparoscopy group. Nevertheless, the crude pregnancy rates and the MFRs were not significantly different for the two groups. Similarly, life-table cumulative pregnancy rates at 1- and 3-year follow-up did not differ significantly between the two groups, being 30% and 52% for the laparoscopy group versus 23% and 46% for the laparotomy group. From these data, we may conclude that in the treatment of endometriosis-associated infertility, comparable results may be expected from laparoscopy or laparotomy, given comparable surgical expertise.[33] For the more severe stages of disease, however, operative laparoscopy appears to yield better pregnancy rates than laparotomy.[30]

Societal and Economic Effect of Laparoscopic Surgery

The generally reported advantages of endoscopic surgery over laparotomy include faster recovery, cost savings, and decreased morbidity.[23,24,35] In 1985, Levine reported an average reduction of 49% in hospital costs when ovarian reconstructive surgery was performed by pelviscopy instead of laparotomy.[34] Brumsted and co-workers, in comparing the treatment of ectopic pregnancy by laparoscopy versus laparotomy, reported shorter periods of convalescence and reduced postoperative analgesia requirements in the patients treated by laparoscopy.[35] The extent of cost savings and reduced recovery time for endometriosis patients treated by laparoscopy has recently been reported.[23] In this 1992 study, hospital cost, hospital stay, and days of convalescence were significantly less for patients with AFS-r stages III and IV endometriosis who underwent laser laparoscopy than for patients treated by laparotomy (Table 20.2).

Table 20.2. Patients with AFS-r stages III and IV endometriosis treated with operative laparoscopy or laparotomy.

	Laparoscopy (Mean ± SD)	Laparotomy (Mean ± SD)
Days in hospital	1.2 ± 0.1	4.2 ± 0.9
Days of convalescence	3.6 ± 1.5	21.4 ± 3.2
Physician charge	$1900 ± 136	$3007 ± 177
Hospital charge	$1821 ± 120	$4068 ± 574

Conclusion

Laparoscopic treatment of endometriosis-associated pain and/or infertility, particularly for moderate and severe disease, gives therapeutic results at least as good as, and in some cases better than, those obtained with laparotomy. As endoscopic surgery use widens and as health-care costs continue to draw attention, it is likely that surgical treatment of endometriosis in the future will be primarily through the laparoscope. Given the high degree of patient acceptance and the decreased morbidity, discomfort, and cost associated with laparoscopic surgery, operative laparoscopy has become a skill necessary for all reproductive surgeons.

References

1. Sampson JA. Perforating hemorrhage (chocolate) cysts of the ovary: their importancee and especially their relation to pelvic adenomas of endometrial type ("adenomyoma" of the uterus, rectovaginal septum, sigmoid, etc.). Arch Surg 1921;3:245.
2. Candiani GB, Vercelli P, Fedele L, et al. Mild endometriosis infertility: a critical review of epidemiologic data, diagnostic pitfalls, and classification limits. Obstet Gynecol Surv 1991;46:490.
3. Cook AS, Rock JA. Role of laparoscopy in the treatment of endometriosis. Fertil Steril 1991;4:663.
4. Nezhat C, Crowgey S, Garrison CP. Surgical treatment of endometriosis via laser laparoscopy. Fertil Steril 1986;45: 778–83.
5. Redwine DB. The distribution of endometriosis in the pelvis by age groups and fertility. Fertil Steril 1987;47: 173.
6. Ballweg ML. Endometriosis: the patient's perspective. Infertil Reprod Med Clin North America, Olive DL (Guest Editor), 1992;3(3):747.
7. Luciano AA, Pitkin RM. Endometriosis, approaches to diagnosis and treatment. Surgery Annual 1984 (Lloyd M. Nyhus, ed.), Norwalk, CT, Appleton-Century-Crofts, 1984, pp 297–312.
8. Redwine DB. Treatment of endometriosis-associated pain. Infertil Reprod Med Clin North America, Olive DL (Guest Editor), 1992;3(3):697.
9. Metzger DA, Olive DL, Haney AF. Limited hormonal responsiveness of ectopic endometrium: histologic correlation with intrauterine endometrium. Hum Pathol 1988;19:1417.
10. Olive DL. Future directions for endometriosis research. Infertil Reprod Med Clin North America, Olive DL (Guest Editor), 1992;3(3):763.
11. Schenken SR, Malinack RL. Reoperation after initial treatment of endometriosis with conservative surgery. Am J Obstet Gynecol 1978;131:416.
12. Tjaden B, Schlaff WD, Kimball A. The efficacy of presacral neurectomy for the relief of midline dysmenorrhea. Obstet Gynecol 1990;76:89.
13. Nezhat C, Nezhat F. A simplified method of laparoscopic presacral neurectomy for the treatment of central pain due to endometriosis. Brit J Obstet Gynecol 1992;99:659.
14. Redwine DB. Conservative laparoscopic excision of endometriosis by sharp dissection: life table analysis of reoperation and persistent or recurrent disease. Fertil Steril 1991;56:628.
15. Wheeler JM, Malinak LR. Recurrent endometriosis. Contrib Gynecol Obstet 1987;16:13.
16. Olive DL, Haney AF. Endometriosis associated infertility: a critical review of therapeutic approaches. Obstetrical and Gynecological Survey 1986;41:538.
17. Strathy JH, Molgaard CA, Coulam CB, et al. Endometriosis and infertility: a laparoscopic study of endometriosis among fertile and infertile women. Fertil Steril 1982;38:667.
18. Jensen RPS. Minimal endometriosis and reduced fecundabililty: Prospective evidence from an artificial insemination by donor program. Fertil Steril 1987;47:40.
19. Adamson DG, Subak LL, Pasta DJ, et al. Comparison of CO_2 laser laparoscopy with laparotomy for the treatment of endometriomata. Fertil Steril 1992;57:965.
20. Nezhat C, Crowgey S, Nezhat F. Videolaseroscopy for the treatment of endometriosis associated infertility. Fertil Steril 1989;51:23.
21. Martin DC. CO_2 laser laparoscopy for the treatment of endometriosis associated with infertility. J Reprod Med 1985;30:409.
22. Dlugi AM, Saleh WA, Jacobsen G. KTP/532 laser laparoscopy in the treatment of endometriosis-associated infertility. Fertil Steril 1992;57:1186.
23. Luciano AA, Lowney J, Jacobs SL. Endoscopic treatment of endometriosis-associated infertility: therapeutic, economic and social benefits. J Reprod Med 1992;37:573.
24. Muhmood TA, Templeton A. The impact of treatment on the natural history of endometriosis. Hum Reprod 1990; 5:965.
25. Luciano AA, Metzger DA. Endometriosis—What can medical therapy offer? Brit J Clin Practice Suppl 72, 1991; 45:14.
26. Buttram VC. Conservative surgery for endometriosis in the infertile female: a study of 206 patients with implications for both medical and surgical therapy. Fertil Steril 1979;31:117.
27. Hammond CB, Rock JA, Parker RT. Conservative treatment of endometriosis: the effects of limited surgery and hormonal pseudopregnancy. Fertil Steril 1976;27:756.
28. Leridon H, Spira A. Problems in measuring the effectiveness of infertility therapy. Fertil Steril 1989;41:58.
29. Wilcox AJ, Weinberg CR, O'Connor JF, et al. Incidence of early pregnancy loss. N Engl J Med 1988;319:189.
30. Olive D, Martin D. Treatment of endometriosis-associated infertility with CO_2 laser laparoscopy: the use of one- and two-parameter exponential models. Fertil Steril 1987; 48:18.
31. Fayes JA, Collazo LM. Comparison between laparotomy and operative laparoscopy in the treatment of moderate and severe endometriosis. Int J Fertil 1990;35:272.
32. Chong AP, Luciano AA, O'Shaughnessy AM. Laser laparoscopy versus laparotomy in the treatment of infertility patients with severe endometriosis. J Gynecol Surg 1990;6:179.

33. Adamson GD, Hurd SJ, Pasta DJ, et al. Laparoscopic endometriosis treatment: is it better. Fertil Steril 1993; 59:35.
34. Levine RL. Economic impact off pelviscopic surgery. J Reprod Med 1985;30:665.
35. Brumstead J, Kessler C, Gibson C. A comparison of laparoscopy and laparotomy for the treatment of ectopic pregnancy. Obstet Gynecol 1988;71:889.
36. DeCherney AH. The leader of the band is tired. Fertil Steril 1985;44:299.
37. Rock JA, Guzick DS, Sengos C, et al. The conservative surgical treatment of endometriosis: Evaluation of pregnancy success with respect to the extent of disease as categorized using contemporary classification systems. Fertil Steril 1981;35:131.
38. Rantala ML, Kahanpaa KV, Koskimies AL, et al. Fertility prognosis after surgical treatment of pelvic endometriosis. Acta Obstet Gynecol Scand 1983;62:11.
39. Gordts S, Boeckx W, Brosens I. Microsurgery of endometriosis in infertile patients. Fertil Steril 1984;42:520.
40. Olive DL, Lee KL. Analysis of sequential treatment protocols for endometriosis associated infertility. Am J Obstet Gynecol 1986;154:613.
41. Feste JR. Laser laparoscopy: a new modality. J Reprod Med 1985;30:413.

21
Operative Laparoscopy: Preventing and Managing Complications

Farr Nezhat, Ceana Nezhat, and Camran Nezhat

The dictum guiding every provider of medical care is that of Hippocrates: first, do no harm. But regardless of the care and caution exercised, complications can occur. An essential prerequisite of proper management is timely recognition of complications. As laparoscopic surgery becomes more commonplace yet more complex, practitioners must be prepared to diagnose and treat complications.

Before the results of large series of advanced operative laparoscopy became available, reports on diagnostic laparoscopy and laparoscopic tubal sterilization served as the yardstick for comparison. Although the overall risk of such procedures is generally low, surgical inexperience, deviation from the standard technique, or performance of complex procedures can all increase the relative risk. Rates of specific major intraoperative and postoperative complications have been reported to be 1% or less (Table 21.1). These figures, however, may underestimate the overall experience nationally because it is based on reports from experienced endoscopists—those with large practices with considerable experience, American Association of Gynecologic Laparoscopists (AAGL) members, and physicians at tertiary referral clinics.[1–4] The actual complication rates of operative laparoscopy in the hands of the average gynecologist is probably higher.

From July 1982 to December 1993 at the Center for Special Pelvic Surgery (CSPS) in Atlanta, Georgia and Stanford University in Palo Alto, California, we performed 6,949 advanced operative laparoscopies with a combined intraoperative and postoperative complication rate of 3.08%.[1] The most common complication was abdominal wall vascular injury (inferior epigastric vessels) (Table 21.2). Intestinal and urinary tract injuries were the second most common complications. Severe adhesions and endometriosis were the main contributing factors for these injuries; most were unavoidable and occurred during the excision and treatment of endometriosis involving the urinary tract and the rectosigmoid colon. Laparotomy was required to manage the complications in only 16 (0.2%) of all patients in the series; most laparotomies occurred early in our experience with operative laparoscopy.

The incidence of complications relates not only to the experience of the laparoscopist but also to the severity of pelvic and abdominal pathology. Adhesions and endometriosis are contributing factors to urinary tract and intestinal injury. Certain complications are not preventable, and laparoscopic surgeons must be prepared to manage them either by laparotomy or laparoscopy. The incidence of conversion to laparotomy to manage complications or complete a procedure tends to be higher early in one's experience.[5] In a study encompassing 17,521 diagnostic and operative procedures performed at seven French centers, an overall complication rate of 3.2 per 1,000 was reported.[6] The rates per 1,000 were .5 and 1.7 for minor operative and diagnostic procedures, and 8.4 and 8.9 for major and advanced operations (Table 21.3). Laparotomies were performed for hemorrhage (17) or visceral injuries (40), which were most common after extensive adhesiolysis and advanced laparoscopic surgery; one fatality was reported.

In the situations we cite, the risk of complication is high. The techniques described should help you avoid, minimize, recognize, and manage these possible complications.

Prevention

At CSPS, we have adopted the well-known dictum "an ounce of prevention is worth a pound of cure." We find

Table 21.1. Major complications of laparoscopic operations.

	Rate per 1000
By instrument	
Verres needle	2.7
Large trocar	2.4–2.7
Accessory trocar	2.5–6.0
Electrocautery	0.5–2.8
Laser	1.2
Pneumoperitoneum	7.4
By site of injury	
Vessels/bleeding	2.6–11.0
Bowel	0.6–2.0
GU	0.6–1.6
Nerve	6.1
Uterine perforation	3.7
Other indicators	
Death	0.05–0.3
Hospitalization >72 h	4.2–27.0
Hospital readmission	3.1–5.0
Persistent beta HCG titers	63.2–144.0
Infection	1.4–6.5
Febrile	2.0

Sources: Peterson et al[3] and Lehmann-Willebrodi et al[4].

this rule as applicable to laparoscopy as to any other field of medicine.

Complications may occur even during the simplest of procedures. Furthermore, they tend to occur when least expected. The endoscopic surgeon, therefore, must always expect complications and be prepared to deal with them promptly. The endoscopic surgeon's most important tools are thorough preoperative evaluation, proper patient selection, and detailed consultation with patients and colleagues. These measures will serve to minimize injury and to prevent possible subsequent legal action.

The responsible endoscopic surgeon must possess a thorough knowledge of normal and abnormal anatomy, understand the disease processes responsible for the patient's condition, and master the instrumentation and energy sources available. Before performing endoscopic

surgery, the neophyte must train under the supervision of a qualified surgeon and make sure that the OR staff has had appropriate training and is equipped to meet the challenges of endoscopic surgery.

Early experience with diagnostic laparoscopy and tubal ligation indicates that expertise of the operator greatly influences the risk of complications. Most complications have occurred during training. The time required to gain sufficient expertise depends on the number of procedures performed. In a study performed in 1973, the complication rate for laparoscopic sterilization was higher among physicians who had performed 100 procedures or less and the rate decreased after 200 operations.[7]

The learning curve of operative laparoscopy differs distinctly from that of mastering the skills necessary for classic laparotomy. Most surgeons acquire their knowledge of laparotomy during residency programs. At present, advanced operative laparoscopic procedures are being learned, and performed, in clinical practice. With few experienced endoscopic surgeons available for teaching, and an increasing number of physicians wishing to attempt laparoscopic procedures, it is crucial that these skills be developed in properly supervised settings. It is also the case that whereas in residency the novice gynecologist learned from "esteemed elders," older surgeons interested in mastering operative laparoscopy may have to learn from and be supervised by younger colleagues, possibly their own former residents.

The learning curve for laparoscopic surgery is long; it has been estimated that it takes four to seven years to acquire sufficient laparoscopic skills for advanced operative procedures.[8] While the risk of complications is greatest early in a surgeon's experience, with the basic technique, it rises again when new procedures are attempted or new pieces of equipment are introduced. Complications associated with operator inexperience

Table 21.2. Summary of complications and method of treatment.

Complication	Vascular		Gastrointestinal		Genitourinary		
	Abdominal wall	Intra abdominal	Small bowel	Large bowel	Bladder	Ureter	Other*
Intraoperative	117	6	22	9	8	3	3
Laparoscopy	116	2	15	8	5	2	0
Minilaparotomy	1	0	3	1	0	0	0
Laparotomy	0	4	4	0	2	0	0
Medical	0	0	0	0	1	1	3
Postoperative	12	5	6	5†	3	1	17
Laparoscopy	6	2	1	1	1	1	3
Laparotomy	1	2	1	3	0	0	3
Medical	5	1	4	1	2	0	12

*Other includes pelvic infection, subcutaneous emphysema, pulmonary edema, incisional hernia, deep vein thrombosis, pleural effusion, vaginal cuff dehiscence and severe dehydration.
†Some patients had a combination of laparoscopy and laparotomy or laparoscopy and medical treatment.

Table 21.3. Complications of gynecologic laparoscopic surgery.

Types of laparoscopies	Laparoscopic Procedures	Laparotomies for complications	Rate per 1000
Diagnostic	4,130	7	1.7
Minor	4,213	2	0.5
Major extensive adhesiolysis	1,910	16	8.4
Advanced	898	8	8.9

Source: Querleu et al.[6]

can be minimized by becoming thoroughly familiar with all equipment, observing and scrubbing with an experienced laparoscopist, and performing procedures under the supervision of an experienced surgeon before doing so independently.

Contraindications

We believe there are few absolute contraindications to operative laparoscopy (Table 21.4). Nevertheless, it is the surgeon's responsibility to recognize the selected cases for which operative laparoscopy is not advisable. An inexperienced laparoscopic surgeon may view some or all of the relative contraindications as absolute. However, there are certain medical conditions that make operative laparoscopy inadvisable, even in the best equipped hospital with the most experienced team. If there is no clear advantage in performing operative laparoscopy, and the possible benefits are overshadowed by possible risks, don't attempt laparoscopy. Generalized peritonitis is a contraindication because the bowel is frequently matted together and adherent to the abdominal wall, and the risk of bowel perforation enhanced. However, if peritonitis is confined to the pelvis, this condition can be appropriately diagnosed and treated laparoscopically. While suspected intraabdominal bleeding due to a ruptured ectopic pregnancy or a bleeding corpus luteum can usually be safely diagnosed and treated at laparoscopy, marked hemoperitoneum in an unstable patient is an indication for laparotomy. If the surgeon presumes (in view of experience, the equipment available, or any other

Table 21.4. Contraindications to laparoscopic surgery.

Absolute
  Generalized peritonitis
  Class IV cardiac disease

Relative
  Large pelvic or abdominal mass > 26 weeks pregnancy
  Intrauterine pregnancy >16 weeks
  Hypovolemic shock
  Intestinal obstruction
  Diaphragmatic hernia
  Chronic pulmonary disease

reason) that the bleeding source will be difficult to locate and treat laparoscopically, laparotomy is preferable.

Intestinal obstruction is often associated with a dilated bowel, which leads to a significantly increased risk of perforation at laparoscopy. The surgeon must keep in mind that intestinal obstruction may be diagnosed noninvasively and may resolve without surgical intervention. If surgical intervention is necessary, it may not be amenable to laparoscopic treatment. Class III cardiac patients may safely undergo short laparoscopic procedures. However, this approach requires a highly skilled anesthesia team experienced in the management of high-risk patients at laparoscopy. Patients with class IV cardiac disease may experience cardiac arrhythmias and irreversible cardiac failure as a result of Trendelenburg positioning. Such risks remain even for relatively short periods and despite proper anesthetic precautions. Attempt laparoscopy in these patients only after carefully considering the possible risks.

Procedural Failure Leading to Complications

Operative laparoscopy instruments and procedures are associated with a variety of complications that may result in mechanical trauma and vascular, electrical, and laser injuries. Meticulous adherence to proper technique in conjunction with appropriate training and operator experience are essential to prevent these complications.

Gomel and co-workers demonstrated that establishing a standardized protocol for laparoscopic tubal ligations led to a tenfold reduction in complications.[9] It is important for each surgeon to develop and adopt a standardized approach to operative laparoscopy and avoid deviating from this protocol unless conditions clearly indicate an alteration is necessary.

Sometimes, laparoscopic surgery needs to be converted to laparotomy. While this is often termed "failed laparoscopy," this step should not be considered a failure. It is better to complete a procedure by laparotomy rather than risk injury to the patient, or be forced to proceed with emergency laparotomy because of a complication. It is valuable to undertake a retrospective evaluation of any case ending in laparotomy so as to assess the adequacy of the presurgical evaluation, the patient informed consent, and the level of surgical skill and anesthetic skill. It is not always possible for surgeons to foresee that certain cases are beyond their laparoscopic capacity. A certain rate of conversion to laparotomy during a laparoscopic procedure is definitely acceptable.

Most major complications of laparoscopy are associated with induction of pneumoperitoneum or trocar insertion. Insertion of the Verres needle and the primary or secondary trocars may be more hazardous in patients who have had previous laparotomies or who are obese or very thin. If the preoperative evaluation shows an increased probability of bowel injury, a complete bowel preparation should be administered prior to laparoscopy. The presence of a large pelvic mass, such as a myomatous uterus or an ovarian cyst, may necessitate changing the insertion sites for the Verres needle and the trocars or converting to laparotomy.

Verres Needle

Though the safety and efficacy of direct trocar insertion have been proven, many operators still prefer the traditional method for induction of pneumoperitoneum, via the Verres needle. This "blind" procedure may cause injury to internal organs or fail to enter the peritoneal cavity. While the needle puncture itself rarely causes serious injury, vascular instillation of CO_2 through the misplaced needle can have serious sequelae.

Preventing Complications

Factors that increase the risk of perforation or laceration from insertion of the Verres needle include bowel adhesions, lateral displacement of the needle during insertion, too steep an insertion angle, or uncontrolled, sudden entry. The patient should be horizontal so that the sacral promontory and sacral curve are identified easily. Premature Trendelenburg positioning should be avoided.

When the Verres needle is inserted in an upper abdominal site, it may puncture the pleural cavity, stomach, liver, or spleen. After prolonged manual ventilation with a mask or difficult endotracheal intubation, the stomach may become distended and displace the transverse colon toward the lower abdomen. In this case, puncture of the stomach may occur, even with umbilical placement, and the probability of intestinal puncture is increased. Placing a nasogastric tube minimizes the risk of gastric distension. Similarly, an overdistended bladder is more prone to injury; a Foley catheter should be routinely placed before the procedure.

Recognizing Problems

Misplacement of the Verres needle is generally not recognized until CO_2 insufflation is attempted, and abnormally high insufflation pressures are encountered, or at the time of laparoscope insertion. Because Verres needle misplacement is not always apparent, it is most important during the initial examination of the pelvis to survey the mid- and upper abdomen for such signs of needle-induced trauma as hematomas, needle punctures, and collections of gas.

Management Strategies

Puncture of a hollow viscus with the Verres needle generally does not require more than a careful examination of the puncture site for bleeding or leakage and through irrigation of the abdominal and pelvic cavity. If no damage is recognized upon examination, the patient can be discharged as scheduled with instructions to consult the physician in case of increasing abdominal pain or fever. If Verres needle puncture results in laceration of a viscus, repair is indicated. The method depends on the organ involved (small or large bowel, bladder, stomach, or major blood vessels), the nature of the fluid leaking, and operator's experience. Though very experienced endoscopists will be able to repair most injuries laparoscopically, those with less endoscopic expertise may prefer immediate laparotomy for repair and adequate irrigation of the abdomen.

Establishing a Pneumoperitoneum

The complications resulting from insufflation of a space other than the abdominal cavity vary. They depend on the structure punctured and the amount of CO_2 instilled before this dangerous situation is recognized.

Prevention

Intraabdominal structures such as the bladder, stomach, or bowel may be punctured by the Verres needle. Routine placement of a nasogastric tube and a Foley catheter before surgery will prevent puncture of these organs. The "syringe test" generally facilitates early recognition of puncture with aspiration of gastrointestinal content, urine, or blood. However, this method is not infallible. When you suspect insufflation into a viscus, failure to aspirate content should not cause this suspicion to be disregarded when there is asymmetric abdominal distension, belching, or passing of flatus. If these signs develop, the gas should be allowed to escape. Once a proper pneumoperitoneum has been established, insert the laparoscope and examine the suspected perforation site.

Recognition

Failure of the Verres needle to enter the peritoneal cavity or its misplacement into a viscus are generally first apparent upon instillation of CO_2. The most common extraperitoneal site to be insufflated is the preperitoneal space. Signs of faulty positioning of the Verres needle include elevated CO_2 filling pressures, continued liver dullness after instillation of 1 L of CO_2, subcutaneous crepitation, belching, passing flatus, asymmetric abdominal distension, hematuria or air bubbles in the Foley catheter line, a sudden drop in blood pressure, tachycardia, cardiac arrest, or difficulty in ventilating the patient. However, the absence of these signs does not guarantee proper placement. Preperitoneal placement of the Verres needle with sufficient insufflation of CO_2 leads to the disappearance of liver dullness. If preperitoneal insufflation is not recognized early and sufficient gas is instilled, you will see a spider-web appearance of the tissue after trocar placement and introduction of the laparoscope. Bowel puncture may not be immediately recognized because the large capacity of the bowel allows low filling pressures. Puncture of the omentum with the Verres needle may be associated with higher than normal filling pressures.

Even though the Verres needle may be placed correctly, the increased abdominal pressure and peritoneal irritation associated with instillation of CO_2 may result in bradycardia and hypotension. These signs respond readily to supportive measures.

Management

If the initial CO_2 flow rate is low or intraabdominal pressure is high (indicating improper Verres needle position), raising the abdominal wall may correct placement, particularly if it was initially placed within the omentum. If the pressure does not immediately fall to normal levels, withdraw the Verres needle and examine it to ensure that the spring-action of the device is working properly and that there is no tissue in the port in the tip. If a second placement attempt fails, consider inserting the Verres needle at another site using open laparoscopy or direct trocar entry.

If you recognize preperitoneal insufflation before trocar insertion, disconnect the CO_2 line and allow the gas to escape. Then remove the Verres needle and reinsert it, paying particular attention to the "pop" that occurs when the needle pierces the peritoneum. If sufficient gas is instilled into the preperitoneal space to allow trocar placement, you will discover this only after introduction of the laparoscope. Allow as much gas as possible to escape before attempting to reinsert the Verres needle. Preperitoneal insufflation can extend to the mediastinum and compromise cardiac function. If this occurs, abandon the laparoscopy and allow the gas to escape.

Pneumo-omentum is a relatively common and benign occurrence unless a vessel is lacerated. Slight withdrawal of the needle or traction on the abdominal wall may release the omentum. Because this occurs frequently, make a point of examining the omentum and other structures in the path of the Verres needle and the trocar at initial exploration of the pelvis to rule out omental laceration. If entry of the Verres needle into a large vessel goes unnoticed, intravascular insufflation with CO_2 may lead to gas embolism.[9] Gas embolism initially presents as cardiorespiratory distress associated with a classic "mill wheel" murmur. Once recognized, the patient needs to be placed in the left lateral decubitus position so that immediate cardiac puncture can release the gas.

Laparoscopic Trocar

The insertion of the principal trocar may cause serious punctures or lacerations of pelvic structures because of its large diameter and sharp tip.

Prevention

Establishing a large pneumoperitoneum and elevating the abdominal wall to increase the distance between the abdominal wall and viscera can decrease the chance of bowel and vessel injury. The syringe test before trocar insertion may indicate the presence of adhesions. However, these measures may not be effective and cannot guarantee against internal injury during trocar insertion. Indeed, we have demonstrated that preliminary Verres needle insertion is no safer than direct insertion of the umbilical trocar without prior pneumoperitoneum.[10] Faulty technique or adherent bowel is usually the cause of trocar injuries.[11] Uncontrolled sudden entry of the trocar, lateral displacement during insertion, or too steep an angle of placement increases the risk of injury. An inadequate umbilical incision, a dull trocar, or the presence of scar tissue can lead the surgeon to apply excessive force, which can result in uncontrolled trocar entry. The trocar should be pyramidal-tipped and sharp to penetrate muscle and fascia. Even with meticulous technique, abdominal wall bleeding, hollow viscus perforation, blood vessel laceration, or liver and spleen injury can occur.

Theoretically, the disposable trocar, with its permanently sharp tip that provides controlled entry should decrease the risk of injury to intraabdominal muscles.[11] However, no large-scale clinical trial has established its advantage over reusable trocars. We recommend inserting the first trocar with the patient in a horizontal position because Trendelenburg can alter the relationship of the sacral promontory and sacral hollow. The abdominal wall is elevated on both sides of the umbilicus. The trocar is inserted and advanced toward the sacral hollow to provide the greatest distance between the trocar tip and solid tissue. Using this technique, the bowel slides away from the advancing trocar.

In the obese patient, the trocar is angled close to the vertical so that the distance between the sacral promontory, blood vessels, and trocar is relatively large. In these patients, the distance between the anterior abdominal wall and sacral promontory is small and the force required to introduce the trocar is often less than anticipated so that controlled, angled entry is essential.[12]

A distended bowel increases the risk for trocar injury. This condition may be iatrogenic, resulting from intraluminal placement of the Verres needle. Because of its large capacity, filling pressure of the small bowel may be the same as that of the abdominal cavity. Therefore, the surgeon may be unaware of this complication.

Recognition

Injury during trocar insertion can be recognized by active bleeding from the trocar sleeve, fecal material on the trocar, or a fecal odor. In such instances, the laparoscope must be immediately inserted for evaluation of the suspected injury. If the laparoscope enters the bowel lumen, the instrument should be left in place to prevent escape of bowel contents and to help identify the injury. In the presence of excessive bleeding, immediate laparotomy may be indicated.

Management

The management of bleeding and bowel injuries is discussed below.

Accessory Trocar Insertion

Intraabdominal injury is less likely to occur during insertion of the accessory trocars because they are inserted under direct observation. The structures most frequently injured are the inferior epigastric vessels, which run lateral to the rectus muscles.[13] We have found that the most common complication of multipuncture operative laparoscopy was inferior epigastric vessel injury (Table 21.2).[1] Three factors play a role in avoiding injury to these vessels: (1) possessing a detailed understanding of abdominal wall anatomy; (2) ascertaining the position of the superficial vessels by transillumination of the abdominal wall, particularly in thin women; and (3) noting the course of the inferior epigastric vessels, which can be seen through the parietal peritoneum laparoscopically. Placing the ancillary trocars 2 to 3 cm lateral to the border of the rectus anterior muscles may also be beneficial in preventing inferior epigastric vessel injury. As the trocar is advanced through the abdominal wall, the direction of the trocar can be altered to avoid laceration.

Recognition

Despite safeguards, the inferior epigastric vessels can be injured intraoperatively. Lengthy procedures associated with frequent repositioning of the trocar sleeve, exchange of the 5 mm trocar sleeve for a 10 mm sleeve, inserting endoscopic instruments directly through the incision sites, or enlarging the incision in order to remove bulky tissue pieces may all damage the anterior abdominal wall vessels. If a vessel is damaged, you may notice blood running down the cannula or see an abdominal wall hematoma. The trocar sleeve may tamponade bleeding from a small laceration, which will not become apparent until the trocar sleeve is removed. If the injury is overlooked at that time, severe postoperative abdominal wall ecchymosis may develop. Profuse bleeding may be observed from the incisional site or significant local swelling may be observed postoperatively.

The risk of internal injury increases if the trocar is not aimed toward the sacral hollow; it may go down the pelvic sidewall or puncture the posterior peritoneum. Injuries to iliac vessels are associated with profuse hemorrhage or a rapidly enlarging retroperitoneal hematoma. Both may require immediate laparotomy. Retroperitoneal bleeding may spread and accumulate before being recognized. This injury is most likely to occur in patients who are thin, have had previous abdominal surgery, or who have lax abdominal walls.

Though the accessory trocars are inserted under direct vision, sudden uncontrolled entry or the use of excessive force may lacerate the bladder, uterus, or bowel. Uterine lacerations are not life threatening, and the bleeding is usually easy to control. Bladder injury can occur if an accessory trocar is placed less than 4 cm above the pubic symphysis or if the bladder is displaced because of incomplete drainage or a previous laparotomy.

Management

Inferior epigastric vessel bleeding can be controlled by suture placement, electrocoagulation, or local pressure application. Without removing the trocar, place a figure eight (0 absorbable suture on a CT-1 needle) on either side of the trocar. Tie the suture above the incision over a 4 × 4 sponge, and remove it 24 hours later. If suture placement does not control bleeding, extend the trocar incision and apply a suture under direct vision.

Grasping forceps may be used to apply pressure to the inferior epigastric artery to help identify the bleeding point. Direct pressure can be applied to the bleeding point via a blunt instrument placed through a contralateral accessory trocar. Bleeding can also be controlled by bipolar forceps introduced through a contralateral accessory trocar. Local pressure can be applied either via a Foley catheter or an expandable trocar. The Foley catheter is inserted through the involved trocar sleeve, the sleeve is then pulled up, and the catheter bulb inflated. Apply upward traction and maintain it by clamping a Kelly clamp to the catheter close to the skin and removing the upper part of the catheter. Or, place an expandable trocar and apply pressure to the skin and parietal surfaces.

Anesthesia

These complications are usually related to the elevated intraabdominal pressure caused by the pneumoperitoneum, the systemic absorption of CO_2, fluid overload from peritoneal absorption of irrigation fluid, and Trendelenburg positioning. The increased intraabdominal pressure and Trendelenburg positioning can cause difficulties in ventilation, especially in the obese patient. Excess CO_2 absorption and pressure on the peritoneum can precipitate vagal reactions resulting in tachycardia, bradycardia, and cardiac arrhythmias such as junctional rhythm, bigeminy, and asystole. Preoperative atropine may help avoid these complications.

Fluid overload can be associated with hydrodissection, copious irrigation, or the use of high-molecular-weight dextran as a distension medium for hysteroscopy. Careful intraoperative measurement of input and output should enable personnel to recognize possible complications of fluid overload such as pulmonary edema. Hypothermia can develop after lavage with large volumes of fluid. Therefore, use of a heating blanket is advisable. Hypothermia can be avoided by keeping irrigation fluid at body temperature.

Electrosurgical Equipment

Complications associated with electrosurgical equipment may involve equipment problems such as improper visualization, electrical failure of the electrocoagulator, or malfunction. Though equipment malfunction and failure can cause considerable delay, they are rarely the direct cause of injury. Rather, the more common case is unfamiliarity with the equipment and the use of incompatible components. Often, the first response to electrosurgical equipment failure is to increase the current, which further increases the risk of patient injury. If the equipment malfunctions, systematically check each component to pinpoint the problem before continuing with its use.

Using bipolar or unipolar forceps for tissue desiccation or for control of hemorrhage may result in damage to neighboring structures. Always identify bowel, bladder, ureter, and large vessels and make sure they are not in contact with the forceps. Some injuries may become evident intraoperatively, but others may become clinically apparent only postoperatively.

When unipolar current is used, apply a grounding pad. Also, avoid mixed trocars (half plastic and half metal) because their use may contribute to burns caused by capacitating coupling.

Bleeding

Most emergency laparotomies are performed to control hemorrhage. Although the surgeon should not hesitate to convert to laparotomy when severe hemorrhage may lead to an unstable hemodynamic state, most bleeding can be adequately managed at laparoscopy if the laparoscopist is highly experienced. We reported, for example, laparoscopic management of an injury to the hypogastric artery with bipolar electrodesiccation.[1] In our first 2,000 cases, we performed three laparotomies to control bleeding after treatment of dense adhesions. However, in 5,000 subsequent operations, only one was converted to laparotomy. Bleeding may occur during sharp dissection of adhesions, transection of vessels during laser excision or dissection (the laser effectively coagulates very small vessels), and uterosacral ablation, or because of rough handling of tissues. Lacerations of the oviduct, mesosalpinx, and infundibulopelvic ligament can bleed profusely. Proper equipment and agents to control bleeding (unipolar and/or bipolar electrocoagulator, vasopressin, clips, sutures, and loop ligatures) must be immediately available to the operative field. The mode of control depends on the surgeon's preference. Most bleeding can be controlled with bipolar forceps. In patients with infertility problems, apply fine bipolar forceps to minimize thermal damage and subsequent adhesions. Direct pressure applied with a blunt instrument or grasping forceps minimizes blood loss until the necessary equipment can be assembled to permit evacuation of blood for better visualization.

The increased intraabdominal pressure from CO_2 insufflation, the decreased venous pressure caused by Trendelenburg position, and retroperitoneal hematoma can tamponade bleeding from small or large vessels. When pressure gradients return to normal, bleeding into the retroperitoneal space may begin and eventually lead to hematoma and hypovolemic shock. At the end of the procedure, with the patient supine and intraabdominal pressure reduced, evaluate all exposed vessels.[14] Evacuate pelvic sidewall blood clots before confirming complete hemostasis.

Complications Involving Specific Organs

Uterus

Cervical lacerations or uterine perforation may occur during sounding of the uterine cavity or from use of the uterine dilator or uterine manipulator. Manage cervical lacerations with pressure from a sponge stick or suture. Carefully observe bleeding from uterine perforations and, if necessary, control it with bipolar electrocoagulation. Occasionally, the uterus is repaired using laparoscopic suturing. The uterine serosa can be lacerated by the CO_2 laser beam laser; therefore, don't use the uterus as a backstop.

Bladder Injuries

Prevention

Bladder injury is rare and usually occurs in patients with previous laparotomies or incomplete drainage of the bladder.[3,15] Sharp instruments such as trocars and uterine anteverters can perforate or lacerate the bladder; the Verres needle can puncture a distended bladder; electricity and lasers can cause thermal injury; and blunt instruments can lacerate the bladder. A misplaced Rubin's cannula can perforate the vagina and bladder with upward pressure.[16] Accessory trocar insertion can injure the bladder if it is distended or distorted by previous pelvic surgery, endometriosis, or adhesions. There may also be a problem if insertion is performed less than 4 cm above the pubic symphysis.

Coagulation or laser ablation of endometriosis implants or adhesiolysis in the anterior cul-de-sac can predispose the patient to bladder injury unless hydrodissection or a backstop is used with the CO_2 laser. During a hysterectomy by operative laparoscopy, the bladder may be lacerated or torn if blunt dissection is used to free the bladder from the pubocervical fascia, particularly in women with prior cesarean section, severe endometriosis, or lower segment myomas. Also, bladder injury can occur while entering and dissecting the space of Retzius before laparoscopic bladder neck suspension.

To prevent bladder injuries, drain the bladder preoperatively with a Foley catheter and leave it in place for the duration of the procedure. Assess the position and boundaries of the bladder during the initial laparoscopic examination. If you can't see the boundaries clearly, particularly when pelvic anatomy is distorted, fill the bladder with 350 mL of normal saline to delineate its position. Take care when performing hysterectomy; have the assistant push the uterus down during bladder dissection.

Recognition

Intraoperative recognition of bladder injury is instrumental in preventing long-term sequelae. Signs of intraoperative bladder injury include: (1) air in the urinary catheter and bag during insufflation; (2) the bladder appearing to be pushed by the accessory trocar as it is advanced through the abdominal wall; (3) hematuria; (4) urine drainage from the accessory trocar incision; and (5) intraoperative leakage of indigo carmine from the injured site. Since trocar injury often involves entry and exit punctures, locating both is important.

Some bladder complications become apparent only postoperatively, particularly those caused by electrocoagulation. Signs and symptoms include urinary retention, decreased urinary output, hematuria, suprapubic bruising, the presence of a mass in the abdominal wall or pelvis, abdominal swelling, azotemia, or peritonitis. If you suspect a bladder injury postoperatively, perform a retrograde cystogram.

Management

Small perforations generally heal without sequelae. However, injuries of 5 mm or more (trocar injuries) to the bladder dome require closure followed by urinary drainage for 5 to 7 days. Drainage promotes healing, encourages spontaneous closure, and minimizes further complications.

Lacerations to the bladder can be repaired laparoscopically by experienced laparoscopists. After identifying the injury and removing any associated endometriosis, adhesions, or necrotic tissue, repair the laceration in one layer, using 0 polyglactin (Vicryl,

Ethicon) or chromic suture. Place the suture through the serosa, muscularis, and mucosa. Small injuries (less than .5 cm) may be repaired by placing an Endoloop around the injury. Perform cystoscopy to be sure there is no damage to the ureteral orifices and that the repair is watertight.

In a series of eight intraoperative bladder injuries, five were repaired laparoscopically using one layer suturing (Table 21.2).

We reported successful laparoscopic partial resection and repair of the bladder wall for severe vesical endometriosis.[17] We have also treated a case of perforation of the anterior and posterior wall of the bladder dome conservatively. Intraoperative cystoscopy revealed that the ureteral orifices were not injured and there was no bleeding. A Foley catheter was inserted and left in situ for 7 days. Prophylactic antibiotics were administered. A cystogram 7 days later revealed complete healing.

Ureter Injury

The ureter develops embryologically in association with the genital tract. This close association, which persists postnatally, predisposes women to ureteral injury. The intrapelvic segment of the ureter, situated near the broad ligament, ovaries, and uterosacral ligaments, is often injured during surgical treatment of these organs (Table 21.5).[18]

Prevention

Knowledge of the ureter's path through the pelvis and its vulnerable points are key to preventing injuries. The surgeon should identify the course of the ureter through the transparency of the peritoneum. Endometriosis and severe pelvic adhesions can thicken the peritoneum and obscure the location of the ureter, especially near the uterosacral ligaments. If the ureter cannot be clearly identified through the peritoneum, it must be located by retroperitoneal dissection.

Until recently, most reported cases of ureteral injury during laparoscopic procedures involved electro-

Table 21.5. Laparoscopic procedures associated with increased risk of ureteral injury.

Infundibulopelvic ligament/ovarian fossa
    Oophorectomy
    Pelvic sidewall adhesions
    Presacral neurectomy
    Endometriosis ablation
    Severe bowel adhesions

Ureteric canal
    Uterosacral nerve transection
    Uterosacral plication
    Hysterectomy

Cardinal ligament
    Hysterectomy
    Vaginal cuff closure

coagulation, the most reliable technique to arrest bleeding. However, with the introduction of stapling devices, additional injuries to the ureters have been reported.[19–21]

Ureteral injury can occur during sharp dissection of adhesions to the pelvic sidewall, uterosacral transection, transection of the uterine arteries, removal of endometriotic implants or fibrosis over the ureter, or during coagulation of blood vessels adjacent to the ureter.[22–24] We reported six cases of ureter injuries, five involving endometriosis and fibrosis and one involving adhesions.[1] Of these, four were performed intentionally in order to treat partial or complete obstruction; two occurred during treatment of severe endometriosis bordering the ureter. Unrecognized anomalies in ureter location may predispose the patient to injury.[25] Meticulous and continuous attention to the location of the ureter, as well as careful identification of any tissue prior to desiccation and/or removal, will reduce complications.

Methods to protect the ureter include using hydrodissection and resecting affected peritoneum.[26] Make a horizontal incision in the peritoneum midway between the ovary and uterosacral ligament. Inject 50 to 100 mL of lactated Ringer's along the course of the ureter. This displaces the ureter laterally, providing a plane for safe ablation of endometriotic implants, lysis of adhesions, or resection of the involved peritoneum. The fluid also absorbs the laser energy and deceases the risk of thermal damage to underlying tissue.[27] This procedure is applicable only when the peritoneum is not densely adherent to the underlying ureter. If the peritoneum is involved with endometriosis and there is retroperitoneal fibrosis, the ureter may be attached to the peritoneum. Extend the horizontal incision in the peritoneum as necessary. During uterosacral transection, a backstop can be placed between the lateral aspect of the uterosacral ligament and ureter. Before using the bipolar forceps during adnexectomy, the infundibulopelvic ligament must be put under traction to identify the ureter and avoid thermal damage.

The routine use of preoperative intravenous pyelography is controversial. No prospective study substantiates that IVP prevents ureteral injury. However, for selected patients, it may help diagnose ureteral obstruction and allow appropriate surgical planning. The routine use of ureteral catheters is not warranted, but it might be useful in cases of severe endometriosis and adhesions.

Recognition

It is reported that a favorite quotation of Dr. Thomas Green of Boston was, "The venial sin is injury to the ureter; the mortal sin is failure of recognition."[28] Early recognition is critical to successful management. Suspect intraoperative ureter damage when urine leakage or blood-tinged urine is noted and when indigo carmine dye is spilled intraperitoneally after intravenous administration. When surgical procedures involve the ureter, postoperative ureteral integrity can be ascertained by cystoscopy, ureteral catheterization, or intravenous retrograde pyelogram. Stenting of the ureter or repair by laparotomy is generally indicated, but laparoscopic repair of partial and full-thickness injuries is an option for some experienced laparoscopists.[23,25]

Unfortunately, the diagnosis of ureteral injury is usually made postoperatively by intravenous pyelography.[18] Fever, flank pain, peritonitis, and abdominal distension within 48 to 72 hours postoperatively should alert the clinician to possible ureteral injury. Leukocytosis and hematuria may be present. Since the patient's symptoms may be indistinguishable from those of ileus or bowel injury, IVP is indispensable for differential diagnosis.

Management

Whether the discovery of ureteral complications is immediate or delayed, consult a urologist. If the IVP indicates ureteral injury, initial therapy should involve attempts at either retrograde or antegrade stenting. Therapeutic options include ureteroureterostomy and ureteroneocystostomy, classically performed by laparotomy. There have been several recent reports of conservative management of ureteral injuries as well as laparoscopic management. Winslow and co-workers reported the successful conservative management of a patient who sustained an electrical burn injury to the left ureter at diagnostic laparoscopy.[29] Gomel reported the laparoscopic repair of a ureteral laceration that occurred during needle electrosurgical ablation of the left uterosacral ligament.[25]

We managed a case of long-term ureteral obstruction caused by endometriosis with laparoscopic partial resection and anastomosis of the ureter.[30] Anastomosis was also performed in another case after resection of a 1.5 cm segment of the ureter during the treatment of severe pelvic wall endometriosis.[23] We also reported four cases of partial resection of the ureter, of which three were repaired by laparoscopic suturing and one by stent insertion. A surgeon familiar with delicate laparoscopic suturing can repair ureteral injuries laparoscopically with good results.

Small Bowel

Small bowel injuries, whether discovered intraoperatively or several days after surgery, can result in unplanned laparotomy, serous morbidity, and even death.[3] Though the bowel can be injured during Verres needle or trocar insertion, bowel manipulation, or enterolysis, direct mechanical injury is less common than electrical injury. Stray laser beams and electrosurgery can result in unrecognized thermal injuries to the bowel. The risk of injury is higher when adhesions are dense and tissue planes poorly defined. Traction on the bowel with serrated graspers may also produce abrasions and lacerations. A case of inadvertent small bowel biopsy, unfortunately diagnosed by the pathologists, has been reported.[31]

Prevention

Such manipulation of the bowel as displacement from the pelvis with a blunt metal probe should be performed with care. Blunt dissection should be avoided. The bowel can be trapped in incisions and as trocars are withdrawn. The patient, then, is at risk for a small bowel obstruction.[32] For this reason, some advocate opening the valve of the umbilical trocar as it is withdrawn to prevent a vacuum that may draw the bowel into the incision. Using a Z-track insertion may eliminate this complication.[33]

Adhesions between the small bowel and anterior abdominal wall are associated with a risk of trocar injury, especially among patients who have had a bowel resection or exploratory laparotomy for trauma. Women who undergo a second-look laparoscopy after treatment for ovarian carcinoma by laparotomy may have adhesions from previous abdominal surgery. Generally, they have had an omentectomy and debulking with adhesion formation.[34]

Despite the use of open laparoscopy, bowel lacerations can occur when the instruments enter the peritoneum.[35] It is difficult to determine which patients should have an open laparoscopy. In our series, all 22 patients who had small bowel injuries also had previous laparotomies and small bowel adhesions. Seven were due to trocar injuries, 13 occurred during adhesiolysis, and two during open laparoscopy (Table 21.2).

When a patient is at risk for bowel adhesions, it is prudent to prepare her with a mechanical and antibiotic bowel preparation preoperatively to eliminate bowel contents, decompress the bowel, and minimize the risk of infection.

Recognition

The presence of bleeding or hematoma should alert the operator to possible bowel trauma. Meticulous inspection should follow sharp dissection of the bowel from neighboring structures. Electrical injuries to the bowel are not always apparent intraoperatively and, when apparent, may not reflect the full depth of injury. This situation may mislead the surgeon in choosing conservative management. Most intestinal burns less than 5 mm in diameter can be managed expectantly. If the area of blanching on the intestinal serosa exceeds 5 cm, the extent of thermal damage will probably exceed

the apparent damage. Therapy should be instituted immediately. The actual area of injury can extend up to 5 cm from the apparent injury.[36]

If the small bowel has been lacerated by a trocar, the surgeon may initially see a mucosal surface or notice a foul smell when the laparoscope is inserted. Small bowel contents may be observed leaking from a laceration or a hematoma may be present on the small bowel serosa.

If the small bowel injury is not recognized intraoperatively, the patient generally presents on the third or fourth postoperative day with lower abdominal pain, mild fever, slight nausea, and anorexia. By the fifth or sixth postoperative day, symptoms include fever, severe abdominal pain, nausea, vomiting, constipation, increased white blood cell count, and peritonitis.[36] Radiographs reveal multiple air/fluid levels or air under the diaphragm.

Management

Complications from small bowel injury are related to the extent of damage and the time elapsed before the injury is discovered. Sharp trocar injuries to the bowel may be limited to the serosa or can be deep involving the entire wall. Small punctures or superficial lacerations seal readily and require no further treatment if careful inspection of the affected bowel reveals no leakage of bowel contents or bleeding. Small (<5 mm) superficial lacerations must be inspected to assure that only the serosa is involved. In these cases, the patient may be treated conservatively and discharged the day of surgery with instructions to report any untoward reaction.

In patients with obvious peritoneal soiling, the bowel should be inspected on both sides to detect through-and-through injuries, especially if they are produced by a trocar. If only one of the two injured sites is found and repaired, peritonitis may develop postoperatively. If the laparoscope has been inserted through the bowel laceration and laparotomy is performed, the defect should be identified and closed by a purse-string suture as the laparoscope is withdrawn to minimize peritoneal contamination.[37,38]

Small bowel should be repaired in one or two layers by placing an initial row of interrupted sutures of 3-0 chromic catgut to approximate the mucosa and muscularis. A reinforcing layer of 3-0 silk Lembert sutures is used to approximate the muscularis and serosa edges.[39] All lacerations should be closed transversely to minimize the occurrence of stenosis of the bowel lumen. This closure is appropriate only if the laceration is less than one half the diameter of the bowel. If the laceration exceeds one half the diameter of the lumen, segmental resection and anastomosis should be performed. If the mesenteric blood supply is interrupted by the puncture, regardless of the size or the length of the laceration, a resection of that particular segment of bowel must be performed.[37] Intraoperative consultation with a general surgeon is appropriate whenever significant bowel trauma occurs. Small bowel injuries caused by trocars or the CO_2 laser can be repaired in one layer using 3-0 silk or 4-0 polydioxanone without complication or laparotomy.[40] Injuries less than 2 cm (small or large bowel) may be repaired transversely or longitudinally; however, injuries over 2 cm should be repaired transversely.

Here is a simple technique to repair bowel injuries of less than 1 cm caused by sharp instruments or the CO_2 laser. After the edge of the perforation is thoroughly clean of any debris, use a 4-0 polydioxanone or 0 polyglactin Endoloop suture to bring the perforation inside the loop and tie it around the perforation. To evaluate the repair, fill the abdomen and posterior cul-de-sac with lactated Ringer's. Use a sigmoidoscope to insufflate the bowel, which is pushed under the fluid.[40] The presence of air bubbles indicates inadequate repair. We have used this technique to repair 12 cases of small and large bowel injuries without complication.

After repair of a bowel laceration, the entire abdomen is irrigated. A nasogastric tube may be placed and removed when drainage has decreased, indicating that bowel function has resumed. The patient is not given solid food by mouth until she passes flatus.

When possible bowel laceration is suspected postoperatively, conservative management is usually successful in patients who have not developed peritonitis.[36] In-hospital management consists of hydration, nothing by mouth, and close observation with white blood count and physical exam every six hours. Wheeless reported that over one half the patients treated conservatively required no surgical intervention.[36] Those whose condition deteriorated during observation underwent laparotomy and had no complications attributable to delayed surgery.

Immediate surgical intervention and possible laparotomy may be indicated in patients who present with fever, severe abdominal pain, nausea, vomiting, obstipation, or peritonitis, or in those whose clinical condition worsens. Surgical considerations for managing bowel injuries discovered postoperatively differ somewhat from those discovered and managed intraoperatively. The damaged bowel must be repaired or resected. Resection of all necrotic tissue in the pelvis is also mandatory, even if this requires a hysterectomy and bilateral salpingo-oophorectomy. If burned or necrotic tissue that has been bathed in intestinal contents, blood, or serum is not excised, a pelvic abscess may develop.[36]

Wheeless presented the following 7-point plan to manage patients with peritonitis secondary to bowel perforation: (1) preoperative stabilization with fluids, electrolytes, and suction; (2) exploratory laparotomy with repair or resection of the injured bowel; (3) resection of all necrotic tissue; (4) copious and repeated saline lavage of the abdomen; (5) pelvic drainage through the vagina using a closed drainage system; (6) aggressive antibiotic therapy; and (7) embolus prophylaxis with mini-dose heparin (5,000 units TID).

In our series, we had six postoperative admissions due to small bowel complications (Table 21.2). Only one required laparotomy. This patient developed peritonitis one day after laparoscopic treatment of endometriosis and adhesions. Exploratory laparotomy showed a severe bowel strangulation due to a congenital malrotation of the mesentery, but no bowel perforation. She required bowel resection and postoperative dietary adjustment.

Three patients with small bowel ileus were managed by conservative therapy and one underwent laparoscopy to rule out pelvic infection. One patient was admitted for hydration and antibiotic therapy for severe gastroenteritis.

In a recent AAGL membership poll, the two deaths reported from 36,928 procedures were attributed to bowel injuries. In one instance, the patient had extensive adhesions from the abdominal wall to the bowel. Although the bowel injury was recognized and repaired, the patient developed a persistent postoperative ileus and died of peritonitis. The second death was attributable to sepsis after an unrecognized small bowel perforation.[3]

Large Bowel

Colon entry is a major complication of laparoscopy, particularly if the bowel is unprepared or if the injury is not recognized. Even small perforations, such as those from the Verres needle, require attention because the high bacterial concentration of minor leaks can cause infection and abscesses.

Prevention

Factors that contribute to an increased risk of large bowel injuries include: (1) failure to establish an adequate pneumoperitoneum; (2) use of dull trocars requiring excessive force; (3) uncontrolled, sudden entry of sharp instruments; and (4) gastric distension. Poorly controlled or sudden trocar entry can cause rectosigmoid laceration. Gastric distension can displace the transverse colon toward the pelvis, where it can be punctured by the Verres needle or lacerated with the trocar. This complication can be prevented by using a nasogastric tube intraoperatively.

The rectosigmoid can be injured if the depth of penetration by endometriosis is underestimated or the cul-de-sac is obliterated. When the rectum adheres to the posterior aspect of the cervix or uterosacral ligaments, blunt dissection may pierce the rectum. We recommend sharp dissection with scissors or the CO_2 laser. The combination of high-power superpulse or ultrapulse CO_2 laser and hydrodissection is relatively safe for working around the bowel.

When the cul-de-sac is dissected, identification of the vagina and rectum is facilitated by placing a probe or an assistant's finger in both the vagina and rectum. Dissection should begin lateral to the uterosacral ligaments, where anatomy is less distorted, and proceed toward the obliterated cul-de-sac.[41,42] Similarly, when posterior culdotomy is performed for tissue removal or during laparoscopic hysterectomy, correct identification of vagina and rectum is important.[19,43]

When a difficult pelvic operation is contemplated, such as cul-de-sac nodularity in a patient with endometriosis or a history suggesting significant pelvic adhesions, preoperative bowel preparation is indicated.

Recognition

Perforation of the large bowel with the Verres needle can sometimes be recognized by the saline aspiration test; recovery of brownish fluid is pathognomonic. Fecal odor may be detected. If large bowel entry is suspected because of either of these two tests, the needle should be promptly withdrawn, and another sterile Verres needle reinserted. Once the laparoscope is inserted, the entry site should be sought and examined. Because of the high bacterial concentration, minor leaks of fecal material into the peritoneal cavity can be the source of serious infection. The underwater examination is recommended after the treatment of severe endometriosis and adhesions of the rectum and rectosigmoid colon.

Large bowel injuries can be serious because they may not be recognized at surgery. Under these circumstances, the patient generally presents on the third or fourth postoperative day with lower abdominal pain, mild fever, slight nausea, and anorexia. By the fifth or sixth postoperative day, these symptoms progress to include fever, severe abdominal pain, nausea, vomiting, obstipation, increased WBC, and peritonitis.[36] An upright x-ray may show changes consistent with an ileus.[44] The patient appears ill with no clear explanation for the symptoms.

Management

For small colonic wounds associated with minimal contamination, primary suture closure at laparoscopy has been the accepted therapy. Copious lavage of the peritoneal cavity, broad-spectrum antibiotics, and drainage also help minimize the risk of infection. We performed this procedure in 25 of 26 large bowel injuries without complication. Copious irrigation and antibiotic coverage are essential.

Electrical injury to the ascending colon is managed by resecting the injured segment and primary an-

astomosis. Diverting ileostomy facilitates healing and reduces morbidity and mortality. Injury to the descending colon, sigmoid, or rectum in unprepared bowel is not amenable to primary closure or resection with primary anastomosis. Diverting colostomy with resection of the injured portion is recommended.[45]

Colonic lacerations in prepared bowel can be repaired laparoscopically after excising endometriosis nodules and identifying the extent of the laceration. A single-layered repair using 4-0 silk, 4-0 polydioxanone, or 0 polyglactin sutures is used.[40]

In a series of more than 50 rectosigmoid colon planned and unplanned enterotomies, repair was completed with single layer suture or an endoloop. Complications included one fistula, one pelvic infection and abscess. The fistula was managed by drainage under CT scan guidance and antibiotic therapy. The pelvic abscess was managed by drainage under CT scan guidance and laparoscopy after failed treatment with antibiotic therapy. Neither patient required laparotomy. Both patients underwent anterior bowel disk excision for full thickness endometriosis. We now know that the bowel can be repaired successfully by laparoscopic techniques in the properly prepared patient. This should increase the confidence of the surgeon operating in the deep pelvis.

Postoperative Complications

Bleeding

Hemorrhage may go unnoticed before closure because of the combined effects of Trendelenburg position, high intraabdominal pressures, and relative supine hypotension. However, once the patient resumes an upright position, in the absence of pneumoperitoneum, an injured blood vessel may resume bleeding. Therefore, if the hypotensive patient does not respond postoperatively to IV hydration, perform a repeat hematocrit. If the hematocrit level is decreasing or if the physical exam reveals abdominal distension, suspect intraabdominal bleeding. Repeat laparoscopy may be necessary.

In our series, there were 17 complications involving postoperative bleeding. Only three patients required laparotomy. Location of the bleeding included eight from the anterior abdominal wall (six from the suprapubic incisions and two from the umbilical incision), three from the vaginal cuff post laparoscopic and laparoscopic assisted vaginal hysterectomy, and five cases of intra-abdominal bleeding (Table 21.2). Vaginal cuff bleeding was managed by vaginal repair and packing without re-exploration or transfusion. Two cases were attributable to blood coagulation disorders. One was caused by a persistent ectopic pregnancy subsequent to surgery at another center. Another patient who had storage pool disease presented with intraabdominal bleeding 24 hours postoperatively. At laparoscopy, we were unable to locate the source of bleeding. Therefore, laparotomy was performed. However, laparotomy also failed to reveal the site. It was generalized oozing from the pelvic cavity. Postoperatively, she was treated with blood products and coagulation factors. In one patient, no obvious reason for bleeding could be identified at laparoscopy. Postoperative evaluation including hematologic evaluation showed no abnormality. All patients presented within 48 hours of surgery.

Large Bowel

Postoperative large bowel complications occurred after unrecognized intraoperative bowel injuries, delayed necrosis caused by excessive thermal damage and ischemia after enterotomy and bowel resection.. Postoperative abdominal pain, fever, constipation, and peritoneal signs should alert the physician. Patients who had excessive posterior cul-de-sac dissection, treatment of endometriosis and lysis of severe large bowel adhesions should be given specific instructions regarding the avoidance of constipation and not using an enema which can contribute to bowel perforation.

In our series, we encountered five postoperative complications involving the large bowel (Table 21.2). All patients had a history of rectum and rectosigmoid colon endometriosis and underwent different techniques of bowel resection. Two women developed leaks and pelvic infections. One required laparoscopic temporary colostomy with subsequent take down and repair. One was managed by prolonged drainage under CT scan guidance and antibiotic therapy. One woman had a bowel stricture after complete segmental resection requiring resection and reanastomosis. One patient developed a pelvic abscess and subsequently underwent right salpingo-oophorectomy. The abscess was drained laparoscopically and under CT scan guidance. One patient with a history of endometriosis and constipation underwent anterior wedge resection of rectal endometriosis had an immediate postoperative rectal prolapse which was reduced without surgical management. Her bowel symptoms persisted and she subsequently had a colectomy.

Bladder and Ureter

Postoperative genitourinary complications can present with peritoneal signs such as small bowel ileus, peritonitis, abdominal and flank pain, or fistula formation. Through postoperative evaluation including IVP and cystogram, pelvic ultrasound or CT scan should be implemented if injury is suspected.

In our series we had four significant genitourinary complications including one ureteral injury. One patient with a history of previous cervical conization underwent total laparoscopic hysterectomy and bilateral salpingo-oophorectomy. Three days postoperatively, she presented with right hydroureter and hydronephrosis with a ureterovaginal fistula.

After placement of ureteral stents failed, she underwent laparoscopic evaluation. At that time, it was found that the distal portion of the right ureter had been obstructed by conization hemostasis suture. The suture apparently became loose and a fistula formed. Laparoscopic adhesiolysis and uterolysis was performed and the injury site was identified close to the bladder. After a ureteral stent was inserted cystoscopically, ureteroureterostomy was performed using 4-0 PDS. An abdominal drain was inserted and the patient was treated with antibiotic therapy. There were no postoperative complications. Follow-up studies showed mild stricture of the distal portion of the ureter which responded to the conservative ureteral dilatation.

Two patients developed vesicovaginal fistulas. One patient underwent extensive pelvic adhesiolysis and removal of ovarian remnant from the rectum, right ureter and bladder. Partial cystectomy had been performed to remove the entire lesion. The bladder was repaired and drained with an indwelling Foley catheter. Unfortunately, the patient discontinued the Foley catheter less than a week postoperatively and she developed a vesicovaginal fistula one week later. The patient did not respond to prolonged bladder drainage and underwent laparoscopic vesicovaginal fistula repair successfully. She has been doing well since. The other woman developed a vesicovaginal fistula two weeks after total laparoscopic hysterectomy. She was managed with two weeks of bladder drainage and antibiotic therapy without any sequelae.

One patient had severe urinary retention which required several months of bladder catheterization. She had undergone laparoscopic hysterectomy and bilateral salpingo-oophorectomy with pelvic lymphadenectomy for early cervical cancer and laparoscopic urethropexy for stress urinary incontinence urinary retention finally resolved spontaneously several months later.

Nerve Injuries

Common postoperative neurologic syndromes include sciatic nerve injury, brachial palsy (shoulder–hand syndrome), and perineal nerve palsy. Allowing the buttocks to protrude too far off the end of the operating table may cause back injury. At CSPS, we have had no cases of brachial, sciatic or femoral nerve palsy. We pay meticulous attention to the placement of the patient's hands and legs prior to surgery.

Shoulder Pain

The CO_2 commonly used for insufflation is a peritoneal irritant. Intraoperatively, this irritation can manifest itself as a vasovagal reaction. Postoperatively, residual gas accumulates under the diaphragm and irritates it when an upright position is maintained. The pain is referred to the shoulder by the phrenic nerve.

Complete removal of intraabdominal CO_2 is difficult, but problems may be minimized by exerting pressure on the abdomen toward the symphysis and expressing the gas in the lower abdomen through the umbilical or suprapubic trocars at the end of surgery. If pain develops postoperatively, the patient should be instructed to lie down and use a pillow to elevate the lower abdomen. This position allows gas to accumulate in the pelvis.

Infection

Postoperative infection is unusual after laparoscopic procedures, although the risk appears higher with prolonged, multiple puncture procedures. Most infections are limited to skin or stitch abscesses that require incision and drainage. Occasionally, a pelvic infection occurs following tubal surgery, but it is unclear whether this is caused by a preexisting condition or contamination, or if it results from tissue destruction and necrosis. Urinary tract infections can be caused by instrumentation or asymptomatic bacteria.

In our series, we had six pelvic infections. Only two required surgical management. All infections occurred in patients who had bowel surgery for treatment of severe endometriosis, bowel adhesions, appendectomy and bowel resection.

Incisional Hernia

Herniation of the omentum or small bowel at the umbilical incision site has been reported with 7 mm or larger trocars. Patients at increased risk are those who are very thin (especially elderly patients), have chronic coughs, or have a history of hernias or connective tissue disorder. Possible preventative measures, although not proven, include Z-track insertion, avoiding trocar insertion directly through the umbilicus, and careful withdrawal of the umbilical trocar.

A subclinical hernia with adhesions between the peritoneal incision site and bowel may place a patient at high risk of bowel perforation should she require another surgical intervention. Some surgeons advocate removing the umbilical trocar under laparoscopic observation to avoid trapping the bowel. Another option is to remove the trocar with the valve open to avoid negative pressure, which could draw omentum or small bowel into the defect. In our series of more than 7000 cases, we had two incisional hernias. One involved the omentum, and the other involved the small bowel. Neither required bowel resection.

Death Rates with Procedure

The AAGL 1979 membership survey, which involved primarily diagnostic laparoscopic procedures for tubal ligation, reported two deaths in 88,986 procedures.[2]

Peterson's team identified 29 deaths (3.6 per 100,000) associated with tubal sterilization: eleven resulted from anesthesia, seven were caused by sepsis after unrecognized bowel injury, four to hemorrhage following major vessel laceration, three to myocardial infarction, and four were related to other causes.[46] Some deaths might have been prevented by using endotracheal intubation for general anesthesia, safer use of unipolar coagulation or use of alternative techniques, and careful insertion of the Verres needle and trocar.

As laparoscopic surgery has increased in complexity, the associated mortality rate increased to 5.5 per 100,000 procedures.[3] The 1988 AAGL membership survey, which concentrated on operative laparoscopic experience, reported two deaths in 36,298 procedures. In one instance, the patient had extensive adhesions from the abdominal wall to the bowel. Although a bowel injury was recognized and repaired, the patient developed a persistent postoperative ileus and died of peritonitis. The second death was attributed to sepsis after an unrecognized small bowel perforation. We report no deaths in our series of more than 7000 cases.

References

1. Nezhat F, Nezhat C, Nezhat CH. Complications of gynecologic operative laparoscopy in 6,949 patients. Presented at the Society of Laparoendoscopic Surgeons meeting, Seattle, WA, June 10–11, 1994.
2. Phillips JM, Hulka JF, Hulka B, et al. 1979 AAGL membership survey. J Reprod Med 1981;26:529.
3. Peterson HB, Hulka JF, Phillips JM. American Association of Gynecologic Laparoscopists' 1988 membership survey on operative laparoscopy. J Reprod Med 1990;35:587.
4. Lehmann-Willenbrock E, Riedel HH, Mecke H, et al. Pelviscopy/laparoscopy and its complications in Germany 1949–1988. J Reprod Med 1992;37:671.
5. Levinson CJ, Hulka JF, Richardson DC. Laparoscopy. In Schaefer G, Graber EA, eds. Complication in Obstetric and Gynecologic Surgery. Harper & Row, Philadelphia, 1981, p 281.
6. Querleu D, Chapron C, Chevallier L, et al. Complications of gynecologic laparoscopic surgery—a French multicenter collaborative study (letter). N Engl J Med 1993;328:1355.
7. Soderstrom RM, Butler JC. A critical evaluation of complications in laparoscopy. J Reprod Med 1973;10:245.
8. Nezhat C, Nezhat F, Nezhat CH. Operative laparoscopy (minimally invasive surgery): State of the art. J Gynecol Surg 1992;8:111–141.
9. Gomel V, Taylor PJ, Yuzpee AA, et al. Laparoscopy and hysteroscopy in gynecologic practice. Chicago, Yearbook Medical Publishers, Inc., 1986, p 56.
10. Nezhat FR, Silfen SL, Evans D, et al. Comparison of direct insertion of disposable and standard reusable laparoscopic trocars and previous pneumoperitoneum with Verres needle. Obstet Gynecol 1991;78:148.
11. Corson SL, Batzer FR, Gocial B, et al. Measurement of the force necessary to laparoscopic trocar entry. J Reprod Med 1989;34:282.

12. Metzger DA. Trocar injuries to the small intestine. In Corfman RS, Diamond WP, DeCherney AH, eds. Intraabdominal Endoscopic Complications: Prevention, Recognition and Management. Cambridge, Blackwell Scientific Publications, 1993, p 50.

13. Pring DW. Inferior epigastric hemorrhage, an avoidable complication of laparoscopic clip sterilization. Br J Obstet Gynaecol 1983;90:480.

14. Nezhat C, Nezhat F, Winer W. Salpingectomy via laparoscopy: A new surgical approach. J Lap Surg 1991; 1:91–95.

15. Georgy FM, Fetterman HH, Chefetz MD. Complication of laparoscopy: Two cases of perforated urinary bladder. Am J Obstet Gynecol 1974;120:1121.

16. Sherer DM. Inadvertent transvaginal cystotomy during laparoscopy. Int J Gynecol Obstet 1990;32:77.

17. Nezhat F, Nezhat C. Laparoscopic segmental bladder resection for endometriosis: A report of two cases. Obstet Gynecol 1993;81:882–884.

18. Granger DA, Soderstrom RM, Schiff SF, et al. Ureteral injuries at laparoscopy: Insights into diagnosis, management and prevention. Obstet Gynecol 1990;75:839.

19. Nezhat C, Nezhat F, Gordon S, et al. Laparoscopic versus abdominal hysterectomy. J Reprod Med 1992;37:247–250.

20. Woodland MB. Ureter injury during laparoscopy-assisted vaginal hysterectomy with the endoscopic linear stapler. Am J Obstet Gynecol 1992;176:756–757.

21. Nezhat C, Nezhat F, Bess O, et al. Injuries associated with the use of a linear stapler during operative laparoscopy: review of diagnosis, management and prevention. J Gynecol Endosc, in press, 1993.

22. Cheng YS. Ureteral injury resulting from laparoscopic fulguration of endometriotic implant. Am J Obstet Gynecol 1976;126:1045.

23. Nezhat C, Nezhat F. Laparoscopic repair of resected ureter during operative laparoscopy to treat endometriosis. A case report. Obstet Gynecol 1992;80:543–544.

24. Chaffkin L, Luciano A. Ureteral injuries. In Corfman RS, Diamond WP, DeCherney AH, eds. Complications of Laparoscopy and Hysteroscopy. Cambridge MA, Blackwell Scientific Publications, 1993, p 134.

25. Gomel V, James C. Intraoperative management of ureteral injury during operative laparoscopy. Fertil Steril 1991;55:416.

26. Nezhat C, Nezhat F. Safe laser excision or vaporization of peritoneal endometriosis. Fertil Steril 1989;52:1:149–51.

27. Cook AS, Rock JA. The role of laparoscopy in the treatment of endometriosis. Fertil Steril 1991;55:663.

28. Nichols DH. Clinical Problems, Injuries and Complications of Gynecologic Surgery, 2nd ed. Baltimore, Williams & Wilkins, 1988, p 181.

29. Winslow PH, Kreger R, Effesson B, et al. Conservative management of electrical burn injury of ureter secondary to laparoscopy. Urology 1986;27:60.

30. Nezhat C, Nezhat F, Green B. Laparoscopic treatment of obstructed ureter due to endometriosis by resection and ureteroureterostomy. A case report. J Urol 1992;148:865–868.

31. Gentile GP, Siegler AM. Inadvertent intentional biopsy during laparoscopy and hysteroscopy: A report of two cases. Fertil Steril 1981;36:402.

32. Sauer M, Jarrett JC. Small bowel obstruction following diagnostic laparoscopy. Fertil Steril 1984;42:653.

33. Corson SL, Bolognese RJ. Laparoscopy overview and results of a large series. J Reprod Med 1972;9:148.

34. Loffer FD, Pent D. Indications, contraindications and complications of laparoscopy. Obstet Gynecol Survey 1975;30:407.

35. Penfield AJ. How to prevent complications of open laparoscopy. J Reprod Med 1985;30:660.

36. Wheeless CR. Gastrointestinal injuries associated with laparoscopy. In Phillips JM, ed. Endoscopy in Gynecology. AAGL, Ca, 1978, p 317.

37. DeCherney AH. Laparoscopy with unexpected viscus penetration. In Nichols DH, ed. Clinical Problems, Injuries and Complications of Gynecologic Surgery. Williams & Wilkins, Baltimore 1988.

38. Corson SO, Batzer FR, Gocial B, et al. Measurement of the force necessary for laparoscopic trocar entry. J Reprod Med 1989;34:282.

39. Borton M. In Laparoscopic Complication: Prevention and Management. Philadelphia, BC Decker, Inc., 1986.

40. Nezhat C, Nezhat F, Ambroze W, et al. Laparoscopic repair of small bowel, colon, and rectal endometriosis: a report of twenty-six cases. Surg Endosc 1993;7:88–89.

41. Nezhat C, Nezhat F, Pennington E. Laparoscopic treatment of lower colorectal and infiltrative rectovaginal septum endometriosis by the technique of videolaseroscopy. Br J Obstet Gynaecol 1992;99:664–667.

42. Redwine D. Laparoscopic en bloc resection for treatment of the obliterated cul-de-sac in endometriosis. J Reprod Med 1992;37:696.

43. Nezhat F, Brill AI, Nezhat CH, et al. Adhesion formation after endoscopic posterior colpotomy. J Reprod Med 1993;38:534–536.

44. Thompson BH, Wheeless CR Jr. Gastrointestinal complications of laparoscopic sterilization. Obstet Gynecol 1973;41:669.

45. Kirkpatrick JR, Rajpal SG. The injured colon: Therapeutic considerations. Am J Surg 1975;129:187.

46. Peterson HB, DeStefano F, Rubin GL, et al. Deaths attributable to tubal sterilization in the United States, 1977 to 1981. Am J Obstet Gynecol 1983;146:135.

22

Operative Laparoscopy: Other Issues

Camran Nezhat, Farr Nezhat, Ceana Nezhat, and Dahlia Admon

The efforts of international and interdisciplinary talent have contributed to the evolution of diagnostic and operative laparoscopy. The underlying concepts have been reviewed by Semm, Cuschieri and Buess, Murphy, Gomel, and Nezhat and co-workers, among others.[1-5] Topics have included essential instrumention, the value of multiple puncture sites, insufflation equipment, light sources, endoscopic photography, and video monitors and their applications in endoscopic procedures. The Nezhat team has emphasized the accelerated emergence of videolaparoscopy and videolaseroscopy as a safe alternative to surgical laparotomy.[5] Since the late 1970s, improvements in light sources, optics, video cameras, monitors, electrosurgery, and laser technology have allowed surgeons and assistants to work with advanced equipment. Comfortably standing up, they can watch a magnified video monitor that gives a view of the surgical field sensed by a "mini" camera coupled to a CO_2 laser laparoscope, which incorporates a helium-beam guide light.[5]

The surgeon who enters this field must master a number of motor skills in order to optimize the options available. For example, when four puncture sleeves house a laparoscope, grasper, suction-irrigator, and bipolar electrocoagulator, a new dexterity is required. The surgeon may control the laparoscope with one hand using the laser for small-vessel hemostasis, for vaporizing lesions, or as a long knife for cutting and dissection. The other hand may be needed to select instruments as needed. Alternatively, with an assistant holding the laparoscope, the surgeon may use instruments in both hands for other coordinated, essential procedures. To carry out such manipulations, the surgeon must learn to be comfortable using monocular depth perception. Proficient videolaparoscopists work successfully in three dimensions using cues displayed on a two-dimensional screen. Loss of depth perception does not hamper performance. Such may be the case, however, initially, for trainees and for experienced videolaparoscopists who are asked to evaluate new, experimental video equipment purporting to provide binocular depth perception.[2] Such a development would require that they master yet another set of visual cues to achieve a safe performance.

Appropriate use of the laparoscopist's feet is an important part of the learning process. Commonly, activation of a left-foot floor switch fires the laser and a right-foot switch energizes the bipolar coagulator. It is essential that switching be timely because lasers and electrocoagulators are potentially hazardous. Habitually using one can lead to complications when a switch is made to the other. Shorter hospitalization, less postoperative pain and morbidity, and shorter return-to-work times are associated with proper laparoscopic procedures when compared with open surgery.[1-5] Reviewers also point out that in laparotomy, postoperative pain and morbidity, among other factors, are a function of incision location and length. However, they also highlight the fact that findings arising during diagnostic endoscopy or intraoperative complications such as severe hemorrhage may require immediate laparotomy. Patients, therefore, should be informed and give appropriate preoperative consent.[6] Furthermore, all laparoscopic surgeons should be qualified for open surgery or have such competence at hand for backup as may be needed. This is particularly important for personnel in training.

With the increasing use of videolaparoscopy, much has been made of "learning" curves. However, one reads little or nothing about "forgetting" curves. Gaining, maintaining, achieving, and losing surgical proficiency depends upon a variety of variables such as the difficulty and number of procedures involved, the frequency with which they are repeated, and the manual dexterity, patience, motivation, dedication, and clinical acumen of the surgeon. We have few data for assessing positive and negative learning (conditioning and deconditioning) in such multifactorial situations. Findings are often elusive and hampered by sparse information about neurophysiologic alterations that accompany variations in both long- and short-term memory. Learning is accompanied by structural and chemical changes in the nervous system.[7] Some skills are more time-dependent and durable than others. Relations between practice sessions and improved performance vary; that is, some learning occurs early and is little influenced by subsequent training, whereas other skills require more repetition over long periods.

Somewhat similar time-related findings are reported for visual learning.[8] Processes serving learning can occur after practice sessions over periods of several hours so that performance is enhanced. Such data suggest collaborative opportunities for experienced gynecologic surgeons, neurophysiologists, and other biomedical personnel to aid in teaching complicated procedures to physicians who choose to become proficient in both open and videolaparoscopic surgery. Basic memory and learning information has been applied to the design of training aids and equipment that stimulate various specific videolaseroscopic techniques and procedures. Semm's "Pelvi-Trainer" and the Tübingen trainer (a closed anatomic phantom) are examples.[2] Their role in training, along with teaching specific endoscopic operations such as appendectomy or cholecystectomy have been described.[2] Another article emphasizes how hands-on simulation exercises featuring eye-hand coordination are beneficial particularly when used early in teaching residents operative endoscopy.[9]

Learning curves for both conventional and endoscopic surgery change over time and differ for relatively simple or more complex interventions. Also, for each procedure, the complication rate will fall as proficiency is achieved. The overall complication rate will be a function of the expertise of the operator at the time any technique is initially used, particularly if it is innovative. As one team using videolaparoscopy in appendiceal surgery reported on the first 50 cases: "Our lack of experience with the method made it difficult to deal with bleeding (three cases), adhesions (three cases) or abnormal position of the appendix (four cases)."[10] Adiposity (three cases), perforation (one case), and abscess (three cases) also required laparotomy. There were no deaths or severe complications. Operative time was 15 to 20 minutes. Patients were "generally discharged one week after operation." The authors concluded: "Our experience shows that laparoscopic appendectomy with the described modification is a safe, practical method of removing the veriform process; last but not least, it can be learned quickly. Within 1½

years, four of the seven surgeons at our hospital have learned this operative technique."

Relevant to these results are the 100 incidental appendectomies following the treatment of other pathology reported by Nezhat and Nezhat, who were already proficient in videolaparoscopy when the study was initiated.[11] Except for a fever, which resolved in 24 hours in one patient, and mild periumbilical ecchymosis, there were no intra- or postoperative complications. Appendectomy time ranged from 4 to 21 minutes. All patients were discharged within 24 hours of surgery.

While these data have general application to learning curves, they only indirectly address the issue of whether laparotomy or either videoendoscopy or videolaseroscopy is the preferred option for appendectomy. Many, but not all, of the relevant, difficult, and complicated questions are addressed in a randomized prospective trial involving 140 patients equally divided between open appendectomy (OA) and laparoscopic appendectomy (LA).[12] The investigators reported no significant difference in the postoperative course between the two groups. They noted the higher-than-expected conversion to OA was probably 50% experience related. However, they reviewed other studies with contrary findings. Thus, the LA–OA issue remains controversial. These authors stated ". . . the ability to perform a diagnostic laparoscopy should be advantageous in the longer term and there should be a reduction in wound infection rates; we believe these are major benefits that justify a laparoscopic approach."

For may more complex surgical problems, particularly where laparotomy incisions are severalfold longer than the standard approach for uncomplicated appendectomy, future randomized trials are unlikely for ethical reasons. Among them are procedures to treat gallbladder disease and intractable midline pelvic pain. In the former instance, the benefits of laparoscopic cholecystectomy are compellingly clear both to patients and physicians.[13]

Credentialing

While most of the data we have cited thus far were evolving, much surgical endoscopy (followed by videoendoscopy and videolaseroscopy) was emerging as a consequence of patient demand for minimally traumatic and stressful procedures. These procedures became available through the efforts of innovative private practitioners. For example, in 1986 Nezhat reported results of 600 cases of endometriosis treated with videolaseroscopy. Subsequent progress, aided by a brisk referral practice and availability of an improved camera-CO_2 laser-laparoscope, encompassed laparoscopic surgery in over 1,000 patients including many with extensive endometriosis.[5,14–16]

Academic teaching centers appeared uninterested initially in what were regarded as improved procedures. Until recently, these institutions and certifying specialty boards were of little help in supporting hospital staff and administration who were responsible for granting endoscopy privileges. They relied on training courses given at selected medical centers and sometimes sponsored by local or regional branches of several national associations. Eventually, the Committee on Gynecologic Practice of the American College of Obstetricians and Gynecologists (ACOG) released credentialing guidelines for operative laparoscopy.[17] These stimulated interest in a requirement by the American Board of Obstetricians and Gynecology that training include documentation that residents were trained in endoscopic procedures of proven value.[18] The realization that such data were not fully available and that the need for changes in training was pressing was highlighted in a survey undertaken by the Council on Resident Education in Obstetrics and Gynecology (CREOG) of junior fellows of ACOG who had finished their residencies between 1987 and 1992.[19] Over half regarded their training in advanced surgical techniques, including endoscopic procedures, as not adequate. Also, CREOG noted that there was no consensus on how best to train surgeons simultaneously in both open and endoscopic techniques because the latter should include advanced video and laser technology. It was realized the staff for such teaching was not broadly available. Two other conclusions were unavoidable. First, that it would be necessary to "teach the teachers" and, second, an experimental training program would have to be conceived and implemented. This was done at the Furman Medical Center in Kansas City.[9] No doubt, other centers have similarly upgraded resident training.

Fortunately, the necessity of incorporating the recent advances achieved by innovative surgeons to improve residency training continues to receive vigorous attention and is advancing on a procedure-by-procedure basis. A July 28, 1993 memo concerning laparoscopic hysterectomy to the Advisory Council of the ACOG is relevant and illustrative.[20] CREOG was asked to consider guidelines for diagnostic laparoscopy (level I), minor operative laparoscopy (level II), moderately advanced laparoscopy (level III), and advanced operative laparoscopy (level IV). Although specific training and performance criteria have not been determined, a number of human cases done under supervision and a list of complications over 2 years were laid out. Final action will evolve through a consensus process that will be greatly influenced by the experience of established open and endoscopic surgeons.

Currently, opinions regarding time to competence vary. Nezhat recently noted: "It takes four or seven years at least to become really proficient, so it is important to disseminate this technology in a carefully taught manner."[21] For a relatively simple laparoscopic appendectomy, Gotz and co-workers noted 1½ years in their experience was a reasonable learning time.[10] In the future, more specific criteria, recognizing the relationship between the number and difficulty of cases, frequency of performance, documented complications encountered, and periodic assessment by peer review, will evolve to refine credentialing guidelines. Thus far, preceptor judgement of proficiency in hands-on human surgery has been and is paramount. That preceptor competence is essential highlights the necessity of assuring the availability of such talent. Hospital administrations and medical board agencies should recognize and give periodic attention to the relationship between supply and demand. Referrals to regional centers specializing in operative videolaparoscopy to achieve an optimal balance between caseload and proficiency has been encouraging.

It is interesting that training and evaluation of endoscopic skills for gastroenterologists have recently been published.[22] Training was done using videoendoscopes. Learning curves for esophagogastroduodenoscopy and colonoscopy were developed showing percent success as a function of procedure number. Cecal intubation success was 84% after 100 trials. Comparable figures for upper GI endoscopy was 90% after 100 procedures. Beyond emphasizing that proficiency in GI endoscopy required more than 100 supervised procedures, the authors noted that the relationship between experience and competence in mastery and using cognitive and technical skills has been inadequately researched. Certainly all physicians and surgeons hope this area encompassing how, where, and why clinical judgment evolves during the training (learning) process will be investigated so it can be better understood.

No doubt, those concerned with the currently changing "balance" between open and videolaparoscopic surgery are also examining a number of options for the future. Rather than emphasizing laparotomy, on the one hand, or videolaparoscopy, on the other, it is clear that competent surgeons will have to master both. Video technology, which offers magnification, excellent visibility, and taping procedures for the record, for enhancing patient rapport, and for teaching purposes already is a major element in surgical training of residents. That available models and simulators can improve teaching efficiency is appreciated, but the optimal use of such assistance is not yet clear.

Academic medicine thrives best when there is healthy communication between clinical and research personnel. Had the laparoscopic revolution been stimulated by teaching centers, appropriate innovations and improvements would have altered resident training programs. A cadre of competent surgeons would now be available and we would not be hampered by the shortage of such skilled people.

Some believe universities are the proper places to encourage the interdisciplinary competence in all the sciences underlying medical progress. But, it is not always an option. Modern medicine, including surgery, has benefited from the contributions of technology experts working both within and outside academic centers. The most successful efforts avoid bureaucratic and political pitfalls. Often success is a matter of chance—being at the right place at the right time.

A valuable aid for those participating in the reorientation of surgical methodology and practice, which often involves the introduction of new and potentially controversial procedures, is the 1978 Belmont Report on ethical principles of research.[23] First, this Department of Health, Education and Welfare report addresses the "fuzzy" interface between practice and research. Second, it highlights three principles: respect for persons, beneficence, and justice. These principles have a critical impact on decisions concerning the role of randomized trials. For example, a paper assessing the relative merits of open versus laparoscopic cholecystectomy noted that patients have the right to make their own decisions about therapy (principle of autonomy) and embodies informed consent.[13] Also, the authors wrote: "Accepting the ethical principle of autonomy means that randomized control trials have become obsolete for alternative treatments that are of concern to the patient. The randomized control trial then joins other obsolete controlled trials. . . ."[13]

Finally, all the videolaparoscopic procedures included in this and future texts will have laparotomy counterparts. Determining the preferred modality will involve application of the noted surgical principles, along with proper consideration of indications and contraindications for either surgical approach determined on a case-by-case basis.

References

1. Semm K. Operative manual: Endoscopic abdominal surgery. Chicago, Yearbook Medical Publishers, 1987.
2. Cuschieri A, Buess G. Introduction and historical aspects. In Cuschieri A, Buess G, Perissat J, eds. Operative manual of endoscopic surgery, Berlin, Springer Verlag, 1992, pp 1–5.
3. Murphy AA. Diagnostic and operative laparoscopy. In Thompson JD, Rock JA, eds. TeLinde's Operative Gynecology, 7th ed. Philadelphia, JB Lippincott Co., 1992, pp 361–384.
4. Gomel V. Operative laparoscopy: time for acceptance. Fertil Steril 1989;52:1–11.
5. Nezhat C, Nezhat F, Nezhat C. Operative laparoscopy (minimally invasive surgery): state of the art. J Gynecol Surg 1992;8:111–141.
6. Donovan JF, Van Voorhis BI. Legal issues in operative laparoscopy. Contemp Obstet Gynecol, August 1993, pp 31–39.
7. Thompson RF, Berger TW, Madden J. Cellular processes of learning and memory in the mammalian CNS. Am Rev Neuro Sci 1983;6:447–491.
8. Karni A, Sagi D. The time course of learning a visual skill. Nature 1993;365:250–252.
9. Summarco MJ, Youngblood. A resident teaching program in operative endoscopy. Obstet Gynecol 1993;81:463–466.
10. Götz F, Pier A, Bacher C. Modified laparoscopic appendectomy in surgery. Surg Endosc 1990;4:6–9.
11. Nezhat C, Nezhat F. Incidental appendectomy during videolaseroscopy. Am J Obstet Gynecol 1991;165:559–564.
12. Tate JTT, Dawson JW, Chung SCS, et al. Laparoscopic versus open appendectomy: prospective randomized trial. Lancet 1992;342:633–637.
13. Neugebauer E, Troidl H, Dierich A, et al. Conventional versus laparoscpic cholecystectomy and the randomized trial. Br J Surg 1991;78:150–154.
14. Nezhat C. Videolaseroscopy: a new modality for the treatment of endometriosis and other diseases of reproductive organs. Colposc Gynecol Laser Surg 1986;2:221–224.
15. Nezhat C, Crowgey SR, Garrison DP. Surgical treatment of endometriosis via laser laparoscopy. Fertil Steril 1986;45:778.
16. Nezhat C, Crowgey S, Nezhat F. Videolaseroscopy for the treatment of endometriosis associated with infertility. Fertil Steril 1989;51:237–240.
17. Committee on Gynecologic Practice, Credentialing guidelines for operative laparoscopy. ACOG Committee Opinion No. 106, April 1992.
18. Youngblood JP. Advanced surgical techniques in obstetrics and gynecology. Correspondence released by the Council on Resident Education in Obstetrics and Gynecology, 409 12th Street SW, Washington.
19. Youngblood JP. Correspondence dated November 18, 1992. Released by the Council on Resident Education in Obstetrics and Gynecology.
20. Nusbaum ML. Memorandum to the Advisory Council of the American College of Obstetricians and Gynecologists regarding laparoscopic hysterectomy. District II NYS, 152 Washington Avenue, Albany, NY 12210. July 28, 1993.
21. Nezhat C. Stanford University Hospital Medical Staff Update 1993;17:3.
22. Cass OW, Freeman ML, Craig JP, et al. Objective evaluation of endoscopy skills during training. Annals Internal Ed 1993;118:40–44.
23. National Commission for the Protection of Human Subjects of Biomedical and Behavioral Research. The Belmont Report: Ethical Principles and Guidelines for the Protection of Human Subjects of Research. Washington, DC: DHEW Publication (05) 78–0012, 1978.

Part 3
Other Management Techniques and Special Issues

23

The Role of Medical Management in the Treatment of Endometriosis

W. Paul Dmowski

Endometriosis is second only to uterine fibroids as the most frequent cause of surgical procedures in premenopausal women.[1] The disease can be diagnosed and its extent can be evaluated only at the time of surgical exploration via laparoscopy or laparotomy. Surgery, therefore, has traditionally been the principal method of treatment.

Prior to the advent of laparoscopy, resection of advanced endometriosis during exploratory surgery was the only method of treatment. Introduction of diagnostic laparoscopy in the 1960s allowed much earlier diagnosis of endometriotic lesions and permitted medical management of limited disease when laparotomy seemed unnecessary. Thus, through the 1980s, estrogen/progestogen-induced pseudopregnancy, danazolinduced pseudomenopause, and gonadotropin-releasing hormone agonist (GnRH-a)-induced medical hypophysectomy, became alternative methods of treatment. Advances in operative laparoscopy during the past decade, and especially introduction of several laparoscopic laser techniques, have been followed by a new trend in the management of endometriosis. Early endometriotic lesions can now be ablated by most laparoscopists at the time of diagnostic laparoscopy, while all stages of the disease can be resected by experienced laparoscopic surgeons. Procedures such as resection of large ovarian endometriomas, extensive adhesiolysis, adnexectomy, presacral neurectomy, and even such complex operations as resection of endometriosis from the rectovaginal septum, bowel or ureters, which may require bowel or ureteral reanastomosis, and which only a few years ago required laparotomy, are now performed laparoscopically on an outpatient basis. Laparoscopic laser surgery has been popularized by the media as a new, futuristic trend. Such procedures are not only accepted, but frequently requested by patients, leading an increasing number of surgeons to offer advanced laparoscopic surgery in spite of the scorn and reservations of the medical establishment.[2]

In view of these developments, the role of medical management in the contemporary treatment of endometriosis is becoming less clear.

What Is Endometriosis? Is Surgery the Optimal Method of Treatment?

It is not clear what type of a disease is endometriosis. Before the 1920s, endometriosis was considered a form of neoplastic disease. Terms such as adenomyoma, cystadenoma, cystomyoma, cystic adenofibroma, or endometrioma were commonly used when referring to endometriotic lesions. In 1925, John Sampson argued that "... a variety of lesions is produced by misplaced endometrial or Müllerian tissue and it is difficult to classify all of them as true tumors. The term endometriosis müllerianosis would possibly be more correct" wrote Sampson, introducing the term "endometriosis" which subsequently became generally accepted.[3] Since then, and until recently, endometriosis was considered a local, nonneoplastic, gynecologic disease that develops in response to abnormal dissemination of the endometrial cells outside of their physiologic location. Recent data indicate that, contrary to these concepts, endometriosis may be a systemic disease, with alterations in the immune system and manifestations primarily, but not exclusively, in the female pelvis.[4] According to this concept, some of the endometrial cells shed during menses are transported through fallopian tubes as well as lymphatic and vascular channels into ectopic locations. This phenomenon seems to be common to all menstruating women. In most women, misplaced endometrial cells are recognized and destroyed by the cells of the immune system, such as natural killer (NK) cells, cytotoxic T lymphocytes (CTL), and monocytes/macrophages. In approximately 10% of women, alterations in immune function allow misplaced endometrial cells to implant, multiply, and spread to other locations giving origin to endometriosis. Autoantibodies against endometrial cells or cell-derived factors and functional changes in monocytes/macrophages, NK cells, and CTL have been implicated in the process.

Interestingly, suppression of the immune system may be followed by the development of endometriosis, at least in rhesus monkeys. Three independent studies indicate that the severity, or frequency and severity of endometriosis in rhesus monkeys were significantly increased several years after exposure to polychlorinated biphenyls (PCBs), dioxin or proton radiation, all of which can suppress immune function.[5-7] Dioxin and PCBs are some of the major environmental pollutants in the industrialized nations.

Thus, it appears that for the development of endometriosis at least three components are necessary: (1) menstrual function, (2) cyclic estrogen/progesterone stimulation, and (3) a genetically or environmentally altered immune response. If alterations in immune function play a role in the development of endometriosis, endometriotic lesions may represent only a manifestation of the underlying disorder, not unlike lesions of lupus erythematosus. Surgical resection or ablation of such lesions may, therefore, have only a debulking effect and not change the course of the disease.

It is well established that microscopic foci composed of endometrial cells are the earliest endometriotic lesions.[8,9] They are not visible to the naked eye or through the laparoscope. As endometriotic cells multiply, the implants become visible and form a variety of lesions characteristic of endometriosis. Some may contain blood or blood-derived pigments. The response from the surrounding tissue results in a variable degree of scar formation. Advanced lesions may take the form of cystic structures (endometriomas) that may become adherent to or invade other organs. Although endometriotic implants are typically visible on peritoneal surfaces, many lesions are subperitoneal or deeply invading. Thus, surgical resection may be incomplete. Endometriotic microfoci, deep subperitoneal lesions or lesions involving vital organs are left behind and give origin to subsequent recurrence. After surgical resection of endometriosis, the process of recurrence begins probably with restoration of menstrual cyclicity. Cyclic secretion of ovarian estrogen and progesterone stimulates the cycle of endometrial proliferation, secretion, and shedding and induces similar changes in residual endometriotic lesions. It is quite likely that a major role in this process is played by estradiol, which fluctuates between 20 pg/mL during menses and as high as 400 pg/mL at midcycle. Certainly estradiol levels at midcycle are directly related to the thickness of the uterine endometrium, and perhaps also to proliferation of the endometriotic lesions. Thus, surgical treatment does not change basic pathophysiologic mechanisms leading to the recurrence of endometriosis. There is no agreement at this time whether stage I or II endometriosis, which is asymptomatic and coincidentally diagnosed, should be treated, irrespective of the choice of therapy. Although endometriosis is a progressive disease, its natural course is variable. In some women, it may remain static for many years. Recurrent endometriotic lesions may require repeat surgical resection. This raises the question of the number and frequency of procedures that could be safely performed in the same patient for the same disease. The question is valid even if the surgery is only "laparoscopic ablation of lesions". These concerns make it imperative that the need for treatment, the choice of therapy, and the necessity and frequency of subsequent retreatments are carefully considered and justified by: (a) the presence of symptoms, (b) clear association between symptoms and lesions, and/or (c) the presence of advanced lesions. Thus in all cases, prior to the initiation of therapy, treatment objectives should be clearly defined.

Objectives in the Treatment of Endometriosis

In the absence of cause-directed treatment, control of symptoms and resection or suppression of advanced endometriotic lesions are the objectives of management (Table 23.1). Most patients present with one or more components of chronic pelvic pain syndrome as their chief complaint.[10] The primary objective of treatment in this group is control of the pelvic symptoms. Occasionally, endometriotic lesions may not be the cause, and other pelvic or abdominal diseases may be responsible for the symptoms. To exclude other causes of pelvic pain and to assess the degree to which endometriosis contributes to the pelvic symptoms, I recommend a trial of ovarian suppression with either GnRH-a or danazol.

About 30% to 50% of endometriosis patients complain of infertility, with or without associated pelvic pain syndrome.[11] The primary objective in this group is to improve reproductive performance. The presence of endometriosis does not exclude other causes of infertility and the couples require complete and thorough evaluation. All identifiable causes of infertility need to be treated and a sufficient period of time allowed (usually three to six cycles) for conception. If endometriosis is assumed to be the cause of infertility, treatment options should be discussed with the couple, and the optimal one selected. I usually recommend the least invasive treatment method that offers a good

Table 23.1. Treatment objectives.

I. Control of chronic pelvic pain syndrome
  1. Exclude other causes of pelvic pain.
  2. If in doubt, use a trial of ovarian suppression with GnRH-analog.
  3. If no symptomatic response to ovarian suppression, perform GI, urological, neurological, and/or other evaluation appropriate to the individual case.
  4. Identify treatment options.
  5. Select and implement most acceptable treatment method.
  6. If symptoms persist, select alternative approach.
II. Management of infertility
  1. Identify and correct other causes of infertility.
  2. Identify treatment options.
  3. Select least invasive treatment method.
  4. Advance to next more complex treatment if pregnancy is not achieved in three to six cycles.
III. Management of ovarian endometriomas larger than 3 cm
  1. Rule out ovarian neoplasia.
  2. Resect endometrioma with or without prior ovarian suppression.
  3. In young, and especially infertile women, preserve all healthy ovarian tissue.
IV. Management of extragenital or extrapelvic lesions
  1. Surgical resection.
  2. Hormonal suppression.
V. Prevention of recurrence and management of asymptomatic endometriosis
  1. In patients who conceive after treatment of endometriosis, recommend breastfeeding and close spacing of pregnancies.
  2. In patients not planning to conceive, consider cyclic, strongly progestational oral contraceptives.
  3. Asymptomatic, limited (stages I and II) and coincidentally diagnosed endometriosis probably does not require treatment.

chance for success, and continue this approach for approximately three to six cycles. If pregnancy is not achieved, the next more complex treatment is selected. Assisted reproductive techniques (ART), such as in vitro fertilization-embryo transfer (IVF-ET) or IVF-tubal embryo transfer (IVF-TET), are generally the last approach. However, in couples of advanced age, ART procedures may be selected earlier. About 10% to 15% of women with endometriosis present with pelvic endometriomas 3 cm or larger, with or without other symptoms. In such patients, the primary objective is to rule out ovarian neoplasia. Prior medical history, sonographic appearance of the lesion, CA-125 levels, and other markers of ovarian neoplasia are helpful in the preliminary evaluation. However, definitive diagnosis can be made only through resection and histologic examination of the lesion. If endometrioma is diagnosed, the options are usually limited to surgical resection via laparoscopy or laparotomy. Prior to surgery, I recommend medical therapy to decrease the size of the cyst and facilitate resection. Although this approach requires diagnostic laparoscopy followed later on by laparoscopic surgery, I believe the results are better, and more ovarian tissue can be preserved, which is of importance in infertile patients.

Women with extragenital or extrapelvic endometriosis usually complain of pain, abnormal bleeding, and symptoms originating from outside the reproductive system. Most commonly these involve the gastrointestinal, urinary, musculoskeletal, or respiratory systems. In such cases, pelvic endometriosis may or may not be present. The diagnosis is usually made during exploratory surgery and confirmed by histologic examination of the specimen. Resection and/or medical suppression of such lesions is the primary objective. Treatment of pelvic endometriosis, if present, should be included in the therapeutic plan.

In all women following treatment of endometriosis, regardless of the presenting symptoms, and regardless of the treatment used, prevention of recurrent disease should be the major objective. Unfortunately, there are no proven methods to accomplish this goal. In women who conceive after treatment, pregnancy and postpartum lactation may have ameliorating effects on the disease. I recommend breastfeeding and close spacing of pregnancies as a way of hopefully delaying or preventing recurrence.

In women who are not planning to conceive after treatment, I recommend cyclic birth control pills (combination estrogen/progestogen), especially those with predominantly progestational properties. The aim is to induce a hypoestrogenic or high progestational/low estrogenic environment, which decreases endometrial proliferation and may also prevent reactivation of endometriosis. Although there are no confirmatory studies, it is my clinical impression that such regimens delay recurrence of endometriosis. The goal is to decrease the amount and length of the menstrual flow by at least 50%.

There is no agreement whether asymptomatic, limited (stage I or II), and coincidentally diagnosed endometriosis should be treated. Periodic evaluation of the patient is perhaps all that is required.

Medical Treatment Options

Medical management of endometriosis includes symptomatic and hormonal therapy. Symptomatic treatment may be appropriate in women with limited (stage I or II) endometriosis and chronic pelvic pain syndrome who are not planning to conceive. This approach may suffice unless symptoms are difficult to control, the disease becomes more advanced, or infertility becomes a problem. Of the hormonal treatment methods, those that induce endometrial atrophy rather than decidual transformation are most effective.

Symptomatic Management

Chronic pelvic pain of cyclic character as well as other components of the pelvic pain syndrome such as dysmenorrhea, dyspareunia, dysuria, and dyschezia are characteristic of, although not unique to, endometriosis.

In most patients, the severity of pain is correlated with the extent of the disease and with deep pelvic lesions.[12,13] However, the association between symptoms and endometriotic lesions may be difficult to establish. Some women with extensive disease may be asymptomatic, whereas others with minimal lesions may have incapacitating symptoms. Furthermore, other pelvic and abdominal diseases coexisting with endometriosis can be responsible for pelvic symptoms commonly referred to as "chronic pelvic pain." It is not unusual for a patient to undergo repeat surgical procedures, including hysterectomy, for endometriosis coexisting with intestinal, musculoskeletal, neurologic, or urinary tract disease which may be responsible for the chronic pelvic pain.

The patient needs to be carefully evaluated to identify the etiology of pelvic pain. Thorough medical history, physical examination, and, if necessary, gastroenterological, urological, neurological, or orthopedic consultation may be required. The cyclicity of symptoms is not enough to exclude other possible causes of pain. The symptoms of irritable bowel syndrome, colitis, or other pelvic diseases may exacerbate at midcycle or around the time of menses. Pelvic adhesions, especially those restricting ovarian or tubal mobility, which may or may not be associated with active endometriotic lesions, may also aggravate pelvic symptoms during ovulation or menses.

To exclude other causes of pelvic pain, a trial of ovarian suppression with either GnRH-a or danazol may be used. For this purpose, I prefer rapid ovarian suppression with a GnRH-analog. If endometriosis is the cause of pelvic symptoms, most patients will report symptomatic improvement after the first month of amenorrhea. If the frequency and intensity of symptoms are unchanged, further workup is indicated.

Symptomatic management of the pelvic pain syndrome, to be effective, requires close collaboration between the patient and her physician. Patients who are well informed, and who thoroughly understand their condition, respond better to symptomatic management. Support groups, counseling, and education are extremely helpful. Many women find marked symptomatic relief through a regular program of physical exercise. It is possible that endogenous endorphins released during exercise block central nervous system (CNS) perception of pelvic symptoms. According to a recent study, beta endorphin concentration in peripheral monocytes is decreased in women with endometriosis, and especially those with pelvic pain.[14] We know that hypothalamic and plasma endorphin levels increase with stress and/or pain, and that secretion of beta endorphin by the CNS and peripheral monocytes is modulated in a parallel fashion.[15] Therefore, it could be postulated that increased pain perception (decreased pain threshold) in women with endometriosis results from low CNS beta endorphin levels.

Dysmenorrhea, and other chronic pelvic pain symptoms in women with endometriosis, may be related to abnormal prostaglandin production by several cell types. Uterine and ectopic endometrium, peritoneal macrophages, and peritoneal mesothelium have been implicated, but the results of studies are conflicting.[11,16] Nevertheless, analgesics and especially various types of prostaglandin synthetase inhibitors (PgSIs) can effectively control dysmenorrhea and pelvic pain in endometriosis.[17] The response is variable. Several PgSIs may have to be tried. To achieve the best response, treatment with PgSIs should begin a day or two before the onset of symptoms (usually related to menses) and continue for three to seven days (usually through the duration of menstrual flow). Analgesic therapy is most effective when administered on a time-rather than pain-contingent basis. The customary recommendation "as needed for pain," may actually increase pain perception in some women. Other forms of pain management including stronger analgesics, nerve blocks, or acupuncture may be beneficial in more difficult cases. Laparoscopic uterosacral nerve ablation and/or presacral neurectomy will benefit some patients.[18]

Women with endometriosis report a decrease in dysmenorrhea and pelvic pain while taking strongly progestational, cyclic oral contraceptives. This effect is probably due to reduced endometrial proliferation and prostaglandin synthesis. Low estrogenic/high progestational preparations that reduce the amount and duration of the uterine bleeding by at least 50%, are most effective. Oral contraceptives may also control bleeding abnormalities reported by some women with endometriosis which are most likely related to adenomyotic changes.

Danazol-Induced Pseudomenopause

Danazol was introduced into the management of endometriosis in the mid-1970s. Until recently, it has been the mainstay of hormonal therapy for this disease. Biologic properties of this compound, clinical applications, and effectiveness in endometriosis have been reviewed in several publications.[19-21] The drug is a steroid derivative, structurally related to the synthetic androgen, 17α-ethinyl testosterone (ethisterone). Danazol is rapidly absorbed from the gastrointestinal system and rapidly metabolized. Its plasma levels reach maximum concentrations of just over 200 ng/mL about 2 hours after a single oral dose of 400 mg. The average half life is about 28 hours and plasma levels decline to a mean of 27.5 ng/mL 60 hours after the last 400 mg dose. The drug is metabolized by the cleavage of the isoxazol ring to four major and at least 25 minor metabolites, and is excreted about equally in the urine and feces. As a steroid, danazol binds to multiple receptor proteins and can cause a multitude of effects. In the peripheral circulation, danazol displaces testosterone and estradiol from the sex hormone-binding globulin (SHBG) and suppresses SHBG levels through its effect on the liver. As a result, the free testosterone fraction is increased.

Danazol can also displace progesterone and cortisol from the corticosteroid-binding globulin (CBG) in vitro. In the target cells, danazol binds to androgen receptors, leading to translocation of the danazol-receptor complex to the nucleus and ultimately initiation of new protein synthesis. Danazol may also bind to intracellular progesterone and glucocorticoid receptors. However, the biologic significance of this binding is unclear. Danazol does not bind to intracellular estrogen receptors. In vitro, danazol has been shown to inhibit multiple enzymes of steroidogenesis in the adrenal and gonadal cells. To exert this effect, danazol either competes with steroid substrates for the active enzymatic sites or binds to androgen receptors and blocks the synthesis of enzymes. At the hypothalmo-pituitary level, danazol inhibits the midcycle FSH and LH surge and lowers basal FSH and LH levels. A decrease in the frequency of LH pulses observed with this compound indicates an effect on the hypothalamus, whereas an increase in the pulse amplitude suggests a pituitary effect of danazol or danazol-induced hypoestrogenism. Suppression of FSH and LH, as well as the direct effect on the ovary, result in the suppression of ovarian steroidogenesis and in the lowering of peripheral estrogen and progesterone concentrations. Without cyclic estrogenic and progestational stimulation, endometrium, both uterine and ectopic, undergoes atrophy. However, the mechanisms through which danazol resolves endometriosis may be more complex than gonadal suppression alone. It has been suggested that atrophy of the ectopic endometrium may be further enhanced by the direct binding of danazol to endometrial androgen or progesterone receptors. The result is suppression of endometrial cell proliferation.

If changes in the immune system are linked to the pathogenesis of endometriosis, as suggested by several studies, the immunomodulatory effect of danazol may contribute to its therapeutic effectiveness.[4,22,23] This effect has been observed both in vivo and in vitro and involves humoral as well as cell-mediated immunity. In vitro, danazol can suppress macrophage-dependent T-cell activation of B cells, as well as IgG production by the B cells.[24,25] A corresponding in vivo effect leads to suppression of abnormal autoantibody production and clinical improvement in several autoimmune diseases. About 50% of women with endometriosis produce autoantibodies against endometrial cells or cell derived antigens. These autoantibodies may play a role in the pathogenesis of endometriosis or may alter reproductive performance through interference with fertilization and/or implantation. Treatment with danazol decreases immunoglobulin levels and suppresses autoantibodies in patients with endometriosis.[26] Studies by many investigators indicate that cell-mediated immunity is also altered in endometriosis. Functional changes in peripheral lymphocytes, in natural killer cells, and especially in monocytes/macrophages may represent a basic pathogenetic mechanism that may lead to the development of the disease. Danazol treatment can reverse these changes both in vitro and in vivo.[27,28] This finding has led to the suggestion that the immunomodulatory properties of danazol, at least to some degree, may play a role in its effect on endometriosis.

Pseudomenopause is induced with danazol administered in a dose of 200 mg four times daily or approximately 12 mg/kg/day for a period of four to nine months, initiated on the first day of menstruation. In some patients, the dose of danazol may be lowered to 600 mg/day after the onset of amenorrhea. However, lower dose regimens and less frequent administration schedules result in a less complete suppression of ovarian function and less consistent clinical improvement. At the full dose, danazol maintains serum estradiol levels between 20 to 50 pg/mL. This is the result of both direct (through suppression of the ovarian enzymes) and indirect (through suppression of pituitary gonadotropins) inhibition of ovarian steroidogenesis.

The length of danazol therapy should be adjusted individually on the basis of the initial stage of the disease and the clinical response. In patients with peritoneal implants but no endometriomas, a three- to four-month course of amenorrhea is usually adequate. The lesions usually regress completely and there is little or no evidence of residual disease. If small (less than 3 cm) endometriomas are present, the patient may require a longer (about six months) course of therapy. In women with large endometriomas, the lesions regress during six to nine months of treatment but do not disappear completely. Surgical resection may be necessary at the end of medical treatment. At light and electron microscopic examination, atrophic and degenerative changes in the ectopic endometrium are observed.[29,30]

Symptomatic improvement usually begins during the first month of danazol treatment, along with the onset of amenorrhea. Complete relief of symptoms has been reported in more than 90% of patients and clinical improvement in more than 80%. Laparoscopic resolution of endometriosis has been observed in 70% to 90% of cases. However, clinical response to danazol therapy depends on the dose and frequency with which the drug is administered and is directly related to the degree of ovarian suppression as reflected by the serum estradiol levels.

Posttreatment pregnancy rates also depend on the adequacy of ovarian suppression. With the 800 mg/day regimen, rates in the range of 50% to 83% have been reported; whereas with the lower doses, have been significantly lower. Disease recurrence rates are highest (23%) during the first year after discontinuation of treatment, indicating perhaps an incomplete resolution of the disease and persistence of endometriotic lesions; during the following years these rates vary between 5% and 9% annually.

The frequency of danazol side effects tends to be overreported. Signs of ovarian suppression, which are the goal of treatment, such as hot flashes, other menopausal symptoms, or vaginal dryness are frequently lumped together with true side effects, such as anabolic or androgenic manifestations. When the efficacy of danazol was compared with that of mestranol-norethynodrel in a prospective, randomized trial, only 4% of danazol patients but 41% of controls discontinued therapy because of side effects.[31] Side effects of danazol can be categorized as hypoestrogenic, androgenic/anabolic, and general (Table 23.2).

Androgenic/anabolic side effects are the net result of (1) changes in SHBG and free testosterone levels; (2) androgenecity of danazol and its metabolites; and (3) competition between danazol and androgens for the receptor binding sites. The androgenic/anabolic side effects paradoxically appear to be more frequent and more intense at the lower dose of the drug. On a low-dose regimen, because of incomplete suppression, ovarian steroidogenesis continues. In the peripheral circulation, testosterone originating from ovarian secretion, as well as peripheral conversion, is displaced from the SHBG by danazol. With an increase in a free testosterone fraction, androgenic side effects are increased. Thus, a common practice of lowering the

dose of danazol, to decrease the intensity of side effects, has the opposite effect and lowers the clinical effectiveness of the drug.

Because of its immunomodulatory effects, danazol should be considered as preferable to other treatment methods in women with endometriosis and infertility or recurrent miscarriages who have elevated autoantibodies. It probably should not be recommended to patients with extensive acne or hirsutism or to those for whom weight gain, deepening of the voice, or other androgenic/anabolic side effects may not be acceptable. Danazol should be avoided in women with a history of liver disease, elevated liver enzymes, atherosclerosis, or abnormal lipid metabolism. There is no contraindication to repeated courses of danazol. However, if the drug was not optimally effective, or had disturbing side effects, other methods of treatment should be considered.

Gonadotropin Releasing Hormone Agonists (GnRH-a)-Induced Medical Hypophysectomy

GnRH-a are synthetic derivatives of the decapeptide GnRH. Multiple compounds varying in potency have been synthesized by substitution of amino acids in positions 6, 10, or both. Those with a half-life longer than that of native GnRH, when administered continuously, downregulate pituitary GnRH receptors within five to ten days, and induce a state of profound pituitary suppression at times referred to as "medical hypophysectomy." Before suppression of FSH and LH, there is usually a brief period of gonadotropin release, the so-called "flare effect." GnRH-a are not active orally and need to be administered intranasally (IN), subcutaneously (SC), or intramuscularly (IM). Several reviews on the efficacy of GnRH-a in the management of endometriosis have been published recently.[32–34]

The degree of hypoestrogenism induced with GnRH-a varies and depends on the analog, its dose, and the route of administration. With some regimens, estradiol levels can be maintained in the range of 20 to 50 pg/mL. With others, and especially with the depot preparations, estrogens are suppressed to a castrate range. The initiation of GnRH-a therapy is usually recommended in the midluteal phase or with the onset of menses. Midluteal administration reduces the flare effect and facilitates ovarian suppression. There is, however, a risk that the drug could be administered during early pregnancy and contraception should be recommended during the entire cycle.

Leuprolide acetate (Lupron) is available in the injectable form only. It can be administered SC 1 mg/day or as IM 3.75 mg/month injections of lyophilized leuprolide acetate in microspheres incorporated into a biodegradable copolymer of polylactic and polyglycose acids. Gradual degradation provides for a slow release of the GnRH-a. Nafarelin acetate (Synarel) is available

Table 23.2. Side effects of danazol.

General side effects
Alterations in lipoprotein metabolism
Alteration in liver function
Breakthrough bleeding
Dizziness, headache
Edema
Muscle cramps, myalgia
Nausea, indigestion
Skin rash

Hypoestrogenic manifestations
Decreased breast size
Depression, mood changes
Hot flashes
Insomnia, irritability
Night sweats
Vaginal dryness

Anabolic/androgenic manifestations
Acne
Androgenicity to the fetus
Hirsutism
Increased appetite
Oiliness of skin/hair
Voice change
Weight gain

as an IN 200 µg per spray solution. It is recommended in a twice-daily dose of 200 µg sprayed into the nostrils by a metered dose pump. Nafarelin is readily absorbed through the nasal mucosa and has a half-life of four hours. Goserelin (Zoladex), can be administered monthly in the form of an SC pellet through a 16-gauge needle. The site of the injection in the lower abdominal wall may be prepared with a local anesthetic. The agonist has a sustained release from a biodegradable matrix containing 3.6 mg of goserelin. Buserelin can be administered either IN in a divided dose of 900 to 1200 µg/day, or SC in a daily dose of 200 to 400 µg of buserelin acetate. The response to these regimens may not be consistent, and some patients may require a higher dose. This is especially so with IN preparations, absorption of which may be affected by nasal congestion. The degree of GnRH-a-induced ovarian suppression may need to be evaluated periodically with serum estradiol levels, and, if necessary, the dose of the GnRH-a can be adjusted. It is not clear to what level endogenous estrogens need to be suppressed for the optimal response and whether better clinical effects could be achieved with severe hypoestrogenism. Studies with danazol and observations on the response of the uterine endometrium indicate that serum estradiol levels during treatment should remain below 60 pg/mL, yet above 20 pg/mL to avoid undesirable side effects. It is possible that different tissues respond to different estrogen thresholds, as suggested recently by Barbieri.[35] The currently recommended length of treatment with GnRH-a is six months, based on prior studies with other regimens. It is possible that a shorter course of treatment, especially when a severe hypoestrogenic state is induced, may be adequate.

Treatment of endometriosis with GnRH-a effectively improves the symptoms of endometriosis and reduces the size of the lesions. Complete resolution of pelvic pain symptoms is usually observed in more than 50% of patients and a significant decrease in the frequency and intensity of symptoms in over 90%. There is a decrease in the size of endometriotic lesions and a decline in laparoscopic score of endometriosis by about 50%. All GnRH-a appear to be equally effective in this respect.[36–39] Several comparative studies of GnRH-a and danazol indicate similar degrees of clinical effectiveness. A somewhat earlier symptomatic improvement with GnRH-a was suggested by one report.[36]

Side effects of GnRH-a are primarily the result of the hypoestrogenic state. Hot flashes, night sweats, vasomotor instability, decreased breast size, and vaginal dryness are the most common and can be expected in as many as 90% of patients treated. They actually indicate the effectiveness of the regimen in inducing ovarian suppression. In patients predisposed to depression or migraine headaches, these symptoms may become more severe. However, side effects are rarely severe enough to cause discontinuation of therapy. Severe hypoestrogenism (estradiol levels consistently below 20 pg/mL) may be associated with increased calcium mobilization from the bones and may result in osteoporosis. However, it is not clear how serious the risk is. Several studies indicate no change in bone density while others reported a minimal, readily reversible bone loss.[40,41]

GnRH-a are of particular advantage if side effects of steroidal preparations are not acceptable, or if profound estradiol suppression is desired (for example, in a patient with endometriosis and uterine fibroids). It is unclear whether such profound ovarian suppression could reduce the length of treatment set arbitrarily for GnRH-a, as for danazol at six months. GnRH-a should not be used in women with osteoporosis. Caution should be exercised regarding possible bone loss if prolonged treatment or repeated courses are contemplated. GnRH-a are not recommended in patients with a history of depression or severe migraine headache since exacerbation of symptoms may occur.

Estrogen/Progestogen-Induced Pseudopregnancy

Continuous administration of estrogens with progestogens in high doses induces a state of hyperhormonal amenorrhea and along with it a multitude of symptoms and findings resembling changes that occur during normal pregnancy. This method of treatment for endometriosis, introduced by Kistner in 1958,[42] has been referred to as "pseudopregnancy."

Various oral contraceptives have been recommended for induction of pseudopregnancy. Those found most effective have strong progestational properties, such as norgestrel 0.5 mg with ethinyl estradiol 0.05 mg (Ovral). The usual therapeutic regimen consists of one tablet daily continuously for six to nine months with an increase by one tablet for each episode of breakthrough bleeding (BTB). In this way, the lowest effective dose is determined for each patient. During pseudopregnancy, pituitary and ovarian function are suppressed more profoundly than during pseudomenopause. Both midcycle and baseline FSH and LH concentrations are low, as are ovarian estradiol and progesterone. However, exogenous estrogens and progestogens, administered as the pseudopregnancy regimen, bind to estrogen and progesterone receptors in the uterine and ectopic endometrium, inducing initial stimulation hypertrophy, vascular congestion, edema, and decidual transformation. Only later during the course of treatment have necrobiosis and resorption of endometriotic lesions been observed.

Symptomatic improvement during pseudopregnancy is variable and depends on the induction of amenorrhea. In some patients, especially at the beginning of treatment, symptoms of endometriosis may exacerbate when endometriotic lesions enlarge. Clinically, estrogens/ progestogens are considered less effective than regimens inducing endometrial atrophy such as danazol or GnRH-a. Side effects, risks, and contraindications to pseudopregnancy are the same as for oral contraceptives.

Oral or Parenteral Progestogens

A form of pseudopregnancy may be induced with synthetic progestogens alone. Exogenous progestogens act synergistically with endogenous estrogens, suppressing ovarian function and inducing hyperhormonal amenorrhea and decidual endometrial changes that are similar to those observed with estrogen/progestogens.[43] However, ovarian suppression is rather inconsistent, with variable estradiol levels and breakthrough bleeding (BTB) is a frequent occurrence. To control BTB, some clinicians recommend supplemental use of low-dose estrogens, thus converting to a typical pseudopregnancy regimen. Progestogens recommended for the treatment of endometriosis include: medroxyprogesterone acetate (MPA), in its oral or depot form; norethindrone; and norethindrone acetate, and gestrinone (not available in the U.S.). The dose, as with estrogen/progestogen preparations, is individually determined in a stepwise fashion. Amenorrhea is usually achieved with 40 mg/ day of oral MPA, 30 mg/day of norethindrone, or 15 mg/day of norethindrone acetate. Depot MPA has been found effective in a dose of 100 to 200 mg monthly in patients with extensive endometriosis who are not interested in pregnancy and in whom surgery is contraindicated. Side effects of progestogens alone are fewer and generally better tolerated than those of estrogen/progestogen preparations. Depot MPA has variable, prolonged absorption and delayed clearance. Progestogens alone may be recommended as an alternative to pseudopregnancy, when contraindications to the use of GnRH-a or danazol exist. Depot MPA may have an advantage in women with residual ovarian function and recurrent endometriosis following hysterectomy, who are not candidates for another surgery.[44] However, depot MPA should not be recommended in women who plan to conceive after a course of treatment.

New Therapeutic Agents

Future developments in the medical management of endometriosis should lead to more effective and shorter courses of treatment. Several approaches are currently being investigated. One involves the use of GnRH analogs with antagonistic properties. These hormones are capable of inducing immediate and more profound pituitary suppression, without the initial flare effect characteristic of GnRH agonists. Although earlier antagonists had unacceptable side effects, newer

products appear to be well tolerated and are currently entering clinical trials. GnRH antagonists may shorten the course of treatment and offer other advantages in the management of endometriosis. Another approach may involve a combination of hormones rather than a single regimen, to maximize the therapeutic effect and to decrease the frequency and intensity of side effects. A new class of hormonal preparations with antiprogestational properties is currently being developed and some have entered clinical trials. It is possible that antiprogestogens may be able to induce endometrial atrophy and have beneficial effect on endometriosis either alone or in combination with other hormones.

Another possible future approach in the management of endometriosis may involve an entirely new class of therapeutic agents, the immunomodulators. If endometriosis is a disease of the immune system, or if infertility associated with endometriosis is the result of immune alterations, as suggested by recent studies, drugs with immunomodulatory properties may have potential therapeutic application. It is possible that some of the therapeutic effectiveness of danazol is secondary to its immunomodulatory properties. Another immunomodulator, pentoxiphylline, when used in animal studies, was able to suppress activated macrophages and reverse the antifertility effects of these cells.[45] Thus, the immunotherapeutic approach may offer a completely new strategy for the management of endometriosis and/or associated infertility.

Selection of Treatment

A variety of therapeutic approaches currently available in the management of endometriosis may present a challenge to some physicians, but offer to the patient a chance for a more individualized approach. Thus, physicians who advocate only one method of treatment, regardless of how effective, probably provide a disservice to at least some of their patients. I prefer to individualize the management of patients with endometriosis, depending on the presenting

Table 23.3. Symptomatic management.

Advantages	Disadvantages
Simple	
Avoids medical or surgical intervention	No effect on the disease
Benefits	Risks/side effects
Symptomatic improvement	Progression of the disease
Little or no interference with reproductive function	Drug dependence
Specific indications	Specific contraindications
Stage I or II disease	Stage III or IV disease
No infertility problems	Unproven diagnosis
Prior to or between pregnancies	

symptoms and taking into consideration their intensity. Factors such as extent of the disease, family status, presence of infertility, desire for the preservation of the reproductive potential, previous treatment history, and age of the patient are also considered. Prior to the selection of treatment, I discuss with the patient alternative therapeutic approaches, both medical and surgical, their advantages and disadvantages, as well as indications, contraindications, side effects, and risks of each method (Tables 23.3 to 23.7). The patient should not only be aware of the rationale for the selection of the specific treatment but should also actively participate in the decision-making process.

Table 23.5. GnRH-A therapy.

Advantages	Disadvantages
Simple	Long treatment
Cost effective	Partial effect on large lesions
Affects microfoci	No effect on adhesions
Suppresses uterine fibroids	
Benefits	Risks/side effects
Symptomatic improvement	Estrogen deficiency symptoms
Regression of lesions	Hypoestrogenic changes
May improve fertility	Osteoporosis
May prevent surgery	Depression
Prevents postop adhesions	Migraine
Specific indications	Specific contraindications
Uterine fibroids	Decreased bone density
Menometrorrhagia	History of depression
Contraindication to surgery	History of migraine
	Unproven diagnosis

Role of Medical Management

There is no cause-directed treatment of endometriosis, because the etiology of this disease is unknown. Surgical resection is limited to visible and accessible lesions. It leaves behind endometriotic microfoci, deep subperitoneal lesions, and lesions on vital organs that the surgeon for obvious reasons is reluctant to resect. Unresected endometriotic lesions, as well as uncorrected pathophysiologic mechanisms, give origin to subsequent recurrence. How frequently a patient can undergo repeat resection or ablation of endometriosis, even if the surgery is minimally invasive, is an unanswered question. We should not forget that even minimally invasive surgery carries risks to the patient. Postoperative adhesions may contribute to infertility or pelvic pain, symptoms that the patient might have presented with initially. It is unclear to what extent laser ablation of ovarian endometriosis, performed by many laparoscopists, contributes to the destruction of

germ cells and may shorten the reproductive life span of the patient.

For these reasons, medical treatment is frequently superior to surgery. It affects all endometriotic lesions, including microfoci, lesions deep under the peritoneum, or outside of the pelvis, and lesions involving vital organs, not suitable for surgical excision. The effectiveness of medical therapy in terms of symptomatic relief, frequency of subsequent recurrence, and posttreatment pregnancy rates is comparable, at least in limited disease, with results achieved with the surgical approach. Furthermore, medical treatment is simple, does not require special skills or sophisticated equipment, and is cost effective when compared with surgery. There is no destruction of ovarian tissue and no postoperative adhesion formation.

There are also disadvantages of the medical approach. The treatment is usually long and there are side effects and risks associated with various regimens. Furthermore, contrary to common misconceptions,

Table 23.4. Danazol therapy.

Advantages	Disadvantages
Simple	Long treatment
Cost effective	Partial effect on large lesions
Affects microfoci	No effect on adhesions
Immunomodulatory effect	
Benefits	Risks/side effects
Symptomatic improvement	Androgenic manifestations
Regression of lesions	Menopausal symptoms
Improved fertility	Weight gain
May prevent surgery	Liver cell damage
Prevents postop adhesions	Atherosclerosis
Specific indications	Specific contraindications
Immune factor infertility	History of liver disease
Autoimmune changes	Elevated liver enzymes
Menometrorrhagia	Obesity
Low weight	Hyperandrogenism
Contraindication to surgery	Atherosclerosis
	Lipid disorders
	Unproven diagnosis

Table 23.6. Estrogen/progestogen therapy.

Advantages	Disadvantages
Simple	Long treatment
Cost effective	No effect on large lesions
Affects microfoci	No effect on adhesions
	Stimulates uterine fibroids
	Less effective than other medical regimens
Benefits	Risks/side effects
Symptomatic improvement	Increased blood coagulability
Regression of lesions	Increased symptoms/lesions
May prevent surgery	Spontaneous endometrioma rupture
Prevents postop adhesions	Breakthrough bleeding
	Other side effects of E/P
Specific indications	Specific contraindications
Contraindication to surgery	Same as for oral contraceptives
Contraindication to other medical regimens	Uterine fibroids
	Unproven diagnosis

Table 23.7. Progestogen therapy.

Advantages	Disadvantages
Simple	Long treatment
Cost effective	No effect on large lesions
Affects microfoci	No effect on adhesions
	Less effective than other medical regimens
Benefits	**Risks/side effects**
Symptomatic improvement	Increased symptoms/lesions
Regression of lesions	Spontaneous endometrioma rupture
May prevent surgery	Breakthrough bleeding
Prevents postop adhesions	Prolonged absorption of MPA
	Side effects of progestogens
Specific indications	**Specific contrainidcations**
Contraindications to surgery	Same as for progestogens
Contraindication to other medical regimens	Uterine fibroids
Endometriosis after TAH	Unproven diagnosis

there is no drug currently known that can "eradicate" endometriosis. All hormonal treatment methods modulate the endocrine environment and suppress cyclic secretion of ovarian estrogens and progesterone. In the hypoestrogenic or hyperprogestational state induced with these regimens, uterine and ectopic endometrium undergo atrophy or decidual changes. The patient develops amenorrhea and endometriotic lesions resolve. Because of the indirect effect of hormonal regimens, it takes several months to achieve a complete regression of the lesions. Also, the effects in advanced endometriosis are limited and there is no beneficial effect on existing adhesions. A combination of medical treatment, followed by surgical reselection, offers advantages and decreases disadvantages of both approaches, and may be a preferred treatment method in advanced endometriosis.

Table 23.8 presents advantages and disadvantages of medical treatment followed by laparoscopic surgery.

Table 23.8. Medical treatment followed by laparoscopic surgery.

Advantages	Disadvantages
Affects microfoci	Long treatment
Facilitates surgery	Requires complex equipment
Effective in advanced disease with adhesions	Requires expert surgical skills
Benefits	**Risks/side effects**
Improved results	Postoperative adhesions
Minor surgery	Surgical complications
	Surgical risks
	Risks of medical therapy
Specific indications	**Specific contraindications**
Extensive disease	As for medical treatment alone
Failed prior treatments	As for surgical treatment alone
Long infertility	Suspected neoplasia
Contraindication to major surgery	

Alternatively, surgical resection of endometriosis may be followed by a course of medical therapy. However, in the latter approach the advantages of performing surgery during the state of ovarian suppression are lost, the resection is more extensive, and the risk of postoperative adhesions may be increased.

Because none of the currently available therapeutic approaches in endometriosis alters basic pathophysiologic mechanisms, none is curative and none is uniformly effective. Each treatment method offers specific advantages and disadvantages. Surgical and medical options should be considered in each case and both the patient and her physician should carefully evaluate specific indications and contraindications as well as weigh the risks and benefits of each option.

Physicians specializing in the management of endometriosis face multiple challenges. Besides possessing traditional surgical skills, they must be experienced laparoscopic surgeons, with access to and expertise in newer laser techniques. They must also be familiar with a variety of hormonal preparations, each one with a somewhat different mode of action. Furthermore, patients today want to know the risks, side effects, alternative approaches as well as indications and contraindications of each method of treatment. It appears likely that the future management of endometriosis will include immunomodulatory drugs or techniques that will modify the immune response. It also appears likely that the therapeutic agents of the future will be selected after specific in vitro testing similar to the current selection process for antimicrobial or antineoplastic treatment.

References

1. Wheeler JM. Epidemiology and prevalence of endometriosis. In Olive DL, ed. Infertility and Reproductive Medicine Clinics of North America. Philadelphia. WB Saunders, 1992, pp 545–549.
2. Pitkin RM. Operative laparoscopy: surgical advance or technical gimmick? Obstet Gynecol 1992;79:441–442.
3. Sampson JA. Heterotropic or misplaced endometrial tissue. Am J Obstet Gynecol 1925;10:649–668.
4. Dmowski WP, Braun D, Gebel H. The immune system in endometriosis. In Rock J, ed. Modern Approaches to Endometriosis. Lancaster, U.K., Kluwer Publishers, 1991, pp 97–111.
5. Wood DH, Yochmowitz MG, Salmon YL, Eason RL, Boster RA. Proton irradiation and endometriosis. Aviat Space Environ Med 1983;54:718–724.
6. Campbell JS, Wong J, Tryphonas L, Arnold DL, Nera E, Cross B, LaBossiere E. Is simian endometriosis an effect of immunotoxicity? Proceedings of Forty-Eighth Annual Meeting, The Ontario Association of Pathologists, London, Ontario, October 1985. Abstract #12, Health Protection Branch, Health & Welfare Canada, Tunney's Pasture, Ottawa, Canada.
7. Rier SE, Martin DC, Bowman RE, Dmowski WP, Becker JL. Endometriosis in Rhesus Monkeys (Macaca

mulatta) Following Chronic Exposure to 2,3,7,8,-Tetrachlorodibenzo-p-dioxin. Fundam Appl Toxicol 1993; 21:433–441.

8. Murphy AA, Green WR, Bobbie D, Cruz ZC, Rock JA. Unsuspected endometriosis documented by scanning electron microscopy in visually normal peritoneum. Fertil Steril 1986;46:522–524.
9. Vasquez G, Cornillie F, Brosens IA. Peritoneal endometriosis: scanning electron microscopy and histology of minimal pelvic endometriotic lesions. Fertil Steril 1984; 42:696–703.
10. Buttram VC, Reiter RC. Endometriosis. In Brown CL, ed. Surgical Treatment of the Infertile Female. Baltimore, Williams & Wilkins, 1985, pp 89–147.
11. Christman GM, Halme JK. Pathophysiology of endometriosis-associated symptoms. In Olive DL, ed. Infertility and Reproductive Medicine Clinics of North America. Philadelphia, WB Saunders, 1992, pp 551–564.
12. Koninckx PR, Meuleman C, Demeyere S, Lesaffre E, Cornillie FJ. Suggestive evidence that pelvic endometriosis is a progressive disease, whereas deeply infiltrating endometriosis is associated with pelvic pain. Fertil Steril 1991;55:759–765.
13. Fedele L, Bianchi S, Bocciolone L, DiNola G, Parazzini F. Pain symptoms associated with endometriosis. Obstet Gynecol 1992;79:767–769.
14. Vercellini P, Sacerdote P, Panerai AE, Manfredi B, Bocciolone L, Crosignani PG. Mononuclear cell B-endorphin concentration in women with and without endometriosis. Obstet Gynecol 1992;79:743–746.
15. Sacerdote P, Rubboli F, Locatelli L, Ciciliato I, Mantegazza P, Panerai AE. Pharmacological modulation of neuropeptides in peripheral mononuclear cells. J Neuroimmunol 1991;32:35–41.
16. Willman EA, Collins WP, Clayton G. Studies in the involvement of prostaglandins in uterine symptomatology and pathology. Br J Obstet Gynaecol 1976;83:337–341.
17. Kauppila A, Ronnberg L. Naproxen sodium in dysmenorrhea secondary to endometriosis. Obstet Gynecol 1985; 65:379–383.
18. Candiani GB, Fedele L, Vercellini P, Bianchi S, DiNola G. Presacral neurectomy for the treatment of pelvic pain associated with endometriosis: a controlled study. Am J Obstet Gynecol 1992;167:100–103.
19. Barbieri RL, Ryan KJ. Danazol: endocrine pharmacology and therapeutic applications. Am J Obstet Gynecol 1981; 141:453–463.
20. Dmowski WP. Danazol-induced pseudomenopause in the management of endometriosis. Clin Obstet Gynecol 1988; 31:829–839.
21. Dmowski WP. Danazol—a synthetic steroid with diverse biologic effects. J Reprod Med 1990;35:69–75.
22. Hill JA. Immunologic factors in endometriosis and endometriosis-associated reproductive failure. In Olive D, ed. Infertility and Reproductive Medicine Clinics of North America. Philadelphia: WB Saunders, 1992, pp 583–596.
23. Dmowski WP, Gebel H, Braun DP. The role of cell-mediated immunity in pathogenesis of endometriosis. Acta Obstet Gynecol Scand 1994;159(S):7–14.
24. Hill JA, Barbieri RL, Anderson DJ. Immunosuppressive effects of danazol in vitro. Fertil Steril 1987;48:414–418.
25. Gebel H, Braun DP, Rotman C, Rana N, Dmowski WP. Mitogen induced production of polyclonal IgG is decreased in women with severe endometriosis. Am J Reprod Immunol 1993;29:124–130.

26. El-Roeiy A, Dmowski WP, Gleicher N, Radwanska E, Harlow L, Binor Z, Tummon I, Rawlins R. Danazol but not gonadotropin-releasing hormone agonists suppresses autoantibodies in endometriosis. Fertil Steril 1988;50: 864–871.
27. Braun DP, Gebel H, Rotman C, Rana N, Dmowski WP. The development of cytotoxicity in peritoneal macrophages from women with endometriosis. Fertil Steril 1992;57:1203–1210.
28. Braun DP, Muriana A, Gebel H, Rotman C, Rana N, Dmowski WP. Monocyte-mediated enhancement of endometrial cell proliferation in women with endometriosis. Fertil Steril 1994;61:78–84.
29. Dmowski WP, Cohen MR. Treatment of endometriosis with an antigonadotropin, danazol: a laparoscopic and histologic evaluation. Obstet Gynecol 1975;46:147–154.
30. Schweppe KW, Dmowski WP, Wynn RM. Ultrastructural changes in endometriotic tissue during danazol treatment. Fertil Steril 1981;36:20–26.
31. Noble AD, Letchworth AT. Medical treatment of endometriosis: a comparative trial. Postgrad Med J 1979; 55(5):37–39.
32. Henzl MR. Gonadotropin-releasing hormone (GnRH) agonists in the management of endometriosis: a review. In Rebar RW, ed. Clinical Obstetrics and Gynecology. Philadelphia, JB Lippincott Company, 1988, pp 840–856.
33. Erickson LD, Ory SJ. GnRH analogues in the treatment of endometriosis. In Rock JA, ed. Obstetrics and Gynecology Clinics of North America. Philadelphia, WB Saunders Co., 1989, pp 123–145.
34. Hurst BS, Schlaff WD. Treatment options for endometriosis. In Olive DL, ed. Infertility and Reproductive Medicine Clinics of North America. Philadelphia: WB Saunders Co., 1992, pp 645–655.
35. Barbieri RL. Hormone treatment of endometriosis: The estrogen threshold hypothesis. Am J Obstet Gynecol 1992;166:740–745.
36. Wheeler JM, Knitte JD, Miller JD. Depot leuprolide versus danazol in treatment of women with symptomatic endometriosis. Am J Obstet Gynecol 1992;167: 1367–1371.
37. Shaw RW. An open randomized comparative study of the effect of goserelin depot and danazol in the treatment of endometriosis. Fertil Steril 1992;58:265–272.
38. Henzl MR, Corson SL, Moghissi K, Buttram VC, Berqvist C, Jacobson J. Administration of nasal nafarelin as compared with oral danazol for endometriosis. N Engl J Med, 1988;318:485–489.
39. Dmowski WP. Comparative study of buserelin versus danazol in the management of endometriosis. Gynecol Endocrinol 1989;3(S2):21–31.
40. Dawood MY. Impact of medical treatment of endometriosis on bone mass. Am J Obstet Gynecol 1993;168: 674–684.
41. Tummon I, Ali A, Pepping ME, Radwanska E, Binor Z, Dmowski WP. Bone mineral density in women with endometriosis before and during ovarian suppression with gonadotropin-releasing hormone agonists or danazol. Fertil Steril 1988;49:792–796.
42. Kistner RW. The use of newer progestins in the treatment of endometriosis. Am J Obstet Gynecol 1958;75:264–278.
43. Gunning JE, Moyer D. The effect of medroxyprogesterone acetate on endometriosis in the human female. Fertil Steril 1967;18:759–774.
44. Dmowski WP, Radwanska E, Rana N. Recurrent endometriosis following hysterectomy and oophorectomy: the

role of residual ovarian fragments. Int J Gynecol Obstet 1988;26:93–103.

45. Steinleitner A, Lambert H, Suzarez M, Serpa N, Roy S. Immunomodulation in the treatment of endometriosis-associated subfertility: use of pentoxifylline to reverse the inhibition of fertilization by surgically induced endometriosis in a rodent model. Fertil Steril 1991; 56:975–979.

Chapter 24

Rationale for Combined Medical and Surgical Treatment of Endometriosis

Veasy C. Buttram, Jr.

Three modes of therapy are available for conservative management of endometriosis: surgery, medical suppression, and a combination of surgery and medical suppression. The mode chosen generally depends on symptoms (for example infertility, dysmenorrhea, dyspareunia) and severity of the disease. Laparoscopic surgery is currently the primary conservative approach to the treatment of all cases of minimal, most cases of mild, and many cases of moderate or severe endometriosis (AFS-r Classification of Endometriosis). However, I believe many endometriosis patients need combined medical and surgical treatment.

Surgical Routes

Until recently, the usual treatment of endometriosis had been surgery. Normal anatomy was restored by excision, laser ablation, or cauterization of implants or endometriomas. Often, adhesions were lysed. During the past decade, the surgical route has been modified by using techniques that allow much of the surgery to be performed endoscopically.

There are several reasons why surgery alone may not be the best method of treatment:

- Postoperative adhesions can cause infertility.[1]
- Endometriosis may not be removed because of fear of injury to a vital organ.
- Nonvisualized endometriosis (microscopic disease) is left unattended.
- Health risks and pain may be too great.
- Expense is a major consideration.

Medical Suppression

Many drugs have been used in the treatment of endometriosis: androgens, progestins, estrogen-progestin combinations, danazol, gestrionone, and, more recently GnRH agonists. There are several reasons why medical therapy alone may not be as effective as desired:

- Endometrial implants and endometriomas tend to recur shortly after medical therapy has been discontinued.[2]
- Improvement of fertility is questionable.[3]
- Dense adhesions (part of the pathology of endometriosis) are unaffected.
- Response varies (not all patients respond in the same way).[4]
- Occasionally, there are intolerable or possibly harmful side effects to the patient.[4]
- Expense may be high.

Combined Medical Suppression and Surgery

Pre- and postoperative medical suppression have been used for many years in the treatment of endometriosis.[1–5] There are several reasons, besides those listed for surgery or drugs, why combined therapy may not give optimal results:

- This mode generally requires two surgical procedures: diagnostic laparoscopy followed by laparoscopic surgery or laparotomy after completion of medical suppression for 3 to 6 months. Therefore, this approach to treatment must be justified.
- To date, no convincing study has documented that medical suppression alone enhances the pregnancy rates, regardless of the stage of the disease.[6]
- In several studies, laparoscopic surgery and laparotomy have been shown to enhance conception rates. The degree of surgical success depends on the disease stage.[7]

- When surgery has been unsuccessful, repeat laparoscopy often reveals persistent or new endometriosis. There is no way of preventing new implants, but meticulous surgery reduces persistent disease. Repeat laparoscopy often reveals severe adnexal adhesions, often a result of the initial surgery.

The development of postoperative adhesions is the main reason surgery for endometriosis is less effective than desired. One way to reduce the risk of adhesions is to treat the patient with medical suppression prior to surgery. This approach is particularly effective for patients with moderate or severe disease.

Why Adhesions Form

To understand why preoperative medical suppression is useful, a review of the pathophysiology of adhesions formation is helpful. The peritoneum is composed of two layers: a superficial layer of polygonal mesothelial cells and the submesothelial stromal layer composed of connective tissue, collagen, and reticular and elastic fibers containing abundant vasculature and lymphatic structures (Fig. 24.1). Anything that causes peritoneal tissue to be injured or inflamed can produce pelvic adhesions. Thus, surgical trauma, infection, or a variety of conditions including endometriosis can cause adhesions. Injuries to the peritoneal surface may disrupt stromal mast cells and cause release of histamine and vasoactive kinins (Fig. 24.2). These substances increase capillary permeability, which leads to the formation of a serosanguinous exudate. This matter produces fibrin deposits. Under normal conditions, a plasminogen activator causes a release of plasmin that results in fibrinolysis. Normal healing then occurs without adhesion formation.

In a hypoxic state, the release of plasminogen activator is reduced.[8] With less plasminogen activator and plasmin, fibrinolysis is decreased. Instead, fibrin matrix develops. The fibroblasts and capillaries proliferate within the matrix in the usual manner of tissue healing and produce scars. Such adhesions become permanent. More injury or inflammation results in additional fibrin deposition. The severity of the inflammation or injury determines the amount and intensity of the adhesions.

With an understanding of pelvic adhesion formation, we gain some insight into the etiology of adhesions associated with endometriosis. Theoretically, the inflammation associated with endometriosis could initiate the exudative process that causes fibrin deposition. It has been demonstrated, for example, that the amount of serosanguinous peritoneal fluid in patients with endometriosis is significantly greater than that among control subjects.[8-10] It is possible that the fibrin deposition is greater in patients with inflammation secondary to endometriosis because the normal fibrinolytic mechanisms are overwhelmed. Although this hypothesis is plausible, it has not been examined critically.

Preoperative Use of Medical Suppression

In a study conducted nearly 20 years ago, a preoperative pseudopregnancy regimen was combined with surgery in an attempt to increase the pregnancy rates of patients with infertility attributed to endometriosis.[11] The pregnancy rates, however, were reduced. Although the exact reasons for the results remain unknown, the regimen may have created a pelvic environment prone to postoperative adhesions. This pseudopregnancy state may result in increased capillary proliferation or vasodilatation, conditions conducive to trauma and increased fibrin deposition.

In 1982, my colleagues and I published a report on the efficacy of danazol for treating endometriosis.[12] We noted that after 6 months of therapy, peritoneal disease tended to regress by about two thirds. Some patients (41%) had total resolution of the disease, whereas others (7%) experienced no beneficial effects. Ovarian disease regressed, but to a lesser extent than did peritoneal disease. Large endometriomas were reduced minimally, but those less than 1 cm in diameter were also decreased by approximately two thirds.

One finding from this study is clear: 6 months of preoperative danazol treatment creates a pelvic environment much different from that of a pseudopregnant or normal ovulatory state. There is much less hyperemia in a hypoestrogenic state. Capillaries are less abundant and less dilated. The reduced inflammatory reaction makes identification and removal of endometrial implants and endometriomas easier.

I do not agree with those who postulate that preoperative suppression therapy reduces endometrial implants to the extent that they or their remnants cannot be visualized. At initial laparoscopy, the endometriosis should be documented, preferably by schematic pictures

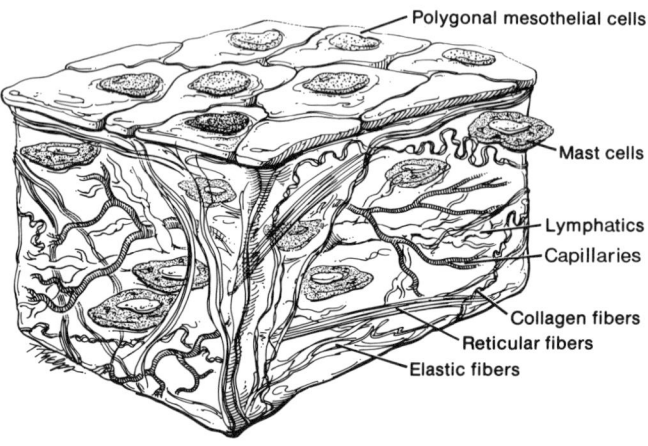

Figure 24.1. Composition of peritoneum.

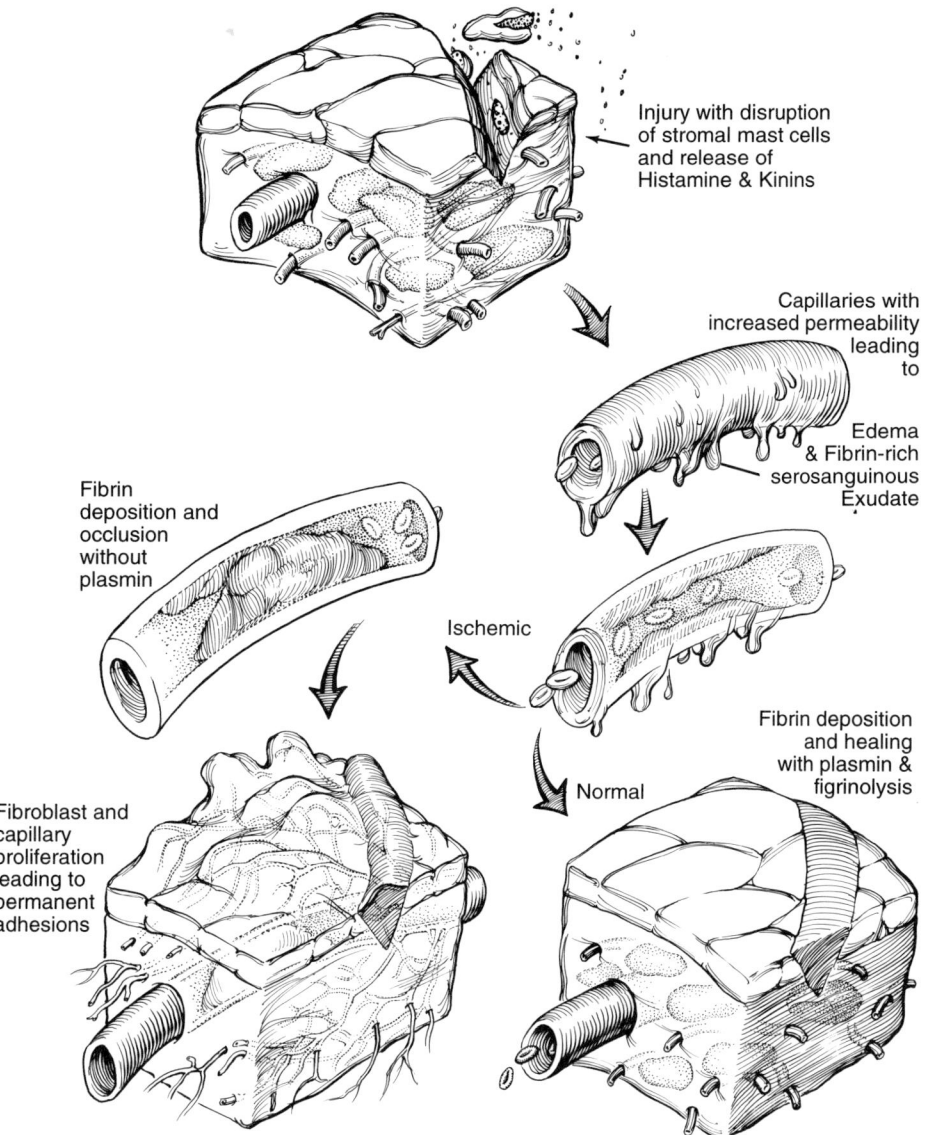

Injury with disruption
of stromal mast cells
and release of
Histamine & Kinins

Capillaries with
increased permeability
leading
to

Edema
& Fibrin-rich
serosanguinous
Exudate

Fibrin
deposition and
occlusion
without
plasmin

Ischemic

Fibrin deposition
and healing
with plasmin &
figrinolysis

Fibroblast and
capillary
proliferation
leading to
permanent
adhesions

Normal

Figure 24.2. Pathophysiology of adhesion formation.

and photographs. After suppressive treatment, peritoneal fluids are not only diminished in quantity but also appear clear. This suggests less fibrin content. The ovaries are inactive. Easily traumatized functional cysts are absent. Endometriomas of the ovaries are easier to remove because they can often be enucleated, thus causing less trauma to the ovary than with an excisive procedure. Adhesions also seem easier to lyse without trauma to adjacent tissue.

It appears preoperative suppression creates a pelvic environment that markedly reduces the risk of postoperative adhesions. Although randomized control trials have not been performed to establish this contention, I am confident it is the case. As others have observed, filmy adhesions often disappear in patients taking danazol for 6 months. It is possible danazol reduces the

inflammatory process and that the motion of pelvic viscera lyses filmy adhesions.[13]

In 1985, our group reported that 6 months of preoperative danazol therapy resulted in improvement in pregnancy rates after surgery for mild, moderate, and severe endometriosis compared with surgery alone (Table 24.1).[4] I believe the increase in pregnancy rates was attributable to the improved pelvic environment and reduction in postoperative adhesion formation.

GnRH agonists produce a hypoestrogenic state (probably more than does danazol). Agonists seem to have the same effect on the pelvic environment as does danazol. They also have a similar effect on endometrial implants, endometriomas, and adhesions. Currently, data substantiating higher pregnancy rates with the use of preoperative GnRH agonists over surgery alone are

Table 24.1. Pregnancy rates achieved following surgery only and combined treatment.

Acosta classification	Pregnancy rates	
	Surgery only	Combined Treatment*
Mild	73%	85%
Moderate	56%	69%
Severe	40%	53%

*Surgery after preoperative danazol (800 mg/d, 96 patients; 400 mg/d, 107 patients).

not available. However, studies on this subject will probably be forthcoming in the near future.

Length of Medical Treatment

How long should danazol or GnRH agonists be used to create a pelvic environment that reduces the risk of postoperative adhesions? This question has been studied for years. Although a clear conclusion has not been reached, I believe that an improved pelvic environment is created after 3 months of therapy. However, there is less resolution of disease after treatment for 3 months compared with after 6 months.

Postoperative Medical Suppression Therapy

Some practitioners believe that medical suppressive therapy should be used postoperatively. In 1981, one team retrospectively analyzed surgical treatment of endometriosis with and without 3 to 6 months of danazol used postoperatively.[5] The patients who received danazol had a higher cumulative pregnancy rate than those who did not receive the drug. The investigators concluded that postoperative danazol suppressed disease that was not completely removed at the time of surgery. However, we know that medical therapy does not eradicate the disease and that temporary suppressive therapy will result in recurrence of the disease. The use of medical therapy preoperatively seems more advantageous since it creates a pelvis more amenable to surgical correction of endometriosis, without as much risk of postoperative adhesions. It also has a suppressive effect upon endometriosis, as does postoperative therapy.

Conclusion

In all cases of minimal and most cases of mild endometriosis, the disease can be eradicated through the laparoscope using a laser or cautery device. The risk of postoperative adhesions is probably not sufficient to warrant medical suppressive therapy and a second surgical procedure. However, in some infertile patients with mild disease and those with moderate or severe disease, I believe that medical suppressive treatment followed by a second operation will result in an improved pregnancy rate.

References

1. Buttram VC, Vacquero C. Post-ovarian wedge resection adhesive disease. Fertil Steril 1975;26:874.
2. Evers JHL. The second-look laparoscopy for evaluation of the result of medical treatment of endometriosis should not be performed during ovarian suppression. Fertil Steril 1987;47:502.
3. Buttram VC. Use of danazol in conservative surgery. J Reprod Med (Supplement) 1990;35:82.
4. Buttram VC, Reiter RC, Ward SM. Treatment of endometriosis with danazol: Report of a six year prospective study. Fertil Steril 1985;43:353.
5. Wheeler J, Malinak LR. Postoperative danazol therapy in infertility patients with severe endometriosis. Fertil Steril 1981;36:460.
6. Seibel MM, Berger MJ, Weinstein FG, Taymor ML. The effectiveness of danazol on subsequent fertility in minimal endometriosis. Fertil Steril 1982;38:534.
7. Buttram VC. Conservative surgery for endometriosis in the infertile female: A study of 206 patients with implications for both medical and surgical therapy. Fertil Steril 1979;31:117.
8. Buttram VC, Reiter RC. Surgical Treatment of the Infertile Female. Baltimore, Williams & Wilkins Publishers, 1985.
9. Confino E, Harlow BS, Gleicher N. Peritoneal fluid and serum autoantibody levels in patients with endometriosis. Fertil Steril 1980;53:242.
10. Bartosik D, Jacobs S, Kelly L. Endometrial tissue in peritoneal fluid. Fertil Steril 1986;46:796.
11. Andrews WC, Larson GD. Endometriosis treatment with hormonal pseudopregnancy and/or operation. Am J Obstet Gynecol 1974;118:643.
12. Buttram VC, Belue JB, Reiter RC. Interim report of a study of danazol for the treatment of endometriosis. Fertil Steril 1982;37:478.
13. Dmowski WP, Cohen MR. Antigonadotropin (danazol) in the treatment of endometriosis. Am J Obstet Gynecol 1978;130:41.

25

Treatment of Infertility Associated With Endometriosis

Deborah Metzger

Despite many years of investigations and clinical trials, treatment of endometriosis-associated infertility remains controversial. A plethora of therapeutic approaches have been suggested including expectant management, medical intervention, major conservative surgery, and laparoscopic resection.[1]

The nature of the often-mentioned association between endometriosis and infertility remains elusive.[2] Because we have no clear understanding of this relationship, optimal management of patients with endometriosis who desire childbearing is hampered. Hormonal therapy has been advocated in the past as a means of enhancing fertility, but controlled studies fail to demonstrate any efficacy.[3] Medical therapy does not appear to eradicate endometriosis implants.[4-6] Given these limitations, surgery seems the preferred way of managing the disease. Besides eradicating visible endometriosis, surgery also affords the opportunity to lyse adhesions. In cases of moderate and severe disease, pelvic anatomy may be restored to as normal a condition as possible.

Does Endometriosis Cause Infertility?

The frequency of pelvic endometriosis in infertile women is significantly greater than that in fertile women undergoing laparoscopy.[7] Although the disease is clearly associated with the failure to achieve pregnancy, whether it is the cause or the result of nonchildbearing remains uncertain. When extensive scarring is present, it seems logical to attribute infertility to the effect of anatomic distortion. However, a reduction in monthly fecundity has been found even when endometriosis implants are the only finding.[8]

Confounding the issue, investigators have noted a high rate of additional infertility factors in these couples, including male factor, cervical factor, luteal phase defect, and tubal factor.[9-11] Any discussion of possible mechanisms of infertility in women with endometriosis must consider these factors.

Reported cycle fecundity rates in women with untreated endometriosis vary widely from 1% to 11%.[1,12] Women with endometriosis undergoing artificial insemination by donor have a cycle fecundity rate of only 2% compared with 12% in women without endometriosis.[13] When techniques such as in vitro fertilization and hMG superovulation with intrauterine insemination are used, they appear to bypass the fertility deficit in these patients. The reported cycle fecundity rates after these treatments are no different from the rates for women without endometriosis.[14-16]

Mechanisms of Infertility With Endometriosis

There is a paucity of evidence identifying the specific mechanism(s) of infertility in endometriosis. At least three separate factors may play a role: implants, ovarian endometriomas, and adhesions. Each may contribute separately to a reduction in fertility by various mechanisms.

Mechanical Factors

When the ovaries and fallopian tubes are involved in extensive scarring, it is easy to suspect impaired transport of the oocyte-cumulus cell complex. A similar mechanism seems possible when the normal anatomic relationship between the ovary and the oviduct is distorted by large endometriomas. More subtle degrees of ovarian capsular scarring may entrap oocytes.[17] Tubal occlusion because of endometriosis is the exception rather than the rule, even with extensive pelvic adhesions. However, hydrosalpinx formation and uterotubal junction obstruction have been observed as a result of local implants and fibrosis.[18]

Tubal Dysfunction

Alterations in the tubal transport of gamete or conceptus have been suspected as a cause of infertility in women with endometriosis. The link between endometriosis and tubal dysfunction is unclear, but it may be related to a higher than normal concentration of prostaglandins in the peritoneal fluid of women with endometriosis implants.[19-22] The actions of prostaglandins, which mediate tubal muscular contractility, depend on the specific tubal segment, the muscle layer, and the type of prostaglandin.

Studies linking prostaglandins and tubal dysfunction are conflicting. Some fail to confirm these findings; others mention the presence of large numbers of peritoneal macrophages which are known to secrete prostaglandins.[23-25] Furthermore, despite the demonstration of prostaglandin-mediated alteration of tubal function in monkeys, studies performed in women given superactive prostaglandin analogues intravenously have failed to demonstrate tubal dysfunction.[26] The association of endometriosis and tubal dysfunction, therefore, remains tenuous.

Luteal Phase Defect

Although a luteal phase defect (LPD) is often mentioned as a mechanism of infertility in endometriosis, there are few controlled studies which could support a cause-and-effect relationship. LPD appears to be a relatively uncommon primary cause of infertility, affecting no more than 5% of the unselected infertile population. The incidence of LPD does appear, however, somewhat higher in women with endometriosis and infertility.[9,27-29] An intriguing report mentions double luteinizing hormone peaks in women with endometriosis, which were reversed following danazol treatment.[30,31] This suggestion of a more profound endocrine abnormality in these patients awaits confirmation. Until objective data are available which document successful treatment of endometriosis-associated infertility by therapy directed toward luteal insufficiency, it should be considered a possible rather than proven mechanism.

Spontaneous Abortion

Several studies have suggested an increased clinical abortion rate in women with untreated endometriosis.[32] The abortion rates ranged from 10% to 49% before treatment and from 0% to 25% after treatment. However, these retrospective data are flawed by selection bias and "before and after" study design. None used an appropriate control population. Two other studies that included an appropriate control group showed no increase in the spontaneous abortion rate attributable to endometriosis. My own group demonstrated a significant decrease in the spontaneous abortion rate not only following conservative resection but also following diagnosis in expectantly managed patients.[32] Another report showed no significant difference in the spontaneous abortion rate in infertile women with and without laparoscopically diagnosed endometriosis.[33] Thus, there is little evidence to support the hypothesis of an increased rate of spontaneous abortion as a mechanism of infertility in women with endometriosis.

Luteinized Unruptured Follicle (LUF) Syndrome

LUF has been investigated as a cause of infertility in a variety of clinical situations including endometriosis.[34,35] In LUF syndrome, the preovulatory follicle luteinizes but the follicle fails to rupture, thus entrapping the ovum. Because luteinization of the granulosa cells does occur, there are such presumptive signs of ovulation as temperature shifts, elevated serum progesterone levels, and endometrial secretory activity. Diagnosis of LUF is determined by the absence of an ovulatory stigma or corpus luteum by direct visualization, absence of postovulatory follicular collapse on ultrasound, or a decrease in the expected postovulatory steroid levels in peritoneal fluid.[36-39] Some investigators have suggested that as many as 60% of women with endometriosis display this syndrome.[35] Others have found no difference in the incidence of LUF in infertile endometriosis patients compared with other fertile or infertile women without endometriosis.[36,39]

The accuracy of the diagnosis of LUF syndrome is in question. Visual assessment of ovulatory stigma may be highly inaccurate. In one study, only 53% of fertile women undergoing laparoscopic tubal sterilization within several days of their basal body temperature shift had evidence of stigmata.[40] This observation is in contrast with a study using daily ultrasound examination in normal fertile women where LUF was found in only 5% of cycles.[41] Neither of these studies provided confirmation of their results by an independent method. Direct visualization of ovulatory stigma is dependent on the time from ovulation and the speed of ovarian capsular healing.

Based on the available data, LUF cannot be said to be observed more frequently in women with endometriosis.

Alterations in the Immune System

Little is known regarding the immune system and infertility in general, and its relationship to infertility in the presence of endometriosis in particular. Despite speculation about a variety of subtle alterations in the immune system in women with endometriosis, the exact mechanism for such alterations producing infertility is unclear.

Circumstantial evidence has suggested an intense immunologic reaction in the endometrial glandular epithelium of patients with endometriosis because of the presence of complement component C_3.[42] More direct evidence has been provided by the demonstration of antiendometrial antibodies and antiovarian antibodies in women with endometriosis but not in controls.[43–45] Antiendometrial antibodies might interfere with implantation and early embryo development. Antiovarian antibodies could similarly affect follicular development and ovulation. These results have not been duplicated in women with mild endometriosis.[46] Antiendometrial antibodies have also been demonstrated in women who had evidence of prior pelvic inflammatory disease.[44] The relevance of this finding to human reproduction is unclear. In one study an adverse reproductive effect of antibodies directed against endometrial antigens was demonstrated.[47]

The association of endometriosis with autoimmune phenomenon in general has also been reported. Patients with endometriosis exhibit twice the normal risk for developing systemic lupus erythematosis.[48] Another study demonstrated a high proportion of endometriosis patients with antinuclear antibodies or lupus anticoagulant.[49] The significance of these findings is not clear, and the involvement of the immune system in the pathophysiology of endometriosis remains to be more fully elucidated.

Intraperitoneal Inflammatory Response

In women with endometriosis, the peritoneal fluid volume, the number of peritoneal macrophages, and associated soluble factors are increased when compared with infertile women without endometriosis.[24,25,50,51] The most likely explanation for these peritoneal findings is that they represent a localized inflammatory process in response to ectopic endometrial implants.

Macrophages, which represent one line of response in the innate defense mechanism of the body, act as effectors in several kinds of cell-mediated cytotoxicity. Investigations into the origin of peritoneal macrophages also suggest they are related to reproductive function. The number of peritoneal macrophages is low in men and in women after hysterectomy, while taking birth control pills, or after menopause.[52] We know that a genital tract inflammatory response can adversely affect gametes and fertility, because macrophages phagocytize sperm in the lumen of the uterus and thus reduce the numbers of viable sperm in the genital tract.[53] In the presence of inflammation, this normal function of macrophages can adversely affect sperm function. In women without endometriosis, 50% have sperm present in peritoneal fluid following insemination, whereas

sperm are absent in the peritoneal fluid of women with endometriosis.[54] Furthermore, the peritoneal macrophages from women with endometriosis appear to be "activated." They have been shown to phagocytize more sperm than macrophages from women without endometriosis.[24,55] Thus, these findings are compatible with a mechanism of reduced fertility based on cell-mediated gamete injury and support the clinical suspicion that even minimal endometriosis may be associated with infertility.

The activation of macrophages is also associated with release of substances that may have adverse effects on local physiologic functions related to reproduction. Supernatants of macrophage cultures have been reported to inhibit zona-free hamster egg penetration by sperm.[56] Interleukin-1, a mediator of host responses secreted by macrophages, is toxic to mouse embryo development in concentrations similar to those found in the peritoneal fluid of endometriosis patients.[57]

That ectopic endometrium, in general, and hyperactivated macrophages, in particular, are involved in the pathogenesis of endometriosis-associated infertility has been clearly demonstrated by a team that showed immunomodulation with pentoxyphylline reversed the subfertility in hamsters with induced endometriosis.[57] Furthermore, they were able to show that the treatment of isolated hyperactivated macrophages with pentoxyphylline reversed the adverse effects of untreated hyperactivated macrophages on fertility in the hamster.[58] These studies provide a model not only for the study of endometriosis-associated infertility but also may provide a basis for clinical trials to evaluate the efficacy of this approach.

Surgical Therapy

Does Surgery Enhance Conception Rates?

Many studies have reported on pregnancy rates after laparoscopic treatment of endometriosis, but the majority fail to demonstrate efficacy in treated patients compared with a control group. Such information is vital when assessing claims of therapeutic efficacy of laparoscopic surgery over no treatment or relative to other therapeutic modalities. In four studies which have included a control group, laparoscopic treatment of endometriosis was associated with significantly better conception rates when compared with expectant management of minimal and mild disease.[8,59–61] However, when conception rates in untreated controls and patients treated by laparotomy were compared, investigators found significant enhancement of fertility only for patients with severe disease.[62] This discrepancy in therapeutic efficacy between patients treated by laparoscopy versus laparotomy may be related to the method of treatment and risk of de novo adhesion formation, which is reported to be more frequent after lap-

Table 25.1. Pregnancy rates after conservative laparotomy surgery for endometriosis by stage of disease (AFS-r classification).

Author	Stage II (Mild)	Stage III (Moderate)	Stage IV (Severe)
Acosta et al[93]	8 (75%)	60 (50%)	39 (33%)
Garcia & David[94]	3 (67%)	19 (37%)	49 (29%)
Sadigh et al[95]	—	23 (74%)	42 (48%)
Schenken & Malinak[74]	—	36 (33%)	21 (29%)
Buttram[96]	88 (69%)	50 (56%)	68 (47%)
Rock et al[97]	45 (62%)	88 (55%)	81 (48%)
Schenken & Malinak[98]	42 (76%)	—	—
Rantala et al[99]	44 (59%)	39 (56%)	46 (39%)
Gordts et al[100]	20 (40%)	99 (42%)	57 (35%)
Olive & Lee[62]	11 (46%)	43 (51%)	34 (29%)
Total	261 (64%)	457 (50%)	437 (39%)

arotomy.[63–65] These preliminary results suggest that laparoscopic ablation of endometriosis appears to enhance fertility over no treatment.

Olive and Martin applied modeling techniques to pregnancy rates following the use of CO_2 laser laparoscopy, conservative laparotomy surgery, and hormonal therapy in endometriosis-associated infertility.[6] They found laser laparoscopy for treatment of endometriosis-associated infertility to be as efficacious as other therapy. When compared with medical treatment and conservative surgery by laparotomy, there appears to be an early rise in the cumulative pregnancy rate with laser therapy, which plateaus between 12 and 18 months postsurgery.[6] Patients treated with medical therapy or conservative surgery had a slower rise in the pregnancy rate, although all groups, regardless of treatment, achieved the same cumulative pregnancy rate by 30 months.

Pregnancy rates after laparotomy are generally inversely proportional to the stage of disease (Table 25.1).[1] This pattern differs from pregnancy rates after endoscopic laser surgery, which appear independent of the stage of disease (Table 25.2).[1] Pregnancy rates after laparoscopic electrosurgical treatment show a pattern similar to after laparotomy (Table 25.3).

When Surgery Fails to Achieve Pregnancy

For patients afflicted with endometriosis and infertility, a complete and thorough workup of all infertility factors is important. In many infertile couples, endometriosis is not the only problem. For example, in one study 95 (78%) out of 122 couples had one or more factors in addition to endometriosis contributing to their infertility.[10] As might be expected, couples with more than one infertility factor had a lower cumulative probability of pregnancy.[11] Thus, early and continuing evaluation and therapy for all such factors is critical, because detection and treatment of all factors contributes to the best outcome.

Hormonal Therapy

Initial reports of crude pregnancy rates following danazol treatment varied from 30% to 53% with monthly fecundity rates of 2% to 7%.[1] However, these early studies lacked an untreated control group; since these women had several years of infertility prior to seeking medical attention, it was assumed that all pregnancies resulted from treatment. More recent studies, however, suggest that hormonal treatment of mild and moderate endometriosis may not offer any advantage over expectant management with respect to enhancing fertility.[3] The time expended during treatment delays conception, because these hormonal agents are effective contraceptives. Although many hormonal treatments have been effective at suppressing implants, many women have histologic evidence of active implants at the end of therapy, and when cyclic menstrual function resumes, reactivation of endometrial implants and the factors related to infertility return.[5,66,67]

Table 25.2. Pregnancy rates after laparoscopic CO_2 laser treatment of endometriosis (AFS-r classification).

Author	Stage I (Minimal)	Stage II (Mild)	Stage III (Moderate)	Stage IV (Severe)	Follow-up (months)
Kelly & Roberts[101]	3/3 (100%)	3/7 (43%)	—	—	6
Feste[102]	24/47 (51%)	4/6 (67%)	2/5 (40%)	—	12
Martin[103]	25/56 (44%)	22/45 (49%)	9/14 (64%)	—	12
Davis[104]	—	20/31 (65%)*	15/26 (58%)	2/7 (29%)	15
Donnez[105**]	26/42 (62%)	11/21 (52%)	3/7 (43%)	—	18
Sutton & Hill[106†]	15/16 (94%)	17/25 (68%)	11/13 (85%)	2/2 (100%)	6–72
Gast et al[10]	36/70 (51%)	12/33 (36%)	9/19 (47%)	—	10
Fayez et al[59]	27/38 (71%)	33/44 (75%)	—	—	12
Nezhat et al[107]	28/39 (72%)	60/86 (70%)	45/67 (67%)	35/51 (69%)	
Paulson et al[108]	109/140 (78%)	60/88 (68%)	—	—	8–32
Total	293/451 (65%)	242/386 (63%)	94/151 (62%)	39/60 (65%)	

*Minimal and mild combined.
**Ovarian endometrioma limited to 3 cm.
†Patients with additional fertility factors eliminated from study.

Table 25.3. Pregnancy rates after laparoscopic electrosurgical destruction of endometriosis (AFS-r classification).

Author	Stage I (Minimal)	Stage II (Mild)	Stage III (Moderate)	Stage IV (Severe)	Follow-up (months)
Eward[109]	4/7 (57%)	10/18 (56%)	—	—	13
Sulewski et al[110]	—	20/42 (48%)	20/58 (35%)	—	37
Seiler et al[111]	—	20/45 (44%)	—	—	7
Nowroozi et al[60]	—	42/69 (61%)	—	—	—
Murphy et al[11]	24/36 (67%)	18/36 (50%)	2/7 (29%)	0/30 (0%)	8
Total	28/43 (65%)	110/210 (57%)	22/65 (34%)	0/30 (0%)	

Preoperative Hormonal Therapy

Some authorities favor a combined medical-surgical approach for optimal treatment. Those who favor preoperative medical therapy reason that shrinkage and fibrosis of the implants may lead to decreased intraoperative blood loss, lessen the need for extensive tissue dissection, and reduce the risk of preoperative adhesions.[68] Moreover, the risk of performing unnecessary ovarian cystectomies on hemorrhagic corpus luteum cysts (which may be confused with endometriomas) is reduced. But preoperative hormonal therapy makes the endometriosis less visible and may increase the risk of leaving disease behind that will reactivate with resumption of ovarian steroid secretion.[67] Further, the induced fibrosis may make surgical dissection and excision of residual disease more difficult. Finally, endometriomas larger than 1 cm generally do not respond to hormonal therapy. There is even some evidence that medical therapy may increase the propensity of endometriomas to rupture. Few studies have reported pregnancy rates following preoperative hormonal therapy and fewer still have compared results with a control group. Despite the paucity of data, some trends can be gleaned. It appears that neither preoperative nor postoperative hormonal therapy is effective for the treatment of infertility associated with endometriosis.[68] The only study that compared preoperative use with postoperative use in a significant number of patients demonstrated relative superiority of preoperative danazol.[69] However, no control group was included in the study to determine if preoperative hormonal therapy had any benefit over no hormonal therapy. Similarly, in a study in which preoperative GnRH agonist therapy was shown to be superior to other preoperative therapies, no control group was included to determine if it had any benefit over no hormonal therapy.[70] Table 25.4 shows crude pregnancy rates after preoperative hormonal therapy combined with surgery.

Postoperative Hormonal Therapy

Proponents of postoperative hormonal therapy believe that surgical debulking of disease followed by medical therapy eliminates both macroscopic and microscopic disease. However, uncontrolled studies fail to demonstrate higher pregnancy rates in patients treated with postoperative hormonal therapy after surgery (Table 25.5) when compared with preoperative hormonal therapy (Table 25.4), surgical treatment alone (Tables 25.1, 25.2, 25.3), or with appropriate control groups.[71,72]

Repeat Surgery

If one believes that debulking of endometriosis enhances fertility, it would seem logical to do a surgical procedure to remove endometriosis that has recurred or developed since the last operation. Moreover, if the

Table 25.4. Pregnancy rates after preoperative medical therapy combined with surgery for endometriosis (AFS-r classification).*

Author	Regimen	Stage of pretreatment disease		
		Stage II (Mild)	Stage III (Moderate)	Stage IV (Severe)
Daniell & Christianson[112]	Danazol, 800 mg/day	—	—	1/5 (20%)
Barbieri et al[113]	Danazol, 800 mg/day	4/16 (25%)	4/11 (36%)	4/7 (57%)
Donnez et al[114]	Lynestrenol, 5 mg/day	—	21/35 (60%)	7/15 (47%)
Buttram et al[69]	Danazol, 400–800 mg/day	15/18 (83%)	18/27 (67%)	15/30 (50%)
Donnez et al[70]	Danazol, 600 mg/day	—	13/27 (48%)	5/13 (38%)
Donnez et al[70]	Lynestrenol, 5 mg/day	—	20/35 (57%)	5/12 (42%)
Donnez et al[70]	Gestrinone, 2.5 mg 3×/week	—	15/31 (48%)	3/7 (43%)
Donnez et al[70]	Buserelin, 300 mg 3×/day	—	21/35 (60%)	8/15 (53%)
Total		19/34 (56%)	112/201 (56%)	48/104 (46%)

* All patients were treated preoperatively for 6 to 9 months.

Table 25.5. Pregnancy rates after surgery combined with postoperative medical therapy for endometriosis (AFS-r classification).

Author	Regimen	Stage II (Mild)	Stage III (Moderate)	Stage IV (Severe)
Andrews & Larsen[115]	Enovid	—	—	—
Hammond et al[116]	Enovid	3/3 (100%)	4/16 (25%)	1/7 (14%)
Hammond et al[117]	Methyltestosterone	0/3 (0%)	2/3 (67%)	0/5 (0%)
Audebert et al[118]	Danazol	—	—	—
Wheeler & Malinak[119]	Danazol	—	—	—
Daniell & Christianson[112]	Danazol	20/35 (57%)	14/25 (56%)	—
Chong & Baggish[120]	Danazol	11/13 (85%)	—	—
Chong[121]	Danazol	21/32 (66%)	—	—
Ronnberg & Javiner[122]	Danazol	—	—	14/44 (32%)
Mettler & Semm[123]	Danazol	—	—	—
	Gestrinone	—	—	—
	Lynestrenol	—	—	—
Buttram et al[69]	Danazol	1/1 (100%)	1/3 (33%)	6/20 (30%)
Total		56/87 (64%)	21/47 (45%)	21/76 (27%)

original surgical procedure produced adhesions, a repeat laparoscopic procedure may restore normal anatomic relationships and thus improve the chances of pregnancy in some cases. The efficacy, however, of repetitive conservative surgeries has not been well studied. Only four studies have reported follow-up results.[67,73–75] Crude pregnancy rates ranged from 20% to 47%. Such an approach offers one infertility treatment option; another is advanced reproductive technologies.

Superovulation and Intrauterine Insemination

Superovulation and intrauterine insemination (IUI) have been used recently in treating endometriosis-associated infertility. Several factors may account for the efficacy of this type of treatment, regardless of the apparent etiology for the infertility. First, the number and concentration of sperm in the upper genital tract are increased at the same time as more oocytes are available. Second, this approach may improve chances of fertilization when a gametotoxic effect may be present, as has been suggested for endometriosis-associated infertility.[76] Third, occult ovulatory disturbances may be corrected and barriers to sperm that may be present in the cervical mucus are bypassed. Fourth, the procedure also offers the technical benefit of improving the timing of insemination relative to ovulation.

CC and Intrauterine Insemination

While human menopausal gonadotropins have traditionally been administered for controlled ovarian hyperstimulation combined with IUI, this treatment is expensive and associated with important risks. Treatment with clomiphene citrate (CC) and IUI has been reported to improve fecundity over periovulatory intercourse in couples with either unexplained infertility or surgically corrected endometriosis.[77] In a randomized study, cycle fecundity rates were 10% for treated patients and 3% for controls.

We have studied the efficacy of CC/IUI for a variety of infertility factors.[78] We enrolled 85 infertile patients and followed them up for a total of 25 cycles. Ovulatory women with surgically treated endometriosis, a history of pelvic adhesive disease, male factor, unexplained infertility, or luteal phase deficiency were randomized to receive 50 to 100 mg CC for 5 days starting on either day 2 or day 5. Vaginal ultrasound scans starting on day 10 were used to determine timing of hCG administration when the average follicular diameter reached 20 mm. IUI was performed 36 hours after hCG administration. Endometrial biopsy was performed during the first cycle of treatment and progesterone suppositories were added if the biopsy was out of phase by more than 2 days from onset of the next menses. The overall cycle fecundity rate (f) for all couples was 11%. Although f was not affected by the start of CC (day 2, 10%; day 5, 12%, NS), the miscarriage rate was significantly higher in those who began CC later in the cycle (18% vs 44%, $p < .0001$) and was associated with increased age (25–29, 17%; 30–34, 33%; 35–39, 30%, 40+, 50% NS). Fecundity and miscarriage rates for diagnostic categories were: male factor (11%, 18%), endometriosis (7%, 40%), adhesions (6%, 33%), unexplained infertility (17%, 20%), and luteal phase deficiency (22%, 71%). These data suggest that CC/IUI may be a useful treatment for a variety of infertility diagnoses, although its use for enhancement of fertility in cases of endometriosis and adhesions is questionable.

hMG and Intrauterine Insemination

Human menopausal gonadotropin (hMG) superovulation combined with IUI is being used increasingly for a variety of infertility factors, including endometriosis.[16,79] The efficacy appears to be stage specific. In our experience, the cycle fecundity remains fairly constant for stages I to III but drops precipitously for stage IV disease (8%, 11%, 14%, 0%, respectively). This variation may reflect the fact that superovulation with IUI depends on an intact ovum pickup mechanism, which may be altered by adhesions in severe disease.

To determine the optimal timing of hMG/IUI therapy relative to conservative laparoscopic surgery for endometriosis, we studied 68 women over 921 months following laparoscopic surgery alone (SURG) and 157 patients who were treated with 496 cycles of hMG/IUI (hMG/IUI) administered every other month beginning at various times following surgery.[80] Cycle fecundity rates (f) for the surgery alone group progressively declined from a high of 7% within 3 months of surgery to 0% at 36 months. In contrast, f remained constant (mean 12.6% ± 2.7) for hMG/IUI regardless of the time since surgery (up to 60 months).

Cumulative pregnancy rates were determined by life-table analysis comparing pregnancy rates in patients who began hMG/IUI within 3 months of surgery (Fig. 25.1A). At 12 months after surgery, 55% of the SURG group and 65% of the hMG/IUI-treated group had achieved a pregnancy (not a statistically significant difference). However, when hMG/IUI was initiated at least 12 months from the time of surgery, cumulative pregnancy rates were significantly higher for the hMG/IUI group than the SURG group; 89% vs 67% when started at 12 months, 93% vs 70% when started at 18 months, and 94% vs 70% when started at 24 months.

When patients were categorized by age groups (≤29, 30–34, 35–39, ≥40), f progressively decreased after surgery with age (6%, 5%, 2%, 2%). In contrast, the hMG/IUI group demonstrated consistent f until after age 40 (11%, 13%, 14%, 3%). These results agree with results of other studies examining the effect of age on response to hMG superovulation.[81] By 12 months after surgery 57% of women under 35, and 33% of those 35 and over had conceived. By 24 months, 77% of those younger than 35 conceived, while 39% of women 35 or older conceived (Fig. 25.1B). When hMG/IUI was initiated 6 months after surgery in women 35 and over, 81% achieved pregnancy within 16 months of surgery. In contrast, when hMG/IUI was started 12 months from surgery in women younger than 35, 88% achieved pregnancy compared with 77% of patients not treated with hMG/IUI.

These results indicate that, overall, hMG/IUI improves treatment of infertility associated with endometriosis taking into account time since surgery, age, and stage of disease. Women 35 years and older and women with moderate and severe disease appear to benefit the most from hMG/IUI soon after surgery.

The results of this study are important for two reasons: (1) all of the women in the study represent a group of treatment "failures" because they had

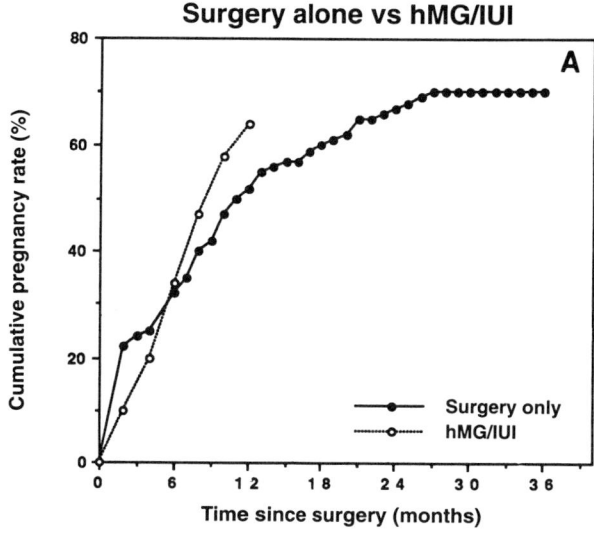

Surgery alone vs hMG/IUI

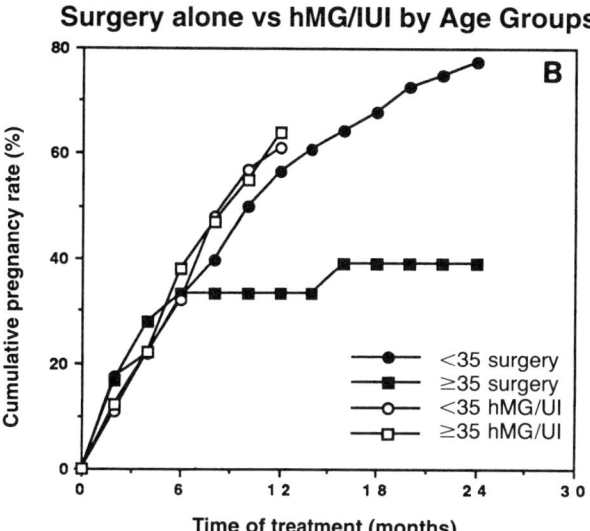

Surgery alone vs hMG/IUI by Age Groups

Figure 25.1. A. Cumulative pregnancy rates after surgery alone versus surgery and superovulation with intrauterine insemination. **B.** Cumulative pregnancy rates by age groups after surgery alone versus surgery and superovulation with intrauterine insemination.

undergone laparoscopic laser surgery as initial treatment for their endometriosis and failed to conceive within 6 to 24 months after treatment; and (2) the cycle fecundity rates observed with combined hMG/IUI were two to six times higher than reported with expectant management or hormonal therapy and two times that observed with hMG alone. Thus, these results suggest that combined hMG/IUI therapy may be an effective alternative to more complex assisted reproductive technologies (GIFT, ZIFT, IVF) for treating infertility associated with endometriosis.

If there is an initial enhancement of fertility after laparoscopic surgery, it seems reasonable to give the patient the benefit of hMG/IUI before instituting additional fertility-enhancing therapy, particularly when the treatment is expensive, and subjects the patient to the risks of ovarian hyperstimulation and multiple pregnancy. Initiated too early, hMG/IUI appears to have no effect on the enhancement of fertility over and above that observed with laparoscopic surgery alone. Unless timing is accurate, patients are subjected unnecessarily to the risks and expense of hMG superovulation. However, when administered at a time when the fertility-enhancing effects of laparoscopic surgery have waned, hMG/IUI therapy can markedly improve the chances of conception over and above that observed with expectant management alone.

GIFT

Gamete intrafallopian transfer results in the insertion of both male and female gametes into the fallopian tube. A pregnancy rate of 27% has been reported for the general population of infertile couples treated by this method.[82] Patients with endometriosis have a reported pregnancy rate of 24% after GIFT.[83] Because laparoscopy is used for egg retrieval and gamete placement, some centers combine GIFT with concurrent laparoscopic treatment of endometriosis. One reported a 45% pregnancy rate for endometriosis patients treated concurrently with laser and 36% in women not receiving any concurrent treatment; another reported a 65% pregnancy rate in women treated at the time of GIFT compared with a 34% rate in women not treated.[84,85]

Another study compared conception rates after GIFT involving women with minimal and mild endometriosis receiving a short course of GnRH analog starting with administration of hMG (group 1), a 6-month course preceding hMG (group 2), and a group receiving hMG alone (group 3).[86] The pregnancy rates were higher in the patients treated by GnRH prior to hMG stimulation (55%), compared with the other 2 groups (32% and 33%). The higher pregnancy rate following prolonged suppression with GnRH perhaps might be related to improvement in the peritoneal milieu or suppression of antiendometrial antibody production.

IVF

IVF is appropriate in women with tubal damage, in situations where assessment of fertilizing capacity of the gametes is indicated, and when other less complicated treatments have failed.

Some reports indicate that women with endometriosis, particularly those with severe disease, do not fare as well with IVF as do women with other indications for the procedure.[87-89] Other reports, however, indicate that women with endometriosis, regardless of the stage of disease, have pregnancy rates comparable to those with other diagnoses when treated with IVF.[14,90,91]

Furthermore, Damewood's group found that of women who underwent concurrent surgical treatment of endometriosis at the time of oocyte retrieval but did not conceive, 28% subsequently conceived on their own within 10 months of the operative laparoscopic procedure.[91]

We assessed the value of IVF in a small group of women with the sole diagnosis of endometriosis who failed to conceive during at least four cycles of hMG/IUI. Women with stages I and II disease had a combined cycle fecundity rate of 0% (N = 17). In contrast, women with stages III and IV disease have a cycle fecundity rate of 55% (N = 11).[92] Based on these small numbers, it appears that the fertility limiting factor in stages I and II disease in women failing hMG/IUI is not overcome by IVF. Perhaps this factor is related to endometrial receptivity, because ovarian stimulation, fertilization, and pre-embryo development do not appear to be impaired. In contrast, with stages III and IV disease, persistent anatomic distortion may well be the fertility limiting factor, which is effectively overcome by IVF, but not by hMG/IUI.

References

1. Olive DL, Haney AF. Endometriosis-associated infertility: A critical review of therapeutic approaches. Obstet Gynecol Surv 1986;41:538.
2. Metzger DA, Haney AF. Endometriosis: Etiology and pathophysiology of infertility. Clin Obstet Gynecol 1988; 31:801.
3. Metzger DA, Luciano AA. Hormonal therapy of endometriosis. Obstet Gynecol Clin NA 1989;16:105.
4. Evers JLH. The second-look laparoscopy for evaluation of the results of medical treatment of endometriosis should not be performed during ovarian suppression. Fertil Steril 1987;47:502–504.
5. Nisolle-Pochet M, Casanas-Roux F, Donnez J. Histologic study of ovarian endometriosis after hormonal therapy. Fertil Steril 1988;49:423.
6. Olive DL, Martin DC. Treatment of endometriosis-associated infertility with CO_2 laser laparoscopy: the use of one- and two-parameter exponential models. Fertil Steril 1987;48:18.
7. Strathy JH, Molgaard CA, Coulam CB, et al. Endometriosis and infertility: a laparoscopic study of endometriosis among fertile and infertile women. Fertil Steril 1982;38:66.
8. Tulandi T, Mouchawar M. Treatment-dependent and treatment-independent pregnancy in women with minimal and mild endometriosis. Fertil Steril 1991;56:790.
9. Grant A. Additional sterility factors in endometriosis. Fertil Steril 1966;17:514.
10. Gast MJ, Tobler R, Strickler RC, et al. Laser vaporization of endometriosis in an infertile population: the role of complicating infertility factors. Fertil Steril 1988;49:32.
11. Murphy AA, Schlaff WD, Hassiakos D, et al. Laparoscopic cautery in the treatment of endometriosis-related infertility. Fertil Steril 1991;55:246.
12. Portuondo JA, Eschanojauregui AD, Herran C. Early conception in patients with untreated mild endometriosis. Fertil Steril 1983;39:22.

13. Jansen RPS. Minimal endometriosis and reduced fecundability: prospective evidence from an artificial insemination by donor program. Fertil Steril 1986;46:141.
14. Jones HW, Anibal AA, Andrews MC, et al. Three years of in vitro fertilization at Norfolk. Fertil Steril 1984; 42:826.
15. Dodson WC, Whitesides DB, Hughes CL Jr, et al. Superovulation with intrauterine insemination in the treatment of infertility: a possible alternative to gamete intrafallopian transfer and in vitro fertilization. Fertil Steril 1987;48:441.
16. Chaffkin LM, Nulsen JC, Luciano AA, et al. A comparative analysis of the cycle fecundity rates associated with combined human menopausal gonadotropin (hMG) and intrauterine insemination (IUI) versus either hMG or IUI alone. Fertil Steril 1991;55:252.
17. Luciano AA, Marana R, Kratka S, et al. Ovarian function after incision of the ovary by scalpel, CO_2 laser and microelectrode. Fertil Steril 1991;56:349.
18. Fortier KJ, Haney AF. The pathologic spectrum of uterotubal unction obstruction. Obstet Gynecol 1985; 65:93.
19. Moon YS, Leung PCS, Yuen BH, et al. Prostaglandin F in human endometriotic tissue. Am J Obstet Gynecol 1981;141:344.
20. Badawy SZA, Marshall L, Gabal AA, et al. The concentration of 13, 14-dihydro-15-keto prostaglandin F_2 and prostaglandin E_2 in peritoneal fluid of infertile patients with and without endometriosis. Fertil Steril 1982;38:166.
21. Drake TS, O'Brien WF, Ramwell PW. Peritoneal fluid thromboxane B_2 and 6-ketoprostaglandin F_1 in endometriosis. Am J Obstet Gynecol 1981;140:401.
22. Dawood MY, Khan-Dawood FS, Wilson L. Peritoneal fluid prostaglandins and prostanoids in women with endometriosis, chronic pelvic inflammatory disease and pelvic pain. Am J Obstet Gynecol 1984;148:391.
23. Rock JA, Dubin NH, Ghodgaonkar RB, et al. Cul-de-sac fluid in women with endometriosis: fluid volume and prostanoid concentration during the proliferative phase of the cycle days 8 to 12. Fertil Steril 1982;37:747.
24. Halme J, Becker S, Hammond MG, et al. Increased activation of pelvic macrophages in infertile women with mild endometriosis. Am J Obstet Gynecol 1983;145:333.
25. Haney AF, Muscato JJ, Weinberg JB. Peritoneal fluid cell populations in infertility patients. Fertil Steril 1981; 35:696.
26. Croxatto HB, Ortiz ME, Guiloff E, et al. Effect of 15 (s)-15-methyl-prostaglandin F_2 on human oviductal motility and ovum transport. Fertil Steril 1978;30:408.
27. Pittaway DE, Maxson W, Daniell J, et al. Luteal phase defects in infertility patients with endometriosis. Fertil Steril 1983;39:712.
28. Winkel CA, Opsahl MS, Cowan BD. Clomiphene citrate treatment failures in women with endometriosis and luteal dysfunction. Fertil Steril 1984;41:645.
29. Schenken RS, Asch RH, Williams RF, et al. Etiology of infertility in monkeys with endometriosis: luteinized unruptured follicles, luteal phase defects, pelvic adhesions and spontaneous abortions. Fertil Steril 1984; 41:122.
30. Cheesman KL, Cheesman SD, Chatterton RT, et al. Alterations in progesterone metabolism and luteal function in infertile women with endometriosis. Fertil Steril 1983;43:590.
31. Cheesman KL, Ben-Nun I, Chatterton RT, et al. Relationship of luteinizing hormone, pregnanediol-3-glucouronide and estriol-16-glucouronide in urine of infertile women with endometriosis. Fertil Steril 1982; 38:542.
32. Metzger DA, Olive DL, Stohs GF, et al. Association of endometriosis and spontaneous abortion: effect of control group selection. Fertil Steril 1986;45:18.
33. FitzSimmons J, Stahl R, Gocial B, et al. Spontaneous abortion and endometriosis. Fertil Steril 1987;47:696.
34. Donnez J, Langerock S, Thomas K. Peritoneal fluid volume, 17 beta-estradiol and progesterone concentrations in women with endometriosis and/or luteinized unruptured follicle syndrome. Gynecol Obstet Invest 1983;16:210.
35. Marik J, Hulka J. Luteinized unruptured follicle syndrome: a subtle case of infertility. Fertil Steril 1978; 29:270.
36. Dmowski WP, Rao R, Scommegna A. The luteinized unruptured follicle syndrome and endometriosis. Fertil Steril 1980;33:30.
37. Daly DC, Soto-Albors C, Walters C, et al. Ultrasonographic assessment of luteinized unruptured folilcle syndrome in unexplained infertility. Fertil Steril 1985; 43:62.
38. Brosens IA, Koninckx PR, Corveleyn PA. A study of plasma progesterone, oestradiol-17B, prolactin, and LH levels and of the luteal-phase appearance of the ovaries in patients with endometriosis and infertility. Br J Obstet Gynaecol 1978;85:246.
39. Koninckx PR, Ide P, Vandebrouke W, et al. New aspects of the pathophysiology of endometriosis and associated infertility. J Reprod Med 1980;24:257.
40. Vanrell JA, Belasch J, Fuster JS, et al. Ovulation stigma in fertile women. Fertil Steril 1982;37:712.
41. Kerin JF, Kirby C, Morris D, et al. Incidence of the luteinized unruptured follicle syndrome in cycling women. Fertil Steril 1983;40:620–626.
42. Weed JC, Arquembourg PC. Endometriosis: can it produce an autoimmune response resulting in infertility? Clin Obstet Gynecol 1988;23:885.
43. Mathur S, Peress MR, Williamson HO, et al. Autoimmunity in endometrium and ovary in endometriosis. Clin Exp Immunol 1982;50:259.
44. Kreiner D, Frommowitz FB, Richardson DA. Endometrial immunofluorescence associated with endometriosis and pelvic inflammatory disease. Fertil Steril 1986; 46:243.
45. Wild RA, Shivers CA. Antiendometrial antibodies in patients with endometriosis. Am J Reprod Immunol Microbiol 1985;8:84.
46. Halme J, Mathur S. Local autoimmunity in mild endometriosis. Int J Fertil 1987;32:309.
47. Saifuddin A, Buckley CH, Fox H. Immunoglobulin content of the endometrium in women with endometriosis. Int J Gynecol Path 1983;2:255.
48. Grimes DA, LeBolt SA, Grimes KR, et al. Systemic lupus erythematosus and reproductive function: A case-control study. Am J Obstet Gynecol 1985;153:179.
49. Gleicher N, El-Roliy A, Confino E, et al. Is endometriosis an autoimmune disease? Obstet Gyencol 1987; 70:115.
50. Drake T, O'Brien W, Grunert G, et al. Peritoneal fluid volume in endometriosis. Fertil Steril 190;34:280.
51. Fakih H. Baggett B, Holtz G, et al. Interleukin-1: a possible role in the fertility associated with endometriosis. Fertil Steril 1987;47:213.
52. VanFurth R, Raeburn JA, van Zwet TI. Characteristics of human mononuclear phagocytes. Blood 1979;54:485.

53. Austin CR. Fate of spermatozoa in the female genital tract. J Reprod Fertil 1960;1:151.

54. Hoxsey RJ, Rao R, Scommegna A. Sperm recovery in peritoneal fluid of endometriosis versus "normal" infertile patients. Fertil Steril 1984;41:395.

55. Muscato JJ, Haney AF, Weinberg JB. Sperm phagocytosis by human peritoneal macrophages: a possible cause of infertility in endometriosis. Am J Obstet Gynecol 1982;144:503.

56. Chacho KJ, Chacho MS, Anderson PJ, et al. Peritoneal fluid in patients with and without endometriosis: prostanoids and macrophages and their effect on the spermatozoa penetration assay. Am J Obstet Gynecol 1986; 154:1290.

57. Steinleitner A, Lambert H, Suarez M, et al. Immunomodulation in the treatment of endometriosis-associated subfertility: use of pentoxifylline to reverse the inhibition of fertilization by surgically induced endometriosis in a rodent model. Fertil Steril 1991a;56:975.

58. Steinleitner A, Lambert H, Roy S. Immunomodulation with pentoxifylline abrogates macrophage-mediated infertility in an in vivo model: a paradigm novel approach to the treatment of endometriosis-associated subfertility. Fertil Steril 1991b;55:26.

59. Fayez JA, Collazo LM, Vernon C, et al. Comparison of different modalities of treatment for minimal and mild endometriosis. Am J Obstet Gynecol 1988;159:927.

60. Nowroozi K, Chase JS, Check JH, et al. The importance of laparoscopic coagulation of mild endometriosis in infertile women. Int J Fertil 1987;32:442.

61. Adamson GD, Lu J, Subak LL. Laparoscopic CO_2 laser vaporization of endometriosis compared with traditional treatments. Fertil Steril 1988;50:704.

62. Olive DL, Lee KL. Analysis of sequential treatment protocols for endometriosis-associated infertility. Am J Obstet Gynecol 1986;154:613.

63. Diamond MP and the Adhesion Study Group. Postoperative adhesion development after operative laparoscopy: evaluation at early second-look procedures. Fertil Steril 1991;55:700.

64. Diamond MP, Daniell JF, Feste J, et al. Adhesion reformation and de novo adhesion formation after reproductive surgery. Fertil Steril 1987;47:864.

65. Nezhat C, Nezhat F, Metzger DA, et al. Adhesion reformation following reproductive surgery by videolaseroscopy. Fertil Steril 1990;53:1008.

66. Luciano AA, Turksoy RN, Carleo J. Evaluation of oral medroxyprogesterone acetate in the treatment of endometriosis. Obstet Gynecol 1988;72:323.

67. Evers JLH, Dunselman GAJ, Land JA, et al. Endometriosis: The management of recurrent disease. In Shaw RW, ed. Endometriosis. Carnforth, Parthenon 1990, pp 93–105.

68. Silverberg KM. Combination therapy for endometriosis. Infertil Reprod Med Clin NA 1992;3:683.

69. Buttram VC, Reiter RC, Ward S. Treatment of endometriosis with danazol: Report of a 6 year prospective study. Fertil Steril 1985;43:353.

70. Donnez J, Nisolle M, Clerckx F, et al. Evaluation of peroperative use of danazol, gestrinone, lynestrenol, buserelin spray and buserelin implant in the treatment of endometriosis-associated infertility. Prog Clin Biol Res 1990;323:427.

71. Telimmaa S, Puolakka J, Ronnberg L, et al. Placebo-controlled comparison of danazol and high-dose medroxy- progesterone acetate in the treatment of endometriosis. Gynecol Endocrinol 1987;1:13.

72. Chong AP, Koene ME, Thornton NL. Comparison of three modes of treatment for infertility patients with minimal pelvic endometriosis. Fertil Steril 1990;53:40.

73. Wheeler JM, Malinak LR. Recurrent endometriosis: Incidence, management and prognosis. Am J Obstet Gynecol 1983;146:247.

74. Schenken RS, Malinak LR. Reoperation after initial treatment of endometriosis with conservative surgery. Am J Obstet Gynecol 1978;131:416.

75. Candiani GB, Fedele L, Vercellini P, et al. Repetitive conservative surgery for recurrence of endometriosis. Obstet Gynecol 1991;77:421.

76. Syrop CH, Halme J. Peritoneal fluid environment and infertility. Fertil Steril 1987;48:1.

77. Deaton JL, Gibson M, Blackmer KM, et al. A randomized, controlled trial of clomiphene citrate and intrauterine insemination in couples with unexplained infertility or surgically corrected endometriosis. Fertil Steril 1990; 54:1083.

78. Metzger DA, Robbins B, Tortora A, et al. Clomiphene citrate (CC) and intrauterine insemination (IUI) for the treatment of infertility. Society for Gynecologic Investigation, April 1–3, 1993, Toronto, Canada, Abstract #347.

79. Nulsen JC, Dumez S, Metzger DA. A randomized prospective trial of human menopausal gonadotropin (hMG) with intrauterine insemination (IUI) versus IUI alone in the treatment of endometriosis, male factor infertility and unexplained infertility. Obstet Gynecol (in press).

80. Metzger DA, Scott L, Nulsen JC, et al. Optimal use of human menopausal gonadotropin (hMG) superovulation combined with intrauterine insemination (IUI) as an adjunct to conservative laparoscopic surgery for the treatment of infertility associated with endometriosis. The American Association of Gynecologic Laparoscopists, 20th Annual Meeting, Las Vegas, NV, Nov. 13–17, 1991.

81. Jacobs SL, Metzger DA, Dodson WC, Haney AF. Effect of age on response to human menopausal gonadotropin stimulation. J Clin Endo Metab 1990;71:1525.

82. IVF Registry, 1991. Fertil Steril 1993;59:956.

83. Hulme VA, van der Merwe JP, Kruger TF. Gamete intrafallopian transfer as treatment for infertility associated with endometriosis. Fertil Steril 1990;53(6): 1095–1096.

84. Corson SL, Batzer FR, Gocial B, et al. Surgical treatment of endometriosis at the time of gamete intrafallopian transfer. J Repro Med 1991; 36(4):274–278.

85. Batzofin J, Tran C, Tan T, et al. Laser laparoscopy as an adjunct to assisted reproductive treatments in women with pelvic adhesions and endometriosis. J Gynecol Surg 1989;5:273.

86. Remorgida V, Anserini P, Croce S, et al. Comparison of different ovarian stimulation protocols for gamete intrafallopian transfer in patients with minimal and mild endometriosis. Fertil Steril 1990;53:1060.

87. Matson PL, Yovick JL. The treatment of infertility associated with endometriosis by in vitro fertilization. Fertil Steril 1986;46:432.

88. Yovick JL, Matson PL, Richardson PA, Hilliard C. Hormonal profiles and embryo quality in women with severe endometriosis treated by in vitro fertilization and embryo transfer. Fertil Steril 1988;50:308.

89. Chillik CF, Acosta AA, Garcia JE, et al. The role of in vitro fertilization in infertile patients with endometriosis. Fertil Steril 1985;44:56.

90. Oehninger S, Rosenwaks A. In vitro fertilization and embryo transfer: an established and successful therapy for endometriosis. Prog Clin Biol Res 1990;323:319.
91. Damewood MD, Rock JA. Treatment independent pregnancy with operative laparoscopy for endometriosis in an in vitro fertilization program. Fertil Steril 1988; 50:463.
92. Manzi DM, Metzger DA, Luciano AA, et al. The efficacy of IVF as a treatment modality for individuals with endometriosis previously failing hMG/IUI superovulation therapy (in preparation).
93. Classification of endometriosis. American Fertility Society. Fertil Steril 1979;32:633.
94. Garcia CR, David SS. Pelvic endometriosis: infertility and pelvic pain. Am J Obstet Gynecol 1977;129:740.
95. Sadigh H, Naples JD, Batt RE. Conservative surgery for endometriosis in the infertile couple. Obstet Gynecol 1977;49:562.
96. Buttram VC. Conservative surgery for endometriosis in the infertile female: a study of 206 patients with implications for both medical and surgical therapy. Fertil Steril 1979;31:117.
97. Rock JA, Guzick DS, Sengoes C, et al. The conservative surgical treatment of endometriosis: evaluation of pregnancy success with respect to the extent of disease as categorized using contemporary classification systems. Fertil Steril 1981;35:131.
98. Schenken RS, Malinak LR. Conservative surgery versus expectant management for the infertile patient with mild endometriosis. Fertil Steril 1982;37:183.
99. Rantala ML, Kahanpaa KV, Koskimies A, et al. Fertility prognosis after surgical treatment of pelvic endometriosis. Acta Obstet Gynecol Scand 1983;61:11.
100. Gordts S, Boeckx W, Brosens I. Microsurgery of endometriosis in infertile patients. Fertil Steril 1984;42:520.
101. Kelly RW, Roberts DK. CO_2 laparoscopy. A potential alternative to danazol in the treatment of stage I and II endometriosis. J Reprod Med 1983;28:638.
102. Feste JR. Laser laparoscopy: a new modality. J Reprod Med 1985;30:413.
103. Martin DC. CO_2 laser laparoscopy for endometriosis associated with infertility. J Reprod Med 1986;31:1089.
104. Davis GD. Management of endometriosis and its associated adhesions with the CO_2 laser laparoscope. Obstet Gynecol 1986;68:422.
105. Donnez J. CO_2 laser laparoscopy in infertile women with endometriosis and women with adnexal adhesions. Fertil Steril 1987;48:390.
106. Sutton C, Hill D. Laser laparoscopy in the treatment of endometriosis. A 5-year study. Br J Obstet Gynaecol 1990;97:181.
107. Nezhat C, Crowgey S, Nezhat F. Videolaseroscopy for the treatment of endometriosis associated with infertility. Fertil Steril 1989;51:237.
108. Paulson JD, Asmar P, Saffan DS. Mild and moderate endometriosis. Comparison of treatment modalities for infertile couples. J Reprod Med 1991;36:151.
109. Eward RD. Cauterization of stages I and II endometriosis and the resulting pregnancy rate. In Philips JM, ed. Endoscopy in Gynecology: the Proceedings of the Third International Congress on Gynecologic Endoscopy. Downey, CA, American Association of Gynecologic Laparoscopists, 1978, p 276.
110. Sulewski JM, Curcio FD, Bronitsky C, et al. The treatment of endometriosis at laparoscopy for infertility. Am J Obstet Gynecol 1980;138:128.
111. Seiler JC, Gidwani G, Ballard L. Laparoscopic cauterization of endometriosis for fertility: a controlled study. Fertil Steril 1986;46:1098.
112. Daniell JF, Christianson C. Combined laparoscopic surgery and danazol therapy for pelvic endometriosis. Fertil Steril 1981;35:521.
113. Barbieri RL, Evans S, Kistner RW. Danazol in the treatment of endometriosis: Analysis of 100 cases with a 4-year follow-up. Fertil Steril 1982;37:737.
114. Donnez J, Lemaire-Rubbers M, Karaman Y, et al. Combination (hormonal and microsurgical) therapy in infertile women with endometriosis. Fertil Steril 1987; 48:239.
115. Andrews WC, Larsen DC. Endometriosis: Treatment with hormonal psuedopregnancy and/or operation. Am J Obstet Gynecol 1974;118:643.
116. Hammond CB, Rock JA, Parker RT. Conservative treatment of endometriosis: The effects of limited surgery and hormonal pseudopregnancy. Fertil Steril 1976; 27:756.
117. Hammond MG, Hammond CB, Parker RT. Conservative treatment of endometriosis extera: The effects of methyltestosterone therapy. Fertil Steril 1978;29:651.
118. Audebert AJM, Larrue-Charlus S, Emperaire JC. Endometriosis and infertility. A reveiw of sixty-two patients treated with danazol. Postgrad Med J 1979; 55(Suppl. 5):10.
119. Wheeler JM, Malinak LR. Postoperative danazol therapy in infertility patients with severe endometriosis. Fertil Steril 1981;36:460.
120. Chong AP, Baggish MS. Management of pelvic endometriosis by means of intraabdominal carbon dioxide laser. Fertil Steril 1984;41:14.
121. Chong AP. Danazol versus carbon dioxide laser plus postoperative danazol: Treatment of infertility due to mild pelvic endometriosis. Lasers Surg Med 1985;5: 571.
122. Ronnberg L, Javiner PA. Pregnancy rates following various therapy modes for endometriosis in infertile patients. Acta Obstet Gynecol Scan Suppl 1984;123: 69.
123. Mettler L, Semm K. Three-step therapy of genital endometriosis in cases of human infertility with lynestrenol, danazol, or gestrinone administration in the second step. In Raynaud JP, ed. Medical Management of Endometriosis. New York, Raven Press, 1984, pp 233–248.

26
Adenomyosis

Paul Devroey and Guy Verhulst

Since Rokitansky described adenomyosis in 1860, there has been little progress in understanding this condition. Incidence, pathogenesis, and pathophysiology still remain unclear. As endometriosis, it is an ectopic presence of endometrium (Fig. 26.1). Sometimes the clinical features can overlap, and frequently the two pathologies coexist. Hysterectomy has been the traditional method for treatment. This chapter provides a review of the literature and evaluates procedures that might be used for making an accurate diagnosis and for treating the disease in a noninvasive way.

Two Distinct Forms

Adenomyosis may appear in two distinct forms, focal or diffuse, and these forms may coexist (Fig. 26.2 and color plate 26.2).[1-3]

Diffuse adenomyosis is the invasion of endometrial glands and/or stroma within the myometrium. The intramural islands generally have the histologic appearance of the basalis of the endometrium. In focal adenomyosis, adenomyomata are present. These are defined as circumscribed tumors, made up of endometrium and muscle tissue. The diagnosis is based mainly upon the finding of endometrial islands deep beneath the endometrial surface within the muscular layer.

Anatomo-pathologic criteria divide the disease into "superficial" and "nonsuperficial" adenomyosis. For the diagnosis of "nonsuperficial" adenomyosis, the area must extend into the myometrium at least two low power fields (8 mm) from the basalis, according to the criteria of Benson and Sneeden.[4] Less strict criteria state that adenomyosis foci must be at least the distance of one high-power field below the basal endometrium. Other criteria have also been used, such as the invasion of endometrial glands and stroma of the myometrium for at least one third of the thickness of the latter or a minimal distance at least of 3 mm below the endometrial surface. In premenopausal women, the presence of smooth muscle hypertrophy around the foci of endometrial invasion is needed to make the diagnosis.

Criteria for "superficial" adenomyosis are unclear and confusing. Some pathologists even deny the existence of a superficial form of adenomyosis, because of the physiologic invaginations of the endometrial basal lamina.

The presence of blood or hemosiderin in adenomyosis is rare. Metaplasia or Müllerian elements have no prognostic importance. Adenomyosis occurs rarely in the region of the uterine cornua, but in these cases the differential diagnosis from salpingitis isthmica nodosa (SIN) can be difficult, especially when stroma is absent. The epithelium of adenomyosis often occurs in clusters and the epithelium is taller, whereas with SIN, the epithelium is arranged sparsely.

Subserosal adenomyosis is a variant of adenomyosis in which ectopic endometrial tissue is distributed in an area distant from the eutopic endometrium. Sakamoto described 15 cases and proposed subserosal adenomyosis as a form of pelvic endometriosis.[5] The distribution of the ectopic endometrium, the young age of the patients, and the presence of concomitant endometriosis are suggestive. Because lymphatic permeation could not be confirmed in these cases, there are no convincing arguments for migration of endometrial tissue via lymphatic channels.[6]

Clinical Findings

In 60% to 80% of the cases of adenomyosis, the uterus is enlarged.[3,7] This enlargement rarely exceeds 12 weeks of gestation and is more or less symmetrical. The in-

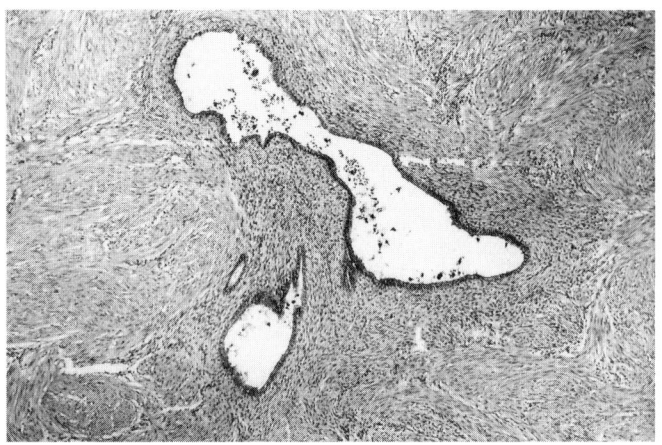

Figure 26.1. Adenomyotic foci composed of dilated glands, surrounded by stroma and hypertrophic smooth muscle tissue (HES, ×630).

crease in size never reaches the large proportions seen so often in myomatosus uteri. As classically described, the uterus is likely to be more enlarged in the anterior-posterior dimension, which reflects the more prominent involvement of the posterior wall. The color of the uterus may vary throughout the cycle, but usually suggests hyperemia and/or congestion.

The cut surface reveals a coarse trabecular pattern, due to crisscrossing fascicles of thickened smooth muscle. Sometimes small cysts or pinpoint bleeding reveal the endometrial tissue within the myometrium. There is no tendency of the involved endometrium to form circumscribed nodules. The striking feature is the diffuse increase of the myometrial wall, which is relatively symmetrical, although often located more at the posterior side of the muscular wall. Occasionally, endometrial extensions have been followed throughout the full thickness of the myometrium to the serosal

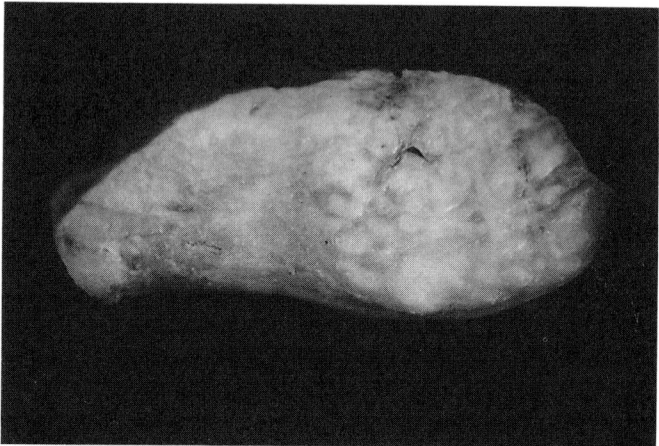

Figure 26.2. Cut surfaces of a uterus with diffuse and focal adenomyosis. See also color plate.

surface of the uterus. In some cases, dark hemorrhagic or chocolate-colored areas, variable in diameter, are scattered diffusely in the musculature.

In cases of focal adenomyosis, the uterus may be irregular and asymmetrical. Adenomyomata are often difficult to differentiate clinically from leiomyomata. Mostly, they can be distinguished because they do not bulge out of the cut surface as myomata tend to do, and they offer resistance to "shelling out." They are situated mainly in the uterine wall, but occasionally they present as submucosal tumors, which distort the shape of the uterine cavity.

Prevalence

A wide variation in prevalence rates in women undergoing hysterectomy exists (<20% and >50%). The histologic diagnosis varies in relation to the number of tissue sections analyzed; Bird and co-workers found a variation of 30% to 60% in hysterectomy specimens.[8] A comparison of prevalence rates in hysterectomy specimens in patients with and without symptoms would provide important information, but no such study has been reported.

The distribution of cases of adenomyosis is age-related; most patients are in their fourth to sixth decade, the range being from 27 to 85.[9] Adenomyosis appears to be much more common in parous than in nulliparous women; perhaps pregnancy is a promoting factor. One recent case report described the presence of adenomyosis in a young infertile woman.[10]

Symptoms

Adenomyosis may produce symptoms or may be silent. In one study, about 35% of patients with adenomyotic uteri had not reported any symptoms.[7] McCausland cautioned that the percentage of asymptomatic adenomyosis is overestimated.[11] Data are limited to studies of patients who had hysterectomies. Menstrual disorders were not always reported or asked for in patients who had had a hysterectomy for reasons other than abnormal bleeding.

There is a correlation between the frequency and intensity of symptoms and the degree of adenomyotic extension.[4] In most cases, symptomatic patients with isolated adenomyosis complain of menstrual bleeding disorders such as menorrhagia (40% to 50%), dysmenorrhea (15% to 30%), and metrorrhagia (10% to 12%). Dyspareunia has also been reported in 7% of patients with adenomyosis.[12] Symptoms often also reflect coexisting pathology, such as endometriosis and/or myomata.

The reason why patients with adenomyosis develop menorrhagia is unknown. Several factors might contribute to this pattern. A greater endometrial surface, as a result of uterine enlargement with or without the presence of submucous adenomyomata, can increase blood loss. Also, the presence of endometriotic tissue within the myometrium may cause an inadequate muscular contraction pattern during menstrual periods. The bleeding could occur because of a dysfunctional endometrium. Frazer measured the amount of blood loss in patients with adenomyosis, which was reduced by a prostaglandin synthesis inhibitor.[13] This finding suggests the possible role of prostaglandins in menorrhagia. The dominant product in adenomyosis is PGI_2, a potent vasodilator and inhibitor of platelet aggregation.[14] This prostaglandin has an inhibitory effect on isolated human myometrium and a relaxing effect on uterine arteries. There is a correlation between the depth of penetration and the amount of blood loss.[11] This action could also be a factor in menorrhagia, but even minimal endometrial penetration can cause menorrhagia.

Nishida studied the relationship between the onset of dysmenorrhea and histologic evidence of adenomyosis.[15] A group of patients with dysmenorrhea had significantly increased numbers of islands of adenomyosis. The depth of invasion was also greater among patients with dysmenorrhea. When 80% of the thickness of the muscular wall is invaded by endometrial tissue, dysmenorrhea occurs. Koike and co-workers investigated the production of eicosanoids in adenomyosis and other gynecologic pathologies.[16] They found the production of 6-keto-PGF1α significantly higher in adenomyotic tissue compared with normal endometrium, myometrium, and myomata, especially in the menstrual period. This product could be responsible for uterine contractions in dysmenorrheic women observed at the end of the menstrual cycle and during menstruation. The same authors found a correlation between the degree of dysmenorrhea and prostaglandin production in adenomyotic tissue.

Jen's team studied the possible association of adenomyosis and infertility in 100 cases of adenomyosis diagnosed from hysterectomic specimens.[17] They reported that if the patients had no coexisting gynecologic pathology, no fertility problems were observed.

Diagnostic Techniques

Ultrasound

Transvaginal or transabdominal ultrasound is noninvasive, relatively inexpensive, and takes little time. The value of this examination in the diagnosis of adenomyosis has been reported in a few patients. Most studies refer to the use of transabdominal ultrasound. In nine patients, Walsh and co-workers detected characteristic irregular cystic spaces of 5 to 7 mm disrupting the normal fine, speckled echo pattern of the uterus (honeycomb image).[18] Pathologic examination was available

for four of the patients and showed the presence of blood-containing cavities. But these findings have not been confirmed by other investigators. Buli's team found no correlation between ultrasound findings and the histologic diagnosis of adenomyosis.[19] When Bohlman analyzed retrospectively the ultrasound findings of seven cases of pathologically proven extensive adenomyosis, he found an enlarged uterus in all cases and a widened posterior uterine wall with displacement of the endometrial cavity in five cases.[20] Six out of seven cases showed a slight decrease in uterine echogenecity. One case revealed no ultrasonographic anomalies, and one was suggestive of a calcified leiomyomata.

Siedler and co-workers used ultrasound to analyze the condition of 80 patients presenting with either adenomyomata or leiomyomata.[21] They found a sensitivity of 63%, a specificity of 97%, and a positive predictive value of 71%. Criteria for diagnosis were as follows: a diffusely enlarged uterus with normal myometrial texture, contour, and central cavity. The low sensitivity can be explained by the cases of adenomyomata, which had obvious focal contour anomalies. When leiomyomata are associated with adenomyosis, the diagnosis of the latter is difficult. This problem is important because there is a frequent association of the two conditions.

Fedele recently reported a series using transvaginal ultrasonography in 49 patients who had undergone hysterectomy for menorrhagia.[22] Ultrasonic diagnosis of adenomyosis was made in 22. Of these, 16 (73%) had pathologic confirmation of this diagnosis. The sensitivity of transvaginal ultrasound was 80%, the specificity 74%.

The diagnosis of adenomyosis cannot be made conclusively by ultrasound, although it can be suggestive for this disease. So far, no hard data are available to demonstrate the superiority of transvaginal ultrasound versus transabdominal ultrasound.

Magnetic Resonance

Magnetic resonance imaging (MRI) is the ideal procedure for therapeutic evaluation of leiomyomata, because the number, size, location, and extent of degeneration can be extremely well documented.[23] Although the differential diagnosis between adenomyomata and myomata often remains difficult, adenomyomata can be diagnosed accurately by MRI.

T_2-weighted images are normally used to diagnose adenomyosis. When image analysis included a single enhanced T_1-weighted sequence, investigators found results of lesion detection significantly inferior to those obtained with T_2-weighted images. Contrast-enhanced T_1- and/or T_2-weighted images do not improve the assessment of leiomyomata or adenomyomata.[24] The appearance of diffuse adenomyosis on MRI has the following characteristics: a low signal intensity band surrounding the normal high-intensity endometrium, focally or diffusely. A band of uneven distribution, of more than 5 mm in thickness, is highly suggestive of adenomyosis. If it is less than 5 mm, a second examination should be repeated at another time during the menstrual cycle, because the thickness in cases of diffuse adenomyosis remains the same and that of the normal junctional zone changes. Solitary or multiple small foci of high signal intensity may be present and are detected with T_1- and T_2-weighted images. When these foci occur on both T_1- and T_2-weighted images, they are thought to represent hemorrhage.[25] When they are seen only on T_2-weighted images, however, they may represent endometrial tissue.

Adenomyomata appear as ill-defined areas with indistinct margins and with relatively homogeneous low signal areas. The differential diagnosis between adenomyosis and leiomyomata can be made in most cases. Myomata are well-circumscribed masses, have a broader spectrum of signal intensity, and are more intense than adenomyomata. Usually, myomata are rounder than adenomyosis lesions, which are focally shaped along the long axis of the uterus.

Togashi and co-workers prospectively diagnosed 15 out of 16 cases of adenomyosis and six out of six cases of coexisting adenomyomata and leiomyomata.[26] In one case, the differential diagnosis could not be made. The cause of uterine enlargement was correctly diagnosed with MRI in 92 of 93 cases. MRI is highly accurate in helping to distinguish between adenomyosis and leiomyomata in cases of enlarged uterus. Mark's group could identify all eight cases of adenomyosis in their series.[27]

At MRI, the diagnosis of adenomyosis can be made by an experienced radiologist. The most important use of MRI is the differential diagnosis with myomata if the uterus is enlarged. MRI is a noninvasive, nonionizing radiation procedure, but the disadvantage is that it is costly and time-consuming.

Hysterosalpingography

The use of hysterosalpingography (HSG) as a diagnostic tool for adenomyosis is very limited.[28,29] In order to be visualized at HSG, the abnormally located glands have to communicate with the endometrial lining. In that case, diverticula can be seen, which seem to branch out from the uterine cavity, which in turn is filled by contrast medium, in the myometrium. The spicular projections end in small sacs thought to be endometrial glands. Coarsely irregular margins can also be noted in patients with adenomyosis. In cases of focal adenomyosis where large adenomyomata are present, the image of the cavity can be enlarged and disturbed, producing a shadow. It is impossible to make the differential diagnosis from submucous myomata by HSG alone.

Confusion can occur if interstitial intravasation is present. This phenomenon can be localized or generalized, and is accentuated when there is excessive pressure within the uterine cavity because of injection of contrast material in cases of tubal occlusion or extensive synechiae. Also, after endometrial instrumentation (biopsy, curettage), intravasation of dye may be seen. Nunley reported a 7% rate of intravasation in a series of 593 HSGs.[30]

Myometrial Biopsy

The only way to make an accurate diagnosis without a hysterectomy specimen is to obtain a biopsy of the abnormal myometrium. Adenomyosis has been diagnosed on myometrial biopsies taken at laparoscopy or laparotomy.[10] The disadvantage of this technique is that only extensive forms of diffuse or focal adenomyosis can be diagnosed. If there is minimal endometrial penetration, it is impossible to get an adequate tissue fragment for diagnosis. Hirata reported a case where, during laparotomy, a deep wedge-shaped biopsy of the uterine fundus extending to the anterior wall was performed and the diagnosis of adenomyosis was made.[31] Nelson's team described the diagnosis of adenomyosis made from a frozen section of an enlarged uterus containing two masses of 5 and 6 mm.[10] McCausland used a 27 French operative hysteroscope and took biopsies of the posterior wall with a 5-mm loop electrode, which was completely embedded into the myometrium.[11] Specimens of 1.5 to 3 cm long, 5 mm in width and 5 mm in depth, were obtained during this procedure. This study showed that myometrial biopsy can be an aid to diagnose adenomyosis accurately. McCausland observed no immediate or long-term complications, such as bleeding, perforation, or irrigation fluid absorption syndrome in his series of 90 patients. This technique is contraindicated in postmenopausal women because of their thin uterine walls. Furthermore, the technique of biopsy has to be improved. A biopsy specimen might prove the presence of adenomyosis in extensive lesions. In limited lesions, however, false–negative biopsy specimens have to be taken into account.

Ca-125

It is generally accepted that endometrium is a source of Ca-125. Bischof et al and Weintraub et al were able to demonstrate the release of Ca-125 by endometrial cells in vitro.[32,33] Jacobs et al found particularly high levels of Ca-125 in endometrial extracts.[34] Kabawat and associates also detected Ca-125 on the surface epithelium of the endometrium.[35] Kijima et al showed that Ca-125 was present on the glandular epithelium localized in muscle layers of adenomyosis.[36] Ida et al and Kobayashi et al demonstrated that heterotopic endometrial epithelial cells produced a significantly higher amount of

Ca-125 than the eutopic epithelial cells in vitro (16 and 9 times respectively).[37,38] These authors state that the increase of Ca-125 production by ectopic epithelial endometrial cells may be responsible for the elevated Ca-125 levels observed in adenomyosis. Takahashi et al observed a significantly higher Ca-125 concentration compared to a control group; six out of seven patients had Ca-125 levels greater than 35 U/ml.[39] In all of these patients normal values were observed one month after hysterectomy. He suggested the possible use of serum Ca-125 levels in differentiating adenomyosis from uterine myomata. However, contradictory data have been published by Halila.[40] In his series, eleven patients with histologically proven adenomyosis had normal Ca-125 levels (<35 U/ml).

If ectopic endometrium can indeed produce Ca-125, the serum levels in adenomyotic patients should be higher and therapy should lower the Ca-125 concentrations. The latter would be very useful in monitoring patients who are treated conservatively. So far, the conflicting data in literature cannot be reconciled and should encourage further investigation in this area.

Pathogenesis

The etiology of adenomyosis is still poorly understood. A widely accepted theory posits a direct downgrowth from the lamina basalis of the endometrium into the myometrium. In this view, the endometrium resembles a lava stream, which flows down between the muscle bundles. Cullen demonstrated a direct continuity between the basalis portion of the endometrium and the endometrial islands within the areas of adenomyosis.[41] No matter how deep the ectopic endometrial tissue, a communication with the uterine cavity was shown by performing serial sections. The reason why this downgrowth occurs is unknown; it could be a reaction to a mechanical factor, such as childbirth or curettage that causes endometrial trauma. Lewinsky was able to produce adenomyosis experimentally in pregnant rabbits by doing a curettage in one uterine horn, while the pregnancy in the opposite one continued.[42] Also, in this model, high levels of estradiol, progesterone, and prolactin were present. Besides mechanical trauma, chronic inflammation could damage the endometrial and myometrial borders and facilitate endometrial downgrowth. In such circumstances, endometrial tissue shows a reactive hyperplasia.

Possibly, an unknown growth factor may trigger the endometrial downgrowth. If it exists, it may be hormonal and result from ovarian dysfunction. Since uterine tissues have a common origin, some authors have suggested that foci of adenomyosis can arise de novo in the myometrium as a result of cellular metaplasia. Von Recklinghausen advanced the hypothesis that endometrial islands could arise from Wolffian ducts; this is

associated with the small group of cornual cases.[43] The mechanisms for the development of either diffuse or focal adenomyosis are not known. It is possible these might involve two different pathologic entities.

Role of Prolactin

Animal experiments suggest that prolactin plays an important role in the genesis of adenomyosis. Isologous anterior pituitary transplantation outside the hypothalamic pituitary venous portal system (into the uterine lumen or under the renal capsule) induces an early and high incidence of uterine adenomyosis with subserous nodules in mice.[44,45] This phenomenon was associated with a significant rise in plasma-prolactin levels. The incidence of adenomyosis was higher in the uterine horn containing the pituitary graft. Others have found that prolactin has a general, rather than a local, effect and that the incidence in both uterine horns with and without pituitary grafts is equal.[46] Singtripop's team induced hyperprolactinemia by means of psychotherapeutic or gastroenteric drugs such as sulpride, perphenazine, and metoclopramide.[47] These dopamine receptor blockers act as dopamine antagonists, stimulating prolactin release from the pituitary gland. Treatment with these drugs resulted in a high incidence of adenomyosis in mice.

Mori and co-workers administered prolactin to mice during their neonatal period and adult life and observed development of adenomyosis.[48] The incidence of adenomyosis was reduced after the administration of bromocriptine for more than four weeks and beginning at four weeks of age. If the duration of treatment was less than three weeks, or the start of the treatment was after 11 weeks, it was not effective. This observation suggests a critical period for the inhibitory effect of bromocriptine on the development of adenomyosis later in life. In conditions where prolactin levels were elevated and progesterone levels were reduced, there was a decrease in adenomyosis lesions. This finding indicates an isolated high prolactin level may be insufficient to produce adenomyosis.

Mori's group observed histologic changes in the uterus while inducing adenomyosis.[49,50] Initially, there was an invasion of stromal fibroblasts into the myometrium along the branches of blood vessels. A second step was uterine gland invasion of the myometrium to the serosa. When the muscle layer is functioning optimally, it protects against invasion of proliferating endometrial tissue into the musculature. Different changes in morphology and arrangement of the smooth musculature, such as the irregular shape of muscle cells, reduced size of the cells with resulting wider intercellular space, disintegration of the muscle layer, scantiness of cell organelles, and pyknosis of muscle cells have been observed using electron microscopy in adenomyosis. Myometrial degeneration might be caused by prolonged exposure to high levels of prolactin. This hypothesis is strengthened by a number of observations in different animals. Investigators reported an inhibitory effect of prolactin on oxytocin-induced myometrial contraction.[48–52]

Prolactin undoubtedly plays a major role in the pathogenesis of adenomyosis. Probably the effect is indirect by modulating the production and/or secretion of sex steroids or the number and/or the susceptibility of their receptors. In this way, prolactin might be responsible for the abnormal response of the uterus to female sex steroids that trigger the development of adenomyosis. We know prolactin affects both progesterone production and also the effect of progesterone on periphery target cells.[53,54] There may also be a direct effect on the endometrial-myometrial barrier and/or on the uterine smooth muscle cells, which loosen and allow endometrial expansion.

Role of Sex Steroids

In 1935, Lacassagne reported adenomyosis in mice after long-term (more than 8 months) estrogen therapy.[55] Many researchers used this estrogen treatment to induce adenomyosis in other animals.[56] Prenatal exposure of mice to DES have resulted in a higher incidence of adenomyosis at an advanced age.[57] Some authors have stated that perinatal treatment with estrogen altered the hormonal balance and decreased responsiveness to the growth-promoting effect on the uterus. This finding might explain the low incidence of adenomyosis in advanced age.[58]

Ostrander's team did not find differences in the incidence of adenomyosis between control and DES-treated mice in the neonatal period.[59] Huseby and Thurlow compared BALB/C female mice exposed to DES with controls and found no differences.[60]

Huseby and Thurlow described the histologic pattern of adenomyosis as having a progesteronal response. They reported a significant rise in the serum level of progesterone in addition to that of prolactin in mice with pituitary grafts. Subcutaneous implants of progesterone in mice increased development of adenomyotic lesions. Other experiments in mice suggest that a hormonal imbalance involving high levels of progesterone is needed to develop adenomyosis.[54,59]

Role of Steroid Receptors

Tamaya and co-workers studied different steroid receptors (estrogen, progesterone, and androgen) by Scatchart plot analysis in ten cases of adenomyosis.[61] They found that there were always estrogen receptors in adenomyotic tissue, but in a reduced quantity when compared with corresponding normal myometrium. Progesterone receptors were not always present, and

when present, there were fewer than in normal endometrium. Androgen receptors have also been detected in adenomyotic tissue. Vanderwalt found fewer estrogen receptors and slightly higher progesterone receptor levels.[62] The technique used in these two studies was a biochemical assay, which has the disadvantage of disrupting the tissue during the assay. With this technique, it is impossible to confirm the presence of the lesion or to ensure the absence of nonlesional tissue that may contain steroid receptors. To avoid false–positive results due to the presence of nonlesional tissue, other methods are preferable. Autoradiography or immunohistochemical techniques can be used. In this way, one might demonstrate estrogen receptors in adenomyotic tissue. Further investigation is needed to clarify these contradictory findings.

Role of Immunologic Factors

When compared to patients without gynecologic pathology and patients with endometriosis, Ota and coworkers found a higher incidence of autoantibodies in 28 patients with adenomyosis.[63] They also found a significant increase in IgG, C_3, and C_4 complement deposits in endometriotic tissue in adenomyosis.[64] This observation may suggest an immune response in adenomyosis. These findings appear to suggest the presence of ectopic endometrium as an antigen-evoking activation of macrophages and interaction with T cells. The same authors also analyzed the distribution of tissue macrophages in uterine muscle layers in patients with adenomyosis and found that the number of macrophages was twice that of patients with uterine myomata.[65] The location of these macrophages was not along the glandular epithelium, but in the stromal region, which could mean that there is no cytotoxic effect on endometriotic tissue. After these studies, Ota's group put forward the following hypothesis: ectopic endometrium liberates certain substances, which could act as antigens. These antigens are recognized by macrophages and presented to T cells. Mediation from B cells results in production of antibodies that might possibly bind to the surface of the glandular epithelium and fix complement.

Adenomyosis and Endometrial Cancer

Endometrial hyperplasia arising in adenomyosis is common. However, the type of hyperplasia that occurs in these cases has not been specified in most reports. The incidence of atypical hyperplasia arising in adenomyosis seems to be low.[9] In rare cases where adenocarcinoma develops, the diagnosis is extremely difficult. Symptoms are lacking and there is no diagnostic tool other than hysterectomy. However, Woodruff's team found cytologic malignant cells in cervical smears from such patients.[66] Ultrastructural findings in adenomyotic tissue were studied by Hayata and co-workers.[67] There were some similarities to differentiated endometrial adenocarcinoma. No data suggest these findings predispose to malignant degeneration. It may be a reflection of the ectopic growth of endometrium.

Different authors have commented on the high prevalence of adenomyosis in patients with endometrial cancer. Giammalvo and Kaplan examined 120 cases of endometrial cancer and 264 controls; adenomyosis was present in 33% of those with endometrial cancer, but in only 18% in the control group.[68] Marcus also observed a higher prevalence of adenomyosis in patients with endometrial adenocarcinoma than in a control group (60% versus 39%).[69] In the same report, a significantly higher percentage of endometrial hyperplasia within adenomyosis lesions was noted; 39 (65%) out of 60 versus 7 (18%) out of 39 in the control group. In 100 adenomyosis lesions, he observed no malignant transformation of the adenomyotic glandular epithelium.

Hayata studied 30 uterine body cancers; eight (27%) were associated with adenomyosis.[70] In a series of 175 cases of endometrial carcinoma reported by Greenwood, adenomyosis was present in 19%.[71] In a comparison group of 203 women who underwent hysterectomy and who did not have endometrial carcinoma, 17% had adenomyosis. There was no significant difference between the affected and the control group. Johnson and Roddick studied pathology slides from 100 women with endometrial adenocarcinoma and 100 age-matched controls.[72] They found adenomyosis in 16% of the cases and 28% of the controls. They used strict criteria for the diagnosis of adenomyosis: ectopic endometrial glands and stroma separated from the endometrial mucosa by at least one low-power microscopic field. Hernandez and Woodruff found 21 cases of adenomyosis among 204 patients with endometrial cancer; 30% of the cases revealed malignant alterations in both surface and intramyometrial endometrium.[73]

In cases of simultaneous endometrial adenocarcinoma and adenomyosis, the distinction between adenomyotic involvement by tumor and true myometrial expansion of cancer is critical, but often very difficult to make. Cases of endometrial adenocarcinoma in which myometrial involvement is limited to adenomyosis have a better prognosis than those with true myometrial invasion of adenocarcinoma.[74] The prognosis for patients with endometrial adenocarcinoma, however, appears unaffected by the coexistence of adenomyosis with or without involvement by adenocarcinoma.[75] Peritumoral myometrial changes and desmoplasia are probably the best indicators of myometrial invasion. Benign residual "marker" glands should be carefully searched for within the adenomyotic foci involved. Their presence indicates extension into the adenomyosis rather than direct myometrial invasion.

Therapy Choices

The only available therapy for adenomyosis in the past was hysterectomy. In fact, it was not really therapy because the diagnosis was usually made only at pathologic examination of the operation specimen. With current techniques being used in the clinical setting, the diagnosis can often be suspected. Hysteroscopic biopsies can give us accurate histologic diagnosis. Preoperative diagnoses of adenomyosis is mandatory in order to decide on a correct therapy.

In contrast with the radical treatment of hysterectomy, less invasive approaches can be contemplated. GnRH analogues have been administered to obtain hypoestrogenemia, as is common in cases of endometriosis or myomata. The first case was published by Grow in 1991 in a patient with primary infertility, menorrhagia, premenstrual spotting, and dysmenorrhea.[76] A marked reduction in uterine size was noticed on ultrasound, and concomitant amelioration of symptoms was seen after four months of treatment. However, after six months from discontinuation of the GnRH analogues, symptoms reappeared and worsened progressively to pretreatment severity. The uterine size returned to its initial value within six months after stopping the treatment. Hirata also treated a patient by GnRH analogues with secondary infertility with adenomyosis who conceived after six months of treatment.[31]

Problems with long-term treatment with GnRH analogues are symptoms due to the hypoestrogenemia and accelerated bone demineralization. Bone loss after ovarian suppression therapy is normally reversible, but the length of time needed and the degree of reversibility vary. A future therapy, which has also been proposed for endometriosis, might be the combination of GnRH analogues and hormonal replacement therapy. This therapy should provide enough estrogen to prevent or minimize osteoporosis and subjective symptoms, but not sufficient to stimulate the adenomyotic lesions. This treatment can be offered to women who have no other indications for hysterectomy, women with a high risk or contraindication for surgical procedures, women with a desire for childbearing, or women who want to preserve their uterus for psychological reasons.

Another alternative to radical surgery is hysteroscopic endometrial ablation. This technique can be used in cases with minimal endometrial invasion (<3 mm). However, if endometrial glands are still present after the procedure, they may cause recurrent bleeding and pain. A less frequent disadvantage of persistence of endometrial glands is the delay in diagnosis of endometrial cancer, if the ectopic endometrium becomes malignant. Maybe deeper ablation with electroresection will prove to be more effective than the use of the rollerball alone in patients with adenomyosis.[11]

Oral danazol administration has been used to treat adenomyosis with apparent benefit.[77] Intrauterine danazol treatment with a vaginal ring containing 175 mg of danazol resulted in atrophy of the adenomyosis, and reduction of the uterine size, without inhibiting ovulation and pregnancy. Singtripop demonstrated that experimentally induced adenomyosis in mice was suppressed by subcutaneous danazol administration.[78] It is not known by which mechanism this process is mediated. It could be indirect, by decreasing the levels of gonadotropic hormones, or a direct effect on endometrial cells. Some studies have demonstrated the presence of local immunologic processes in adenomyosis. We can therefore hypothesize that danazol might have an inhibitory effect on local immunological reactions in patients with adenomyosis.[79]

To sum up, although hysterectomy is still a widespread procedure to treat adenomyosis, one can speculate that early (preoperative) diagnosis will change treatment policy. In the future, the combination of GnRH analogues and HRT may become the preferred treatment.

References

1. Hendrickson MR, Kempson RL. Non-neoplastic conditions of the endometrium and uterine serosa. In Fox H, ed. Haines and Taylor Obstetrical and Gynecological Pathology, 3rd ed. New York, Churchill Livingstone, 1987, pp 405–410.
2. Novak ER, Woodruf JD. Novak's Gynaecologic and Obstetric Pathology. Philadelphia, WB Saunders Co., 1979, pp 280–290.
3. Tindall VR. Jeffcoat Principles of Gynaecology, 5th ed. London: Butterworths, 1987, pp 360–361.
4. Benson RC, Sneeden VD. Adenomyosis: a reappraisal of symptomatology. Am J Obstet Gynecol 1958;76:1044–1061.
5. Sakamoto A. Subserosal adenomyosis: a possible variant of pelvic endometriosis. Am J Obstet Gynecol 1991;165:198–201.
6. Javert CT. Observations on the pathology and spread of endometriosis based on the theory of benign metastasis. Am J Obstet Gynecol 1951;62:477–487.
7. Azziz R. Adenomyosis: Current Perspectives. Obstetrics and Gynecology Clinics of North America 1989;16:221–235.
8. Bird CC, McElin TW, Manalo-Estrella P. The elusive adenomyosis of the uterus. Am J Obstet Gynecol 1972;112:583–593.
9. Molitor JJ. Adenomyosis: a clinical and pathological appraisal. Am J Obstet Gynecol 1971;110:275–84.
10. Nelson JR, Corson SL. Long-term management of adenomyosis with a gonadotropin-releasing hormone agonist: a case report. Fertil Steril 1993;59:441–443.
11. McCausland AM. Hysteroscopic myometrial biopsy: its use in diagnosing adenomyosis and its clinical application. Am J Obstet Gynecol 1992;166:1619–1628.
12. Owolabi TO, Stickler RC. Adenomyosis: a neglected diagnosis. Obstet Gynecol 1977;50:424–430.
13. Frazer JS, McCarron G, Maikham R, et al. Measured menstrual blood loss in women with menorrhagia associated with pelvic disease or coagulation disorder. Obstet Gynecol 1986;69:630–635.
14. Koike H, Egana H, Ohtuka T, et al. Eicosanaids production in endometriosis. Prostaglandins Leukotines and Essential Fatty Acids 1992;45:313–317.
15. Nishida M. Relationship between the onset of dysmenorrhea and histologic findings in adenomyosis. Am J Obstet Gynecol 1991;165:229–231.
16. Koike H, Egana H, Ohtuka T, et al. Correlation between dysmenorrheic severity and prostaglandin production in women with endometriosis. Prostaglandins Leukotines and Essential Fatty Acids 1992;46:133–137.
17. Jen SW, Lim-Tan SK, Wee D, et al. The clinical significance of adenomyosis and its relation to fertility. In Advances in fertility and sterility series, volume 5. London, The Parthenon Publishing Group, 1987, pp 207–212.
18. Walsh JW, Taylor KJM, Rosenfield AT. Gray scale ultrasonography in the diagnosis of endometriosis and endometriosis. Am J Radiol 1979;132:87–90.
19. Buli CM, Kasnar V, Dukovic I. Use of ultrasound in the diagnosis of genital endometriosis. Jugoslav Ginekol Perinatal 1986;26:33–38.
20. Bohlman ME, Ensor RE, Sanders RC. Sonographic findings in adenomyosis of the uterus. Am J Radiol 1987;148:765–766.
21. Siedler D, Laing FC, Jeffrey RB. Uterine adenomyosis: a difficult sonographic diagnosis. J Ultrasound Med 1987;6:345–349.
22. Fedele L, Bianchi S, Dorta M, et al. Transvaginal ultrasonography in the diagnosis of diffuse adenomyosis. Fertil Steril 1992;58:94–97.
23. McCarthy S. Gynecologic applications of MRI. Critical Reviews in Diagnostic Imaging 1990;31:2,263:281.
24. Hricak H, Finck S, Honda G, et al. MR imaging in the evaluation of benign uterine masses: value of gadopentetate dimeglumine-enhanced T_1-weighted images. Am J Radiol 1992;158:1043–1050.
25. Hricak H, Cannagton BM. MRI of the pelvis (a text atlas). Martin Dunitz Ltd., 1991, pp 100–101.
26. Togashi K, Ozasa H, Konishi I, et al. Enlarged uterus: differentiation between adenomyosis and leiomyoma with MR imaging. Radiology 1989;171:531–534.
27. Mark AS, Hricak H, Heinrichs LW, et al. Adenomyosis and leiomyoma: differential diagnosis with MR imaging. Radiology 1987;163:527–529.
28. Hunt RB, Siegler AM. Hysterosalpingography: Techniques and Interpretation. Chicago, Year Book Medical Publishers, Inc., 1990, pp 75–77.
29. Winfield AC, Wentz AC. The uterine cavity in diagnostic imaging in infertility. Baltimore, Williams & Wilkins, 1992, pp 112–115.
30. Nunley MC, Bateman BC, Kitchin JD, et al. Intravasation during hystersalpingography using oil base contrast medium. Obstet Gynecol 1987;70:309–312.
31. Hirata JD, Moghissi KS, Ginsburg KA. Pregnancy after medical therapy of adenomyosis with a gonadotropin-releasing hormone agonist. Fertil Steril 1993;59:444–445.
32. Bischof P, Zseng L, Brioschi PA, et al. Cancer antigen 125 is produced by human endometrial stromal cells. Hum Reprod 1986;1:423–426.
33. Weintraub J, Bischof P, Zseng L, et al. Ca-125 is an excretory product of human endometrial glands. Biol Reprod 1990;42:721–726.
34. Jacobs IJ, Fay TN, Stabile I, et al. The distribution of Ca-125 in the reproductive tract of pregnant and non-pregnant women. Br J Obstet Gynecol 1988;95:1190–1194.
35. Kabawat SE, Bast RC, Bhan AK, et al. Tissue distribution of a coelomic epithelium related antigen recognized by

the monoclonal antibody OC 125. Int Gynecol Pathol 1983;2:275–285.

36. Kijima S, Takahashi K, Kitao M. Expression of Ca-125 in adenomyosis (with 1 color plate). Gynecol Obstet Invest 1987;23:122–123.

37. Ida W, Kobayashi H, Naito Y. An in vitro study on the mechanism of Ca-125 production of endometrial cells—comparison of ectopic and heterotopic endometrium. Nippon-Somka-Fiyinka-Gukhai-Zasshi 1990; 42:1161–1167.

38. Kobayashi H, Ida W, Teiao T, et al. Qualitative assessment and characterization of Ca-125 antigen produced from human endometrial epithelial cells. Nippon-Somka-Fiyinka-Gukhai-Zasshi 1990;44:303–309.

39. Takahashi K, Kijima S, Yoshino K, et al. Differential diagnosis between leiomyomata uteri and adenomyosis using Ca-125 as a new tumor marker of ovarian carinoma. Acta Obstet Gynecol Jap 1985;37:591–595.

40. Halila H, Suikkari AM, Seppala M. The effect of hysterectomy on serum Ca-125 levels in patients with adenomyosis and uterine fibroids. Hum Reprod 1987;2:265–266.

41. Cullen TS. Adenomyoma of the uterus. Philadelphia, WB Saunders Co., 1908.

42. Lewinski H, Esnge LA. The elusive adenomyosis of the uterus. Am J Obstet Gynecol 1962;83:1541–1555.

43. von Recklinghausen F. Die Adenomyose und cystadenoma den Uterus und Zuberwandung: ihne Abkunft von Resten des Wolffschen Korpers. Berlin: August Hirschwald, 1896.

44. Mori T, Nagasana H. Mechanisms of development of prolactin-induced adenomyosis in mice. Acta Anat 1983; 116:46–54.

45. Huseby RA, Soares MJ, Talamantis F. Ectopic pituitary grafts in mice: hormone levels, effects on fertility, and its development of adenomyosis uteri, prolactinomas, and mammary carcinomas. Endocrinology 1985;116:1440–1448.

46. Sakamoto S, Mori T, Singtripop T, et al. Increase of DNA synthesis in uterine adenomyosis in mice with ectopic pituitary isograft. Acta Anat 1992;145:162–166.

47. Singtripop T, Mori T, Kynnnpark M, et al. Development of uterine adenomyosis after treatment with dopamine antagonist in mice. Life Science 1991;49:201–206.

48. Horrobin DF, Lipton A, Muiruri KL, et al. An inhibitory effect of prolactin on the response of rat myometrium to oxytocin. Experienta 1973;29:109–110.

49. Mori T, Nagasana H. Alteration of the development of mammary hyperplastic alveolar nodules and uterine adenomyosis in SHN mice by different schedules of treatment with CB-154. Acta Endocrinologica 1984;107: 245–249.

50. Mori T, Ohta Y, Nagasawa H. Ultrastructural changes in uterine myometrium of mice with experimentally-induced adenomyosis. Experientia 1984;40:1385–1387.

51. Mati JKG, Mugambi M, Muriuki PB, et al. Effect of prolactin on isolated rabbit myometrium. J Endocr 1974; 60:379–380.

52. Lipton A, Leah J, Parkington HC. Effects of ovarian steroids and prolactin on the contractibility and sodium pomp site density of guinea-pig myometrium. J Endocr 1978;77:43–48.

53. Armstrong DT, King ER. Uterine progesteron metabolism and progestational response: effects of estrogens and prolactin. Endocrinology 1971;89:191–197.

54. Lipschultz A, Iglesias R, Panasevich V, et al. Pathological changes in the uterus of mice with the prolonged administration of progesteron and 19-m-contraceptives. Br J Cancer 1967;21:160–165.

55. Lacassagne A. Modifications progressives de l'uterus de la souris sous l'action prolongée de l'oestrogène. CR Séances Soc Biol 1935;120:1156–1158.

56. Mori T, Singtripop T, Kawashima S. Animal models of uterine adenomyosis: is prolactin a potent inducer of adenomyosis in mice? Am J Obstet Gynecol 1991;165: 232–235.

57. Walker BE. Uterine tumors in old female mice exposed prenatally to diethylstilbestrol. J Natl Cancer Inst 1983; 70:477–484.

58. Mori T. Abnormalities in the reproductive system of aged mice after neonatal estradiol exposure. J Endocrinol Invest 1986;9:397–402.

59. Ostrander PL, Mills KT, Bern HA. Long-term responses of the mose uterus to later sex hormone exposure. J Natl Cancer Inst. 1983;74:121–135.

60. Huseby RA, Thurlow S. Effets to prenatal exposure of mice to "low-dose" diethylstilbestrol and the development of adenomyosis associated with evidence of hyperprolactinemia. Am J Obstet Gynecol 1982;144:939–949.

61. Tamaya T, Motoyama T, Ohono Y. Steroid receptor levels and histology of endometriosis and adenomyosis. Fertil Steril 1979;31:396–400.

62. Van der Walt LA, Sanfilippo JS, Siegel JC, et al. Estrogen and progestin receptors in human uterus: reference ranges of clinical conditions. Clin Physiol Biochem 1986;4:217–220.

63. Ota H, Maki M. Content of immunoglobulin G and complement components C3 and C4 in endometriotic tissue or endometrium in women with adenomyosis or endometriosis. Med Sci Res 1990;18:727–728.

64. Ota H, Maki M. Evaluation of autoantibody and Ca-125 in the diagnosis of endometriosis or adenomyosis. Med Sci Res 1990;18:309–310.

65. Ota H, Igarashi S, Maki M. Distribution of tissue macrophages in uterine muscle layers in patients with adenomyosis. Med Sci Res 1991;19:473–474.

66. Woodruff JD, Erozam YS, Genadry R. Adenocarcinoma arising in adenomyosis detected by atypical cytology. Obstet Gynecol 1986;67:145–148.

67. Hayata T. Ultrastructural study of glandular epithelium in adenomyosis in comparison with those of proliferative endometrium and well-differentiated endometrial cancer. Am J Obstet Gynecol 1991;165:225–228.

68. Giammalvo JJ, Kaplan K. The incidence of endometriosis interna in 120 cases of carcinoma of the endometrium. Am J Obstet Gynecol 1958;75:161–165.

69. Marcus CC. Relationship of adenomyosis uteri to endometrial hyperplasia and endometrial carcinoma. Am J Obstet Gynecol 1961;82:408–16.

70. Hayata T, Korwashima Y. Clinicopathologic study of eight cases of uterine body cancers associated with endometriosis interna (uterine adenomyosis). Am J Obstet Gynecol 1987;156:663–666.

71. Greenwood SM. The relation of adenomyosis uteri to coexistent endometrial carcinoma and endometrial hyperplasia. Obstet Gynecol 1976;48:68–72.

72. Johnson RV, Roddick JW Jr. Incidence of adenomyosis in patients with endometrial adenocarcinoma. A study of 100 patients. Am J Obstet Gynecol 1961;81:268–271.

73. Hernandez E, Woodruff JF. Endometrial adenocarcinoma arising in adenomyosis. Am J Obstet Gynecol 1980;138: 827–832.

74. Jacques SM, Lawrence DW. Endometrial adenocarcinoma with variable-level myometrial involvement limited to adenomyosis: a clinicopathologic study of 23 cases. Gynecol Oncol 1990;37:401–407.

75. Hall JB, Young RH, Nelson JH. The prognostic significance of adenomyosis in endometrial carcinoma. Gynecol Oncol 1984;17:32–40.

76. Grow DR, Filer RB. Treatment of adenomyosis with long-term GnRH analogues: a case report. Obstet Gynecol 1991;78:538–539.

77. Igarashi M. A new therapy for pelvic endometriosis and uterine adenomyosis: local effect of vaginal and intrauterine danazol application. Asia Oceania J Obstet Gynecol 1990;16:1–12.

78. Singtripop T, Mori T, Sakamoto S, et al. Suppression of the development of uterine adenomyosis by danazol treatment in mice. Life Sci 51:1119–1125.

79. Ota H, Maki M, Shidara Y, et al. Effects of danazol at the immunologic level in patients with adenomyosis with special reference to autoantibodies: a multi-centre cooperative study. Am J Obstet Gynecol 1992;167:481–486.

27

Psychological Aspects of Chronic Pelvic Pain in Women With Endometriosis

Mary Casey Jacob

For many women with endometriosis, chronic pain is the most challenging aspect of the disease. Because the illness is invisible to the casual observer, and generally isn't life threatening, the woman with endometriosis and those around her may struggle to know how much attention and worry to accord it. It can be very difficult to accept that having so much pain does not imply an emergency. Chronic pain is a significant challenge to the physician as well as the patient. Physicians want to relieve suffering, and yet with chronic pain their task is sometimes to say, "I can't fix it."

In approaching the woman with chronic pain, three questions are helpful initially: "Am I able to identify the reasons this woman has pain? If I can identify some of the reasons, can I do anything about them? If I am unable to cure the problem, or alter her experience of pain, do I know who might be able to help her?"

Three additional questions can be asked when working with women with endometriosis: "Do I think the disease is now in control? Can I offer this woman anything else *now*? Do I want to recommend to her that she also work with specialists who may help her live with her residual pain for now?"

Why are these questions pertinent for a surgeon to ask? Clinically significant symptoms, including pain, are so common they are often considered "normal" by those who have them.[1,2] Frequently, people with symptoms do not consult physicians.[3] Given these facts, it is important to consider what brings our patients to us. Why do some patients with pelvic pain consult us when others with pain don't?

One medical sociologist has identified critical stimuli that lead people to consult doctors.[2] First, people go to the doctor when a symptom disrupts normal functioning, for example when pain prevents attending school or work. Second, people consult doctors when a symptom interferes with social functioning; for example, when pain makes intercourse too uncomfortable, or makes a woman afraid to have a sexual relationship. Third, people consult doctors when the symptoms last "too long." We all have commonsense understandings of what kind of pain is "normal" and what is not, and when pelvic pain begins to last for more and more days each month, a woman may seek help. Fourth, doctors are consulted when symptoms change rather suddenly, for example, if the pain moves to a new location. Fifth, people go to the doctor when the opinions of others, or one's lay referral system, tell them to. Many women, for example, tolerate extraordinary pelvic pain because their mothers or sisters tell them it is normal. If one's mother suggests that the symptoms have gone beyond the norm, or one's best friend tells of going to the doctor for similar pain and getting effective help, then one might go to the doctor oneself. Sixth, people also go to the doctor when major life events occur; for example, before marriage or attempting conception, women may consult physicians to see if they can obtain pain relief.

Helping patients requires that we not only do what we can to reduce or eliminate symptoms, but also that we attend to the questions, anxiety, or other needs that convinced them to make the appointment. Even when our power to completely relieve the symptoms is limited, we can still address their concerns.

Often there is not a clear relationship between pain and recognizable organic pathology. Studies have shown a lack of correlation between organic findings and reports of back pain, and between adhesions and other organic findings, and reports of pelvic pain.[4-9] Investigators have reported that pelvic pain intensity cannot be predicted from the presence or absence of endometriosis or severity of adhesions.[10,11] These reports tell

267

us not only that many people have pain for reasons we don't understand, but also that many people we would expect to have significant pain do not. Thus, physical findings are not the only variables that influence pain perception.

Pain

Models of Pain

Historically, *somatic models* of pain, implying a linear relationship between structural tissue damage and pain intensity, have driven treatment planning. However, because somatic models do not adequately account for the lack of correlation between organic findings and pain perception, pain specialists have sought a more sophisticated and useful understanding of the pain experience. Such an understanding requires the recognition of a range of psychological and environmental variables that influence pain perception. These include factors as varied as attention and distraction, beliefs about pain, gender and age, mood, personality traits or disposition, styles of thinking, and ways of coping.[12-20]

Another limitation of somatic models of chronic pain is that they do not address the common concomitant clinical and social problems of our patients. These problems include affective distress, family dysfunction, relationship problems, substance and alcohol abuse, unemployment, and underemployment.[21-24] The prevalence of these additional life problems highlights the need to plan treatments with the patient as the focus, rather than the pain.[25,26]

Central models of chronic pain take nociception into account, but also highlight the critical roles of the central nervous system and psychological factors in the perception and perpetuation of pain, and the determination of disability and distress. Most research on the central models has been cross-sectional, however, and while relationships between neurobiological and psychosocial variables can be examined, such research does not accommodate the historical context in which the chronic pain occurs. For example, a relationship has been found between chronic pain and maladaptive ways of thinking.[14] However, it isn't known if idiosyncratic ways of thinking are sequelae of chronic pain, or if they precede and possibly contribute to its development.

The *diathesis-stress model* of chronic pain attempts to address the deficits in somatic and central models by integrating contemporary neurobiological and psychosocial perspectives.[27] This model suggests that some people have preexisting congenital or learned *vulnerabilities* that heighten their risk for developing chronic pain. These vulnerabilities may be in cognitive (for example, maladaptive thinking), affective (for example, trait anger), or behavioral (for example, always resting when having pain) domains, or present in the individual's social milieu (when for example, a girl's mother predictably says, "Stay home from school if you have cramps"). The diathesis-stress model emphasizes the temporal and social contexts in which pain becomes chronic, and explicitly suggests that the experience of pain may persist and become associated with disability and distress when there is a match between a preexisting vulnerability and a specific *challenge* associated with acute pain. Three examples of challenges are (1) physical impairment, (2) activation of central monoamine and endorphin systems, and (3) fear. Finally, the model emphasizes the likely moderating role of social support. As an example of the vulnerability/challenge relationship, consider how dysfunctional family relationships (a preexisting vulnerability) may be challenged by increased pain-contingent attention from a mother to a daughter with severe menstrual pain.

Having such a model of pain in mind may be helpful as you try to understand the experience of pain reported by your patients with endometriosis. Your understanding of each woman's pain will influence the ways you respond to her and help her think about her pain.

Factors Influencing Pain Perception and Requests for Help

People generally assume that pain means something is wrong. Patients often have a specific *worry* in mind (for example, "Is it cancer?"), which should be discovered and addressed. At the same time, patients must be educated to understand that chronic pain does not serve the same important function of alerting a person to get help that acute pain serves.

Learning influences pain perception and reactions to pain. Society teaches that pain means something is wrong, and doctors can diagnose and heal. Family and cultural messages are also an important influence. One investigator, for example, has found differences in medical utilization between different European-American ethnic groups.[3] Life experiences also teach us: we may like the attention we get when we report our pain, for example. *Expectations*, often learned in the family, that pelvic pain is normal for women, may help women tolerate pain or keep them from asking for help.

Distractions are important in the determination of pain tolerance.[12] Many athletes continue to play after being hurt, without being aware of injury in some cases. Pain is often more intrusive at night while trying to sleep, when other sensory input is at a minimum.

When others help too much, or are too *solicitous*, beliefs that something terrible is wrong and one should take it easy are reinforced. Numerous studies have documented the influence of social interactions on the maintenance of pain and disability.[28,29]

These personal, cultural, social, and situational factors also influence physicians "responses to patients" reports of pain. Many doctors have firm ideas about how much pain should accompany particular conditions, and deviations from the norm may influence how patients are treated.[30]

Clinical Implications of the Diathesis-Stress Model

The diathesis-stress model encourages *inter*disciplinary (not just *multi*disciplinary) collaboration. Given the multifactorial etiology of chronic pain in most patients, involvement of multiple specialists offering integrated and coordinated clinical programs is ideal, particularly for the most puzzling or refractory cases. Consultation among independent practitioners or settings can be useful also *if* communication is active and ongoing, and if treatment planning is collaborative.

Several arguments for this approach can be made. First, the sophistication of different disciplines is often required in order to assess fully all pertinent medical issues. For example, in women with endometriosis, residual chronic pain may be related to the disease, but other conditions may also be present, such as irritable bowel syndrome, abdominal trigger points, urethral syndrome, pelvic neurofibromatosis, multiple sclerosis, reflex sympathetic dystrophy, or interstitial cystitis.[31] Second, other clinical and social problems may coexist with and exacerbate chronic pain.

Assessment and treatment planning should target these and other pertinent problems through the coordinated involvement of physicians, psychologists, acupuncturists, social workers, vocational rehabilitation specialists, and physical and occupational therapists. The efficacy of interdisciplinary pain clinics is well established and has been shown to lead to significant improvements not only in terms of self-reported symptom relief, but also in terms of return to work and appropriate use of the health care system.[25,32,33] Always be clear with the patient about why you are involving other professionals. State explicitly that you are not trying to "get rid of her," but to enhance her treatment and her coping.

Assessment of Patients With Endometriosis and Chronic Pain

An interdisciplinary assessment consists of discipline-specific evaluations, followed by collaborative discussion, and the development of hypotheses about the etiology and maintenance of the pain problem for this particular patient. Participating specialists should vary depending on the characteristics of the pain. Evaluation should focus on further medical diagnosis as well as consideration of pharmacologic, anesthesiologic, surgical, psychologic, and rehabilitation options.

The diathesis-stress model is grounded on the premise that for an individual patient, some particular factors out of many possible ones, will interact over time to contribute to the development and maintenance of chronic pain and associated disability and distress. Therefore, the assessment process should begin with each provider scanning for current problem areas and their possible contributors. As assessment progresses, it should be increasingly focused, behaviorally specific, and quantitative. Such an approach facilitates the examination of possible relationships among pertinent variables. In collaborative discussion, this process generally leads to identification of treatment goals and ideas for a treatment plan.

Generally, the assessment role of the rehabilitation specialists is to discriminate physical impairment (limits on functioning that are directly related to structural pathology and neurological deficits) from functional disability (limits related to avoidance of pain and deconditioning). Although many treatment modalities focus on somatic relief, rehabilitation efforts that emphasize education are most consistent with chronic illness and self-management perspectives.

In an interdisciplinary assessment, the participation of a psychologist is generally accepted as critical. In the last two decades, often in collaboration with medical colleagues, psychologists have developed psychometrically sound and clinically useful strategies for the measurement of pain, pain-related disability, and other important variables. Some of these strategies or instruments require minimal interpretation (for example, pain intensity ratings) and can be used and interpreted by nonpsychologists. For the assessment of variables requiring psychological interpretation (such as personality tests), the involvement of a psychologist with specific expertise in testing and chronic pain assessment is indicated.

Standardized psychological evaluation can provide reliable and quantifiable data on many pertinent variables.[34–36] Psychological assessment may target pain perception; frequency of pain behaviors; impact of the pain on social, family, sexual, and work situations; coping with infertility related to endometriosis or worries about future infertility; beliefs about the pain that might influence participation in or response to treatment; concomitant affective distress; psychiatric history; history of physical, sexual, or emotional abuse; current or past substance abuse or dependence; and current coping skills.

These data can be used to identify targets for intervention (for example, depression, or an incorrect belief that when in pain one should be inactive or further trauma may result); identify contributors to these problems that may be additional targets for intervention (for example, dependence on CNS depressants that may be contributing to depression, inactivity, and deconditioning); and provide a baseline for comparison at reevaluation points.

A comprehensive evaluation also communicates to a woman that the team is serious about helping her to reduce the impact of pain in her life. The psychological evaluation demonstrates this broad interest and concern and begins a dialogue with the patient about how to reduce disability and distress. This approach may enable the patient to learn the importance of a self-management approach.

Affective Distress

Depression coexists with chronic pain, perhaps 50% or more of the time.[37-40] It has been argued that this coexistence is so common, chronic pain and depression are best considered in a single entity, the "depression–pain syndrome."[37] Others, however, have argued that empirical data show the direct link between pain and depression to be weak, and that perceived interference in one's life by the pain, and perceived self-control are significant mediating variables.[41] Depressed chronic pain patients report greater pain intensity, greater interference due to pain, and more frequent pain behaviors.[13] It has also been argued that affective distress is a sequelae of chronic pain. Empirical support for depression as a sequelae to chronic pain has recently been provided.[41,42]

Because of the reciprocal influence that chronic pain, disability, and affective distress appear to have on one another, interventions that relieve pain, disability, or insomnia are believed to positively influence mood and associated symptoms. Pharmacological and psychological therapies that target depression and anxiety are commonly offered. Antidepressants are frequently prescribed for pain and insomnia as well as affective distress. Behavioral treatments for insomnia, stress management, and anxiety reduction are often part of a therapeutic plan. Treatments that target behavioral avoidance resulting from fear of pain and fear of injury have also been successfully applied.[43] Other treatment strategies focus on general social skills training, such as anger management and assertiveness training.[44] Finally, common areas of distress and dysfunction for women with chronic pain are marital and family relationships.[24] In cases of severe dysfunction, marital or family therapies are sometimes indicated. Such interventions may also help alleviate depression or other negative mood states.[38]

Narcotics

Debate continues on the use of narcotics for chronic, nonmalignant pain.[45,46] Because narcotics act on the central nervous system, users often suffer undesired side effects that may contribute to the maintenance of the pain and cause certain aspects of disability. Daily use of narcotics promotes dependency, tolerance, and abuse. This, in turn, may increase dependence on others for coping and may decrease self-esteem. Narcotics often impair concentration and memory, further increasing disability. Regular use may cause or exacerbate depression, and often results in apathy, which can have a negative impact on relationships at home and at work. Daily use may "reinforce" and thus increase, the pain, especially if used on a PRN rather than fixed schedule basis.[47]

These side effects are so significant and debilitating in so many cases, one team has argued that the most useful step taken in many chronic pain clinics is the careful withdrawal of pain medications.[48] Their statement is consistent with my clinical experience. Generally, following such withdrawal, most patients report their pain unchanged.

Most patients with chronic pain do not see themselves as addicted or dependent. When questioned closely but nonjudgmentally, however, many will admit that the medication does not change the pain, it just makes them not care so much about it. Many will also acknowledge that sometimes they take the medication to help with general coping, even when the pain is not too bad. By discussing the links between medication use and decreased performance at work, poor concentration, lack of interest in activities, and relationship difficulties, you may motivate patients to try managing their pain without narcotic medication.

Abuse History

It has been stated that a greater than expected number of pelvic pain patients have histories of physical or sexual abuse.[8,49,50] This can be difficult to substantiate, given the known problem of underreporting. There are also difficulties in comparing abuse incidence rates in a clinical population asking for help and, perhaps, willing to disclose, to rates in a general population, many of whom would be unwilling to disclose their histories to researchers.

A history of abuse is one of many factors influencing the extent of suffering and disability from chronic pain.[31] The literature documents the relationship between a history of abuse and increased risk for depression and anxiety, somatization, alcohol and drug abuse, among other problems. Thus, a history of abuse may be considered one diathesis that can be challenged by a diagnosis of endometriosis and by chronic pain. It is especially pertinent to address issues of abuse within the context of a self-management approach to chronic pain, because having been abused may influence the degree to which a woman is open to strategies of empowerment.[51] Each woman should be carefully asked about any abuse history. Because some will be reluctant to disclose, and some may not remember, all women who deny any history should be told that you are always willing to talk about such issues should they have any questions or concerns later.

Team Treatment Planning

The goal of treatment planning is a plan for intervention based on an integrative understanding of the patient's problems. Consensus building takes time, but is essential if the patient is to be offered clear and consistent information about her problems and a plan for tackling them. Unless the patient understands the rationale for the treatment plan, particularly if it targets disability as well as pain, cooperation and adherence are unlikely. Feedback to the patient should involve discussion and negotiation in an effort to help her make sense of the team's suggestions in the context of her own experiences and beliefs. Treatment goals should include improved quality of life.

Because patients often finally consult the doctor because of worry about a symptom, the first important step is to convey to the patient that you accept what she is saying about her pain and distress. Let her know you will clarify diagnosis and prognosis as much as possible, but it will also be helpful to acknowledge the limits of medical and surgical interventions with regard to chronic pain. Feedback that is heard as "You have to learn to live with your pain" may be seen as gratuitous and uncaring, especially if you offer no guidance and no referral to someone who can guide her in learning to live with pain.

Caring for the patient with chronic pain is a long-term proposition, regardless of the degree of physical findings. Giving the patient a follow-up appointment each time she leaves the office allows her to know that she will have ongoing contact to discuss her problems in living with her endometriosis. Without this, patients often feel they must identify the pain as an emergency in order to get back into medical care.

Emphasize to the patient the positive aspects of the multiple treatment and rehabilitation alternatives and present a credible biobehavioral rationale for each intervention. Develop both short- and long-term goals targeting not only pain relief, but also reduction of disability and alleviation of affective distress. Specific goals should be negotiated with the patient and defined behaviorally and temporally, so that the patient and the team share an understanding of the parameters of each goal and when it should be reached, and will be able to agree on goal attainment. The goals should be critically evaluated with an eye toward making them small enough to be attainable, in order to help the patient develop confidence, hopefulness, and a sense of mastery.

All recommended treatments and rehabilitation efforts should be consistent with a chronic illness self-management perspective. For example, a chronic illness perspective argues against sole reliance on analgesic medication, and procedures such as trigger point injections that target somatic relief alone generally have a disappointing outcome, given the complex and chronic nature of the problem. However, pharmacological or anesthesiological approaches may be quite helpful within the context of a broadly conceived treatment approach. For example, trigger point injections might be applied as the patient begins a physical conditioning program. Any benefit from the injections might help ease the patient into more activity without an increase in pain. A successful increase in activity might shift the patient's focus from the injections to her own efforts.

Treatments that target a problem in one domain may exert effects in other areas as well, positive or negative. For example, antidepressant medications may have important analgesic effects.[52–55] Conversely, medications prescribed for muscle relaxation and pain relief may have depressant effects. Physical exercise and improved conditioning may lead to increased productive and pleasurable activity, and ultimately, improved mood and sleep.[56] The diathesis-stress model provides a structure for considering these interactions and encourages development of a treatment plan that maximizes positive effects in more than one domain.

Antidepressants

Antidepressants are now used for chronic pain, insomnia, generalized anxiety, bulimia, panic attacks, peptic ulcer disease, and tension and vascular headaches as well as depression.[53,57,58] Heterocyclic antidepressants inhibit the reuptake of serotonin and/or norepinephrine. The resultant increase of neurotransmitters may be the mechanism by which depression is relieved. The mechanism of analgesic action is unclear, although it has been argued that chronic pain decreases the circulating levels of brain serotonin.[59] Some investigators believe that analgesia occurs as depression lifts; others argue that analgesia occurs as a separate and isolated effect.[52,54,55] Arguments for direct analgesic action are made from studies finding the onset of pain relief to be more rapid than that expected for antidepressants; studies finding analgesia in the absence of an antidepressant effect and in patients who are not depressed; and laboratory studies showing that an extended availability of serotonin at the neuronal synapse increases the pain threshold.[53]

From a purely academic perspective, the efficacy of antidepressants as analgesic medications is still not clearly established.[53,60–63] Increasingly, however, these medications are among the first pharmacological alternatives to narcotics considered by clinicians, probably as a function of their presumed low potential for abuse and dependence.

The drugs most commonly used and frequently studied have been the heterocyclic antidepressants, particularly doxepin HCL (Sinequan) and amitriptyline HCL (Elavil). These drugs, known to block the reuptake of serotonin, are also sedating, and thus are quite helpful with the sleep disturbance so often a part of chronic pain. A rested patient is generally better able to cope with chronic pain. Antidepressants may also relieve some of the anxiety that frequently accompanies chronic pain.

In selecting an antidepressant, consider any need for sedation to help with sleep; cardiovascular effects; and anticholinergic effects. Doses considerably lower than those used to treat depression are often helpful and thus treatment should begin with a very low dose. Dosage should be very gradually increased, both to decrease uncomfortable side effects (and thus increase adherence), and so that the lowest possible therapeutic dose may be identified. A trial would not be complete, however, until true antidepressant doses have been tried.

Symptom relief may be obtained anywhere from 1 day to 10 weeks, but generally a trial could be considered complete after maintaining a woman on the maximum dose for four to six weeks. Individual reductions in pain perception using antidepressants are truly idiosyncratic, so if the first drug tried is not helpful, try a second and even a third.

Generally, it is best to prescribe the entire dose to be taken at bedtime to capture the sedating effects for sleep enhancement (and to prevent daytime sedation). Also compliance is generally better with a single dose, and one dose reduces any focus on medication as a primary pain management technique.

In introducing the use of an antidepressant medication, take the time to explain the many uses of these medications. Be honest if you are using it with depression in mind as well as pain, and educate about the time frame in which you might expect to see results.

Psychologic and Rehabilitation Treatments

Numerous psychological treatments may result in reduction of pain reports. These include specific techniques such as progressive muscle relaxation, biofeedback, hypnosis, and meditation, as well as individual and group psychotherapies.[64-69]

Rehabilitation efforts target functional disability. These efforts are often initiated by rehabilitation specialists such as physical or occupational therapists, but the psychological aspects of integrating new activities into daily life require the application of psychological principles. Rehabilitation programs may include education in energy conservation (regular, brief rest periods can improve pain tolerance); training in alternative approaches to problems of daily living that compensate for physical limitations posed by underlying structural pathology (for example, sexual intercourse may be less painful if the woman is on top, controlling the amount and direction of penetration); and graded physical exercise and conditioning programs (people with chronic pain have commonly decreased their activity level to the point where they are badly deconditioned).

An increase in activity level and conditioning is almost always a treatment goal. Patients must learn that increased activity does not always mean more pain, and more pain rarely means more medical problems. Increased activity allows patients to resume normal social relationships and responsibilities. Besides targeting physical conditioning, exercise and conditioning programs may target more specific functional activity such as activities of daily living or work hardening. Vocational rehabilitation assessment and counseling is also an option for the unemployed or underemployed patient.

It is helpful to find ways to include family members in treatment efforts. For example, partners can be educated about the chronic illness/rehabilitation approach, and encouraged to support the patient in her efforts. Communication between partners may be examined, and specific patterns of communication that solicit or reinforce "pain behaviors" identified and discouraged.

Conclusion

The diathesis-stress model is a way to make sense of your clinical experience with endometriosis patients with chronic pain. In this context, pain perception and pain reports are understood to be influenced by myriad variables, including many psychosocial variables. Complex patients may benefit from care provided by an interdisciplinary team, or by you as well as some colleagues in other professions with whom you communicate well and easily.

References

1. Patrick DL, Scambler G. Sociology as applied to medicine, 2nd ed. London: Balliere-Tindall, 1982.
2. Zola IK. Pathways to the doctor—From person to patient. Soc Sci Med 1973;7:677–689.
3. Zola IK. Culture and symptoms—An analysis of patients' presenting complaints. Am Sociol Rev 1966;31:615–630.
4. Flor H, Turk DC. Etiological theories and treatments for chronic back pain: I. Somatic models and interventions. Pain 1984;19:105–121.
5. Turk DC, Flor H. Etiological theories and treatments for chronic back pain: II. Psychological models and interventions. Pain 1984;19:209–233.
6. Rapkin AJ. Adhesions and pelvic pain: A retrospective study. Obstet Gynecol 1986;68:13–15.
7. Baker PN, Symonds EM. The resolution of chronic pelvic pain after normal laparoscopy findings. Am J Obstet Gynecol 1992;166:835–836.

8. Walker E, Katon W, Harrop-Griffiths J, et al. Relationship of chronic pelvic pain to psychiatric diagnoses and childhood sexual abuse. Am J Psychiatry 1988;145:75–80.
9. Gillibrand PN. Investigation of pelvic pain. Communication at the Scientific Meeting on Chronic Pelvic Pain—A Gynaecological Headache, Royal College of Obstetricians and Gynaecologists, May 1981.
10. Stout AL, Steege JF, Dodson WC, et al. Relationship of laparoscopic findings to self-report of pelvic pain. Am J Obstet Gynecol 1991;164:73–79.
11. Steege JF, Stout AL. Resolution of chronic pelvic pain after laparoscopic lysis of adhesions. Am J Obstet Gynecol 1991;165:278–283.
12. Beers TM, Karoly P. Cognitive strategies, expectancy, and coping style in the control of pain. J Consult Clin Psychol 1979;47:179–180.
13. Haythornthwaite JA, Sieber WJ, Kerns RD. Depression and the chronic pain experience. Pain 1991;46:177–184.
14. Jensen MP, Turner JA, Romano JM, et al. Coping with chronic pain: A critical review of the literature. Pain 1991;47:249–283.
15. Kashima KJ, McCreary CP. Sex differences in chronic low back pain patients. Paper presented at the annual meeting of the American Psychological Association in New York City, August 1987.
16. McCaul KD, Malott JM. Distraction and coping with pain. Psych Bull 1984;95:516–533.
17. Melding PS. Psychosocial aspects of chronic pain and the elderly. IASP Newsletter 1992;Jan/Feb:2–4.
18. Sachem S, Dar R, Cleeland CS. The relationship of mood state to the severity of clinical pain. Pain 1984;18:187–197.
19. Timmerans G, Sternbach RA. Factors of human chronic pain. An analysis of personality and pain reaction variables. Science 1974;184:806–808.
20. Turk DC, Rudy TE. Assessment of cognitive factors in chronic pain: A worthwhile enterprise? J Consult Clin Psychol 1986;54:760–768.
21. Atkinson JH, Slater MA, Patterson TL, et al. Prevalence, onset, and risk of psychiatric disorders in men with chronic low back pain: A controlled study. Pain 1991;45:111–121.
22. Flor H, Turk DC, Scholz OB. Impact of chronic pain on the spouse: Marital, emotional and physical consequences. J Psychosom Res 1987;31:63–71.
23. Gervais S, Dupuis G, Veronneau F, et al. Predictive model to determine cost/benefit of early detection and intervention in occupational low back pain. J Occup Rehab 1991;1:113–131.
24. Thomas M, Roy R. Pain paients and marital relations. Clin J Pain 1989;5:255–259.
25. Rapkin AJ, Kames LD. The pain management approach to chronic pelvic pain. J Reproductive Med 1987;32:323–327.
26. Fordyce WE. Pain and suffering: A reappraisal. Am Psychol 1988;43:276–283.
27. Kerns RD, Jacob MC. Toward an inegrative diathesis-stress model of chronic pain. In Goreczny AJ, ed. Handbook of Recent Advances in Behavioral Medicine. New York, Plenum, in press.
28. Faucett JA, Levine JD. The contributions of interpersonal conflict to chronic pain in the presence or absence of organic pathology. Pain 1991;44:35–43.
29. Flor H, Kerns RD, Turk DC. The role of spouse reinforcement, perceived pain, and activity levels of chronic pain patients. J Psychosom Res 1987;31:251–259.
30. Gallagher EB, Wrobel S. The sick-role and chronic pain. In Roy R, Tunks E, eds. Chronic pain. Psychosocial factors in rehabilitation. Baltimore, Williams & Wilkins, 1982, pp 36–52.
31. Reiter RC, Milburn A. Exploring effective treatments for chronic pelvic pain: Contemp Obstet Gynecol, in press.
32. Caudill M, Schnable R, Zuttermeister P, et al. Decreased clinic use by chronic pain patients: Response to behavioral medicine intervention. Clin J Pain 1991;7:305–310.
33. Flor H, Fydrich T, Turk DC. Efficacy of multidisciplinary pain treatment centers: A meta-analytic review. Pain 1992;49:221–230.
34. Kerns RD, Jacob MC. Assessment of the psychosocial context of the experience of chronic pain. In Turk DC, Melzack R, eds. Handbook of Pain Assessment. New York, Guilford, 1992, pp 235–253.
35. Turk DC, Kerns RD. Conceptual issues in the assessment of clinical pain. Int J Psych Med 1983;13:52–68.
36. Turk DC, Kerns RD. Assessment in health psychology: A cognitive-behavioral perspective. In Karoly P, ed. Measurement strategies in health pscyhology. New York, Wiley, 1985, pp 335–372.
37. Lindsay PG, Wyckoff M. The depression-pain syndrome and its response to antidepressants. Psychosomatics 1981;22:571–577.
38. Kerns RD, Turk DC. Depression and chronic pain: The mediating role of the spouse. J Marriage Fam 1984;46:845–852.
39. Kramlinger KG, Swanson DW, Murata T. Are patients with chronic pain depressed? Am J Psychiatry 1983;140:747–749.
40. Wilson WP, Blazer DG, Nashold BS. Observations on pain and suffering. Psychosomatics 1976;17:73–76.
41. Rudy TE, Kerns RD, Turk DC. Chronic pain and depression: Toward a cognitive–behavioral mediation model. Pain 1988;35:129–140.
42. Brown GK. A causal analysis of chronic pain and depression. J Abnorm Psychol 1990;99:121–137.
43. Lethem J, Slade PD, Troup JDG, et al. Outline of a fear–avoidance model of exaggerated pain perception—I. Behav Res Ther 1983;21:401–408.
44. Fedoravicius AS, Klein BJ. Social skills training in an outpatient medical setting. In: Holzman AD, Turk DC, eds. Pain management: A handbook of psychological treatment approaches. New York, Pergamon, 1986, pp 86–99.
45. Portenoy RK. Chronic opioid therapy for persistent non-cancer pain: Can we get past the bias? APS Bulletin 1991;1:1–5.
46. Turk DC, Brody MC. Chronic opioid therapy for persistent noncancer pain: Panacea or oxymoron? APS Bulletin 1991;1:1–6.
47. Hanson RW, Gerber KE. Coping with chronic pain. A guide to patient self-management. New York: Guilford Press, 1990.
48. Gildenberg PL, DeVaul RA. The chronic pain patient: Evaluation and management. Basel, Switzerland: S. Karger, 1985.
49. Rapkin AJ, Kames LD, Darke LL, et al. History of physical and sexual abuse in women with chronic pelvic pain. Obstet Gynecol 1990;76:92–96.
50. Reiter RC, Gambone JC. Demographic and historic variables in women with ideopathic chronic pelvic pain. Obstet Gynecol 1990;75:428–432.
51. Karol RL, Micka RG, Kuskowski M. Physical, emotional, and sexual abuse among pain patients and health care providers: Implications for psychologists in multidisciplinary pain treatment centers. Prof Psychol Res Pract 1992;23:480–485.

52. Beresin EV. Imipramine in the treatment of chronic pelvic pain. Psychosomatics 1986;27:294–296.

53. Egbunike IG, Chaffee BJ. Antidepressants in the management of chronic pain syndromes. Pharmacotherapy 1990:10:262–270.

54. Feinmann C. Pain relief by antidepressants: Possible modes of action. Pain 1985;23:1–8.

55. Wang JK. Antinociceptic effect of intrathecally administered serotonin. Anesthesiology 1977;17:269–271.

56. Turner JA, Clancy S, McQuade KJ, et al. Effectiveness of behavior therapy for chronic low back pain: A component analysis. J Consult Clin Psychol 1990;58:573–579.

57. Aronoff GM, Evans WO. Doxepin as an adjunct in the treatment of chronic pain. J Clin Psychiatry 1982;43(8)Sec. 2:42–47.

58. Gitlin MJ. The psychotherapist's guide to psychopharmacology. New York, Free Press, 1990.

59. Sternbach RA. The need for an animal model of chronic pain. Pain 1976;2:2–4.

60. Goodkin K, Guillion CM. Antidepressants for the relief of chronic pain: Do they work? Ann Behav Med 1989;11:83–101.

61. Stimmel GL, Escobar JI. Antidepressants in chronic pain: A review of efficacy. Pharmacotherapy 1986;6:262–267.

62. Walsh TD. Antidepressants in chronic pain. Clin Neuropharmacology 1983;6:271–295.

63. Magni G. The use of antidepressants in the treatment of chronic pain. Drugs 1991;42:730–748.

64. Linton SJ, Melin L. Applied relaxation in the management of chronic pain. Behav Psychother 1983;11:337–350.

65. Keefe FJ, Schapira B, Williams RB, et al. EMG-assisted relaxation training in the management of chronic low back pain. Am J Clin Biofeedback 1981;4:93–103.

66. Hilgard ER, Hilgard JR. Hypnosis in the relief of chronic pain. Los Altos, CA: Kaufman, 1975.

67. Kabat-Zinn J, Lipworth L, Burney R. The clinical use of mindfulness meditation for the self-regulation of chronic pain. J Behav Med 1985;8:163–190.

68. Merskey H. Traditional individual psychotherapy and psychopharmacology. In Holzman AD, Turk DC, eds. Pain management: A handbook of psychological treatment approaches. New York, Pergamon, 1986, pp 51–70.

69. Kerns RD, Hegel MT. Chronic benign pain: Cognitive-behavioral treatment and support groups. In Seligman M, Marshak LE, eds. Group psychotherapy: Interventions with special populations. Needham Heights, MA, Allyn & Bacon, 1990, pp 105–126.

28

The Puzzle of Endometriosis

Mary Lou Ballweg

"Endometriosis remains an enigma to the practicing gynecologist."[1]

"Endometriosis provides a unique clinical and scientific challenge."[2]

"The literature on endometriosis is extensive, but often inadequate or contradictory."[3]

". . . a riddle wrapped in a mystery inside an enigma."[4]

Most people, as a pastime, enjoy a puzzle—be it a jigsaw puzzle, a three-dimensional maze, a magician's sleight-of-hand, a Rubik's cube, a mystery or detective novel or movie. But real life puzzles are not so much fun. No one tells us the answer at the end. People living with the puzzle have no easy way to explain for themselves and everyone around them what is happening to them. And if we must interact professionally with people afflicted by an illness that is a puzzle, the puzzle can deprive us of meeting some basic human needs—to be successful, to understand the things around us, to be able to help those who come to us for help, to be able to make a difference.

Endometriosis has certainly earned a reputation as perhaps the most puzzling entity in gynecology. And, with an estimated 5.5 million women in the United States and Canada with the disease and probably millions more worldwide, there is an overwhelming need to solve the puzzle. Not that people have not been trying. In the past quarter century, over 4,500 articles have been published on endometriosis (although scientific rigor has been applied only recently, according to one authority).[5]

With so much energy going into this endeavor, why do we seem only a little closer to solving the puzzle of this disease? Perhaps, just as with other puzzles in our lives, it may be useful to step back, reframe the problem, rethink the conceptual framework, question assumptions and premises, and ask new questions. Answers could be staring us right in the face.

Endometriosis may resemble those trick pictures in which you can see two pictures, but once you visualize one, it is difficult to see the other until you force yourself *not* to see the first picture. You have to create a blank slate in your mind. If we view endometriosis only as a gynecologic disease tied to endometrial implants, we may miss other, even obvious, ways of seeing the disease.

Just What Is Endometriosis Anyway?

Oh sure, it is these endometrial implants that somehow appear in ectopic locations. But is it? The fact that endometrial implants can be found in more than 40% of women; that symptoms may or may not be associated with these implants; that extent of implants does not correlate with symptoms; that removal or atrophy of the implants does not necessarily improve symptoms or cure the disease; that the classification schemes, tied to extent of implants, tell us little about symptoms or prognosis; that some women undergo repeated laparoscopies for symptoms that any experienced clinician would wager is endometriosis and no implants are found (later laparoscopies sometimes find implants, sometimes not)—all may lead to the conclusion that implants may *not* be the quintessential element, the sine qua non, of the disease.[6-14]

A consortium of European leaders on endometriosis has already defined the disease as more than the mere presence of implants. "Endometriosis is a disease affecting many women during their reproductive life. However, the mere presence of what is defined as endometriosis histologically cannot be equated *per se* to the presence of a disease. Endometriosis as a disease should be defined as 'the presence of ectopic endometrium, in association with evidence of cellular activity in the lesions and of progression, such as the formation of adhesions, or by its interference with normal physiological processes.'"[15]

While lauding the excellent scientific work being done at the cellular level to determine the activity of the implant and its similarities and differences from endometrium, it seems time to also look beyond the endometrial implant. If the puzzle of endometriosis is a systemic immunological, biochemical, or metabolic one, implants could come to be seen as peripheral to the root of the problem, as sequelae which perhaps must also be treated in addition to addressing the underlying disorder.

To continue to equate endometriosis strictly and solely with implants could lead to erroneous conclusions. Some researchers already are concluding that since so many women can be found to have ectopic endometrial tissue, endometriosis is not a disease or that endometriosis (defined as implants) does not cause pain, that women with implants and pain have psychological reasons for their pain since other women with implants have no pain.[16–19] Others, while agreeing that endometriosis causes pain, suggest that pain that continues after thorough surgery (directed at implants) must be from something other than endometriosis.[20] All are blocks in our thinking based on defining endometriosis as implants when all evidence suggests something more is involved. Continuing to equate endometriosis strictly with implants could also mean we harness ourselves to treatments that might be directed only at the tip of the iceberg.

No doubt looking beyond the implant is hard—after all, the definition of endometriosis as ectopic endometrium has been taught since the 1920s. It's human nature to hang on tenaciously to what we think we "know." But, in a case like endometriosis, where so little is *really* known, it's dangerous to hang on to old ideas to the exclusion of new. We dare not laugh at new ideas, though at first glance they may seem outlandish, because we truly do not know where the answers will come from. Remember the lessons of the past—in the Middle Ages, for instance, it was outright heresy to suggest that there might be any cause for disease other than God's will. And later, when Louis Pasteur proposed that "invisible enemies" might be causing disease, he was considered crazy. After discovering the bacteria that cause several diseases and also the method of vaccinating with inoculations to protect against these diseases, he became a hero. But before that, the doctors of his time would not listen to him since he was not a physician and because his ideas were so revolutionary.[21]

Beyond Implants: What Is Endometriosis Associated With Besides Implants? What Else Does This Disease Do?

So, if we need to look beyond the implant, where do we look next? As with all puzzles, we may need to go back to the source–the disease itself, which all can agree, lies somewhere in the patient. If we look at patients closely, listen to them carefully, listen without shutting out symptoms that do not fit our preconceptions, we will find we hear over and over again systemic complaints, complaints that go far beyond the pelvis.

The Endometriosis Association research registry, housed at the Medical College of Wisconsin, consists of over 3,000 case histories of women with confirmed endometriosis. The registry was begun in 1980 by the women who started the Endometriosis Association in order to help answer the many questions we had about the disease. Common symptoms reported by women in the registry include "fatigue, exhaustion, low energy" experienced by 82%; bowel problems by 79%; and a wide range of bodywide symptoms such as muscular aches. A smaller group also report low resistance to infections (39%) and low-grade fever (29%).[22]

In a selected group of these women, those with family histories of endometriosis, we also find a propensity to atopic diseases, including allergies, eczema, and asthma.[23–25] There is also a tendency to infections, and sometimes sore throats, and problems with fungal infections, especially those caused by Candida albicans.[26] These symptoms, repeated in the histories of women with endometriosis which pour into headquarters and the more than 150 chapters and support groups of the Endometriosis Association, point to particular types of immune problems. Candida albicans, for example, is kept in check by cell-mediated immunity which has been speculated to be faulty in women with endometriosis. These symptoms, including the nongynecological ones, may offer important clues to the nature of endometriosis.

Dysmenorrhea is the single most frequent symptom reported by women with endometriosis. Over 96% of the women in the Association registry report it.[22,27] In addition, primary dysmenorrhea seems to precede (or occur simultaneously with) endometriosis in the majority of cases.

Physicians must ask patients about dysmenorrhea as so many believe menstrual pain and menses-associated problems are normal and do not report it. At the Endometriosis Association, we often hear a woman say she first developed symptoms of endometriosis at such and such an age—when questioned about cramps and illness with her period, or bowel problems with her period, or pain with or after sex, she will often say she just has the "usual cramps and things everyone gets."

Granted, many women do experience primary dysmenorrhea in the modern world; however, that does not mean it is normal or healthy or has always been the case. There may be factors in our modern world, environmental, dietary, or others, causing these problems. The Endometriosis Association's recent work with a dioxin-induced endometriosis animal model has brought to light the powerful impact of pollutants on hormones, for example.[28,29]

Despite being the most frequent, and usually the earliest symptom reported in endometriosis, dysmenorrhea has not been studied much, although one multicenter study found primary dysmenorrhea to be a risk factor for endometriosis.[30] Clearly, studies delineating the relationship of primary dysmenorrhea to endometriosis are needed. Where does one end and the other begin or are they on a continuum? What is the natural course of primary dysmenorrhea? Why does primary dysmenorrhea occur in families as does endometriosis? What is the relation of this symptom and others seen in endometriosis (such as allergies) that may also be related to prostaglandin synthesis and fatty acid metabolism?

Physicians have paid more attention to some symptoms associated with endometriosis than others; strangely, the symptoms they most attend to are not the most prevalent ones. In an Australian study, for example, women who reported period pain, heavy bleeding, back pain and bowel pain had longer diagnosis delays than those who did not report these symptoms. Women who reported period pain, the most common symptom of endometriosis, had a diagnosis delay of 4.9 years compared to 2.3 years for those who did not report period pain.[31]

The symptoms girls and women often find most disruptive to their lives are sometimes not the ones physicians address. Patients tend to think in terms of the impact of the symptom on their lives—some symptoms may not even matter to them, while others may be destroying their self-image, their relationships with family or a sexual partner, their ability to work or study. The teenager with life-disruptive dysmenorrhea and her family may care much more about that symptom than her future fertility but find that her physician, while concerned about her future fertility, considers the pain not worth follow-up investigation. (If we were diagnosing and treating the fifteen-year-old with endometriosis and incapacitating pain, perhaps she might not be infertile at twenty-five!)

Pain is the most commonly reported symptom, yet one recent textbook on endometriosis does not even have an index heading for pain.[32,33] As a British physician recently noted: "...there is a definite gulf between the patient and the gynaecologist. The patient actually goes to see the doctor because she has got something that is seriously interfering with her life, which is pain. The gynaecologist, however, is more interested in what is causing the pain and not so much in the interference with her life. If he does not find what is causing the pain he tends to give up at that point, and that produces intense resentment on the patient's part, who after all is not interested particularly in endometriosis—she just wants her pain dealt with. I think pain is poorly taught at medical school, with the result that the histories taken by doctors do not cover the detailed components of pain that may actually lead to a much greater understanding not only of the cause, but of how to relieve it."[34]

Looking at the timing of symptom onset might also help us unravel the puzzle of endometriosis. For instance, over 40% of women in our registry, 42% in an Australian Endometriosis Association study, and 35% in a British Endometriosis Society study report experiencing their first symptoms of endometriosis by age 19. But only 2% to 6% were diagnosed before age 20; 83%, 79%, and 71%, respectively, reported their first symptoms before age 30 but only 52% to 56% were diagnosed before age 30.[35,31] Because of the delay between onset and diagnosis, many clues may be lost by the time diagnosis occurs. Clearly, if we are to solve the puzzle of endometriosis, we will have to try tracking the clues while they are still warm (if not hot). We may even need to look at youngsters before puberty. In families with endometriosis, it is common to hear the same stories over and over of allergies, asthma, low resistance to infections, and problems with Candida albicans long before puberty.

What about infertility? In our registry, 44% of the women report infertility. The history of medical interest in endometriosis in recent decades is that infertility specialists were the first to be concerned about the disease. But the relationship between endometriosis and infertility has been widely questioned in recent years.[36] In our registry, the patients who report no symptoms (3%) invariably are infertility patients.[22]

Selection bias may be inflating the significance that infertility has in endometriosis, since infertility patients are far more likely to be investigated for endometriosis.[37] This selection bias also means that we may be closing our eyes to other symptoms that may offer important clues to the nature of the disease. Women with endometriosis who have bladder symptoms, for instance, are sometimes told they have urinary tract infections or receive a diagnosis of interstitial cystitis.[38] Women with endometriosis with bowel symptoms are sometimes "diagnosed" with irritable bowel syndrome or spastic colon.[39]

Other Health Problems of Women With Endometriosis

The full range of frequently reported health problems in women with endometriosis provides valuable clues. But too often, as specialists, there is a tendency to look only at the pelvic symptoms or at those traditionally associated with endometriosis. The reported association with lupus; atopic diseases; thyroid disease, especially Hashimoto's thyroiditis (an autoimmune disease); mitral valve prolapse; problems with Candida albicans and a susceptibility to chronic fatigue and immune dysfunction syndrome (CFIDS) or fibromyalgia are clues that much more is going on, at least in the most problematic form of endometriosis.[25,40–45] The Endometriosis Association and the nonprofit groups serving those with related problems (including CFIDS, fibromyalgia, and candidiasis) have noted the overlapping nature of these problems. (A report appearing in the Association newsletter on fibromyalgia, following the observation by a member that so many of the women in the Fibromyalgia Network with confirmed fibromyalgia had a history of endometriosis, resulted in more than 600 letters from Association members to the Network, for example.)

The following letters, samples from the hundreds of thousands the Endometriosis Association has received, show the difficulties encountered because of the currently fragmented way of looking at the disease and provide examples of the related health problems noted in our research registry.

Dear Endo Assoc.

. . . I have undergone 3 laparoscopies in 10 months (each with a new doctor familiar with previous treatment) due to extensive endo. In each case I was gripped with pain to a point of having to have surgery.

I also was very put off by my struggle with feeling so ill only to have gyns dissuade me from believing there was an underlying problem in need of further investigation. Finally, after a 3rd surgery and Lupron treatment for severe endo . . . as well as a negative colonoscopy (due to my irritable bowel concerns), done by an internist who allowed the gyn's diagnosis to completely dictate his evaluation, I broke through to an internist specializing in rheumatic diseases. Prior to any lab work, I fit into a description of fibromyalgia. After specialized blood work . . . I have been diagnosed with systemic lupus erythematosis (SLE).

. . . Ablating endo implants is, in my case, a frustrating experience in treating the tip of the iceberg. One specialty doesn't know or want to know about the other and the patient becomes a victim of a medical evaluation system that has more blind spots than truly exist. All the answers are not in, but better and extensive evaluation may do a patient more justice. You can bet I have the last paragraph of p. 205 highlighted in my book [*Overcoming Endometriosis*].[46] What if endometriosis is a symptom of immune system problems rather than a disease itself? How do we educate the medical profession to evaluate the whole patient? . . .

Deborah, California

Dear Mrs. Ballweg:

. . . Over the past 5 years, I have been diagnosed with each of the above medical problems [fibromyalgia, chronic fatigue immunodeficiency syndrome, mitral valve prolapse, candidiasis, and endometriosis]. . . . The latest diagnosis of fibromyalgia came from an autoimmune and connective tissue specialist at the Mayo Clinic in Jacksonville, FL. . . .

. . . While my overall health has improved greatly from the above treatments [for the various conditions] in terms of a reduction of abdominal pain, extreme fatigue, vaginal itching, low-grade fevers, joint and muscle pain, etc., I am still unable to locate a physician who will assist me in pulling each of the diagnosed illnesses together and work with me in treating them collectively. Based on my own experiences and research, I am confident that the illnesses and symptoms are all related but I am very frustrated by the lack of interest and knowledge each Dr. exhibits in regard to my entire medical history. Each doctor who has helped me only wants to concentrate on one aspect of my symptoms (his own area of expertise) and as a result, I feel treatment and improvement are limited. . . .

Margaret, Florida

Dear Mary Lou:

. . . The article in the Vol. 12, No. 3, 1991 newsletter on fibromyalgia sounded hauntingly familiar. For the past six months I have taken between 1,400 and 2,400 mgs of ibuprofen per day to keep symptoms similar to what was described under control. The fatigue I have felt the past two years has been overwhelming, but I kept telling myself it was "all in my head. . . ." I finally got the courage to go back to my gynecologist for a physical. . . . I expected him to say everything is fine, come back in a year. But he ended up biopsying a vaginal lesion he thought was endometriosis. The pathology report stated "chronic inflammation." As I reviewed my pathology report from my hysterectomy, a frequently used word was "chronic inflammation." It seemed to describe everything they removed. . . .

I was sent back to my family doctor for possible lupus or arthritis testing. Some of the other symptoms I frequently experience are aching joints, low-grade fever, general achiness, and sensations of numbness in fingers, toes, and lips. A blood count showed signs of—you guessed it—"chronic inflammation." No wonder my body was so tired all the time—it was chronically inflamed. I pictured little white cells constantly coursing through my system looking for something to attack, and finding nothing, attacking those very cells they were supposed to protect. Needless to say, my allergies have been almost overwhelming over the past few years, and I have frequently been on Hismanal to control sinus problems as well as rashes. . . .

The changes I experienced on the ibuprofen have been dramatic. For the first time in years, I feel alive again. I have energy to do things I haven't done for years. I have discontinued the Hismanal, except for a few weeks of hay fever in the summer. I have decreased my estrogen (Ogen) replacement therapy by half. . . .

Susan, Utah

Dear Madam,

. . . On vacation I returned to my parents' home in London, England, where, despite having just had a laparoscopy which had diagnosed and cauterized my mild endo, I continued to have severe stomach pains, feelings of cystitis and yeast infection, and constant exhaustion—the symptoms that had, finally, led to the laparoscopy. After seeing my local general practitioner and being told that it was an "unspecific virus" that was troubling me (since all tests were negative) I finally found help. . . .

. . . The help came, first, from a Dr. I was referred to for back trouble who said that he thought that I might have food allergies . . . he referred me to an allergy doctor, who decided that I had acute candidiasis and food allergies (for which I'm still being tested). After only 3 days on the diet many of my symptoms improved, and by the end of the week I felt, for the first time in several years, alive, free of pain of all sorts and full of energy.

It's amazing: the past year has been an enormous struggle to get control over endless cystitis and yeast infections, and to get help for the dreadful stomach pains I had for most of my menstrual cycle (they became unbearable one week before and during my period), for the back pains, the migraines and the sudden fevers. . . .

. . . As it is, the year has been a living nightmare, a constant battle simply to get through each day awake, and not to give in to the fury, depression and helplessness provoked by the doctors as much as by my symptoms. . . .

. . . on my mother's side of the family (my grandmother, my mother's twin) there is a history of severe allergies, and my sisters and I used to have allergic reactions to bubble bath, petrol, etc., when we were small (swollen faces, rashes, nausea). . . .

Anabelle, Massachusetts

To Endometriosis Association

. . . I am a DES daughter. My mom died at the age of 37 of ovarian cancer. I have been treated for a yeast infection since I was 8 years old. Many doctors would even accuse me of poor hygiene as to why I suffered from this recurring problem. I had painful periods but my stepmother told me that was normal. At the age of 20 I suffered with a virus that the doctors never could explain. They thought I had mononucleosis but the test was negative. I was married and became pregnant and had a healthy baby boy. At the age 29 I was found to have Hashimoto's disease. I had a large tumor on my thyroid gland. . . .

At age 30 I developed a soreness around my upper abdomen. The doctor told me it was probably a pulled muscle. Then I had a severe attack of pain, diarrhea, fever and they rushed me to the hospital thinking it was my appendix. It wasn't. For the next 6 months I was sent from doctor to doctor thinking it was Crohn's disease. I lost 20 pounds and felt miserable. . . . I have pain constantly in my upper abdomen, fatigue, slight fever at times and twice a month I lie in bed for 2–3 days in severe pain. The pain in my back has become so severe that I am unable to walk.

Just yesterday I went to a gynecologist at B. Hospital in New York. He seemed puzzled by my medical history and didn't offer any help. He said either I take the pill or have a hysterectomy as I am high risk for ovarian cancer. Recently they did find an ovarian cyst, but he told me it was nothing to worry about. I left his office in tears from frustration but also the exam was so painful. . . .

. . . If only you knew what joy it brought me to read your book and newsletters. I have felt so very, very alone with all of this. People close to me don't understand the pain and also feel endo is not a "big deal" . . . I am on welfare now as I have been unable to work. . . .

. . . I have been disabled with this for the past two years and I'd like very much to find a way to become functional again. . . .

Lisa, New York

Gaps in Other Fields Affect Our Understanding of Endometriosis

The gaps in other fields also converge on endometriosis to create more holes in our knowledge. For instance, endometriosis is a disease that clearly involves the female hormones and also appears to involve the immune system. But the interlinking of hormones and the immune system is still a big mystery. As long ago as 1985, *Science* magazine published an article on the interactions between the gonadal steroids and the immune system but the precise nature of this link is still a puzzle.[47,48]

The finding that certain pollutants can cause endometriosis in rhesus monkeys may help us understand this link.[28,29] The toxicology literature is filled with examples of how pollutants such as dioxin appear to act as hormones in the body and at the same time disturb immune response.

In 1992, the Endometriosis Association learned that autopsy results in two monkeys in a reproductive toxicology study showed they had died of intestinal obstruction or kidney failure from ureteral obstruction due to extensive endometriosis. The study colony, which had been exposed to the pollutant TCDD ("dioxin"), had also experienced markedly impaired reproduction. This study echoed a Canadian study in which PCBs, another pollutant toxicologically related to dioxin, reportedly had caused development of severe endometriosis and marked impairment of reproduction.[49] Mild endometriosis occurs in menstruating primates without toxin exposure but no cases of moderate or severe endometriosis have been noted without toxin exposure.[50] In addition, monkeys exposed to radiation developed endometriosis in long-term U.S. Air Force studies.[51]

The Endometriosis Association provided emergency funding for the colony (which was about to be sold and dispersed) and arranged for laparoscopies and immunological work to be carried out on the entire colony (low dose, high dose, and control group). Seventy-nine percent of the animals exposed to dioxin in the study developed endometriosis. Moreover, the disease increased in severity in proportion to the amount of dioxin exposure (Figure 28.1). Control monkeys tended to have minimal disease; exposed monkeys moderate or severe, depending on the amount of dioxin exposure (AFS-r classification).[30,52–55] (The Association invites researchers interested in carrying out studies with the colony to contact us: Endometriosis Association, International Headquarters, 8585 N. 76th Place, Milwaukee, WI 53223.) A newly reported study from Germany also supports the link between certain pollutants and endometriosis. The study found that women with endometriosis and antithyroid antibodies have higher levels of PCBs in their blood.[56]

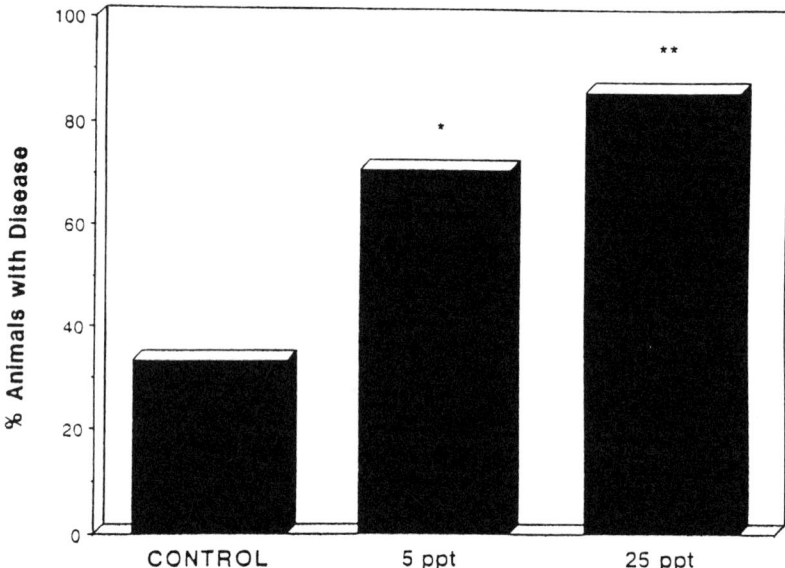

Figure 28.1. Incidence of endometriosis in dioxin-exposed rhesus monkeys. Frequency of disease was increased in dioxin-treated animals compared to animals with no history of dioxin exposure. All groups ($n = 20$), $p < 0.05$, Cochran-Armitage test, Control vs 5 ppt animals (51/169 vs 5/7), $^{*}p < 0.05$, Fisher's exact test. Control vs 25 ppt animals (51/169 vs 6/7), $^{**}p < 0.01$, Fisher's exact test.

There are at least 23 chemical families of pollutants, like dioxins and PCBs, that have known ability to disrupt the endocrine system, according to a consensus statement issued by scientists gathered at a conference, "Endocrine Disrupters in the Environment," held July 1991. The consensus statement also noted:

Many wildlife populations are already affected by these compounds. The impacts include thyroid dysfunction in birds and fish; decreased fertility in birds, fish, shellfish, and mammals; decreased hatching success in birds, fish, and turtles; gross birth deformities in birds, fish, and turtles; metabolic abnormalities in birds, fish, and mammals; behavioral abnormalities in birds, fish, and mammals; demasculinization and feminization of male fish, birds, and mammals; defeminization and masculinization of female fish and birds; and compromised immune systems in birds and mammals. . . .

The mechanisms by which these compounds have their impact vary, but they share the general properties of (1) mimicking the effects of natural hormones by recognizing their binding sites; (2) antagonizing the effect of these hormones by blocking their interaction with their physiological binding sites; (3) reacting directly and indirectly with the hormone in question; (4) altering the natural pattern of synthesis of hormones; or (5) altering hormone receptor levels.[57]

Another example of how gaps in other fields impinge on our ability to understand endometriosis is the lack of understanding of how immune abnormalities, particularly subtle ones, relate to clinical problems. The first report on the dioxin-induced endometriosis monkey colony indicated that despite altered T-cell ratios there was no clinical evidence of immune deficit in the monkeys.[58] Endometriosis had not yet been found in the monkeys—two were to die over the next few years and two others were experiencing pain with their menses and it was difficult for these researchers in immunology to understand the implications of the alterations they found. But the conclusion that there was no clinical evidence of immune deficit, despite their failure to look for such evidence, is the kind of statement that contributes to confusion. Similar statements have been made about women with endometriosis.[59]

Why So Many Myths and Misconceptions?

Medical mysteries are not the only puzzles about endometriosis. There are also sociological ones (which have contributed to keeping endometriosis a medical mystery). One member of the Endometriosis Association recently wrote that her physician said endometriosis is a disease of "overeducated women who wait too long to get pregnant," that she was "too educated for her own good," and that "you don't see Miss (Hispanic name), the fifteen-year-old migrant field worker, having any problems getting pregnant." Her physician's comments are a perfect example of the way myths work—drawing on common biases and prejudices in society to explain puzzles society has not yet resolved.[60]

It appears to be human nature to make up answers when none are forthcoming because it so frustrates us not to have answers. This occurs particularly in the area of taboo subjects, such as the symptoms of endometriosis. The myths take on a life of their own because they pick up the nonconscious ideologies at the heart of society—the unspoken things that everyone just "knows" and does not question. When the nonconscious becomes conscious, spoken, discussed, investigated, true science and change can take place.

We like to believe that medical science is beyond myth and taboo, especially as we approach the 21st century, but just as often deep-seated taboo or myth color science. An example of how mythmaking and taboos taint science is the story behind the myth that black women do not get endometriosis. A leading gynecologist, involved internationally in training gynecologists, confided to me soon after we began the Endometriosis Association in 1980, that gynecologists would almost automatically diagnose a black woman with symptoms of endometriosis as having pelvic inflammatory disease. The underlying reason was an assumption that black women were sexually promiscuous, a contributing factor in contracting PID. Statistical analyses then showed that black women had a lot of PID but not endometriosis, further perpetuating the myth that black women did not get endometriosis but did get PID. Except that the *numbers*, now in the guise of science and separated from their human element, could not so easily be accused of racism! And the numbers, based on racism, reinforced the scientific "truth" that black women did not get endometriosis.

Myths and taboos also make it harder for the physician to do his or her job. Because of the myths and taboos, women and girls are reluctant to share all of their symptoms with the physician or they delay seeking help. Some years ago, when the Endometriosis Association was planning a major advertising campaign to educate women about endometriosis, we carried out focus groups in New York City. We learned from these groups that many women with endometriosis would rather die first than tell a doctor they suffered pain with sex. They feared being labeled frigid or saw the symptom as shameful. Because they were not sharing a complete picture of their symptoms with their physicians, they were making it harder for the physicians to diagnose endometriosis. (Physicians can help patients know they are approachable on endometriosis symptoms by displaying pamphlets, videotapes, and other patient education items in their waiting rooms.)

But why have physicians themselves perpetuated misconceptions about the disease, especially the one that symptoms, particularly dysmenorrhea and pain with sex, are in a woman's head? A study at one endometriosis center found that although women complained of classic symptoms of endometriosis, physicians and other caregivers tended to diagnose their complaints as normal menstrual events. The majority of the women were led to believe they were overreacting to the pain and their symptoms were psychological in origin.[61,62] Another endometriosis treatment center and the Endometriosis Association have found that about three-fourths of women with confirmed endometriosis

were told their symptoms were "in their heads," "stress," due to "nerves," or that they were "frigid." And when researchers first analyzed data from our registry, they were surprised to find that some of the women had been prescribed tranquilizers and told it would take care of their problems!

Few of us today really believe endometriosis is an imaginary disease, but somehow unconscious taboos and subtle training that teach women are not reliable reporters about their bodies, take over in actual encounters with patients.[63] Remember that well-known study in which women and men presented with the same symptoms and the men were referred for medical workup and the women, in much greater proportion, were referred for psychological counseling?[64]

We have all had the experience of thinking we understand something—say divorce, or heart attack, or the loss of a loved one—but when we went through it ourselves realized we really had not. Add to this natural experience the fact that men do not have the organs and cycle that women do, even without a perplexing disease to complicate the picture, and that it is easier to think a girl or woman is exaggerating or that a problem does not exist than to constantly remember that she is describing something one cannot really relate to unless one is very empathetic and willing to put oneself in another's shoes.

This tendency of human nature to define reality as one's *own* reality, as well as the tendency to disbelieve the experience of women's reality, especially when it comes to reporting pain and problems with their reproductive organs, has tended to distort care. For example, the whole category of mental disorders called "somatization disorders," affecting primarily women according to the psychiatric literature, is based on physical symptoms of primarily female disorders (the differential diagnoses include lupus, multiple sclerosis, and should include endometriosis). Why are we not surprised to find obvious symptoms of endometriosis on the list of diagnostic criteria for somatization disorder?! The list includes: pain during intercourse, painful menstruation, irregular menstrual periods, excessive menstrual bleeding, pain during urination, difficulty urinating, abdominal pain (other than when menstruating), diarrhea, intolerance of several different foods, back pain, and other symptoms frequently reported by women with endometriosis.

Somatization disorders are said to affect mostly women and the prevalence is from 0.2% to 2% of women (remarkably close to some of the estimates of how many women have endometriosis).[65,66] The DSM-III-R states, "Menstrual difficulties may be one of the earliest symptoms in females." In an amazingly illogical statement, it also notes, "Although most people without mental disorders at various times have aches and pains and other physical complaints, they rarely bring them to medical attention." (Does this mean that mostly only people with mental disorders seek medical attention? Or that the symptoms of endometriosis, lupus, and multiple sclerosis are trivial "aches and pains"?)

It is a disgrace that such clear symptoms of endometriosis are listed as a "mental" disorder and we call on endometriosis specialists to work to have this changed. The following letter shows some of the distortions in care (and unnecessary costs to the medical system) that result from the myths and taboos surrounding endometriosis.

To whom it may concern:
...I am 28 years old, married for eight years with no children.... My story is typical. I've been sick with stomach problems for 12 years but my doctor kept telling me that there's nothing physically wrong with me. She sent me for all kinds of tests and specialists, but everything came back negative. I was sent to psychiatrists [who] told me to get a job and stop feeling sorry for myself. They said I was a nervous type of person, which they felt caused my stomach problems. For years I really thought it was all in my head, but that didn't make me feel any better. My family believed the doctors, so I had no one to talk to....
My doctor was getting fed up with me going to her and complaining all the time and she even told me so. After about nine years of feeling sick and crazy, my doctor sent me to a gynecologist. [Teresa was diagnosed with endometriosis on her ovaries, appendix, bowel, and cul de sac.]
                                                                            Teresa, Ontario

As dangerous as the idea that these symptoms are part of a mental disorder if complained about, is the idea that they are a *normal* part of being female. To be female is to suffer?

So, if it seems that endometriosis has gathered numerous myths and misconceptions around it, in part because of the taboo nature of many of its symptoms, the next obvious sociological mystery is why are these symptoms taboo? Even normal menstruation and female sexual issues are taboo although they are life elements at the very heart of survival of the human race. It is the nature of taboos to be about the subjects most feared or most involved with the power relationships in a society. Certainly sexuality and reproduction are powerful forces. And the exclusively female nature of menstruation and female sexuality have made them easy targets for myth and taboo in a world that for the past several thousand years has been mostly patriarchal. (Many millennia before that appear to have been predominantly matriarchal.)

A number of modern books have delved, some with sociologically and anthropologically careful science, into the mystery of the taboos surrounding menstruation and female sexuality. Physicians who work in gynecology and fertility will find these volumes of great interest and helpful in their work. Worth mentioning are *The Curse: A Cultural History of Menstruation* and *The Woman In The Body: A Cultural Analysis of Reproduction.*[67,68]

Why Is Endometriosis Not Seen as a Serious Disease?

Finally, there is another sociological myth which perhaps contains seeds of answers to the other puzzles and questions we have addressed. That is, why is endometriosis not seen as a serious disease? How can the same disease that is considered "all in their heads" or "just cramps" by some, end up in hysterectomy and surgical castration for hundreds of thousands of women?[69] The only answer to such a contradiction is that the disease (and women) are not taken seriously. Only if women, their bodies, and their life needs are not taken seriously can one so easily dismiss their complaints. And only if it does not matter (in a society in which women are devalued) whether women have their sexual organs or not, can one so simply remove their female organs if the complaints continue. Whereas most men would react violently to the idea of castration, it is so commonplace in this society for women that few even question the great disparity in the number of women who have had their reproductive organs removed versus the number of men. Are our industrialized societies really that much more civilized about this issue than the African countries which so routinely and crudely carry out female genital mutilation?[70]

Of course, several factors complicate the picture of why it might be difficult to see the disease as serious. First the cyclicity of the symptoms, at least at the beginning, may make it harder to quantify the loss. Second, there's the invisible nature of the illness (although many other invisible illnesses are taken seriously).[71] Third, women may hide the symptoms because they are taboo or they may feel, with shame, that the symptoms reflect poorly on their femininity. Finally, there is the selection bias mentioned earlier, which means that only certain symptoms have been looked at rather than the whole picture of the disease.

Another indication that female status is the problem is the frequent unwillingness, in the woman and her family or in the physician, to help the girl or woman suffering from endometriosis. The following two letters describe situations in which the girl or woman cannot get a pelvic exam until she is sexually active. What clearer statement could there be that women's bodies, especially their sexual organs, belong to males? Can anyone imagine an illness in which a boy or man would be expected to live with severe pain in his sexual organs until he was no longer a virgin? The very idea is ludicrous. It is always easier to see the blindspots in a culture other than our own, especially if more exaggerated, so we are including an excerpt from a letter from an Algerian woman that articulates the same issue.

Dear Sir or Madam:

I am a young girl suffering.... I attempted many treatments, mostly hormonal treatments based on Duphaston and danazol. All were inefficient since I am still suffering, and the disease grows more and more serious as I get older.

Just at the very beginning before undertaking any treatment, doctors found big enlarged ovaries full of cysts in the ultrasonographic examination. Concerning my periods... these are very painful and full of big clots....

If I am addressing you, it is just because you are my only hope which keeps me alive. I am seriously ready to serve for any medical test for new treatments... *there is the problem of virginity*; *all doctors refuse to practice a gynecological examination, which is very vital for me, for fear that they would rupture my hymen....* [emphasis added]

Saker, Algeria

To whom it may concern,

My name is Lorie. I am married and I have an 8 year old son. I'm 24 years old. The baby and marriage came young, but I wouldn't trade that for the world. It sounds as if I should be content and happy, doesn't it? I would be except for one major problem. I have severe endometriosis.

It all started when I was 10 years old and started menstruating. My "time of the month" was a very excruciating week of pain. The doctor said I just had difficult periods. I would scream for hours and if I got out of bed I would faint.

At 13 I made love for the first time, so the doctor could now do a pelvic exam. [emphasis added] I was in his office every month because of my pain. He said I had ovarian cysts which were normal for a girl that age and gave me codeine to help with the pain....

I turned 16 in August, had my baby in September, got married the following June, life was great. Then came my period in November.... The pain was every bit as terrible as before, but more so. I went to my gynecologist and he found a large cyst on my right ovary and said I needed surgery. He removed a softball size cyst and I was released four days later.... In February I was back in the hospital having a cyst removed from each ovary and part of my right ovary removed.

In March I found out I was pregnant and started feeling great. In the last week of June I began having severe cramps and bleeding. I lost my baby and had a D&C.

In September I switched gynecologists and after he removed three grapefruit sized cysts, one from each ovary and one from my intestine, he told me I had endometriosis. I was put on Danocrine, but didn't get any better.

In February, I had a hysterectomy and oophorectomy. I was only seventeen and I was heartbroken. The doctor said that my problems were over.

I was okay for awhile, for about a year and a half. Then the pain was back. I decided to go to a doctor in B. and he did a laparoscopy. I had adhesions and they were removed. I was put on Premarin. He saw no endometrial lesions. I was constantly in pain and nothing was being done. I suffered a nervous breakdown three months later.

I suffered with the pain until August 1990. I was in such severe pain I felt I would die. My doctor in B. couldn't see me for six weeks so I went to a gynecologist here. He did a laparoscopy and found a large cyst on my small intestine. I was sent to a general surgeon who, because I had no money to pay, refused to do the surgery to remove the cyst. I found another surgeon who did emergency surgery and told me I still had endometriosis....

... [My doctor] told me that less than one in a hundred women still have endometriosis after a hysterectomy and I am

that less than one.* I was continued on the Premarin and was also put on Provera. Two months ago the pain got worse and I was back at the doctor. I was told I may have a cyst on the intestine. I am having trouble urinating and was told I possibly have the disease on my bladder and was referred to a urologist. The Premarin and Provera were discontinued pending what he says. I had to wait seven weeks to see him.

... I saw the urologist this Monday after several weeks of pain, urinating every half hour, sometimes in my pants, and not sleeping enough to say so. He performed a cystoscopy and said my bladder is only capable of holding 130 cc of urine and that amount causes pain.... My kidneys are now causing pain, but he didn't do anything yet.... I won't go back to him until October 24th and I don't know if I can take it until then. I'm tired. I hurt. And after 14 years I want some relief.

Through the years I've had lasting and loving support from a lot of friends and my family. I have people who ask how much it takes mentally to deal with this and have been told I'm an extremely strong person. Well, I don't feel strong anymore. I want this over and don't know how. We have no money to pay for all these medical bills and medication and are on the verge of bankruptcy....

... In all these years I feel as if I haven't gotten any better or been helped to understand why this is happening to me. I pray every night for my health back. My husband keeps telling me he thinks I'm going to die because he knows they can't keep taking out my organs one at a time. I can't make him understand any differently because I am also confused. I'm too young to live my life like this. I want energy and just a day without pain. I want a doctor who'll understand my fears and who'll help me feel better without waiting months and possibly getting worse in that time. I want to make love to my husband without pain and I want my sex drive back. I want this to end and I want a life because this isn't living. This is endometriosis and it really is hell....

Lorie, Vermont

Ultimately, perhaps the last sociological puzzle (why the disease has not been seen as serious) is not so mysterious after all—it is directly related to the status of women in society. The bigger mystery is what it will take to change it. As noted by the authors of *The Curse: A Cultural History of Menstruation*, "It is impossible to escape the conclusion that menstrual politics has dominated social and economic relations between the sexes since the beginning of time."[73]

But if we apply ourselves to reframing the questions related to endometriosis (and indirectly to some of the most important things involved in life), we may be able to solve the puzzle. After all, if there were five million young men with endometriosis in the United States, young men whose dreams were in danger of being destroyed by a disease, whose ability to function sexually was at risk, whose fertility was at risk, whose ability to

---

* Hysterectomy and removal of the ovaries have been widely proclaimed as the cure, without any long-term follow-up studies. Recently, the Association conducted one; unfortunately, for about one third of the patients, hysterectomy and removal of the ovaries did not offer a cure or even relief of symptoms. Forty-four percent of those receiving estrogen replacement therapy experienced a return of symptoms.[72]

build a satisfying work life and carry out the normal activities of living were at risk, and who even would face the threat of castration—if this was happening to young men, no one would dare say it was not serious. Men would have banded together long ago, research institutes would have been devoted to it, and by now, it would probably be not only curable but also preventable. The puzzle would be solved. Can we afford to do anything less for women and girls?

References

1. Olive DL. Infertility and Reproductive Medicine Clinics of North America. Philadelphia, WB Saunders Company, 1992;3:3, p xi.
2. Thomas EJ, Rock JA. Modern Approaches to Endometriosis. Lancaster, UK, Kluwer Academic Publishers, 1991, p ix.
3. Schenken R. Endometriosis: Contemporary Concepts in Clinical Management. Philadelphia, JB Lippincott, 1989, p ix.
4. Wilson E. Endometriosis. New York, Alan R. Liss, 1987, p 1.
5. Olive DL, ed. Future Directions for Endometriosis Research. In Infertility and Reproductive Medicine Clinics of North America, Philadelphia, WB Saunders Co., 1992, p 763.
6. Rawson JMR. Prevalence of endometriosis in asymptomatic women. J Reprod Med 1991;36:513,514.
7. Pittaway DE. Diagnosis of Endometriosis. In Infertility and Reproductive Medicine Clinics of North America, Philadelphia, WB Saunders Co., 1992, p 619.
8. Redwine DB. Treatment of Endometriosis-Associated Pain. In Infertility and Reproductive Medicine Clinics of North America, Philadelphia, WB Saunders Co., 1992, pp 701–706, 708–713.
9. Nisolle-Pochet M, Casanas-Roux F, Donnez J. Histologic study of ovarian endometriosis after hormonal therapy. Fertil Steril 1988;49:423–426.
10. Brosens IA. The Endometriotic Implant. In Thomas EJ, Rock JA, eds. Modern Approaches to Endometriosis, Lancaster UK, Kluwer Academic Publishers, 1991, p 30.
11. Olive DL, Haney AF. Associated infertility: A critical review of therapeutic approaches. Ob Gyn Surv 1986; 41:538.
12. Vernon MW, Beard JS, Graves K, et al. Classification of endometriotic implants by morphologic appearance and capacity to synthesize prostaglandin F. Fertil Steril 1986;46:801.
13. Redwine DB. Age-related evolution in color appearance of endometriosis. Fertil Steril 1987;48:1061–1063.
14. Murphy AA, Green WR, Bobbie D, et al. Unsuspected endometriosis documented by scanning electron microscopy in visually normal peritoneum. Fertil Steril 1986;46:522.
15. Audebert A, Bäckstrom T, Barlow DH, et al. Endometriosis 1991: A discussion document. Hum Reprod 1992;7:432–435.
16. Rawson JMR. Prevalence of endometriosis in asymptomatic women. J Reprod Med 1991;36:515.
17. Thomas EJ, Rock JA. The Future. In Thomas EJ, Rock JA, eds. Modern Approaches to Endometriosis, Lancaster UK, Kluwer Academic Publishing, 1991, p 291.
18. Reiter RC, Shakerin RL, Gambone JC, et al. Correlation between sexual abuse and somatization in women with somatic and nonsomatic chronic pelvic pain. Am J Ob Gyn 1991;165:104–109.
19. Gottesfeld I. Chronic Pelvic Pain: Stalking a Clinical Enigma. Today's Woman, October 1991.
20. Redwine DB. Conservative laparoscopic excision of endometriosis by sharp dissection: Life table analysis of reoperation and persistent or recurrent disease. Fertil Steril 1991;56:634.
21. Ballweg ML. Overcoming Endometriosis: New help from the Endometriosis Association. New York, Congdon & Weed, 1987, p 221.
22. Characteristics of women with endometriosis. From Endometriosis Association Research Registry. In Endometriosis Association Newsletter, 1989;10:2, p 2.
23. Lamb K, Hoffmann RG, Nichols TR. Family trait analysis: A case control study of 43 women with endometriosis and their best friends. Am J Ob Gyn 1986;154: 596–601.
24. Lamb K, Nichols TR. Endometriosis: A comparison of associated disease histories. Am J Prev Med 1986;2: 324–329.
25. Nichols TR, Lamb K, Arkins JA. The association of atopic diseases with endometriosis. Ann of All 1987;59: 360–363.
26. Ballweg ML. Overcoming Endometriosis, pp 198–219.
27. Ballweg ML. Data bank results are in! From Endometriosis Association Research Registry. In Endometriosis Association Newsletter, May 1983, p 1.
28. Ballweg ML. Research News—Endometriosis linked to radiation and environmental pollutants in research studies. Endometriosis Association Newsletter, 1992; 13(2)1–2.
29. Ballweg ML. Research News—Exciting findings in dioxin monkey colony. Endometriosis Association Newsletter, 1992;13(3):1–2.
30. Cramer DW, Wilson E, Stillman RJ, et al. The relation of endometriosis to menstrual characteristics, smoking, and exercise. JAMA 1986;255:1904.
31. Wood R. The Pathway to Diagnosis of Women with Endometriosis. Endometriosis Association (Victoria), Melbourne, Australia, Presented at 3rd World Congress on Endometriosis, 1–3 June 1992, Brussels, Belgium.
32. Redwine DB. The distribution of endometriosis in the pelvis by age groups and fertility. Fertil Steril 1987;47: 173.
33. Thomas EJ, Rock JA. Modern Approaches to Endometriosis, p 300.
34. Kennedy S. What is important to the patient with endometriosis? Discussion. Brit J Clin Prac 45:3, Suppl. 72, Autumn 1991, p 11.
35. Ballweg ML. A few comparative findings: Endometriosis Association, British Endometriosis Society and Australian Endometriosis Association. In Overcoming Endometriosis: New Help from the Endometriosis Association. New York, Congdon & Weed, 1987, p 297.
36. Rosen GF. Treatment of endometriosis-associated infertility. In Infertility and Reproductive Medicine Clinics of North America. Philadelphia, WB Saunders Co., 1992, p 721.
37. Haney AF. The pathogenesis and aetiology of endometriosis. In Thomas EJ, Rock JA, eds. Modern Approaches to Endometriosis. Lancaster UK, Kluwer Academic Publishers, 1991, p 4.
38. Yap AL. Endometriosis and the urinary tract: endometriosis of the bladder, bladder and urinary tract symptoms, new directions in understanding and treatment, and related problems. Endometriosis Association Newsletter, 1992;13(1):2–3.

39. Ballweg ML. Endometriosis and the intestines: endometriosis of the bowel, intestinal symptoms, new directions in understanding and treatment. Endometriosis Association Newsletter, 1988;9(1):5.
40. Grimes DA, LeBolt SA, Grimes KRT, et al. Two-fold risk of endometriosis in hospitalized patients with lupus. Am J Ob Gyn 1985;153:179.
41. Brush MG. Increased incidence of thyroid autoimmune problems in women with endometriosis. Endometriosis: A collection of papers written by PGs, researchers, specialists and sufferers about endometriosis. Compiled by the Conventry Branch of the Endometriosis Society, March 1987.
42. Ballweg ML. Overcoming Endometriosis, pp 228–231.
43. Fletcher N. Mitral valve prolapse. Endometriosis Association Newsletter, 1992;13(2):1–2.
44. Jessop C. Clinical features and possible etiology of CFIDS. Chronic Fatigue and Immune Dysfunction Syndrome: Unravelling the mystery conference, Charlotte, North Carolina, November 18, 1990. Summary: The CFIDS Chronicle 1991; Spring:70–73.
45. Ballweg ML. Fibromyalgia/endometriosis link? Endometriosis Association Newsletter, 1991;12(3):6–8.
46. Ballweg ML. Overcoming Endometriosis. New York, Congdon & Weed, 1987, p 205.
47. Science Magazine, January 1985.
48. Ballweg ML. Overcoming Endometriosis, p 219.
49. Campbell J. Is Simian Endometriosis an Effect of Immunotoxicity? Ontario Assocation of Pathologists, October 1985.
50. Cornillie FJ, D'Hooghe TM, Bambra CS, et al. Morphological characteristics of spontaneous endometriosis in the baboon (Papio anubis and Papio cynocephalus). Gyn Obstet Invest 1992;34:225–228.
51. Fanton JW, Golden JG. Radiation-induced endometriosis in Macaca mulatta. Radiation Research 1991;126:141–146.
52. Rier SE, Martin DC, Bowman RE, et al. Endometriosis in rhesus monkeys (Macaca mulatta) following chronic exposure to 2,3,7,8 tetrachlorodibenzo-p-dioxin. Fundamental and Applied Toxicology, 1993;21(4):433–441.
53. Rier SE. Research News—Immunological Findings in Dioxin Monkey Colony. Endometriosis Association Newsletter 1992;13(4):1,6.
54. Martin DC, Rier SE, Bowman DE, et al. Dioxin-induced endometriosis in rhesus monkeys (Macaca mulatta). Abstracts, p 330, Annual Meeting of the Society for Gynecologic Investigation, Toronto, Canada (April 1993).
55. Rier SE, Spangel BL, Martin DC, et al. Production of IL-6 and TNF by peripheral blood mononuclear cells from rhesus monkeys with endometriosis. American Association of Immunology, Denver, Colorado (May 1993).
56. Gerhard I, Runnebaum B. Grenzen der Hormonsubstitution bei Schadstoffbelastung und Fertilitätsstörungen. Zentralblatt für Gynäkologie 1992;114:593–602.
57. Consensus Statement: Chemically induced alterations in sexual development: The Wildlife/Human Connection. Wingspread Conference, Racine, WI, USA, July 26–28, 1991.
58. Hong R, Taylor K, Abonour R. Immune abnormalities associated with chronic TCDD exposure in rhesus. Chemosphere 1989;18(1–6):313–320.
59. Haney AF. The pathogenesis and aetiology of endometriosis. In Thomas EJ, Rock JA, eds. Modern Approaches to Endometriosis. Lancaster UK, Kluwer Academic Publishers, 1991, p 14.
60. Migrant workers have many menstrual problems and endometriosis according to comments of Cesar Chavez. Personal communication from Russell Jaffe, M.D., Ph.D.
61. Halstead L, Pepping P, Dmowski WP. The woman with endometriosis: ignored, dismissed and devalued. Second International Symposium on Endometriosis, Houston, TX, USA, May 1989.
62. Halstead L, Pepping P, Haile L, et al. Women's experiences with endometriosis: delay and disbelief. Abstracts, 3rd World Congress on Endometriosis, June 1992, Brussels, Belgium.
63. Ballweg ML. Endometriosis: the patient's perspective. In Olive DL, ed. Infertility and Reproductive Medicine Clinics of North America. Philadelphia, WB Saunders Co., 1992, pp 747–761.
64. Armitage KJ, Schneiderman LJ, Bass BA. Response of physicians to medical complaints in men and women. JAMA 1979;241:2186–2187.
65. Rasmussen N, Avant R. Somatization disorder in family practice. American Family Practice 1989;40(2):206–212.
66. American Psychiatric Association: Diagnostic and Statistical Manual of Disorders, 3rd ed., rev. Washington, DC, 1987, pp 261–262.
67. Delaney J, Lupton MJ, Toth E. The Curse: A Cultural History of Menstruation. Urbana and Chicago, University of Illinois Press, 1988.
68. Martin E. The Woman in the Body: A Cultural Analysis of Reproduction. Boston, Beacon Press, 1987.
69. Hysterectomies in the United States, 1965–1984. Vital and Health Statistics, U.S. Department of Health and Human Services, Public Health Service, Centers for Disease Control, National Center for Health Statistics, Series 13, No. 92, 1987.
70. Rosenthal AM. Female Genital Torture. New York Times, December 29, 1992.
71. Donoghue PJ, Siegel ME. Sick and Tired of Feeling Sick and Tired: Living with Invisible Chronic Illness. New York, WW Norton & Company, 1992.
72. Lamb K, Breitkopf L, Hamilton K, et al. Does total hysterectomy offer a cure for endometriosis? Endometriosis Association Newsletter, 1991;12(3):1–5.
73. Delaney J, Lupton MJ, Toth E. The Curse: A Cultural History of Menstruation. Urbana, University of Illinois Press, 1988, p 62.

Epilogue

Modern Surgical Management of Endometriosis: "Experience Treacherous, Judgment Difficult"

Gary S. Berger and Camran Nezhat

"Life is short, the art long, opportunity fleeting, experience treacherous, judgment difficult."

This aphorism by Hippocrates over 2400 years old aptly describes the situation today regarding the management of endometriosis. This is apparent from the varying opinions and practices presented by leading authorities in the preceding chapters of this book.

Endometriosis: Advanced Management and Surgical Techniques describes the current state of the art, with emphasis on advanced laparoscopic techniques, made possible by improved endoscopic, video, laser and other surgical instrumentation, as well as a clearer understanding of the early manifestations of the disease visible upon laparoscopic examination.

While the relative advantages and disadvantages of the two primary surgical approaches (laparoscopy versus laparotomy) have been debated, the approaches themselves have evolved. An assumption underlying comparisons between the two has been that laparoscopy is an outpatient procedure and laparotomy an inpatient procedure. But this distinction has become blurred by techniques permitting such advanced surgery through laparoscopy that postoperative hospitalization is necessary, and techniques permitting laparotomy to be performed safely and effectively in the ambulatory setting.[1] The choice of surgical approach, instrumentation, and technique must be based not only upon the clinical situation, but also upon the surgeon's training, experience, and skill in order to best accomplish the surgical objectives while minimizing the risk of complications.

Given the dramatic improvements in modern surgical management, why does experience with endometriosis remain treacherous and judgment difficult? The reasons have not so much to do with the surgical techniques themselves, but with basic limitations in our understanding of the disease and in the ways treatment results are evaluated and reported.

Information about the natural history of the disease is lacking. Although we now recognize that endometriotic lesions change in their appearance over time, it is not clear whether endometriosis is progressive (in the sense of spread of new lesion sites) or static (sites established during early reproductive years with their appearance changing over time). The concept that endometriosis may either progress or resolve spontaneously is based on a study which included 17 placebo-treated women who underwent consecutive laparoscopic examinations.[2] This study was conducted before the subtle, atypical, and invisible forms of endometriosis were appreciated and needs confirmation with larger numbers of patients. If endometriosis resolves spontaneously in some women, an understanding of the natural mechanisms by which this occurs could lead to improved treatment and possibly cure of the disease.

Understanding the natural history of the disease is critical, since it relates to the need for appropriate study methodologies in assessing the efficacy of any treatment, as compared with no treatment at all. It is evident from literature reviews provided throughout the preceding chapters that most existing studies of treatment (whether surgical, medical, or combined) have been uncontrolled case series which report outcome measures based on before-and-after reasoning (for example, the pregnancy rate after treatment of a previously infertile group of patients).

Drawing conclusions about the relative effectiveness of different treatments based on uncontrolled case studies representing the experience of clinicians can be treacherous. The populations of women in different case series are not necessarily comparable, since they are not identical in age, prior reproductive history, stage of disease, and presence of other factors which affect the outcome, independent of the treatment under study. In order to compare the reported results between different groups of patients, these factors must be accounted for. There are various epidemiologic and statistical methods for doing this, but most clinical series report only the overall proportion of patients (crude pregnancy rate) who conceived subsequent to treatment, without accounting for these confounding variables. Furthermore, the effect of passage of time must be properly taken into account in comparing the results of different study populations. This requires actuarial or life-table analysis, which takes into account the interval between treatment and outcome events as well as the varying interval of loss to follow-up for some patients.

The evaluation of treatment effects on infertility at least has the advantage that pregnancy is an objective end point that can be easily measured. Evaluating the effect of differing treatments on pain is much more difficult. Pain is not a discrete variable. It is a subjective experience that varies considerably over time in location, extent, duration, quality, and description by different individuals, and pain is affected by many other factors that are difficult or impossible to measure. There is no uniformly agreed instrument by which to measure pain. It is not surprising, therefore, that the literature is even more confusing to those looking to draw valid conclusions about the effectiveness of different treatments for endometriosis on relieving pain.

Adding to the "puzzle" of endometriosis is that the classic definition of the disease (the presence of ectopic endometrial tissue outside the uterus) may be inadequate as a criterion for treatment. If minimal or mild endometriosis is observed in women with otherwise unexplained infertility, should it be treated or not? We lack experimental evidence that ablation of lesions in these early cases improves fertility. But if endometriosis is a progressive disease, will treatment at early stages avoid progression to more extensive, symptomatic disease later on? This hypothesis, reasonable as it is, needs to be tested in properly designed clinical studies.

Attention is currently focused on the possibility that endometriosis is a systemic disease, and that the endometriotic implants seen at surgery are only one manifestation. While many findings are observed in women with endometriosis which indicate activation of both humoral and cellular immunity, we do not know whether these are responsible for, or consequences of, the growth of ectopic endometrium. Despite increasing understanding of pathophysiologic mechanisms, we cannot yet answer the essential question of why some women develop endometriosis while others do not, even though retrograde menstruation apparently occurs in most women of reproductive age.

Without understanding the cause of endometriosis, we can neither prevent nor cure the disease; *management* is the best option we can offer at present. As the twenty-first century approaches, important advances have been made in both surgical and medical techniques for managing endometriosis. Further progress, however, must lie in advancing our understanding of the cause of this disorder. Only then will it be possible to resolve the puzzle of this most "enigmatic" disease of women.

References

1. Berger GS. Outpatient pelvic laparotomy. J Reprod Med 1994;39:569–574.
2. Thomas EJ, Cooke ID. Impact of gestrinone on the course of asymptomatic endometriosis. Br Med J Clin Res 1987; 294:272–274.

Index